Experimental Procedures in
Life Sciences

(Manual for Biochemistry, Biotechnology, Botany, Genetics, Microbiology, Molecular Biology, Zoology, Nursing, Medicine, DMLT, MLT and also for B.Tech-Biotechnology, Bio-Medical Engg. & Bio Informatics students)

Dr. S. Rajan, M.Sc., Ph.D.,
Assistant Professor
Department of Microbiology
M.R. Government Arts College
Mannargudi - 614 001

Mrs. R. Selvi Christy, M.Sc., M.Phil.
Microbiologist

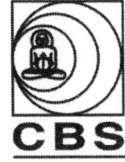

CBS

CBS Publishers & Distributors Pvt Ltd

New Delhi • Bengaluru • Chennai • Kochi • Kolkata • Mumbai
Bhopal • Bhubaneswar • Hyderabad • Jharkhand • Nagpur
• Patna • Pune • Uttarakhand • Dhaka (Bangladesh)

Experimental Procedures in Life Sciences

CBS Reprint: 2018, 2019

First Edition: 2010
Reprint: 2011, 2012, 2015

ISBN 978-93-86478-25-2

Published by Satish Kumar Jain and produced by Varun Jain for

CBS Publishers & Distributors Pvt Ltd
204 FIE, Patparganj Industrial Area, Delhi 110 092
E-mail: delhi@cbspd.com, cbspubs@airtelmail.in

Ph: 4934 4934   Fax: 4934 4935   Website: www.cbspd.com
                                                e-mail: publishing@cbspd.com;
                                                publicity@cbspd.com

Branches

- **Bengaluru:** Seema House 2975, 17th Cross, K.R. Road, Banasankari 2nd Stage, Bengaluru 560 070, Karnataka
  Ph: +91-80-26771678/79   Fax: +91-80-26771680   e-mail: bangalore@cbspd.com
- **Chennai:** 7, Subbaraya Street, Shenoy Nagar, Chennai 600 030, Tamil Nadu
  Ph: +91-44-26260666, 26208620   Fax: +91-44-42032115   e-mail: chennai@cbspd.com
- **Kochi:** 42/1325, 1326, Power House Road, Opp KSEB Power House, Ernakulam 682 018, Kochi, Kerala
  Ph: +91-484-4059061-65   Fax: +91-484-4059065   e-mail: kochi@cbspd.com
- **Kolkata:** No. 6/B, Ground Floor, Rameswar Shaw Road, Kolkata-700014 (West Bengal), India
  Ph: +91-33-2289-1126, 2289-1127, 2289-1128   e-mail: kolkata@cbspd.com
- **Mumbai:** 83-C, Dr E Moses Road, Worli, Mumbai-400018, Maharashtra
  Ph: +91-22-24902340/41   Fax: +91-22-24902342   e-mail: mumbai@cbspd.com

Representatives

- Bhopal   0-8319310552   • Bhubaneswar   0-9911037372   • Hyderabad   0-9885175004
- Jharkhand   0-9811541605   • Nagpur   0-9021734563   • Patna   0-9334159340
- Pune   0-9623451994   • Uttarakhand   0-9716462459
- Dhaka (Bangladesh)   01912-003485

Printed at Chaman Interprises, Daryaganj, India

Foreword

I have a great pleasure in writing this foreword to the book entitled 'Experimental Procedures in Life Sciences', authored by Dr. S. Rajan, Head, Department of Microbiology, Srimad Andavan Arts and Science College, Tiruchirapalli.

An academician of par excellence, Dr. Rajan possesses a vast experience in teaching and research in life sciences, particularly in microbiology. He has already authored four text books and published papers in reputed journals.

Dr. Rajan has made a sincere attempt to write a comprehensive Laboratory Manual covering almost all branches of life sciences (Microbiology, Biochemistry, Biotechnology, Genetics, Botany, Zoology, Medical Laboratory Technology, Nursing etc). 'Experimental Procedures in Life Sciences' is certainly a unique practical manual that has brought over 200 wide range of experiments under one umbrella.

The author has nicely organized the experiments into different categories/chapters, giving due emphasis to different branches of life sciences. For each experiment, adequate information on the principle, procedure, expected results/observations and interpretation has been given. Further, certain *viva* questions have also been included to guide the students to boldly face the examinations. The information given in the appendices (calculations, sources of microorganisms and media, glossary, bibliography) is highly useful for teachers as well as students.

It is worth mentioning here that this book 'Experimental Procedures in Life Sciences' is one among the rare Laboratory Manuals authored by an Indian to cater the needs of several branches of life sciences. It is ultimately for the reader with his/her own specialization in life sciences to do appropriate self-service and enjoy the menu (by choosing required experiments from 'Experimental Procedures in Life Sciences').

Undoubtedly, writing a good practical manual is tougher task compared to writing a textbook. This is for the reason that practical experiments have to be tested in the laboratory (by the author or his group) before writing a manual. It appears that Dr. Rajan has the personal experience of handling majority of the experiments given in the manual.

Dr. Rajan has made a sincere and whole hearted attempt to bring out this manual 'Experimental Procedures in Life Sciences'. I hope that the readers (students and teachers) will utilize the book to the maximum possible and give him feedback (suggestions, critical comments) to further improve it in subsequent editions.

I congratulate Dr. Rajan for bringing out such a comprehensive and unique laboratory manual for the benefit of student community of life sciences. I wish him and his book a great success.

Dr. U. Satyanarayana,
Professor & Head
Department of Biochemistry,
Siddhartha Medical College,
(Dr. NTR University of Health Sciences)
Vijayawada-520008, A.P., India.

Vijayawada
Dt : 09-06-2010.

Preface

Experimental Procedures in Life Sciences is a manual for all life science students belongs to Biochemistry, Biotechnology, Botany, Genetics, Microbiology, Molecular Biology, Zoology, Nursing, Medicine, DMLT, MLT. This book is prepared based on a decade experience on the field experiments of Life Science teaching and research. This book has been written to fulfill the requirements of the syllabus for B. Sc., M. Sc., B. Tech., M. Tech, MLT etc., This book provides ample informations regarding *"aim, principle, background informations, specific procedures, possible observations and results"*. We have also included possible spotters and viva voce questions for all the experiments to reduce fear of the students during their practical examinations. Students make use of this manual for their routine practical, research and writing record notebooks.

This book is divided into 15 prime chapters and 11 appendix part, which provides basic information related to pH, pH indicators, normality and morality calculations, periodic table, glossary, details of spotters, glossary etc., This book covers the practical procedures related to general microbiology, microbial physiology, immunology & immunotechnology, medical microbiology- bacteriology, virology, parasitology, mycology, soil and agricultural microbiology, environmental biotechnology, microbial genetics, molecular biology, microbial biotechnology, industrial biotechnology, general virology, biochemistry, plant tissue culture, animal cell culture, cell biology and genetics. Spotters section provides detailed information about scientific concept of the chapter. Background information of each experiment is prepared in such a way that, the students are able to answer viva questions. This book has been structured in such a way, without sacrificing the completeness or accuracy of information, that students can access information in small, well identifiable steps. A major bit of information within a topic is given as box and table. Illustrations make the subject more interesting and easy to understand. We hope this manual will promote self learning, creates interests and will help the students for quick revision of the practical for their university as well as competitive examinations.

Our First and foremost, duty is to thank our microbiology guru, Dr. T. Thirunalasundari, Professor, Department of Biotechnology, Bharathidasan University, Tiruchirapalli who has been providing constant encouragement to sustain in this field. We should thank profusely Dr. P. Brindha, Dean In Charge, CARISM, SASTRA University, Thajavur, a mam of great wisdom from whom I learnt the skill of sincerity and hard work. We cherish our association with our friends Dr. S. Balakumar, Lecturer, Microbiology, SASTRA University, Kumbakonam, Prof. S. Shanthi, Lecturer, Microbiology, Srimad Andavan Arts and Science College for their constant support. We are highly thankful to Dr. N. Thajuddin, Head, Department of Microbiology, Bharathidasan University for his encouragement and support. We should not forget the support of Shri. V. S. Narasimhan, Former Secretary Srimad Andavan Arts and Science College, in all my endeavors. We would like to place our graditude to Shri N. Kasturirangan, Secretary, Dr. K. Prema, Director, Dr. S. Sivasubramanian, Principal, Srimad Andavan Arts and Science College, who molded my carrier and gave me the confidence that nothing is impossible in life.

We owe our gratitude to all the scientists in the field of life science, without their contribution, genesis of this manual would not have been possible.

We are highly thankful to the Publisher M/s. Anjanaa Book House for their suggestions & encouragements without which this book would not have come in this form. We are also delightful when thanking Mr. P. Raaju, M/s. PRS Associates, for their typesetting and Cover design.

We are highly indebted to our family members for their constant support, cooperation, encouragement throughout our life.

Last but not least, we thank god almighty for making my attempt to reality.

We earnestly invite comments and suggestions from the readers to enable us to improve the book in the subsequent editions, for any suggestions please feel free to contact us through our **E-mail Id : ksrajan_99@yahoo.com**

- Authors

CONTENTS

General Microbiology

1. Introduction

Microbiology is a branch of life science, which deals with the study of microorganisms. All the microorganisms are included under microscopic life. Microorganisms are not visible to the naked eye and are visible or observed only under microscope. Microbiology is a new field, which was emerged from the basic biological sciences like Botany and Zoology. After the discovery of microscope, developments of the Microbiology started at the end of 19th century but advancements were observed in the middle of the 20th century. Bacteria, Virus, Protozoan, micro algae (Cyanobacteria) and Fungi are considered as a microorganism.

Major subdivisions of Microbiology are Bacteriology, Mycology, Virology, Phycology and Protozology. These are based on the type of microbial nature. Microbiology is again classified into various fields of applications. They are Soil Microbiology, Agricultural Microbiology, Food Microbiology, Dairy Microbiology, Medical Microbiology, Environmental Microbiology, Microbial Genetics, Microbial Biotechnology, Industrial Microbiology, Immunology, Pharmaceutical Microbiology etc.. All microorganisms are categorized into two groups. They are Prokaryotes and Eukaryotes. The cells without specific nuclear membrane are called prokaryotes. Prokaryotes has very simple structure. Genetic materials lies as a single piece of DNA (nucleoid) in the cytoplasm. The cell contains simple enzyme system but lacks mitochondria. Prokaryptie cells divide by means of binary fission. E.g., Bacteria and Cyanobacteria. Eukaryotic organisms are larger than prokaryotes and have definite cell structures and shape. Each and every cellular organelle has definite cell membrane. Genetic materials are available within membrane in the form of chromosome. Cell division in Eukaryotes is by mitosis. E.g., Algae, fungi and protozoa (Table 1.1)

Table 1.1: Difference Between Prokaryotes and Eukaryotes

S.No	Character	Prokaryotes	Eukaryotes
1	The membrane bound nucleus	Absent	Present
2	Histones	Absent	Present
3	Nucleolus	Absent	Present
4	Introtes in genes	Rare	Common
5	Number of chromosomes	One except *V.cholerae*	Variable
6	Mitochondria	Absent	Present
7	Chloroplast	Absent	Present
8	Endoplasmic reticulum	Absent	Present
9	Golgi apparatus	Absent	Present
10	Cell wall	Chemically complex with peptidoglycon	Chemically simple lack peptidoglycon
11	Ribosomes	70S	80S
12	Lysosomes	Absent	Present

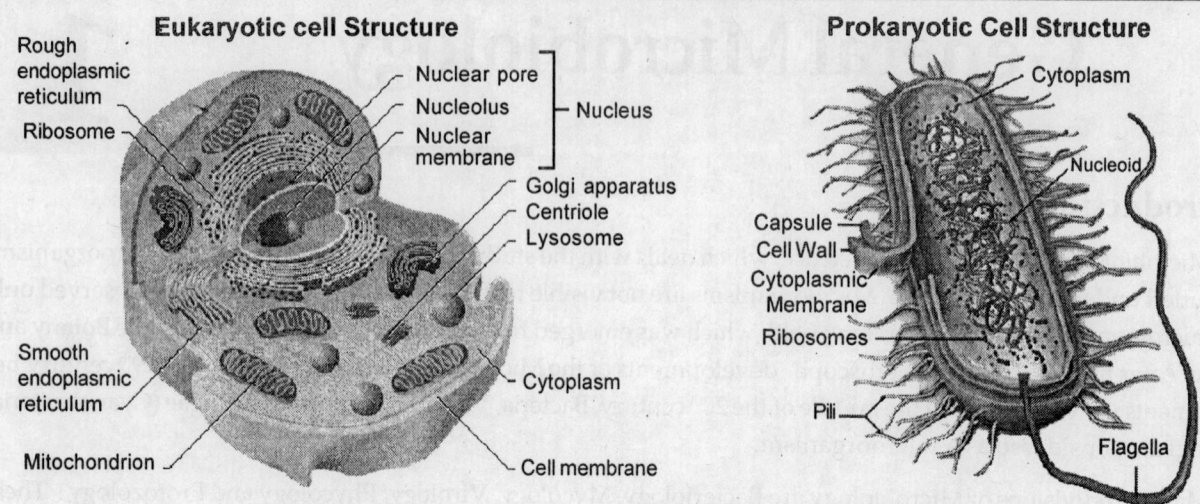

Fig 1.1: Structure of Eukaryotic Cell   Fig 1.2: Structure of Prokaryotic Cell

2. Laboratory Safety Guidelines (Rules and Regulations)

The biology department should provide a safe environment for all. Laboratory safety is a mutual responsibility and requires full participation and cooperation of all involved persons (students and staff).

Common Instructions

- Restrict laboratory access to authorized persons only. Children are not permitted in the laboratory.

- Smoking; eating; drinking; storing food, beverages or tobacco; applying cosmetics or lip balm and handling contact lenses are not permitted in laboratories.

- Wear lab coats (knee length) and safety glasses in laboratories employing chemicals, biohazards or radioisotopes.

- Open shoes, such as cut shoes, should never be worn in the lab.

- Tie back or otherwise restrain long hair when working with chemicals, biohazards, radioisotopes.

- Keep work places clean and free of unwanted chemicals, biological specimens, radioisotopes and idle equipment.

- Avoid leaving reagent bottles, empty or full, on the floor.

- Work only with materials once you know their flammability, reactivity, toxicity, safe handling and storage and emergency procedures.

- Prepare and maintain a chemical inventory for the lab.

- Keep exits and passage ways clear at all times.

- Ensure that access to emergency equipment (eyewashes, safety showers and fire extinguishers) is not blocked.

- Working alone is an unsafe practice at any time.

- Report accidents and dangerous incidents promptly to your supervisor

- Perform procedures that liberate infectious bioaerosols in a biological safety cabinet
- Carefully handle all human blood and body fluids.
- Do not mouth pipette microbial culture.
- Decontaminate the work surfaces at least once a day after spill of viable material.
- Persons should wash their hands after handling infectious materials and animals.
- Decontaminate conduct all procedures carefully to minimize aerosols.
- All contaminated liquid and solid waste before disposal.
- Safety glasses or other protective devices must be worn to protect the eyes and face from the splashes and impacting objects.
- Gloves must be worn for all procedures (especially for medical microbiology practicals).
- All laboratory spills, accidents must be immediately report to the laboratory supervisor.
- All laboratory personels must be vaccinated.
- Laboratory doors must be closed when work is in progress.

After completion of lab work make sure to:

- Turn off gas, water, electricity, vacuum and compression lines and heating apparatus.
- Replace materials, equipment and apparatus in their proper storage locations.
- Label, package and dispose of all waste material properly.
- Remove defective or damaged equipment immediately, and arrange to have it repaired or replaced.
- Decontaminate any equipment or work areas that may have been in contact with hazardous materials.
- Leave behind protective clothing (lab coats, gloves, etc.) while leaving the laboratory.
- Close and lock the door of the laboratory if you are the last one to leave.

Among potential laboratory hazards, be alert for the following:

Chemical products of flammable, toxic, oxidizing , reactive and corrosive materials

Microbiological disease-producing agents and their toxins of viruses, bacteria, parasites, rickettsiae and fungi.

Physical or mechanical hazards like ionizing and non-ionizing radiation, electrical, poor equipment design or work organization and tripping hazards.

Understanding hazard warning information Symbols

Class A Compressed Gas (Fig. 2.1)

Characteristics

- ✓ Gas inside cylinder is under pressure
- ✓ The cylinder may explode if heated or damaged
- ✓ Sudden release of high-pressure gas streams may puncture skin and cause fatal embolis

Precautions

- ✓ Transport and handle with care
- ✓ Make sure cylinders are properly secured
- ✓ Store away from sources of heat or fire
- ✓ Use proper regulator

Class B Flammable and Combustible Material (Fig. 2.1)

Characteristics

- ✓ May burn or explode when exposed to heat, sparks or flames
- ✓ Flammable: burns readily at room temperature
- ✓ Combustible: burns when heated

Precautions

- ✓ Store away from Class C (oxidizing materials)
- ✓ Store away from sources of heat, sparks and flame
- ✓ Do not smoke near these materials

Class C Oxidizing Material (Fig. 2.1)

Characteristics

- ✓ Can cause other materials to burn or explode by providing oxygen
- ✓ May burn skin and eyes on contact

Precautions

- ✓ Store away from Class B (flammable and combustible) materials
- ✓ Store away from sources of heat and ignition
- ✓ Wear the recommended protective equipment and clothing

Class D Poisonous and Infectious Material (Fig. 2.1)

Characteristics

Division 1: *Materials Causing Immediate and Serious Toxic Effects*

May cause immediate death or serious injury if inhaled, swallowed, or absorbed through the skin

Precautions

- ✓ Avoid inhaling gas or vapours
- ✓ Avoid skin and eye contact
- ✓ Wear the recommended protective equipment and clothing
- ✓ Do not eat, drink or smoke near these materials
- ✓ Wash hands after handling

Class D Poisonous and Infectious Material (Fig. 2.1)

Characteristics

Division 2: *Materials Causing Other Toxic Effects*

- ✓ May cause death or permanent injury following repeated or long-term exposure

✓ May irritate eyes, skin and breathing passages: may lead to chronic lung problems and skin sensitivity

✓ May cause liver or kidney damage, cancer, birth defects or sterility

Precautions

✓ Avoid inhaling gas or vapours

✓ Avoid skin and eye contact

✓ Wear the recommended protective equipment and clothing

✓ Do not eat, drink or smoke near these materials

✓ Wash hands after handling

Class D Poisonous and Infectious Material (Fig. 2.1)

Characteristics

Division 3: *Biohazardous Infectious Materials*

Contact with microbiological agents (e.g., bacteria, viruses, fungi and their toxins) may cause illness or death

Precautions

✓ Wear the recommended protective equipment and clothing

✓ Work with these materials in designated areas

✓ Disinfect area after handling

✓ Wash hands after handling

Class E Corrosive Material (Fig. 2.1)

Characteristics

✓ Will burn eyes and skin on contact

✓ Will burn tissues of respiratory tract if inhaled

Precautions

✓ Store acids and bases in separate areas

✓ Avoid inhaling these materials

✓ Avoid contact with skin and eyes

✓ Wear the recommended protective equipment and clothing

Class F Dangerously Reactive Material (Fig. 2.1)

Characteristics

✓ May be unstable, reacting dangerously to jarring, compression, heat or exposure to light

✓ May burn, explode or produce dangerous gases when mixed with incompatible materials

Precautions

✓ Store away from heat

✓ Avoid shock and friction

✓ Wear the recommended protective equipment and clothing

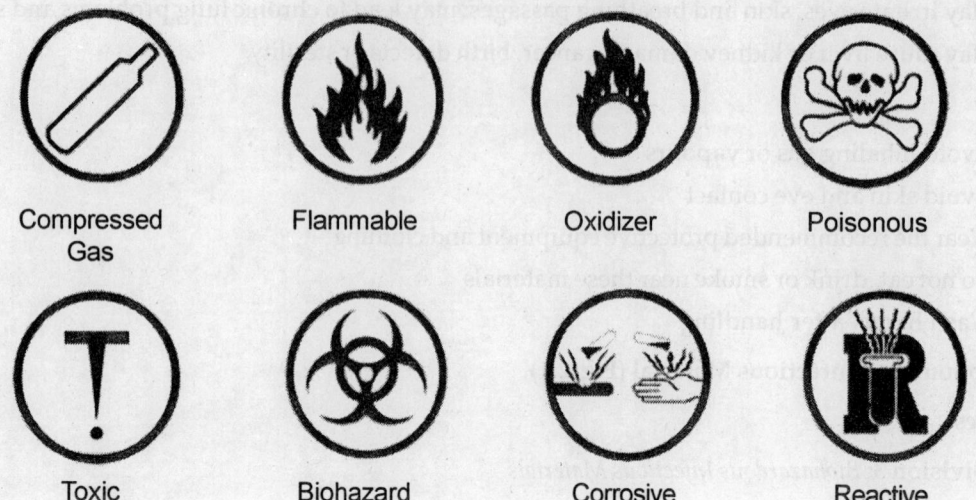

| Compressed Gas | Flammable | Oxidizer | Poisonous |
| Toxic | Biohazard | Corrosive | Reactive |

Fig. 2.1 : Hazard Warning Symbols

Glassware safety

- Use a dustpan and brush, not your hands, to pick up broken glass.
- Discard broken glass in a rigid container and label it appropriately.
- Protect glass that is subject to high pressure or vacuum. Wrapping glass vessels with cloth tape will minimize the possibility of projectiles.
- Glassess are weakened by everyday stresses like heating and bumping hence handle used glassware with extra care.

Lab coats

Appropriate protective clothing (e.g., lab coats, aprons, coveralls) is required in all experimental areas where hazardous materials are handled.

Instructions for selection and use of protective laboratory clothing are as follows:

- Select knee-length lab coats with button or snap closures.
- Wear a solid-front lab coat or gown with back closures and knitted cuffs when working with highly toxic or infectious agents.
- Wear protective aprons for special procedures such as transferring large volumes of corrosive material
- Remove protective clothing while leaving the laboratory.
- Remove protective clothing in the event of visible or suspected contamination

3. Basic Requirements of Biology / Biotechnology Laboratory

Good Biology / biotechnology laboratory should fulfill all basic needs. Both laboratories use microorganisms as a major tool. Different types of microorganisms are present in the world. They are omnipresent and omnipotent in nature. A minimum of 800sq. feet inbuilt area is required for good biology / biotechnology laboratory. Building should be constructed with good standard construction design and should be spacious. Emergency exit, fire safety, ventilators, electrical provisions, water pipelines, gas pipelines, laminar air flow chamber room for bacteriology, virology, mycology, parasitology, tissue culture, washing area, distillation area, sterilization room are the major requirements in the laboratory.

Water is the most important factor in life science laboratory. This is essential for the growth of all organisms. It is used for various purposes like cleaning, media preparation, washing, discarding etc., Salt free water is needed for all kinds of biological work. If the water contains too much of salt it may corrode all instruments and damage glasswares etc., It must be free from any chemicals, which inhibit the bacterial growth. Deionized water or distilled water must be used for the preparation of culture media. Glasswares, instruments, plastic wares and stationary materials are also being a major part of biology laboratories. Good laboratory practices should be followed when handling all these items.

Glasswares like Petri plates, pipettes, test tubes, culture tubes, screw cap tubes, boiling tubes, Pasteur pipettes, conical flask, side arm flask, beaker, standard measuring flask, measuring cylinder, glass spreader, capped glass bottles, BOD bottles, capillary tubes, Durham's tube, microscopic slide, concavity slides, cover slip, burette, glass column and TLC plate are basic needs of a biology laboratory. Similarly, haemocytometer, haemometer stage micrometer, ocular micrometer, microscopes, ESR pipette, ESR stand, Inoculation needle, Nichrome wire, incubator, incubatory shaker, BOD incubator, shaker, autoclave, cooker, hot air oven, microwave oven, thermometer, laminar air flow chamber, colony counter, pH meter, calori meter, UV-VIS Spectro photometer, centrifuge, cooling centrifuge, Balance, Vaccum desicator, Electrophoresis unit, Electrophorator, sonicator, water bath, hot plate, air sampler, agitator, fermenter, ELISA reader, PCR, magnetic stirrer, cuvette are also inevitable equipments of a laboratory.

Cotton, filter paper, glass rod, dettol soap, disinfectants, antiseptics, first aid box with all necessary items, butter paper, spatula, soap oil, Detergent powder, pH paper, Buffer tablets, Sample collector, forceps, needle, scissors, lancet, syringe, Para film, plastic bags, rubber band, match box, apron are some of the stationery items required for basic biology laboratory.

Some important features of instruments, glasswares and other laboratory items are given below.

pH meter (Fig. 3.1)

A **pH meter** is an electronic instrument used to measure the pH of a liquid. A typical pH meter consists of a special measuring probes connected to an electronic meter that measures and displays the pH reading. The first commercial pH meters were built around 1936 by *Radiometer* in Denmark and by *Dr. Arnold Orville Beckman* in the United States. The Danish biochemist Soren Sorensen invented the pH scale in 1909. A standard pH meter has two electrodes, one glass electrode and the other is reference electrode.

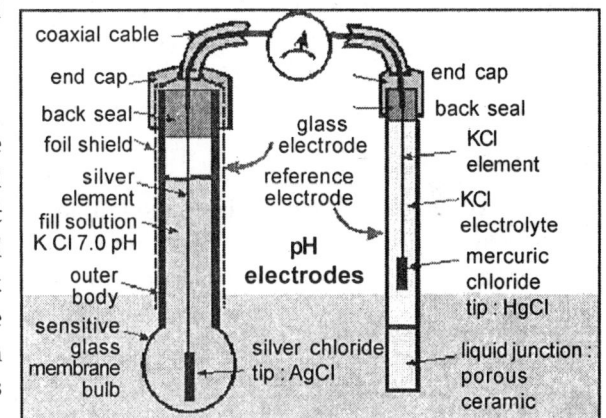

Fig 3.1: pH meter electrodes

The voltage produced by one pH unit (say from pH=7.00 to 8.00) is typically about 60 mV (milli Volt). Present pH meters contain microprocessors that make the necessary corrections for temperature and calibration. The reference electrode, which traditionally used silver chloride (AgCl) and has been superseeded by the *kalomel* (mercurous chloride, $HgCl_2$). This electrode uses mercuric chloride (HgCl) in a potassium chloride (KCl) solution. A pH meter measures essentially the electro-chemical potential between a known liquid inside the glass electrode (membrane) and an unknown liquid outside. The calomel reference electrode consists of a glass tube with a potassium chloride (KCl) electrolyte which is in intimate contact with a mercuric chloride element at the end of a KCL element. It is a fragile construction, joined by a liquid junction tip made of porous ceramic or similar material. This kind of electrode is not easily 'poisoned' by heavy metals and sodium. The glass electrode consists of a sturdy glass tube with a thin glass bulb welded to it. Inside is a known solution of potassium chloride (KCl) buffered at a pH of 7.0. A silver electrode with a silver chloride tip makes contact with the inside solution. To minimise electronic interference, the probe is shielded by a foil shield, often found inside the glass electrode.

Centrifuge (Fig. 3.2)

A centrifuge is an equipment used in all biological laboratories. It is driven by a motor, that puts an object in rotation around a fixed axis, applying force perpendicular to the axis. Simple centrifuges are used in biology and biochemistry for isolating and separating biomolecules, cell organelles or whole cells. They vary widely in speed and capacity. They usually comprise a rotor containing two, four, six, or many more numbered wells within which centrifuge tips or centrifuge tubes may be placed.

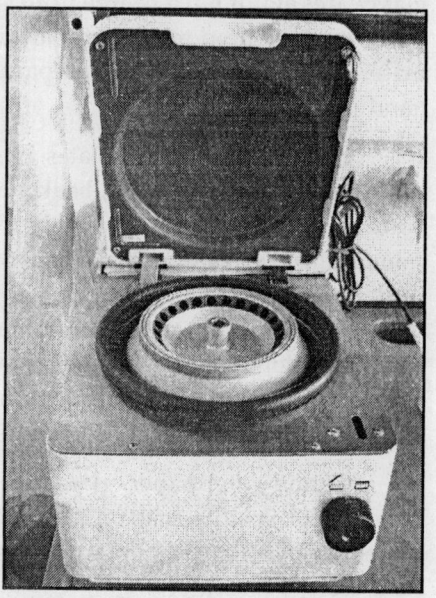

Antonin Prandl invented the first centrifuge. The centrifuge works using the sedimentation principle, where the centripetal acceleration is used to separate substances of greater and lesser density. There are different kinds of centrifuges, including those for very specialised purposes. They are Tabletop/ Clinical/Desktop centrifuge or microcentrifuge, High-speed centrifuge, Cooling centrifuge,Ultra-centrifuge and Gas centrifuge. The rotor is covered by a plastic cover. The cover is usually interlocked to prevent the motor from turning the rotor when it is open, and from allowing the cover to be opened before the rotor stops for several minutes. The cover protects the user from being injured by touching a rapidly spinning rotor. It also protects the user from fragments in case the rotor fails catastrophically. To ensure that the rotor does not turn

Fig. 3.2: Table top centrifuge

unbalancedly, it must be balanced by placing samples or blanks of equal volume opposite each other. Some centrifuges may stop turning when wobbling is detected. The ultra centrifuge was invented in 1925 by **Theodor Svedberg** used for the separation of low molecular weight substances. Gas centrifuges are used in uranium enrichment.

Colony counter (Fig. 3.3)

It is a device used for counting the small closely growing colonies of bacteria on the surface of media. Plate is placed on the counters and marked off with a felt tipped pen on the outer surface of the plate while the operator kept the count manually or electronically.

Bunsen burner (Fig. 3.4)

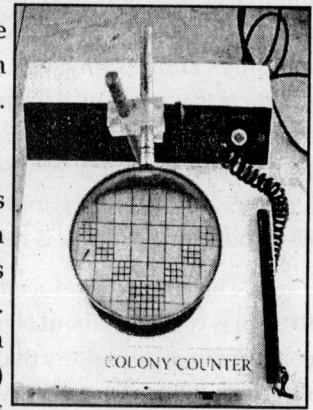

Michael Faraday is the inventer of burner. Improvement of Faradays burner is made in 1855 by Peter Desaga, laboratory assistant of German chemist Robert Wilhelm Bunsen. The name Bunsen burner is given by Robert Wilhelm Bunsen. A Bunsen burner is a common piece of laboratory equipment used for heating, sterilization, and combustion. The latest improved burner is also called a *Tirrill Burner*. The device safely burns a continuous stream of a flammable gas such as natural gas (which is principally methane) or a liquified petroleum gas such as propane, butane or a mixture of both. The burner has a weighted base with a connector for a gas line (hose barb) and a vertical tube (barrel)

Fig. 3.3: Colony counter

rising from it. The hose barb is connected to a gas nozzle on the lab bench with rubber tubing. Most lab benches are equipped with multiple gas nozzles connected to a central gas source, as well as vaccum, nitrogen, and steam nozzles. The gas then flows up through the base through a small hole at the bottom of the barrel and is directed upward. There are open slots in the side of the tube bottom to admit air into the stream via the Venturi effect, and the gas burns at the top of the tube once ignited by a flame or spark. The most common methods of lighting the burner are using a match stick or a spark lighter. The amount of air mixed with the gas stream affects the completeness of the combustion reaction in the flame. All forms of vegetative cells and spores are removed by flaming process. It produces non-luminous flame, the temperature of which reaches $1,860^0$C at its hottest point ie., during flaming of Inoculation loop. Bunsen burner and spirit lamp is used to sterilize inoculation loops/needles. It is also used to sterilize the mouth of the test tubes, media containing flasks etc. Heating of inoculation wires and loops by holding them almost vertically in Bunsen flame until red hot along their whole length, almost to the tip of the metal holder. It is called as red heat.

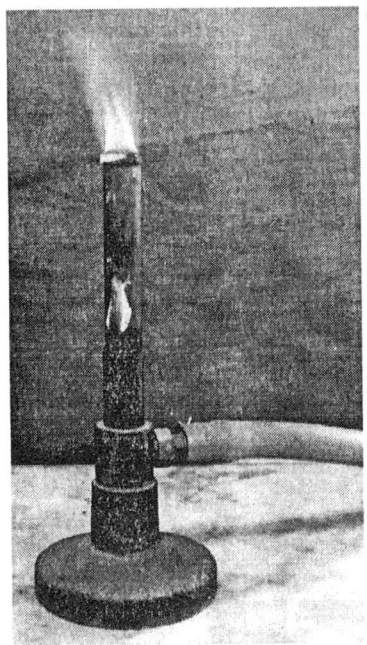

Fig. 3.4: Bunsen Burner

Incubator (Microbiology) (Fig. 3.5)

In microbiology, an incubator is a device for controlling the temperature, humidity and other conditions in which a microbiological culture is being grown. The simplest incubators are insulated boxes with an adjustable heater, typically raising up to 60 to 65°C. More elaborate incubators can also include the ability to lower the temperature (via refrigeration) or the ability to control humidity or CO_2 levels. Most incubators include a timer; some can also be programmed to cycle through different temperatures, humidity levels, etc. Incubators can vary in size from tabletop to the size of small rooms. Incubators also contain certain features such as the shaker, measured by revolutions per minute. Common incubating temperature for the cultivation of bacteria are approximately $36-37^0$C and for the fungus are $25-30^0$C. Incubatory condition may vary with the type of microorganisms.

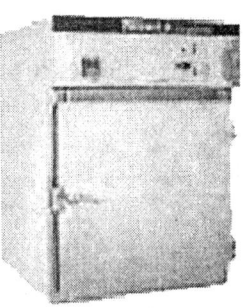

Fig. 3.5: Incubator

Homogenizer (Mortar and Pestle) (Fig. 3.6)

It is a laboratory equipment for the homogenization of various types of material such as tissue, plant, food, soil and many others. Many different models have been developed using various physical technologies for the disruption. Mortar and pestle is one of the most important homogenizer used for thousands of years and still it is a standard tool even in modern laboratories. Most of the solutions are based on blender type of instruments (also known in the kitchen as mixie), bead mills, ultra sonic treatment, high pressure, and many other physical forces. Homogenization is a very common sample preparation step prior to the analysis of nucleic acids, proteins, cells, metabolism, pathogens and many other targets.

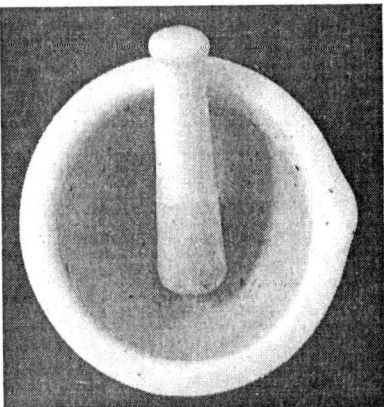

Fig. 3.6: Pestle & Mortar

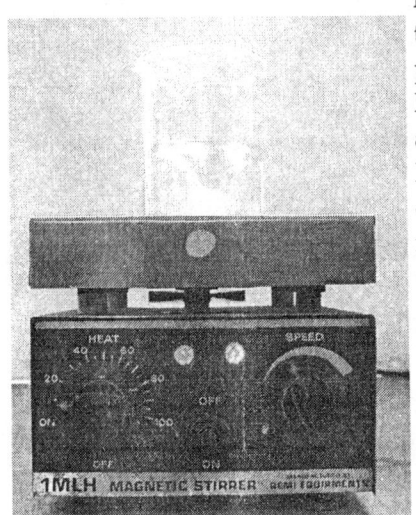

Fig. 3.7: Magnetic stirrer

Magnetic stirrer (Fig. 3.7)

A magnetic stirrer consists of a small bar magnet (or stir bar), which is normally coated in a plastic or stationary electomagnets creating a rotating magnetic field. Often, the plate can also be heated. During operation of a typical magnetic stirrer, the bar magnet (or flea) is placed in a vessel containing a liquid to be stirred. The vessel is set on top of the stand, where the rapidly rotating magnetic field causes the bar magnet to rotate. A stir bar stirring a solution on a magnetic hot plate stirrer. Two knobs are available in the instrument. The left knob controls the stirring rate, the right knob controls heating. The first multipoint magnetic stirrer was developed and patented by **Salvador Bonet** of SBS Company in 1977.

Spectrophotometer (Fig. 3.8)

Spectrophotometry involves the use of a spectrophotometer. A spectrophotometer is a photometer (a device for measuring light intensity) that can measure intensity as a function of the colour or the wavelength of light. There are many kinds of spectrophotometers. Distinctions used to classify the spectrophotometers are the wavelengths they work with, the measurement techniques, how they acquire a spectrum and the sources of intensity variation they are designed to measure. Other important features of spectrophotometers include the spectral bandwidth and linear range. Most common application of spectrophotometer is the measurement of light absorption, but they can be designed to measure diffuse or specular reflectance. There are two major classes

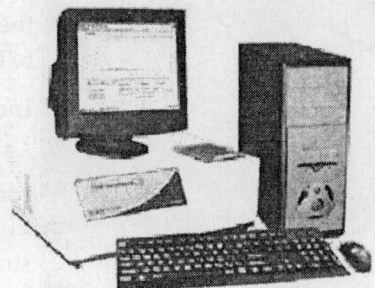

Fig. 3.8: Spectrophotometer

of spectrophotometers; single beam and double beam. A double beam spectrophotometer measures the ratio of the light intensity on two different light paths, and a single beam spectrophotometer measures the absolute light intensity. Although ratio measurements are easier, and generally stabler, single beam instruments have advantages; for instance, they can have a larger dynamic range. **Visible-region spectrophotometers** are similar to colourimeter. Spectrophotometer works under the principle called Beers Lamberts law. Scientists use this machine to measure the amount of compounds in a sample. If the compound is more concentrated more light will be absorbed by the sample. Components of spectrophotometer are 1. The light source shines through the sample. 2. The sample absorbs the light. 3. The detector detects intensity of the light the sample has absorbed. 4. The detector then converts the intensity of light into a number. **UV – VIS spectrophotometers** are the most common spectrophotometers are used in the UV and visible regions of the spectrum. The spectrophotometer measures quantitatively the fraction of light that passes through a given solution. In a spectrophotometer, a light from a lamp in a VIS/UV spectrophotometer (typically a deuterium gas discharge lamp) is guided through a monochromator, which picks light of one particular wavelength out of the continuous spectrum. This light passes through the sample that is being measured. After the sample, the intensity of the remaining light is measured with a photodiode or other light sensor and the transmittance for this wavelength is then calculated.

Microtiter plate (Fig. 3.9)

The microplate has become a standard tool in analytical research and clinical diagnostic testing laboratories. A Microtiter plate is a flat plate with multiple "wells". A very common usage is in the enzyme-linked immunosorbent assay (ELISA). A microtiter plate typically has 6, 24, 96, 384 or even 1536 sample wells arranged in a 2:3 rectangular matrix. Some microplates have even been manufactured with 3456 or even 9600 wells. Each well of a microplate typically holds somewhere between a few to a few hundred microlitres of liquid. The first microplate was created in 1951 by **Dr. G. Takatsky**. **John Liner** in USA had introduced a modified version of micro titre plate.

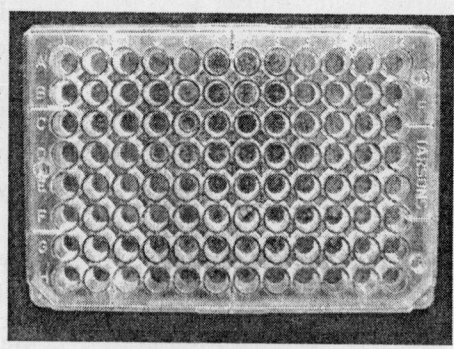

Fig. 3.9 : ELISA plate

Stir bar (Fig. 3.10)

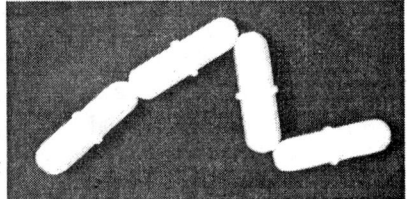

A stir bar (or flea) is a magnetic bar, used to stir a liquids in a laboratory. The stir bar rotates in synch with a separate rotating magnet located beneath the vessel containing the reaction. Glass does not affect a magnetic field appreciably (it is transparent to magnetism) and most chemical reactions take place in glass vessels. This allows the magnetic stir bars to work well in glass vessels. Stir bars are typically coated with teflon, so that they are chemically inert and do not contaminate or react with the reaction mixture they are in.They are bar shaped and often octagonal in cross-section and sometimes circular. Most stir bars have a ridge around the centreon which they rotate. The smallest are only a few

Fig. 3.10 : Stir Bar

millimeters long and the largest a few centimeters. A stir bar retriever is a separate magnet on the end of a long stick, which can be used to get (or fish) stir bars out of the reaction vessel. Most magnetic stirrers today spin their magnets with an electric motor. Stir bars work best for relatively small reactions that are not very viscous. For larger volumes or more viscous liquids, some sort of mechanical stirring is typically needed.

Vortex mixer (Fig. 3.11)

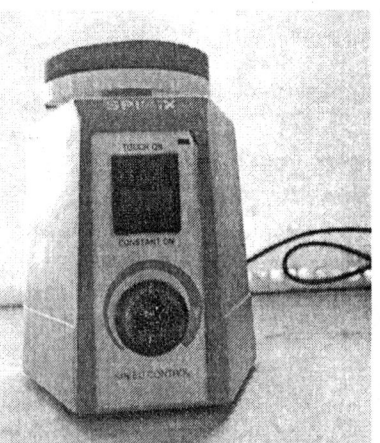

A vortex mixer is a simple device used commonly in laboratories to mix small vials of liquid. It consists of an electric motor with the drive shaft oriented vertically and attached to a cupped rubber piece mounted slightly off-centre. As the motor runs the rubber piece oscillates rapidly in a circular motion. When a test tube or other appropriate container is pressed into the rubber cup (or touched to its edge) the motion is transmitted to the liquid inside and a vortex is created. Most vortex mixers have variable speed settings and can be set to run continuously, or to run only when downward pressure is applied to the rubber piece. Vortex mixers are common in bioscience laboratories. In cell culture and microbiology laboratories they may be used to suspend cells. In a biochemical or analytical laboratory they may be used to mix the reagents of an assay or to mix an experimental sample and a dilutant. An alternative to the electric vortex mixer is the "finger vortex" technique in which a vortex is created manually by striking a test tube in a forward and downward motion with one's finger or thumb. This generally takes longer and often results in an inadequate suspension, although it may be suitable in some cases when a vortex mixer is unavailable or the forces involved in vortexing would damage the sample.

Fig. 3.11 : Vortex Mixer

Petri dish (Fig. 3.12)

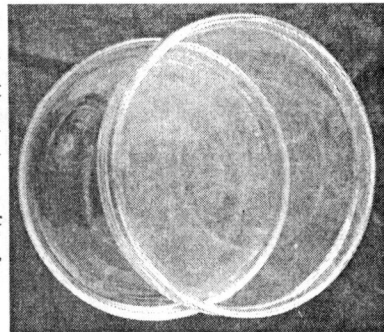

A Petri dish is a shallow glass or plastic cylindrical dish used for the cultivation of microorganisms. It was named after the German bacteriologist Julius Richard Petri (1852–1921) who invented it in 1877 when working as an assistant to Robert Koch. It consists of two shallow glass dishes, the upper half or lid and the lower half or bottom half. Glass petri dishes can be re-cycled after use by dry heating in a hot air oven at 160^{0}C for an hour. Plastic petri-dishes are not recycled. The dish is partially filled with warm liquid agar along with a particular mix of nutrients, salts and amino acids and optionally, antibiotics. After the agar solidifies, the dish is used for microbial inoculation.

Fig. 3.12 : Petriplate

Ocular Micrometer (Fig. 3.13)

The ocular micrometer is a circular disc that is graduated into several small parts. It is placed inside the eyepiece of the microscope. The distance varies according to the objective of the microscope. The distance is easily determined by using a stage micrometer. Occular micrometer is used to measure the accurate dimension of a microorganism, a cell or any microscopic material.

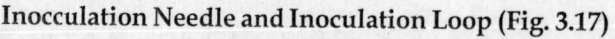

Fig. 3.13: Ocular micrometer

Stage Micrometer (Fig. 3.14)

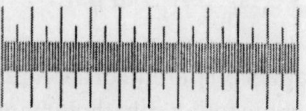

Fig 3.14: Stage micrometer

The stage micrometer is a glass slide graduated in 1mm. ie, the scale measures only 1mm, 0.1mm or 0.01mm depend on the brand. Again it is divided into 10 large divisions and 100 small divisions; one large division is divided into 10 small divisions.These divisions are equally placed. Therefore the least count is 0.01mm. It means that each smaller division of stage micrometer is equal to 10µm. It is used to calibrate the ocular micrometer.

Balance (Fig. 3.15)

Balance is an instrument used for weighing process. For chemical or biological experiments, accurate amount of chemical should be weighed by using a balance. There are several types of balances used for weighing such as single pan, chemical or analytical, and electronic balances. These balances are used according to requirement and the quantity of materials to be weighed. Single pan manual balance is used to weigh the quantity of material more than 100g upto 200g. A chemical or electronic balance is used to weigh 10 mG quantity but its total weighing capacity is 100 g. The ultra micro balance can weigh the materials of 0.01µg to 2 mG quantity.

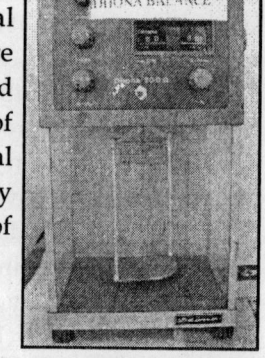

Fig. 3.15: Electronic Balance

Glass Spreader (Fig. 3.16)

Glass spreader is also called L Rod. Glass spreader is made by bending a glass rod and making an L-shaped structure. It is used to spread evenly the microorganisms on agar surface. The long arm is used to hold in hand and the small arm is flame-sterilised and put on agar surface. It is brought forth and back so that the microorganisms inoculated may be distributed or spread evenly on entire surface of the agar. L – Rod is used for spread plate technique.

Fig 3.16: L - Rod

Inocculation Needle and Inoculation Loop (Fig. 3.17)

Inoculation needle and loop are made up of a long nichrome wire fixed into a metallic rod. Inoculation loop is sterilized either by using Bunsen burner or hot heating coil wire till the needle or loop become red. After cooling these are used to transfer or inoculate the culture from one container to the other i.e., from liquid to solid and vice versa. Both loop and needle are to be flamed immediately after use to avoid contamination. Width of the common inoculation loop is 4 mm and it holds about 0.05mL of liquid. During flaming temperature of inoculation loop reaches upto 1860⁰C. Nichrome can immediately be heated and cooled, so it is used in the inoculation loops & needles.

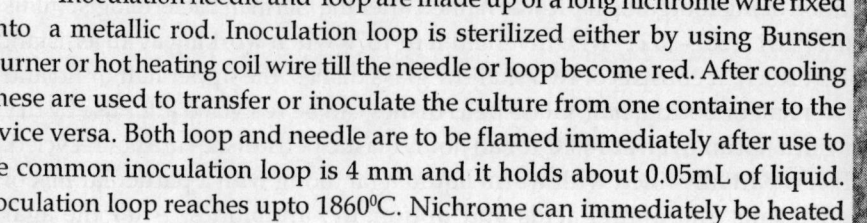
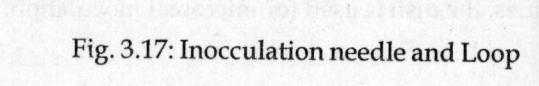

Fig. 3.17: Inocculation needle and Loop

Water Bath (Fig. 3.18)

Water bath is an instrument, used to provide constant temperature to a sample. It consists of an insulating box made up of steel fitted with electrode heating coil. The temperature is controlled by the thermostat. The main use of water-bath is the incubation of samples at a desired and constant temperature. In some of the water-bath, the platform rotates and it is called as water-bath shaker. It is more useful to the microbiologists because it provides a uniform heat to the sample material meant for incubation.

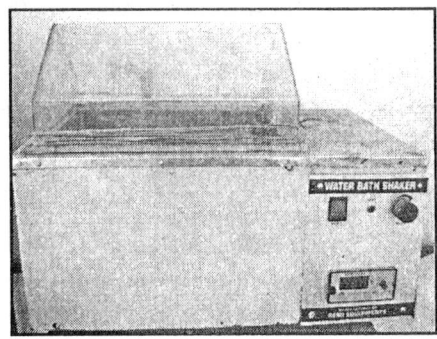

Fig. 3.18: Water bath Shaker

Autoclave - refer Page No. 32 (Fig. 7.1)

Pressure Cooker - refer Page No. 33 (Fig.7.2)

Hot air oven - refer Page No. 34 (Fig. 7.3)

Membrane filter - refer Page No. 35 (Fig. 7.4)

Haemocytometer (Fig. 3.19)

An instrument used for determining the total cell count, viable cell count or spore count. It is mainly used for blood cell count. A grid, etched on the central plateau of the glass block, typically consists of a sqauare of side 1mm divided into 400 squares each $0.0025mm^2$. The distance between grid and coverslip may be 0.1mm. The susbstance is introduced into the space between coverslip and central plateau and cells are allowed to settle for counting. Volume of liquid = $1/4000mm^3$ = $1/4,000,000$. Distance between coverslip and grid 1/10 mm. Each small square in the grid is 1/400. On scanning all 400 small squares 500 cells were counted this would give an average of $500 \div 400 = 1.25$ cells per small square thus since 1.25 cells occur in 1/4,000,000 and the sample must contain 1.25 X 4,000,000 cells per mL. If the sample is diluted before examination the count must be multiplied by the dilution factor.

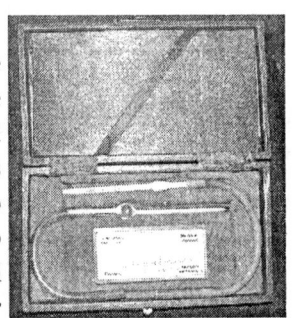

Fig. 3.19: Haemocytometer with counting chamber

Thermometer (Fig. 3.20)

The thermometer is a device that measures the temperature using different principles. The word thermometer is derived from two smaller word fragments: *thermo* from the Greek for heat and *meter* also from Greek,

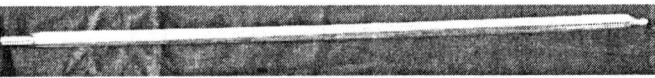

Fig. 3.20: Thermometer

meaning to measure. A thermometer has two important elements that are the temperature sensor (e.g. the bulb on a mercury thermometer) and scale. Industrial thermometers commonly use electronic means to provide a digital display or input to a computer. Thermometers can be divided into two groups according to the level of knowledge about the physical basis of the underlying thermodynamic laws and quantities.

Beaker (Fig. 3.21)

A beaker is a simple container for stirring, mixing and heating liquids. They are commonly used in all laboratories. Beakers are generally cylindrical in shape, with a flat bottom. Beakers are available in a wide range of sizes, from 1 mL to several litres. They may be made of glass (very often borosilicate glass) or of various plastics. Beakers are used for holding solutions of

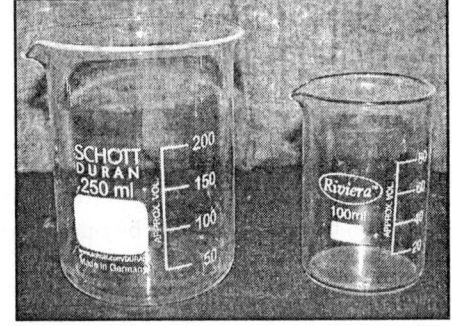

Fig. 3.21: Beaker

corrosive chemicals such as acids or other highly reactive chemicals. They are often made of polytetrafluroethylene or other low reactivity materials. Beakers may be covered, perhaps by a watch glass, to prevent contamination or loss of the contents. Beakers are often *graduated*, marked on the side with lines indicating the volume. The accuracy of these marks can vary from one beaker to another. A beaker is distinguished from a flask by having sides which are straight rather than sloping. In general Chemistry lab beakers are used more often than flasks.

Volumetric flask (Standard Measuring Flask) (Fig. 3.22)

A volumetric flask is a laboratory glassware used in analytical chemistry & biological laboratories media for the preparation of solutions and media. It is made of glass or plastic and consists of a flat bottomed bulb with a long neck, usually fitted with a stopper. The stopper is normally made in a chemically resistant plastic such as polypropylene rather than glass. The neck has a single ring graduation mark and a label. The label should show the nominal volume, tolerance, calibration temperature, class, relevant manufacturing standard and the manufacturer's logo. The glass or plastic is generally clear but may be amber coloured for handling light sensitive compounds such as silver nitrate or vitamin A. Volumetric flasks generally come in two different standards. The higher standard flasks (Class A) are made with a more accurately placed graduation mark, and have a unique serial number for traceability. Class B is used for qualitative or educational work. Volumetric flasks are used for making up solutions to a known volume.

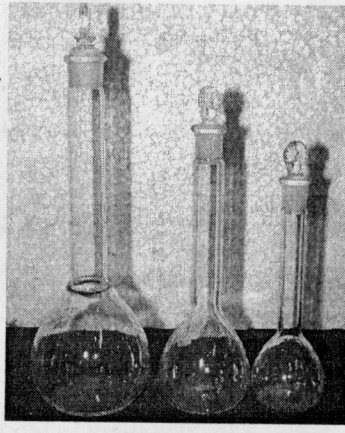

Fig. 3.22: SMF

Pasteur pipettes (Fig. 3.23)

Pasteur pipettes are also known as droppers or eye droppers. They are used to transfer small quantities of liquids. They are usually glass tubes or plastic tubes tapered to a narrow point and fitted with a rubber bulb at the top. Pasteur pipettes come in various lengths. They are sold in boxes of hundreds and are generally considered cheap enough to be disposable. Disinfectants are used to sterilize pasteur pipettes.

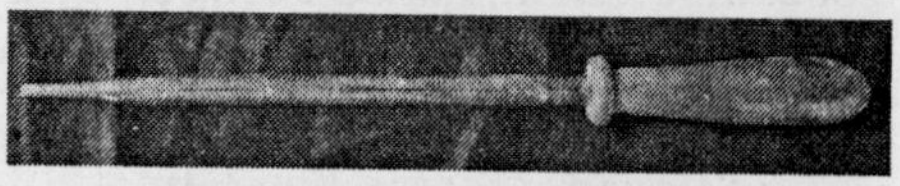

Fig. 3.23:Pasreur Pipettes

Pipette (Fig. 3.24)

A pipette is a laboratory instrument used to measure the volume of a liquid. Pipettes are commonly used in chemistry and biological laboratories. One end of the pipette is tapper and other end is smooth. Pipettes are available in different measuring capacity such as 0.1mL, 0.2mL, 1mL, 2mL, 5mL, 10mL, 25mL etc.,. They are also available in several designs for various purposes with differing levels of accuracy. Nature of pipettes are ranges from single piece glass pipettes to more complex adjustable or electronic pipettes. A pipette works by creating a vaccum above the liquid-holding chamber and selectively releasing this vaccum to draw up and dispense liquid. Pipettes that dispense between 1 and 1000μL are termed as micropipettes. The original pipette is made of glass. The pipette is filled by dipping the tip in the volume to be measured and drawing up the liquid with a pipette filler past the inscribed mark. The volume is then set by releasing the vaccum using the pipette filler or a damp finger. While moving the pipette to the receiving vessel, care must be taken not to shake the pipette because the column of fluid may "bounce". Different types of pipettes are **Pasteur pipettes, Serological pipettes, Mohr pipettes, Dispensable pipettes.** Glass pipettes are sterilized by making use of hot air oven.

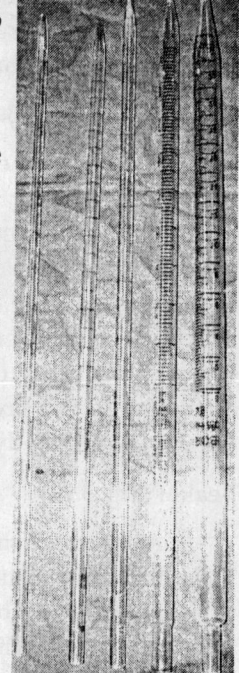

Fig. 3.24: Glass Pipettes

Measuring cylinder (Fig. 3.25)

It is also called graduated cylinder or graduated glass. It is made up of glass or plastic. It is used for measurement of volumes. They are generally more accurate and precise than flasks. Often, the largest graduated cylinders are made of polypropylene (excellent chemical resistance) or polymethylpentane (clarity), Polypropylene is easy to autoclave (sterilize) repeatedly.

Cuvette (Fig. 3.26)

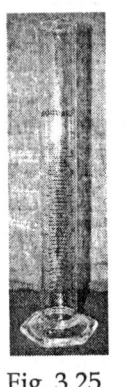

A cuvette is a kind of laboratory glassware, usually a small tube of circular or square cross section. They are sealed at one end and made of plastic, glass or optical grade quartz. It is designed to hold samples for spectroscopic experiments. The best cuvettes are as clear as possible, without impurities. Inexpensive cuvettes are round and look similar to test tubes. Fig. 3.25 Some cuvettes will be clear only on opposite sides, so that they pass a single beam of light through that pair of sides; often the unclear sides have ridges or rough to allow easy handling. Cuvettes used in fluorescence spectroscopy are clear on all four sides.

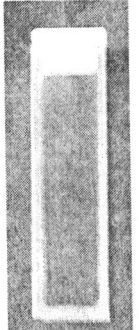

Fig. 3.26: Cuvette

Separating funnel (Fig. 3.27)

A separating funnel is also known as separation funnel or sep funnel. It is a laboratory glassware used in liquid-liquid extractions to separate (*partition*) the components of a mixture between two immiscible solvent phases of different densities. A separating funnel has the shape of a cone mounted by a hemisphere. It has a stopper at the top and stopcock (tap), at the bottom. Separating funnels used in the lab are typically made from borosilicate glass and the stopcocks are made from glass or Teflon. Typical sizes are between 50 mL and 3 L. To use the funnel, the two phases and the mixture to be separated in solution are added through the top with the stopcock at the bottom closed. The funnel is then closed and shaken very strongly to bring the phases into close contact. The funnel is then inverted and the tap carefully opened to release excess vapour pressure. The separating funnel is set aside to allow for the complete separation of the phases. The top and the bottom tap are then opened and the two phases are released by gravitation.

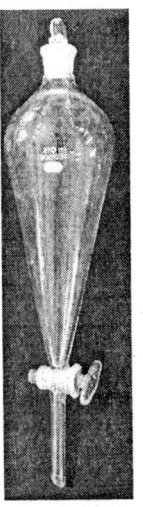

Wash bottle (Fig. 3.28)

A wash bottle is a squeeze bottle with a nozzle, usually used to rinse various glasswares, such as test tubes and round bottom flasks. Usually, wash bottles are filled with deionized water. Wash bottles can also be filled with detergent solutions and rinse solvents such as acetone and ethanol.

Fig. 3.27: Separating Funnel

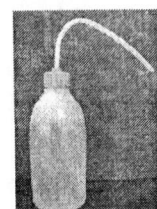

Fig. 3.28: Wash bottle

Soxhlet extractor (Fig. 3.29)

A Soxhlet extractor is invented in 1879 by Franz von Soxhlet . It was originally designed for the extraction of a lipid from a solid material. However, a Soxhlet extractor is not limited to the extraction of lipids. Typically, a Soxhlet extraction is only required where the desired compound has only a limited solubility in a solvent and the impurity is insoluble in that solvent. If the desired compound has a high solubility in a solvent then a simple filtration can be used to separate the compound from the insoluble substance. Normally a solid material containing some of the desired compound is placed inside a thimble made from thick filter paper, which is loaded into the main chamber of the Soxhlet extractor. The Soxhlet extractor is placed onto a flask containing the extraction solvent. The Soxhlet is then equipped with a condenser. The solvent is heated to reflux. The solvent vapour travels up a distillation arm and floods into the chamber housing the thimble of solid. The condenser ensures that any solvent vapour cools, and drips back down into

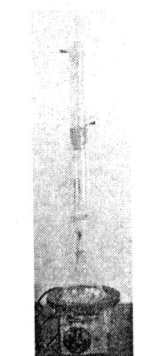

Fig. 3.29: Soxhlet Extractor

the chamber housing the solid material. The chamber containing the solid material slowly fills with warm solvent. Some of the desired compound will then dissolve in the warm solvent. When the Soxhlet chamber is almost full, the chamber is automatically emptied by a siphon side arm, with the solvent running back down to the distillation flask. This cycle may be allowed to repeat many times, over hours or days. During each cycle, a portion of the non-volatile compound dissolves in the solvent. After many cycles the desired compound is concentrated in the distillation flask. The advantage of this system is that instead of many portions of warm solvent being passed through the sample, just one batch of solvent is recycled. After extraction the solvent is removed, typically by means of a rotary evapourator, yielding the extracted compound. The non-soluble portion of the extracted solid remains in the thimble and usually discarded.

Conical flask (Fig. 3.30)

It is named after the German chemist Emil Erlenmeyer, who created it in 1861. An Erlenmeyer flask, commonly known as a conical flask or E-flask. They are usually marked on the side (*graduated*) to indicate the approximate volume of their contents. It has narrow neck. The neck allows the flask to be stoppered using rubber bungs or cotton plugs. The conical shape allows the contents to be swirled or stirred during an experiment; the narrow neck keeps the contents from spilling. Conical flasks are available in different volumes like 10mL, 25mL, 50mL, 100mL, 250mL, 500mL, 1000mL. In some flasks side arm is fitted on the conical flask are used for filteration and are called side arm flask. Erlenmeyer flasks, are used for pH titrations and for the preparation of culture media. Plastic Erlenmeyer flasks used in cell culture are pre-sterilized and feature closures and vented closures to enhance gas exchange during incubation and shaking.

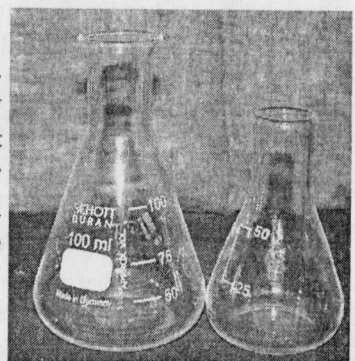
Fig. 3.30: Conical Flask

Boiling tube (Fig. 3.31)

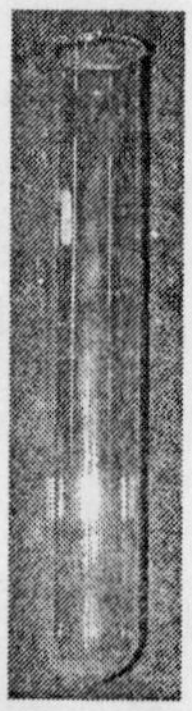

A boiling tube is a large cylindrical vessel like test tube used to heat the substances strongly in the flame of a Bunsen Burner. It is 50% larger than test tube. They are wider than Test tubes and allow substances to boil violently. Some times they can also be used as a general test tube. They are commonly made up of Pyrex glass, which can withstand high temperatures. They can be used as an ignition chamber for gases where their large volume allows for more effective gas air mixture compared to that possible in a test tube.

Test tube (Fig. 3.32)

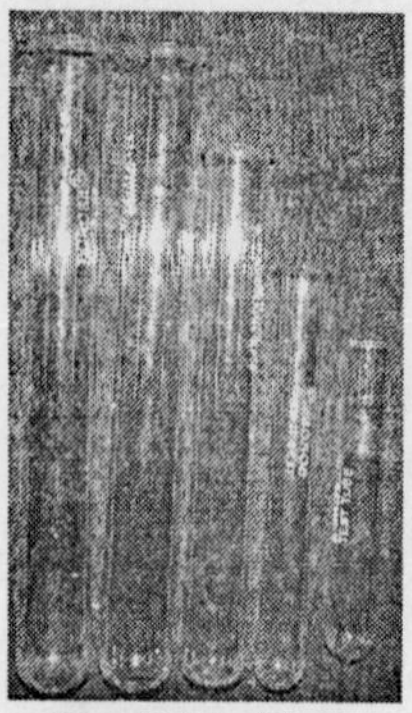

Fig. 3.31: Boiling tube

A test tube is a common laboratory glassware, which is also known as a culture tube. Test tube composed of a finger-like length of glass tubing. It is open at the top, with a rounded U-shaped bottom. Top of the test tube is to aid pouring of a liquid from the test tube to other glasswares or instruments. A tube with a rim is called a test tube and one without a rim is called a culture tube. These glass items are used in microbiology laboratory for performing biochemical tests, broth preparations, serial dilutions etc.,. Cotton plug is inserted on the top of the test tube to maintain sterility. Test tubes are available in various volumes (i.e. 5mL, 7mL, 10mL, 15mL, 20mL, 25mL etc.,). Some test tubes had screw at the top and are called screw capped tube.

Fig. 3.32: Test tube

BOD Bottle (Fig. 3.33)

BOD bottle is a standard 300 mL size clear glass. BOD bottles are fitted with tapered ground glass stopper to prevent air entrapment, flared lip for water seal, and white marking area for identifying sample. B.O.D. Bottles are ideal for incubating diluted samples of sewage, sewage effluents, polluted waters and industrial wastes to determine the amount of oxygen required during the stabilization of the decomposable organic matter by aerobic biochemical action. The 300 mL capacity bottles are recommended for the 5-day B.O.D. test. These B.O.D. bottles have a specially designed shoulder radius that sweeps all air from inside the bottle during filling. The interchangeable stoppers have a tapered bottom that also prevents air entrapment. The bottles have a flared mouth to form a water seal around the stopper that prevents air from being drawn into the bottle during incubation. The stopper joint is compatible with the probes of the leading B.O.D. and D.O. meters. All the bottles are manufactured from Type I borosilicate glass.

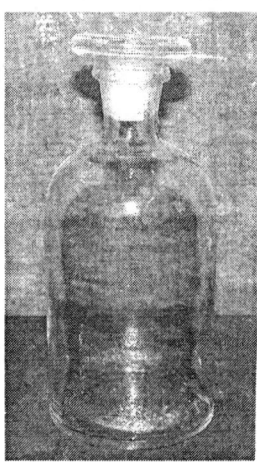

Fig. 3.33: BOD

Capillary Tube is a tube with less internal diameter. It holds liquid by capillary action

Microscope slide

A microscope slide was originally a 'slider' made of ivory or bone. Standardized microscope slides are in the form of a thin sheet of glass used to hold objects for examination under a microscope. A standard microscope slide is 75 x 25 mm (3" X 1") and about 1.0 mm thick.

Coverslip

Smaller sheet of glass is called a cover slip or cover glass, and typically measures between 18 and 25 mm on a side, and 0.085 to 0.25 mm thick. It is shaped into circles, squares or rectangles for covering the specimen. The thickness and refractive index of the glass **coverslip** are important because certain of their values have been assumed by the designer and manufacturer. The cover glass serves two purposes. They are (1) it protects the microscope's objective lens from contacting the specimen and (2) it creates an even thickness (in wet mounts) for viewing. The thickness of the coverslip is crucially important for high-resolution microscopy.

Burette (Fig. 3.34)

An apparatus for delivering measured quantities of liquid or for measuring the quantity of liquid or gas received or discharged. It consists of a graduated glass tube, usually furnished with a small aperture and stopcock. François Antoine Henri Descroizilles developed the first burette in 1791. Joseph Louis Gay-Lussac developed an improved version of the burette that included a side arm, and coined the terms "pipette" and "burette" in a 1824 paper on the standarization of indigo solutions. A major breakthrough in the methodology and popularization of volumetric analysis was achieved by Karl Friedrich Mohr, who redesigned the burette by placing a clamp and a tip at the bottom.

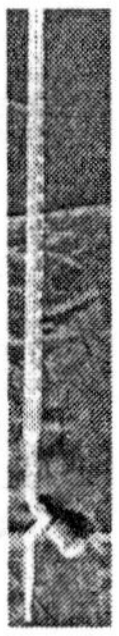

Fig. 3.34: Burette

Refrigerator

A **refrigerator** (often called a "**fridge**") is a cooling appliance comprising a thermally insulated compartment and a mechanism to transfer heat from it to the external environment, cooling the contents to a temperature below ambient. Refrigerators are extensively used to store foods which deteriorate at ambient temperatures; spoilage from bacterial growth. A device described as a "refrigerator" maintains a temperature a few degrees above the freezing point of water; a similar device which maintains a temperature below the freezing point of water is called a "**freezer**". The refrigerator is a relatively modern invention amongst kitchen appliances. It replaced the common icebox which had been placed outside for almost a century and a half.

Haemometer (Fig. 3.35)

It is a compact kit used for detecting the haemoglobin content of the blood by diluting an acidified sample and comparing it with a coloured standard. Its reliability, simplicity and rugged construction makes this kit suitable for simplified services are unavailable. The kit consists of a Sahli haemometer, graduated dilution tube, dropping pipette, brush, glass rod, amber coloured acid vial, a blood pipette and a suction tube.

Chemicals

Good laboratory grade chemicals also required as per experimental requirement. For exact chemical need, refer materials required section of individual practicals and also appendix.

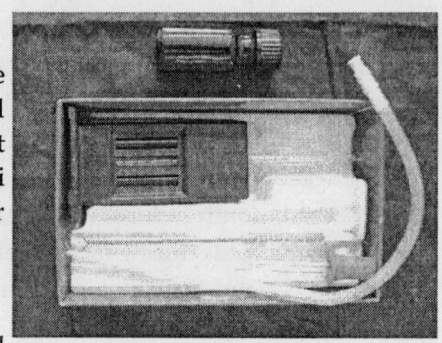

Fig. 3.35: Haemometer

Laboratory instruments, glasswares, plasticwares, chemicals, stationery items only do not satisfy the good performance of the laboratory. Laboratory performances rely only on laboratory chief, workers / students. Laboratory personnels should have the following, Analytical bent of mind, Aptitude for research, Keen power of observations, Mathematical and computational skills, Good at technical and report writing, Mind of Upgradation of knowledge, hard working nature, maintanence of good laboratory practices, following good disposal procedures for disposing chemicals, biological etc.,

When performing experiments students should have the following accessories, clean laboratory coat, record note book, glass marking pencil, glass slide & cover slip, labeling slips, match box, cloth, slide box, scissors, forceps, needle, mask, gloves, scale, eraser etc.,

4. Microscopy

Aim

To understand the nature and types of microscopes.
To know the basic principles and theory of microscopes.
To understand the working procedures of microscope.
To visualize the microorganisms by microscope.

Introduction

The study of Micro organisms / cells requires appropriate methods for observation. Microscopy is the use of a microscope to view objects too small to be visible with the naked eye. Microorganisms are the tiny particles seen through microscope.

In 1676, Antony Von Leuvenhoek observed minute objects and named as animalcules through his ground pieces of glasses. His microscope magnification is around 50 – 300 times. The common initial microscope may be invented by Zacharias Janseen from Netherlands or Galielo Galielei of Italy. Advanced compound microscope was invented by Robert Hook in 18th century.

Two key characteristics of a reliable microscope are *magnification,* or the ability to enlarge objects, and *resolving power* or the ability to show detail. Lenses act like a collection of prisms operating as a unit. When a light source is distant so that the parallel rays of light strikes the lens, a convex lens will focus these rays at a specific point, the focal point. The distance between the centre of the lens and the focal point is called focal length. Many different types of microscopes have been developed over the past two centuries. Each has its own characteristics features that provide it with a specific value in microscopy. Basically there are two kinds of microscopes light and electron.

Light microscope uses light as its source of illumination and has four types. They are (1) Bright field Microscope, (2) Dark field Microscope, (3)Fluorescent Microscope and (4)Phase contrast Microscope. Electron microscopes uses a beam of electrons instead of light waves to produce an image.There are two types of electron microscopes. They are (1)Transmission Electron Microscopes and (2)Scanning Electron Microscope

Compound Microscope (Bright Field) (Fig. 4.1 and 4.2)

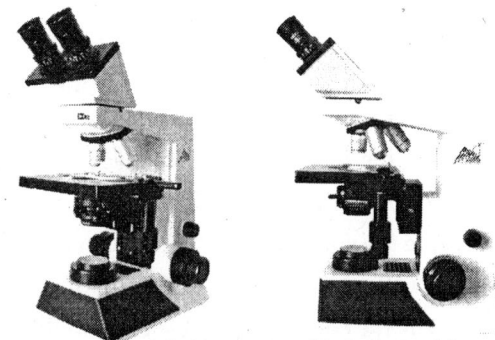

The standard instrument used in the laboratory to observe microorganism is the compound light microscope. This is called compound because it contains two or more sets of lenses. Modern compound microscope has a condenser lens, which focuses light on the objective lenses that are close to the specimen and magnify it, and ocular lenses that are close to eye and further magnify the image.

Light rays passes through the specimen in a bright field microscope. Since objects are seen against the light background and staining of the specimen enhances its contrast against the background. Specimens that are stained and view with the bright field (light field) microscope appear dark against a bright background.

Fig 4.1: Compound Bright Field Binocular Microscope

Parts of microscope.

Ocular lens, Body tube, Movable arm, Nose piece, Objective lens, Body of the microscope, Mechanical stage, Coarse adjustment, Fine adjustment, Condenser, Iris diaphragm, Base, Illuminator lamp.

Resolving power

The ability to distinguish two objects as separate and distinct entities are called resolution. The resolving power of the microscope is determined by three factors i.e., (a). The wavelength of light used for illumination, (b). Numerical aperture of the condenser and (c). Numerical aperture of the objective lens.

Magnification

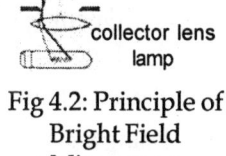

The total magnification of a specimen seen through a compound microscope is determined by multiplying the power of objective lens and ocular lens.

Objective lens X ocular lens =magnification

010   X 10 = 0100
040   X 10 = 0400
100   X 10 = 1000

Fig 4.2: Principle of Bright Field Microscope

The **refractive index** varies with the medium used between the lens and the specimen. Air is generally used as the standard surrounding medium. The refractive index of air is assumed to be 1.00. Since the value of $\sin\theta$ remains constant for any given lens, the numerical aperture of an objective lens can be increased only by inserting a medium with a refractive index higher than 1.00 between the specimen and lenses. Water has a refractive index of 1.33 where as immersion oil- has refractive index of 1.52 by changing the medium from air to oil, the numerical aperture of objective lens has to be increased. Resolving power also depends on condensers numerical aperture. **Abbe condenser** used in student microscopes. This consists of two or more lenses that are not corrected for spherical or chromatic aberration. Other type condenser has 6 elements, which correct aberration and provide neat perfect images of the light source. An adjustable multi leaf **iris diaphragm** is located in the condenser. It controls the diameter of light leaving the condenser and striking the specimen. Adjusting voltage mode of **light source** controls light intensity in microscopy.

Microscope Operation Procedure

- Keep the microscope in correct position and identify the essential parts.
- Clean the eyepieces, objectives, condenser lens, stage and illuminator properly.
- Before switching on the microscope turn the lamp brilliance control to its lowest setting, then increased it to about three-quarters of its power.
- Bring the 10X objective into place.
- Make sure the underside of the specimen slide and surface of the stage is completely dry and clean.
- Place the specimen on the stage in the slide holder
- Focus the specimen with the 10X objective.
- Focus the condenser and leave it in this position for all objectives.
- Examine the specimen with the 10X objective.
- Obtain the best image by
    - Closing the iris about two thirds.
    - Adjusting the lamp brightness control to give illumination with the minimum of glare.
- Use the mechanical stage to examine the specimen systematically
- Examine the specimen with the 40X objective
- Obtain the best image by
    - Opening the iris more
    - Increasing the illumination
- Move the 40X objective to the slide, place a drop of oil on the specimen and bring the 100X objective in to position.
    - Opening iris fully
    - Increasing the illumination
- Turn the lamp brightness control to its lowest setting and switch off the microscope.
- Using a piece of soft tissue or a soft piece of clean cotton cloth, wipe the immersion oil from the 100X objective and its surrounding mount.
- Cover the microscope with its dust cover.

Table 4.1-Differential Properties of microscopic objectives

Character	Low power 10x	High power 40x	Oil immersion 100x
Magnification	100-150	400-450	1000-1500
Numerical aperture	0.25	0.55-0.65	1.25-1.4
Focal length	16mm	4mm	1.8-2mm
Working distance	4-8mm	0.5-0.7mm	0.1mm
Resolving power	0.9mm	0.35m	0.18mm

Note:

Oil has same refractive index as glass. It prevents the loss of light due to bending of light rays as they pass through air. It enhances the resolving power of the microscope. Open diaphragm during the use of oil immersion lens as much as possible. Blue or green filters are used to enhance the resolving power. Only grit free optically safe tissue paper should be used for lens cleaning

Dark Field Microscopy (Fig. 4.3)

It is designed to eliminate the need for staining to achieve contrast between the specimen and background. Instead of normal condenser, dark field microscope uses dark field condenser that contains an opaque disc. The disc blocks light that enters the objective directly. Only light that is reflected off the specimen enters the objective lens. The dark field condenser directs the rays of light into the specimen field at such an angle that only the rays strikes an object in the field are bent, or refracted in to the objective.

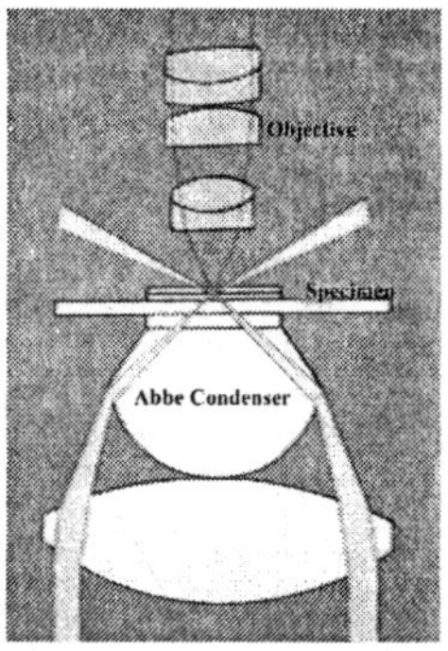

Phase Contrast Microscope (Fig. 4.4)

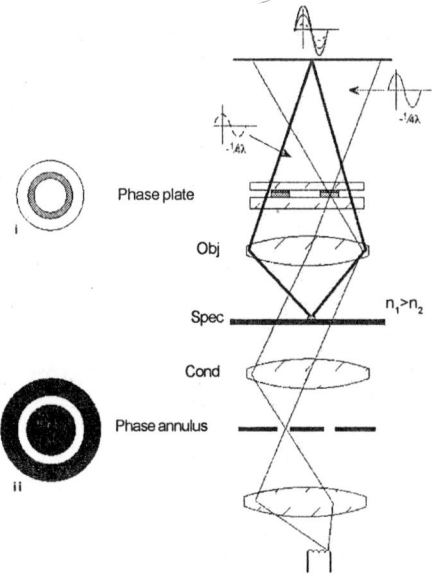

Fig. 4.4: Principle of Phase contrast Microscopy

It is useful because it permits detailed examination of internal structures in living microorganisms. It is not necessary to fix or stain the specimen. The principle of phase contrast microscopy is based on the wave nature of light rays, and the fact that light rays can be in phase or out of phase. If the wave peak of light rays from one source coincides with the wave peak of light rays from another source, rays interact to produce reinforcement (relative brightness). One set of light rays directly from the light source, another set is from light that is reflected or diffracted from the particular structure in the specimen. When the two sets of light rays -direct rays and reflected or diffracted rays are brought together, they form an image of the specimen on the ocular lens, containing areas that are relatively light, through shades of Grey to black. In phase contrast microscope, the internal structures of a cell become sharply defined. This microscope uses special condenser that contains an annular (ring - shaped) diaphram.

Fig. 4.3: Principle of Dark Field Microscopy

Fluorescence Microscope (Fig. 4.5)

It is a light microscopic technique used widely in hospitals and clinical laboratories because it can be adopted to rapid tests that identify disease-causing microbes. A chemical compound is said to be fluorescent if it is capable of absorbing UV light and emitting the energy as visible light. Some fluorescent dyes used in fluorescent microscopy are fluorescine.

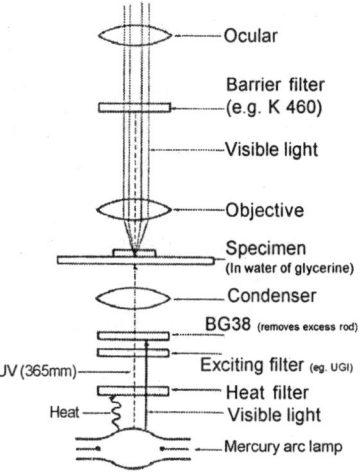

Fig. 4.5: Principles of Fluorescent Microscopy

Electron Microscope

Electron microscopes are scientific instruments that use a beam of highly energetic electrons to examine objects on a very fine scale. It permits much greater resolution and thus obtains higher useful magnification than the light microscope. Electron microscopes functions exactly as their optical counterparts except that they use a focused beam of electrons instead of light to 'image' the specimen and gain information as to its structure and composition.

The basic steps involved in all electron microscopes are

1. A stream of electrons is formed (by the electron source) and accelerated toward the specimen using a positive electrical potential.

2. The stream is confined and focused using metal apertures and magnetic lenses into a thin, focused, monochromatic beam.

3. This beam is focused onto the sample using magnetic lens.

4. Interactions occur inside the irradiated sample, affecting the electron beam.

5. These interactions and effects are detected and transformed into an image.

Total magnification of electron microscope is 10,000 X plus

Two main types of electron microscopes are

    1. Transmission Electron Microscope (TEM)
    2. Scanning Electron Microscope (SEM)

1.Transmission Electron Microscope (TEM) (Fig. 4.6)

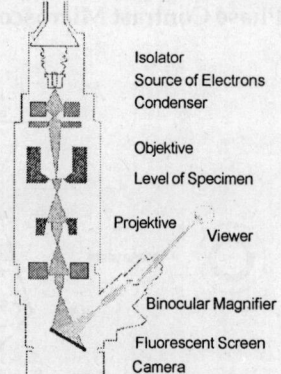

Fig. 4.6: Principles of Transmission Electron Microscopy

- It was the first type of electron microscope.

- Max Knoll and Ernst Ruska in Germany developed it in 1931.

- TEM works much like a slide projector.

- Specimen for TEM is prepared by *shadow casting technique*. This will give three-dimension structure.

- Structures appear after these types of microscopy are called artifacts.

- Electron gun produces a stream of monochromatic electrons.

- This is focused to a small, thin, coherent beam by the use of condenser lenses 1 and 2.

- The beam strikes the specimen and parts of it are transmitted.

- This transmitted portion is focused by the objective lens into an image.

- Optional objective and selected area metal apertures can restrict the beam; the objective aperture enhancing contrast by blocking out high angle diffracted electrons, the selected area aperture enabling the user to examine the periodic diffraction of electrons by ordered arrangements of atoms in the sample.

- The image is passed down the column through the intermediate and projector lenses, being enlarged all the way.

- The image strikes the phosphor image screens and light is generated, allowing the user to see the image. This image represents two areas of the specimen. They are thicker area and thinner area. In thinner area electrons are passed easily.

- Specimens are prepared by sectioned into extremely thin slices (20-100nm) and stained or soaked in metals that will increase image contrast.

Scanning Electron Microscope (SEM) (Fig. 4.7)

The first scanning electron microscope debuted in 1942 with the first commercial instrument around 1965. Its later development is due to the electronics involved in scanning the beam of electrons across the sample.

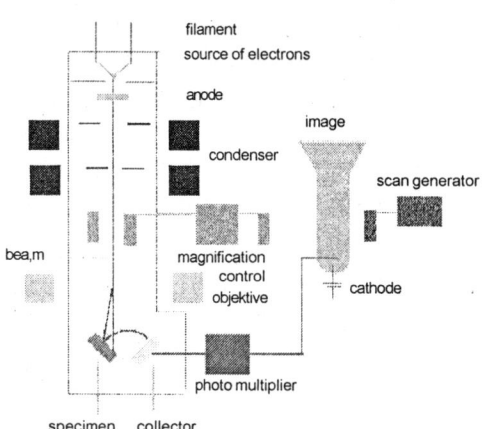

Fig. 4.7: Principles of Scanning Electron microscopy

- Electron gun produces a stream of monochromatic electrons.
- First condenser lens condenses the stream.
- The condenser aperture, eliminating some high angle electrons then constricts the beam.
- The second condenser lens forms the electrons into a thin, tight, coherent beam and is usually controlled by the ' fine probe current knob'
- A user selectable objective aperture further eliminates high angle electrons from the beam.
- A set of coins then scan or sweep the beam in the grid fashion, dwelling on points for a period of time determined by the scan speed.
- The final lens, the objective, focuses the scanning beam onto the part of the specimen desired.
- When the beam strikes the sample interactions occur inside the sample and are detected with various instruments.

Advantages of electron microscope over light microscope

✓ It is useful for the detection of fastidious gastroenteritis viruses such as rota, adeno, astro, norwalk and calici viruses.

✓ It is also used for the detection of herpes infections.

✓ All viral inclusions are detected with electron microscopes.

✓ Internal structures of the viruses are also detected with the help of electron microscopes.

Confocal microscope (Fig. 4.8)

Confocal microscopy is an optical imaging technique used to increase micrograph contrast and/or to reconstruct three-dimensional images by using a spatial pinhole to eliminate out-of-focus light or flare in specimens that are thicker than the focal plane. This technique has been gaining popularity in the scientific and industrial communities. Typical applications include life sciences and semiconductor inspection.

The principle of confocal imaging was patented by Marvin Minsky in 1957. In a conventional (i.e., wide-field) fluorescence microscope, the entire specimen is flooded in light from a light source. Due to the conservation of light intensity transportation, all parts of the specimen throughout the optical path will be excited and the fluorescence detected by a photodetector or a camera. In

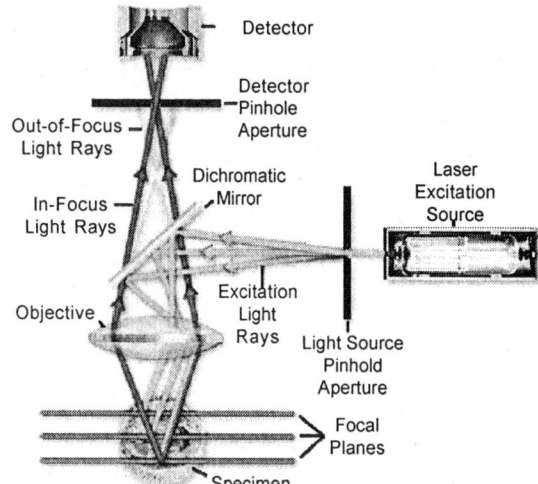

Fig. 4.8: Principles of Confocal Microscopy

contrast, a confocal microscope uses point illumination and a pinhole in an optically conjugate plane in front of the detector to eliminate out-of-focus information. Only the light within the focal plane can be detected, so the image quality is much better than that of wide-field images. As only one point is illuminated at a time in confocal microscopy, 2D or 3D imaging requires scanning over a regular raster (i.e. a rectangular pattern of parallel scanning lines) in the specimen. The thickness of the focal plane is defined mostly by the square of the numerical aperture of the objective lens, and also by the optical properties of the specimen and the ambient index of refraction.

Three types of confocal microscopes are commercially available: Confocal laser scanning microscopes, spinning-disk (Nipkow disk) confocal microscopes and Programmable Array Microscopes (PAM).

Table 4.2: Difference between light and electron microscopes.

Character	Light microscope	Electron microscope
Highest practical magnification	About 1000-15000	Over 100,000
Best resolution	0.2mm	0.5mm
Radiation source	Visible light	Electron beam
Medium of travel	Air	High vaccum
Types of lens	Glass	Electromagnet
Source of contrast	Differential light absorption	Scattering of electrons
Focusing mechanism mechanically	Adjust lens portion	Adjust current to the magnetic lens
Method of changing magnification	Switch the objective lens	Adjust current to the magnetic lens
Specimen mount	Glass slide	Metal grid usually copper

Cleaning of microscopic lences

Xylene, acetone, alcohol are used for cleaning of lenses. Cotton cloth or fine tissue papers are used for cleaning of lens. Should not use hard cloth or other materials to clean lens.

Viva Questions

- Why is oil used while using 100X objective lens?
- Name a specimen preparation method in electron microscope.
- Define resolving power, magnification, numerical aperture, refractive index
- Differentiate between the resolving power and magnifying power of a lens.
- What is meant by the term "parfocal"?
- Why is the low-power objective placed in position when the microscope is stored or carried?
- What is the function of the iris diaphragm? The substage condenser?
- What is meant by the limit of resolution?
- How can you increase the bulb life of your microscope if its voltage is regulated by a rheostat?

- How can you increase the resolution on your microscope?
- What is the principle behind dark-field microscopy?
- When would you use the dark-field microscope?
- Why is the field dark and the specimen bright when a dark-field microscope is used to examine a specimen?
- Differentiate between bright-field and dark-field microscopy.
- What is the function of the Abbé condenser in dark-field microscopy?
- What is the function of the dark-field stop?
- In the phase-contrast microscope, what does the annular diaphragm do?
- When would you use the phase-contrast microscope?
- Explain how the phase plate works in a phase-contrast microscope that produces bright objects   with respect to the background.
- What happens to the phase of diffracted light in comparison to undiffracted light in a phase-contrast microscope?
- What advantage does the phase-contrast microscope have over the ordinary bright-field microscope?
- What is the difference between a bright-phase-contrast and a dark-phase-contrast microscope?
- What is the kind of light used to excite dyes and make microorganisms fluoresce?
- List two fluorochromes that are used in staining bacteria.
- What is a serious hazard one must guard against when working with mercury vapor arc lamps?
- What is the function of each of the following?a. exciter filter b. barrier filter c. heat filter d. mercury vapor arc lamp
- When is fluorescence microscopy used in a clinical laboratory?
- Differentiate between phosphorescence and fluorescence.
- What advantage is there to using fluorescence procedures in ecological studies? Give several examples.

Possible spotters

10X, 40X, 100X objective lens, Photograph of different types of microscopes, Antony Von Leuvenhoek

5. Cleaning and Sterilization of Glasswares

Aim

To clean all glasswares required for the biological laboratory

To sterilize glasswares appropriately.

Background informations

Glassware cleaning and sterilization is an important procedure in the biological laboratories. Improperly cleaned glassware leads to pH alteration. If the pH of the medium is altered the entire work will be wasted. So care must be taken during the preparation of glasswares for sterilization. Sterilization means complete destruction of microbes from an article or freeing of a bacteria and spores from an article. All glasswares must be thoroughly cleaned before use.

Materials required

Glassware cleaning solution Preparation

Add 1.5g potassium dichromate to 100mL of warm water. Cool it and stir slowly, while stirring slowly add 100mL of concentrated sulphuric acid.

Glasswares as per practical requirment, Hot air oven, Pipette can, Petrican, Pipette stand, Detergent powder, Distilled water etc.

Procedure

- Collect required glasswares as per instructions or experimental procedure. (Select only glasswares, which are free from stains and cracks for sterilization.)
- New glasswares are best cleaned by soaking in hot water and detergent and then rinsing with tap water.
- Used glasswares should be cleaned with brush using detergents and acids. Chromic acid is often used for cleaning of glasswares.
- Pipettes are cleaned by using chromic acid solution.
- After wasing with detergent and acid, rinse the glasswares finally with distilled water.
- Air dry all glasswares by inverting them in a water absorbing paper or in a test tube stand or pipette stand before sterilization.
- Arrange petriplates in hot air oven in straight position. Should not place petriplates in inverted position.
- Load air dried glasswares in a Hot Air Oven and sterilize at 180 ° C for 10 minutes or 160 ° C for 1 hour.
- After sterilization dont open the oven immediately because if you open cool air enters inside and it may leads to cracking of glasswares. So wait until the temperature of hot air oven is below 50°C. Pipette can may also used for the sterilization of pipettes.
- Arrange all glasswares in a clean air system (Laminar air flow) before the starting of microbiological work.

Observation

Sterilization of glasswares especially petriplates and other materials used in culturing are checked by making use of control plates.

Viva questions

- How do you prepare glassware-cleaning solution?
- Why is cleaning essential in biological laboratories.
- How do you clean new and old glasswares?
- Why is glassware finally rinsed with distilled water?
- How detergent & acid act on dirty materials?
- How do you check glasswares used in microbiology laboratory are completely sterilized?

Spotters: Detergent, chromic acid , hot air oven.

6. Preparation of Culture Media

Aim

To understand media and its types.

To become familiar with media preparation.

To cultivate microorganisms.

Introduction

Any material that support the growth of organisms are called culture media. It must contain many nutrients. Micronutrients and macronutrients are required for the growth of microorganisms. Microbial culture medium is basically classified into two types. They are Defined medium and Complex medium. Medium, which contains known chemical constituents are called *defined medium*. Eg., Minimal Medium. Those medium which contains unknown chemical constituents are called *complex medium* Eg., Nutrient Agar. Most essential culture media are available commercially in readymade dehydrated form. Simple medium, Enriched and enrichment medium, Selective medium, Differential medium and Transport medium are the types of culture medium.

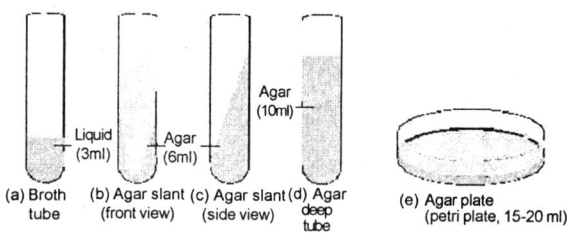

Fig 6.1: Agar deep, Agar Slant and Agar Plate

Simple medium

These are simple nutrient medium that will support the growth of microorganisms that do not require special nutrition. They are often used to prepare enriched media, storing of stock cultures and sub culturing. Eg., Nutrient Agar.

Enriched and enrichment medium

These are the medium that enriched with whole blood, lysed blood, serum, extra peptones, special extracts or vitamins to support the growth of fastidious organisms. Eg., *Haemophillus influenzae* require X and V factor for growth that is given in the form of chocolate agar. The term enrichment is used to describe a fluid medium that increases the number of pathogens by enhancing the growth and discouraging the multiplication of unwanted pathogens or bacteria. Eg., GN broth discourage the growth of Enterobacteriaceae members other than *Salmonella, Shigella* and *Escherichia*.

Selective medium

These are the media, which contains substances that prevent or slowdown the growth of microbes other than pathogens for which the media are intended. Eg. XLD medium selects Salmonella and Shigella. Now a day antimicrobial agents have became increasingly used as selective agents. Eg. New York City Agar medium used to select *Neisseria gonorrhoea* which contains Colistin, Nalidixic acid, Nystatin and Trimethoprim Sulphate. These antibiotics inhibit the growth of all gram positive, gram negative except Neisseria.

Differential medium

This type of the medium is used to differentiate various pathogens. Main differential part of the medium is indicators and dyes. Eg., TCBS medium contain bromo thymol blue which differentiate sucrose fermenting Vibrio from others.

Transport medium

These are mostly semisolid media that contain ingredients to prevent the over growth of commensals and ensure the growth of aerobic and anaerobic pathogens. Eg. Cary Blair medium used for preserving enteric pathogens.

Classification of media based on solidification

Culture media used in three forms they are Solid, Semisolid and Fluid medium.

Solid medium

Medium with agar or gelatin are called solid medium. On solid media culture is grown as colonies. Based on colony morphology on solid medium microbiologist preliminarily identify the organisms. These mediums are used for slant preparation, deep preparation and also for subculturing and stock culture preparation.

Semisolid medium

This media is prepared by adding lower quantities of agar (0.4-0.5%) to the fluid medium, used as transport medium and for motility testing.

Fluid medium

This is prepared without agar. In this, the growth and multiplicaton is described into four stages Lag, Log, Stationary and decline. Growth was shown by turbidity and used as enrichment, biochemical test and blood culture medium.

Microbial growth requirements

Approximately 80% of the living weight of microbial cell is made up of water and of dry weight 2-5% phosphorus remaining part is made up of minerals & combination oxygen, hydrogen and nitrogen containing organic compounds.

Common ingredients of culture media

Peptone

This is a general term for the water-soluble products obtained from the break down of animal or plant protein. The proteins are commonly from meat, milk and soyabean meal. They are hydrolyzed by acids or by enzymes such as pepsin, trypsin and papain. These products are free from aminoacids, peptides and proteases. All forms of peptones are not coagulated by heat. Peptone provides nitrogen for growing microorganisms. Plant protein such as Soya peptone provides carbohydrates. Most peptones contain nucleic acid fractions, minerals and vitamins. Peptone powder should be light in colour, dry and have neutral in pH. The concentration and forms of peptone used depends on the use of individual culture media. Various types of peptones are described on the basis of its nitrogen and sodium chloride concentration.

Mycological peptone	-9.5% nitrogen and 1.1% sodium chloride
Bacteriological peptone	-14% nitrogen and 1.6% sodium chloride
Proteose peptone	-12.7% nitrogen and 8% sodium chloride
Soya peptone	-8.7% nitrogen and 0.4% sodium chloride
Special peptone	-11.7% nitrogen and 3.5% sodium chloride

Meat extracts / Yeast extracts

Beef extracts supply amino acids, vitamins and minerals such as phosphorus and sulfates to the organisms. It is an essential ingredient in most general-purpose culture media.

Trypsin digested meat extract is used for hartley's broth

Mineral salts

Sulphates are required as the sources of sulphur and phosphates are the sources of phosphorus for cell growth. Culture media should also contain traces of magnesium, potassium, iron, calcium and other minerals, which are required for bacterial enzyme activity. Sodium chloride is an essential ingredient in most culture media.

Agar agar

This is an inert polysaccharide and mucopolysaccharide obtained from red- purple seaweed called Gelidium. Gelidium is one of the agarophyte group of marine algae. Agar consists of two main polysaccharides, agarose (70-75%) and agaropectin (20-25%). For use in culture media, agar must be free from pigments and substances toxic to bacteria.

Agar is used as a solidifying agent in all culture media because of gelling strength and its setting temperature of 32-39°C and melting temperature of 90-95°C. Normal concentration of agar in culture media is 1.5 %. If the agar concentration is <1%, the medium is called semi solid media. It acts as a nutrient medium to some marine microorganisms like Pseudomonas, Cytophaga etc. It has two important properties called gelation and solation.

Water

This is highly essential for the growth of all organisms. It must be free from any chemicals, which inhibit the bacterial growth. Deionized water or distilled water must be used for the preparation of culture media.

Steps in media preparation

Media should be prepared carefully for the successful isolation of microorganisms. Each of the following must be performed correctly. They are Weighing, dissolving, Dispensing, pH testing, Sterilization, Addition of heat sensitive materials, Quality control and storage.

Choice of culture medium depends on the following

- The major bacteria to be isolated .
- The nature of specimen.
- The cost, availability and stability of the media.

Instructions for media preparations

☐ Use only ingredients that are suitable for microbial work.

☐ Wear the facemask when weighing toxic chemicals.

☐ When weighing dehydrated media, weigh rapidly and make sure the tops of stock bottles are replaced immediately and tightly because dehydrated media is hygroscopic when exposed to moisture, it absorbs water and becomes unfit for use.

☐ Weigh accurately.

☐ Once the ingredients are weighed, do not delay in making up the medium.

☐ Use completely cleaned glasswares.

☐ The container in which the medium is prepared should have a capacity of atleast twice the volume of the medium being prepared.

☐ Use distilled water obtained from glass distillation unit.

☐ Add powdered ingredients to the water and stir to dissolve. Mix also by rotating the flask.

☐ pH should be checked before the addition of agar agar.

☐ Adjust pH with the help of 0.1N sodium hydroxide if the medium is too acid and 0.1N hydrochloric acid if too alkaline otherwise use acetic acid.

☐ When heat is required to dissolve the medium, stir while heating and control boiling and foaming. Overheating can alter medium nutritional and gelling properties and also its pH.

- ☐ Autoclave the medium only when the ingredients are completely dissolved. Always autoclave at correct temperature.

- ☐ Add heat sensitive materials at correct proportions after sterilization. Aseptic technique should be followed during this procedure.

- ☐ After the completion of media preparation, media should be dispensed to the specific containers such as petri plates, test tubes, culture tubes or screw cap tubes.

Preparation of Nutrient Agar

Materials required

Distilled water, Conical flasks, Cotton, Peptone, Sodium chloride, Yeast extract, Beef extract, Agar agar, pH meter, test tubes, glass rod, petriplates, Hot air oven, Autoclave etc.,

Procedure

Preparation of agar plate

1. Arrange all the required materials in a table
2. Take 100mL of distilled water in 250mL of conical flask.
3. Weight the ingredients of nutrient agar (Appendix A) one by one and dissolve in distilled water.
4. Adjust the pH to 7.2±0.2 by adding few drops of 0.1N acetic acid or 0.1N sodium hydroxide and check using pH meter or pH paper.
5. Add 2g agar agar as a solidifying agent.
6. Completely dissolve media by boiling for few minutes.
7. Sterilize the medium using autoclave at 121°C for 15 minutes.
8. Add *Bacillus steriothermophillus* spores to the autoclave as a quality control agent of autoclaving.
9. Cool the medium after sterilization up to ear bearable temperature and pour 20mL of the medium into petriplates (approximately 45-50°C).
10. Allow the medium to solidify
11. Perform microbial inoculation by spread or streak plate technique.

Preparation of agar slant

1. Perform steps 1, 2,3,4, 5, 6 as per Preparation of agar plate section.
2. Pour 4mL of medium in to 10 mL test tubes and plugged the tube with appropriate cotton.
3. Sterilize the medium using autoclave at 121°C for 15 minutes.
4. Place the tubes in a **slanting position** in the laminar air flow and allowed to solidify. This will create an agar slant. This is used for culture storage and performing biochemical tests etc.,

Preparation of agar deep

1. Perform steps 1, 2,3,4, 5, 6 as per Preparation of agar plate section
2. Pour 4mL of the medium in to 10 mL test tubes and plugged the tube with appropriate cotton.
3. Sterilize the medium using autoclave at 121°C for 15 minutes.
4. Place the tubes in a laminar air flow as **upright** and allow to solidify. This will creates agar deep. This is used for culture storage and performing biochemical tests etc.,.

Preparation of Broth

1. Perform steps 1, 2,3,4 as per preparation of agar plate section (Don't add agar agar).

2. Sterilize the medium using autoclave at 121°C for 15 minutes.

3. Cool the medium up to ear bearable temperature (approximately 40-45°C) and inoculate the culture.

Observation

Observation is made on all the plates, slants, deeps and broths for the growth of bacterium and also contamination of unnecessary microorganisms.

Viva questions

-   Define the following: media, nutrients, defined medium, complex medium, enriched medium, selective medium, differential medium, transport medium, solid medium, semi solid medium, liquid medium.
-   How do you prepare selective medium?
-   What is the purpose of adding antibiotics to the medium ?.
-   What are the needs of indicator in the medium ?.
-   Mention various types of peptone.
-   What is the source of agar agar?.
-   Why are minerals needed in the medium?
-   What is the chemical nature of agar agar?
-   List out agar agar utilizing microorganisms .
-   Is pH checking necessary in media preparation? why?
-   How do you prepare media for the cultivation of fastidious microorganisms?
-   Why is gelatin not used as a solidifying agents.
-   Is nutrient agar a simple medium? explain .
-   How is yeast extract support the growth of the micro organism?

Spotters: Peptone, Sodium chloride, yeast extract, agar agar, nutrient agar, nutrient broth, EMB agar, Mac Conkey agar, blood agar.

7. Sterilization

Aim

To have an idea about specific types of sterilization.

To know about the control of microorganisms.

To differentiate dry heat, moist heat, cold sterilizations etc.,

To understand the principles of sterilization.

To know how some specific articles are sterilized.

Background informations

Sterilization means complete destruction of microbes from an article or freeing of an bacteria and spores from article. Dry heat, Moist heat, Gaseous chemicals, Filtration and Radiations are the some of the methods available for sterilization.

Moist Heat sterilization

Moist heat destroys microorganisms and its spores very effectively than dry heat. Autoclaving, tyndallization and pasteurization are the examples for moist heat sterilization. Moist heat sterilization was first performed by Robert koch.

Autoclaving

Autoclave is an instrument used for the sterilization. It works under the principle of moist heat sterilization. It was first discovered by Charles chamberland. Pressure is used to produce high temperature steam. It is based on the principle that when water is boiled at an increased pressure, the temperature at which it boils and of the steam it forms, rises. Hot saturated steam rapidly penetrates and gives up its latent heat when it condenses cooler objects, it ensures the destruction of bacterial endospores as well as vegetative cells by coagulating and denaturing microbial proteins and enzymes.

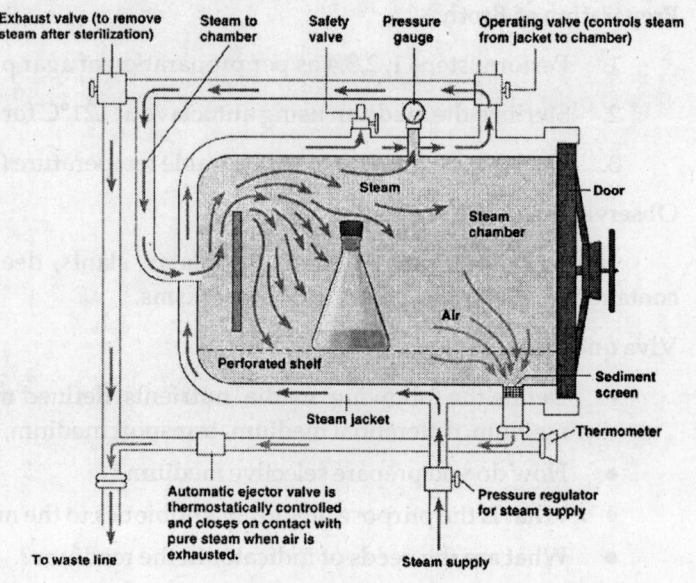

Fig 7.1 : Autoclave

Method of Use

- Add correct volume of water to the autoclave.

- Place all materials to be sterilized in the inner chamber of autoclave.

- Do not over load the autoclave.

- Secure the lid as directed by the manufacturer. Open the air lock (air outlet) and close the draw off knob.

- Apply heat electrically. As the water boils, air and steam will emerge through the aircock.

- When all the water droplets have been expelled and only steam is emerging, wait for 1 minute and then close the airlock. This will cause the pressure to rise.

- When the required pressure has been reached and the excess steam begins to be released from the safety valve, reduce the heat and begin timing.

- Hold all materials at 121⁰C for 15 minutes with 15 psi pressure (Holding time will vary depends on the materials to be sterilized).

- At the end of the sterilization time, turn off the heat and allow the autoclave to cool naturally. This usually takes few hours.

- Check that the pressure gauge is showing zero. When at zero, open airlock and then wait for few minutes before opening the lid to allow time for autoclave to become fully vented.

- Remove all sterilized material from the autoclave and tighten the bottle caps.

Control of autoclaving

A biological method is available to control the performance of an autoclave. It is called bioindicator for sterilization. Spores of *Bacillus stereothermophilus* act as a bioindicator system. Its spore will be destroyed at 121°C for 10 minutes. So people set autoclaving temperature as 121°C for 15 minutes.

Pressure Cooker

It works under the principle moist heat sterilization. It is used in the laboratory instead of autoclave. It is easy to use and require minimum time.

How To Use

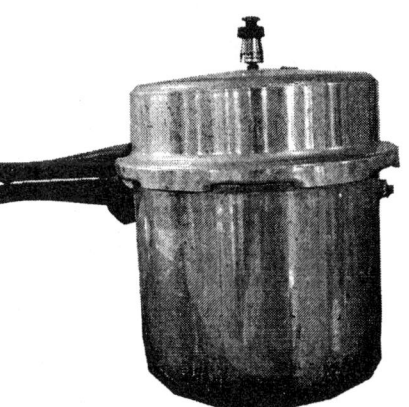

Fig 7.2: Pressure Cooker

- Prepare the articles for sterilization.
- Add correct amount of water to the cooker.
- Check that the lid gasket is correctly located and close the cooker as instructed by the manufacturer.
- Apply heat using gas burner when steams can be seen emerging strongly from the pressure valve. During this time air will be expelled with the steam.
- Push the weight over the nozzle.
- Continuously apply the heat.
- During the heating the pressure of the cooker is increased and steam rise.
- When the steam comes through the pressure weight and gives hissing sound then the pressure inside are 15psi and cooking temperature is rise.
- Allow for 3 continuous hissing sound.
- Then turn the heat to *sim* (bitlow) so that weight may not hiss loudly. Wait for 15 minutes in sim stage.
- At the end of sterilization holding time, turn off the heat and leave the cooker and its contents to cool.
- Remove pressure weight from the nozzle.
- Open the cooker and unload it.

➤ Never remove the pressure weight while processing, sudden changes of pressure in the cooker will spilt the contents of the jar into the pan.

➤ Never fill the cooker more than two third of full.

➤ Never run cold water on to an over heated cooker this may cause it to crack.

Tyndalization

It is used to sterilize media. It consists of steaming on three successive days. On the first day the medium is steamed at 100°C for 30 minutes to kill the vegetative cells. It is then left overnight at room temperature to encourage germination of endospores. The second and third day the medium is steamed for a further 30 minutes to ensure the destruction of the germinated spores.

Pasteurization

Sterilization of heat labile fluids such as milk, beverages may be done by heating for 1 hour at 56°C or for 10 minutes at 65°C - 75°C. This treatment is sufficient to kill mesophilic vegetative bacteria. Vaccines prepared from culture of nonsporing bacteria maybe sterilized at 60°C for 1 hour.

Boiling

Boiling is performed by heating the materials at 100°C. This is a best example for moist heat sterilization. This method is very effective in destroying vegetative forms within 10 minutes where as spores are not destroyed.

Dry Heat Sterilization

Dry heat is suitable for glassware, instruments and articles not affected by very high temperature.

Flaming

It is used to destroy all forms of vegetative cells and also spores by slow passage through Bunsen burner. Bunsen burner (named after R.W. Bunsen) is a type of gas burner. It produces non-luminous flame, the temperature of which reaches 1,860°C at its hottest point. Bunsen burner and spirit lamp is used to sterilize inoculation loops/ needles. It is also used for flaming the mouths of test tubes, media containing flasks. Heating of inoculation wires and loops by holding them almost vertically in Bunsen flame until red not along their whole length, almost to the tip of the metal holder. It is called red hot.

Incineration

Incineration in which all contaminated materials is burned to ashes. Eg., waste media, dressing materials and solid wastes.

Hot air oven (Fig. 7.3)

An oven is based on the principle where dry heat or hot air accomplishes sterilization. The sterilization process in an oven is longer than autoclaving. Dry heat removes water from microorganisms while moist heat adds water to them. In addition, moist heat has greater penetrating power than dry heat.

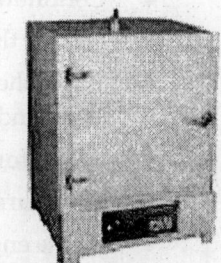

It is used for sterilizing glasswares like petriplates, test tubes, pipettes, metal instruments, oils, powders, waxes etc., Commonly used temperature for hot air oven sterilization is 10 minutes at 180°C, 40 minutes at 170°C, 60 minutes at 160°C, 150 minutes at 150°C,180 minutes at 140°C,480 minutes at 120°C. An oven consists of an insulated cabinet, which is held at a constant temperature by means of an electric heating mechanism and thermostat. It is fitted with a fan to keep the hot air circulating at a constant temperature.

Fig7.3: Hot air Oven

Filtration

Filtration, the process of passing liquid or gases through a filter that retains many microorganisms. It is used to sterilize solutions, which are thermo labile, and to remove particulate matter from the materials. Vaccum or pressure is required for passing solutions through the filters. Basically there are two types of filters. They are Depth filters and Membrane filters.

Depth filters

It consists of fibrous or granular material that are pressed, wound, fired or bound into a maze of flow channels. Various types of depth filters are designated on the basis of its basic components. They are describesd as follows.

Seitz filters

These consist of an asbestos disk inserted into a metal holder, which is connected to a flask. The disks have various degrees of porosity and are known as claryfying, normal and special. The last two donot allow bacteria pass through it.

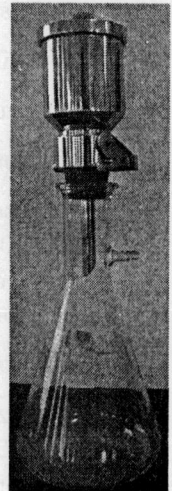

Sintered glass filters

It is similar to seitz filter, but the disks are made of finely ground glass.

Fig7.4:
Filtration
Unit

Barkefeld filters or earthenware filters

These are made from a fossil diatomaceous earth called kiesselguhr. According to the size of the granules forming the substance of filters, there are three grades of porosity, that are V (coarse), W (fine) and N (intermediate). After use, these filters should be brushed with a stiff mail brush and then boiled in distilled water to regenerate for further use.

Chamberland filters

These are made from unglazed porcelin and have various degrees of porocity, the finest type of particles pass only through the membrane.

Membrane filters (Fig. 7.4)

The filter membrane are composed of cellulose nitrate or cellulose acetate. They can be obtained in various diameters (13-293mm) and in porocities from 0.015-12 µm.

- 0.22µm retains *Pseudomonas diminuta*
- 0.45µm retains coliform bacilli.
- 0.8µm retains air borne bio particles.
- 0.1µm filters retains viruses.

Filters are disposable materials. The unit can be sterilized by autoclaving. The filtration is performed by adding the fluid to be filtered into the filter holder of the unit above the filter and apply pressure, then fluid can pass through the filter. Generally negative pressure (vaccum) is applied.

Syringe filters (Fig. 7.5)

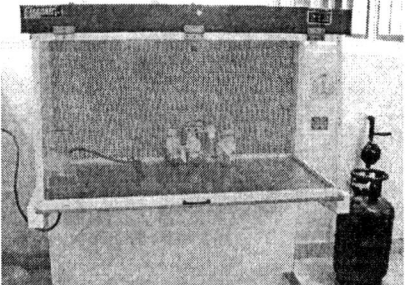

Membranes of 13mm and 25mm diameter can be fitted in syringe like holders of stainless steel or polycarbonate. This is used to sterilize small volume of heat labile fluid. The fluid is forced through the filters by pressing down the piston.

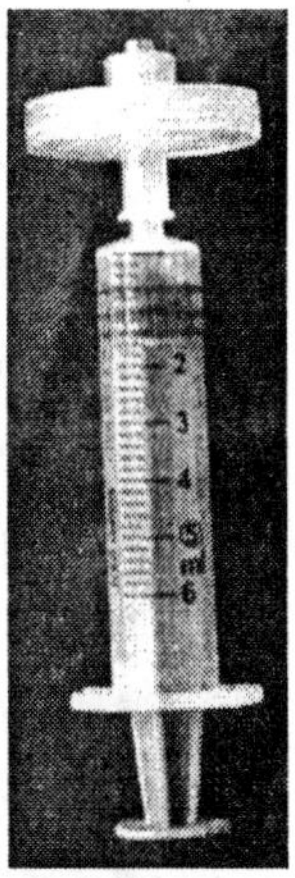

Air filters

Air may be filtered through HEPA (High Efficiency Particle Arrester) filters. HEPA filters are used to decontaminate the air input of the laminar airflow chamber (Fig. 7.6).

Laminar Flow Chamber Operating Procedure

- Turn off UV lamp, turn on fluorescent lamp and check air grilled for obstructions.
- Spray or swab all interior surfaces with appropriate disinfectant & allow to air dry.

Fig 7.5: Syringe Filter

- Arrange only material required for performing the procedure.
- Allow air purge period with no activity inside.
- Do not remove hands from work space until procedures are complete and all article materials secured.
- Remove gloves into disinfectant container.
- Remove protective clothing mask etc., disperse as appropriate and wash hands.
- Spray or swab all interior surfaces with appropriate disinfectant and turn off blower and fluorescent lamp.
- Turn on UV LAMP.

Fig. 7.6 : Laminar air flow

Radiation

Ionizing radiations like gamma rays provides an reliable means of sterilizing plastic and other materials that are liable to be damaged by heat. UV rays effective against nonsporing bacteria. It is used in the biological laboratory to disinfect the internal surfaces of safety cabinets. It is used in operation theaters and sterile room in some factories. Infra red radiations may be employed to sterilize metal instruments and glass syringes in hospitals. The infra red rays are directed from electrically heated elements onto the objects to be sterilized.

Gaseous Chemicals

Medical surgical articles that cannot withstand even heating at 73⁰C can be treated with ethylene oxide. This lethal gas is an alkalating agent and kill microorganism including viruses. Ethylene oxide is toxic and highly explosive

Viva questions

- Define moist heat sterilization & dry heat sterilization.
- What is cold sterilization?
- Give example for moist heat & dry heat sterilizations.
- What are the principle of autoclaving?
- How does moist heat kill microorganisms?
- Why is moist heat sterilization better than dry heat sterilization.
- What is mechanical scrubbing?
- How do you sterilize heat labile materials?
- How do you sterilize petriplates & filter?
- What are the similarities between cooker& autoclave?
- Define Tyndalization, pasteurization, boiling.
- Define flaming, red hot, incineration.
- Who invented autoclave & filter?
- What are the principles of hot air oven?
- What kind of filters are used to remove viruses from heat labile medium?
- What is HEPA? Mention its uses.
- How does radiation kill bacteria?
- How does UV inactivate bacteria?

Spotters: Autoclave, membrane filter, cooker, ethylene oxide, syringe filter , Bunsen burner.

8. Demonstration of Ubiquitous Nature of Microbes

Aim

To demonstrate the ubiquitous nature of microbes experimentally.

To understand omnipresent/omnipotent nature of Microorganisms.

Background Information

Microorganisms are active creators. In an accommodating environment, they are constantly metabolizing, growing in both size and numbers. Microbial concentration can be measured in the laboratory by several methods.

Microorganisms are growing in soil, oceans and other parts of the world. The main aim of this experiment is only analyzing the presence or absence of microorganisms in the environment.

Materials required

Samples chosen for the analysis are Soil, Water, Air, Bench top, Human skin, Plant surface.

Other materials required are Nutrient agar, Rose bengal chloramphenicol agar / Potato Dextrose agar, Petriplates, Cotton swab, Bunson burner, L-Rod etc...

Procedure

Sample preparation

Dissolve soil sample in sterile distilled water before inoculation (1g in 10mL of water).

Water sample is directly used.

Cotton swab is used to collect skin, bench top and plant surface samples.

Inoculation

- Prepare and sterilize nutrient agar and Rose Bengal Chloramphemicol medium or Potato dextrose medium.
- Pour the medium into sterilized petriplate.
- Allow all plates to solidify.
- Spread Soil, water and other samples on the medium directly.
- Expose plate to air for 5 minutes to understand the air microbial nature.
- Incubate all nutrient agar plates at 37^0C for 24 hours and rosebengal / PDA plates at 30^0C for 48 hours.
- Observe plates for growth and record the results.

Observation

S.No	Sample	Observation
1	Soil	
2	Water	
3	Skin	
4	Plant surface	

Result

Either bacteria or fungi are observed in any one of the medium from all samples. This indicated that microorganisms are ubiquitous in nature.

Viva questions

1. Why is microorganism present everywhere?
2. How do you find out microorganism from air?
3. What are the kinds of microorganism present in volcanoes?
4. Which is the kind / group of microorganism large in the world? Why?

9. Aseptic technique and culture inoculation

Aim

- To prevent microbial contamination.
- To prevent wastage of media and other items required for microbiological work.
- To prevent infection of the laboratory worker and the environment.
- To prevent contamination of cultures.

Background informations

Removal of microorganisms from the working environment and performing the techniques without any contamination (unwanted microbes) are called aseptic technique. Aseptic technique is recommended to prevent contamination of cultures and to prevent infection of the laboratory worker and the environment. Aseptic technique was performed during microbial inoculation procedures. Laminar cabinet is used to maintain aseptic condition. UV lamp and the bunsun burner also used in laminar air flow, which prevents microbial contamination. Fumigation (potassium permanganate and formaldehyde) is a process, in which external microbial population is completely removed. It also useful for the creation of aseptic technique.

Materials required

Laminar air flow chamber, UV lamp, Bunsen burner, Potassium permanganate, Formaldehyde, Spirit, Match box etc.,

Procedure

- Clean and fumigate laminar flow chamber / inoculation chamber/ UV chamber in a proper way on the previous day of inoculation (Fumigation is performed by taking 10g of Potassium permanganate in a petriplate lid and pour 10mL of formaldehyde and close the chamber / room immediately).
- Switch on UV lamp for 15 minutes before the experiment commencement.
- Light bunsen burner or spirit lamp before the commencement of experiment.
- Disinfect bench top of Laminar air Flow with Lysol or spirit.
- Sterilize inoculation needle, loop by flaming before and after use.
- Show specimen bottles, conical flasks, culture bottles and tubes mouths on the flame after removing and before replacing caps / cotton.
- Mask and gloves should be used while performing inoculation.
- Inoculate the medium by pour plate, Spread plate or looping out methods.
- Incubate inoculated media under appropriate environment.

Observation

Our aim should be satisfied only when you perform the experiments with strict aseptic condition.

Viva questions

1. What is asepsis & aseptic technique?
2. Define fumigation? How do you perform it?
3. How do you create aseptic technique in laminar airflow?

4. What are the modes of action of fumes generated during fumigation.

5. What is the role of alcohol in maintaining aseptic condition.

Spotters: Laminar airflow, potassium permanganate, formaldehyde.

10. Serial Dilution Technique

Aim

To know microbial population of the given sample.

To study the number of microorganisms present in the environment.

To dilute the sample to get countable number of colonies.

To understand serial dilution technique.

> **Box 10.1: Colony counting**
> Countable colony range
>   – 30 – 300 CFU / Plate
> TLTC – Below 30CFU/Plate
> TNTC – Above 300CFU/Plate
> TLTC – To   Low Too Count
> TNTC – To   Neumerous Too Count

Introduction

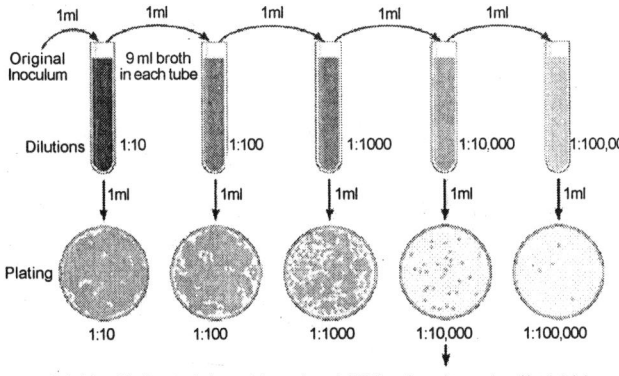

Calculation : Number of colonies on plate x reciprocal of dilution of sample = number of bacteria/ml
(For example, if 32 colonies are on a plate of 1/10,000 dilution, then the count is 32x10,000=320,000/ml in sample).

Fig 10.1: Serial dilution and pour plate

The microbial population in our environment is large and complex. Microbes are isolated from various substrates and sources. Organisms are isolated from various places by using culture media. Each and every environment harbours millions and millions of microorganisms. Number of microorganisms will vary depends on the nature of the environment. To study the number of microorganisms present in the environment or quantitative analysis of microbial load, a specific microbial technique is required. The following technique are used to study the number of microbes present in the given sample. They are Direct microscopic examination, Measuring cell mass, Viable count technique. Cell mass measurement, direct microscopic techniques are called indirect methods. The viable count is used to count accurate number of microorganisms present in the given sample. In the viable count method, cells present in the sample is counted in the form of colonies. Single cell can emerged as a colony. Colony means a group of cells that is emerged from a single cell by continuous transverse fission within prescribed time. Type of colony will vary depends on the nature of microbes. Colony counting is a best method used for the enumeration of microorganisms. If we inoculate the whole sample in to the medium there is a possibility for the non-countable colonies (TNTC). To avoid this type of problems and to obtain countable colonies (between 30- 300 colonies per plate) microbiologists perform **serial dilution technique.**

Dilution Scheme

When one part of culture or sample is mixed with one part of diluent, the result will be 1:2 dilution. One part of culture or sample is placed in nine parts of diluent, the result will be 1:10 dilution.. When one part of the 1:10 dilution was transferred to 9 mL of the diluent the result will be an additional one to ten dilutions. This is because the final dilution is a multiple of all dilution. To determine final dilutions multiply all dilution factors.

$$1/10 \times 1/10 \quad = \quad 1/100$$
$$1/100 \times 1/10 \quad = \quad 1/1000$$

$$1/1000 \times 1/10 \qquad = \qquad 1/10000$$

A single dilution was calculated as

$$\text{Dilution} \qquad = \qquad \frac{\text{Volume of sample}}{\text{Total volume of the sample and diluent}}$$

For example in the initial dilution 1mL of sample was taken.

$$\text{Dilution} \qquad = \qquad \frac{1}{10} = 1{:}10 \text{ or}$$

$$\text{Dilution} \qquad = \qquad \frac{10}{100} = 1{:}10$$

Sample is mixed with large volume of sterile water or saline during serial dilution and is called diluent or dilution blank. Dilutions are usually made in multiples of ten.

Materials Required

9mL water blanks in sterile test tubes, Pipettes, Cotton, Nutrient agar, Potato dextrose agar, Kustars agar, Petriplates, Marker etc…

Procedure

Sample

It may be collected from the environment or from humans or from animals or from plants.

Stock preparation

For solid materials

10 g of the sample is taken and grinded by using mechanical blender and suspended in 100 mL of diluent (1:10)

For liquid materials

1mL is suspended in 9 mL of water (1:10)

Diluent preparation

- Arrange test tubes in a rack.
- Fill the tubes with 9 mL of distilled water or saline
- Insert cotton plug to test tubes.
- Sterilize test tubes with diluents at 121°C for 15 minutes.
- Keep tubes ready for serial dilution.

Preparation of materials requires for dilution (other than diluent)

- Clean glasswares (petriplates, pipettes) and sterilize at 180°C for 10 minutes.

- Workbench of laminar flow chamber should be cleaned properly with disinfectants.
- Turn on UV lamp for 15 minutes before starting experiment.

Performance of serial dilution

- Keep ready and arrange all materials required for the serial dilution in the laminar flow chamber
- Arrange test tubes and label them appropriately (1:100,......1:1000000000 or 10^{-8})
- Add 1 mL of the sample from 1:10 or stock to 1:100 diluent.
- Make up further dilutions up to 10^{-8}
- Perform plating from the appropriate dilution by pour plate method.
- Add one mL of diluted sample to appropriately labeled petriplates after dilution.
- Pour 15-20 mL of media to the petriplates and rotate clockwise and anti clockwise direction for the even distribution of sample.
- Incubate all the plates at appropriate temperature
- Observe plates for growth and record the results.
- Calculate the number of colonies per mL by the following formula.

> **Box 10.2 : Dilution plating and incubation**
> For bacteria isolation
> > Use nutrient agar or plate count agar.
> > Use 10^5, 10^6 and 10^7 dilutions.
> > Incubation temperature is 37°C
> > Incubation time is about 24-48 hours.
> For fungal isolation
> > Use Rose Benal Chloramphenicol Agar.
> > Use 1:10 and 1:100 dilutions.
> > Incubation temperature is 30 ° C
> > Incubation time is about 48 hours
> For actinomycetes isolation
> > Use actinomycetes isolation medium.
> > Use 1:1000 and 1: 10000 dilutions.
> > Incubation temperature is 30 ° C
> > Incubation time is about 72 hours

Calculate the number of colonies per gram by

$$= \frac{\text{Number of colonies X dilution factor}}{\text{Dry weight of the sample}}$$

Note:

- Care must be taken during mixing of sample.
- Specimen should not touch with cotton plug.
- Should follow aseptic technique during serial dilution or decimal dilution.
- Flame the mouth of the pipette and test tubes.
- Pipette accurately.
- Pour plating needs one mL of sample.
- Spread plating requires 0.1 mL of sample.
- Use loop full of culture/ sample for streak plating.
- Triplicates must be performed in each dilutions.

Table 10.1 Observation record table

S. No	Dilution	Dilution Factor	Medium	Colonies		Average
				Original	Replicate	
1	1:10 (10^{-1})	10	Rosebengal chloramphenicol agar			
2	1:100 (10^{-2})	100				
3	1:1000 (10^{-3})	1000	Actinomycetes agar			
4	1:10000 (10^{-4})	10000				
5	1:100000(10^{-5})	100000				
6	1:1000000 (10^{-6})	1000000	Nutrient agar			
7	1:10000000(10^{-7})	10000000				

Result

Calculate number of microorganisms present in the sample. Bacteria present in the sample is – – –CFU/g., Actinomycetes – – – –CFU/g and Fungus – – –CFU/g.

Viva questions

- What is serial dilution?
- What are the needs of serial dilution?
- What is colony?
- Why colour & nature of colony of different bacteria vary?
- What is TLTC and TNTC?
- Give countable colony range of bacteria.
- How do you select dilution for the specific microorganism?
- How much sample is needed for pour plating, spread plating & streak plate technique
- What are the needs of maintaining duplicates in pour plating.

Spotters : Serial dilution picture, diluents.

11. Pure Culture Technique

Aim

- To know procedures for the isolation and purification of microorganisms.
- To understand the principles and procedures of pour, spread and streak plate techniques.
- To isolate and maintain pure culture of Microorganisms.
- To purify single strain of microorganisms from a mixed population.

Background informations

Robert Koch first introduced pure culture technique. Pure culture means a culture contains only one kind of microorganisms. All the pure cultures are free from contamination. The following techniques are used to study quantitative examination and to isolate pure cultures of microorganisms. They are Pour plate technique, Spread plate technique and Streak plate technique.

Combining serial dilution and plating techniques performed isolation and cultivation of microorganisms from the environment. Isolation means the separation of particular microorganisms from the mixed population. The cultivation means the growth of microbial population in culture medium as pure cultures. In solid medium pure cultures are isolated in the form of colonies. These isolates are subjected to identification by using both solid and liquid medium.

Microbiologists have five basic techniques to manipulate, grow, examine and characrcterise the Microorganisms. Basic techniques are, Inoculation, Incubation, Isolation, Inspection and Identification.

To cultivate microbes, inoculate tiny sample (the inoculum) into a container of nutrient medium, which provides an environment for growth. This process is called inoculation. After this process, inoculated plates or tubes are incubated in to a specified chamber (an incubater). After incubation, plates are observed for growth(inspection). Isolates (grown colony) are subjected to identification(isolation and identification). A group of cells arising from the single cell is called **pure culture**.

Table 11.1 - Basic steps in isolation , identification and culturing

Sample	Inoculation	Incubation	Inspection & isolation	Identification
Soil Water Body fluids Biopsy Autopsy Plant materials etc.	Pour plate Spread plate Streak plate	Aerobic Anaerobic Microaerobic	Observation of growth and subculturing	Staining, biochemical tests & Molecular biological techniques

11a. Pour plate technique

Aim

To isolate microorganisms from the sample

To get pure culture of micro organisms.

Principle

Pour plate is a rapid quantitative isolation method. This method is used to isolate bacteria, fungus and Actinomycetes. Original sample is diluted several times to thin out the population sufficiently. Then most diluted sample is mixed with warm agar and poured into petriplates. After the agar has hardened each cell is fixed in place and forms an individual colony. The total number of colonies equals the number of viable microorganisms. Colonies grown on pour plate is carefully transfered on fresh media for identification.

Materials required

Test tubes with 9 mL of diluents, Cotton, Autoclave, Hot air oven, Water bath, Nutrient agar or any one type of medium, Petriplates,Pipettes etc.

Procedure

1. Prepare nutrient agar and PDA medium (one plate needs approximately 15 – 20mL) and sterilize at 121⁰C for 15 minutes.

2. Dilute the sample upto 1:10000000 (10^{-7}) using diluent.

3. Add 1mL of sample from 1:1000 (10^{-3})dilution to appropriately labeled petriplate (10^{-3}).

4. Pour the medium into sample added petriplates.

5. Rotate the petriplates clockwise and anticlockwise direction

6. Allow the plates to solidify.

7. Similarly perform pour plating for other dilutions like 10^{-4}, 10^{-5} and 10^{-6}.

8. Incubate all Nutrient agar plates at 37^0C for 24 hours and PDA plates at 25 - 30^0C for 48 hours and record the results.

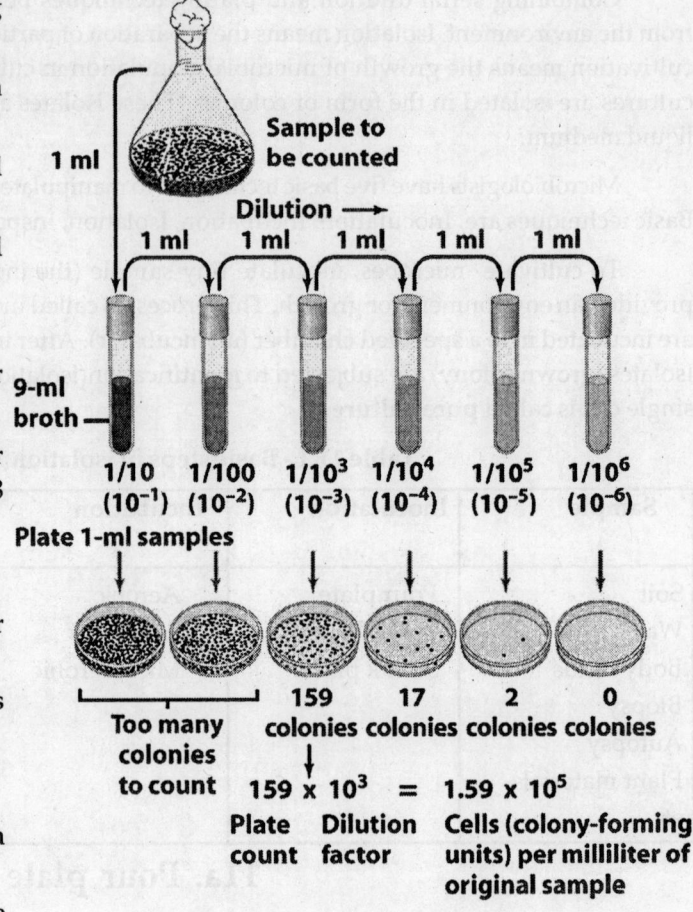

Fig 11.1: Pour plate method

Advantageous

- Need Large volume of sample than other methods.
- Allow the growth of micro aerophiles beneath the surface of the medium.

Disadvantages

- Heat sensitive organisms are destroyed with melted agar.
- Some colonies are formed beneath the surface of the agar, these colonies are not satisfactorily used for identification.

Observation and Results

Individual colonies are noted and calculated number of bacteria present in the sample

11b. Spread plate technique

Aim

- To perform spread plate technique.
- To perform isolation of microorganisms from the sample.
- To isolate mutagenic or converted strains of microorganisms by using differential new procedures.

Principles

A disadvantage of pour plate method is overcome with the help of spread plate method. This method is performed for the assay of chemicals like antibiotics, vitamins etc., This method is called spread because L Rod or cotton swab is used to spread the sample. This techniques also used for the isolation and enumeration of microorganisms from samples with lower populations of bacteria and other microorganisms.

Materials required

Test tubes with 9 mL of diluents, Cotton, Autoclave, Hot air oven, Water bath, Nutrient agar or any one type of medium, Petriplates, Pipettes, L Rod, Spirit etc.

Procedure

1. Prepare nutrient agar medium, sterilize at 121°C and pour in to the petriplates.

2. Dilute the sample up to 1:100000 (10^{-5}).

3. Add 0.1mL of sample from 10^{-3} onto the centre of an agar medium using sterile pipette.

4. Perform similar procedure for for 10^{-4} & 10^{-5} dilutions.

5. Dip the glass spreader (L-rod) into a beaker of ethanol / Spirit.

6. Breafly flame ethanol soaked spreader on Bunsen burner and allowed it to cool.

7. Spread the sample evenly over the agar surface.

8. Incubate all the plates at appropriate temperature (For Bacteria 37°C & for fungus 25-30°C) for 24 to 48 hours.

9. Observe the growth of the microorganisms and record the results.

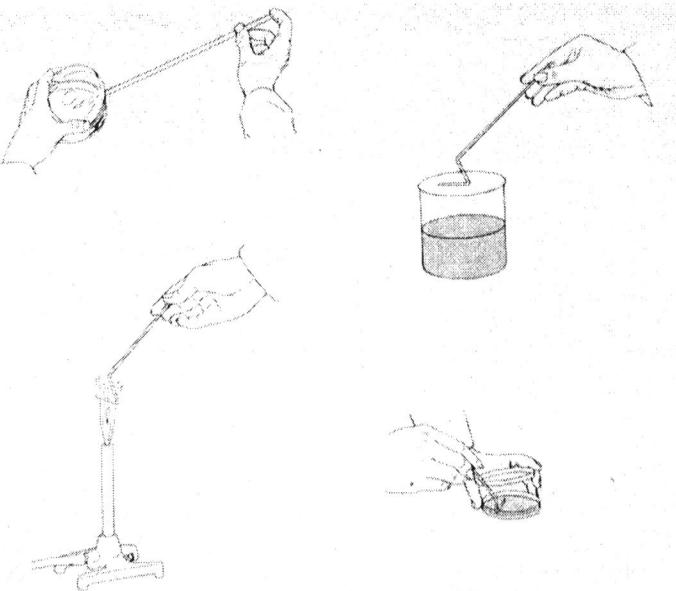

Fig 11.2: Spread plate method

Disadvantage

In this method, only aerobes will grow anaerobes and microaerophiles may be eliminated.

Advantage

Very small quantity sample is enough to enumerate microorganisms.

Observations and Results

Individual colonies are noted at highest dilution and counted properly. This technique also used to perform assay procedures

11c. Streak plate technique

Aim

- To purify microorganisms from a mixed population.

- To learn different types of straking techniques.

Principle

It is also called looping out method. It is not a proper quntitaive method for the isolation and enumeration of bacteria and other microorganisms. It is a good method for microbial purification. This method is called streak because create lines on the surface of the medium like streaking. Inoculation loop is used to transfer inoculum from the sample for streaking and is called looping out technique. Different types of streaking techniques are available, they are T- Streak, Quadrant streak (Fig. 11.3), Simple streak and continuous streak. These techniques are named based on the type of line of streak drawn on the surface of the medium

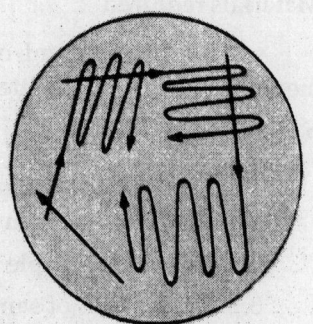

Materials required

Sample of mixed culture, Cotton, Autoclave, Hot air oven, Water bath, Nutrient agar or any one type of medium, Petriplates, Spirit, Inoculation loop etc.

Fig 11.3: Quardent Streak

Procedure

1. Prepare nutrient agar or any required medium and poured in to the petriplates.

2. Allow the plates to solidify.

3. Sterilize the inoculation loop using flaming technique

4. Transfer microbial mixture from a tube to the edge of an agar plate with an inoculation loop as per illustration given in figure(Fig 11.3 for quadrant streak; 11.4 for T streak.

5. Incubate plates at 37⁰C for 24 hours.

Observation and Result

Purified individual colonies are noted. Individual colonies are subjected to identification

Viva questions

- Who is the pioneer of pure culture?
- Define pure culture.
- Why is pure culture needed?
- How do you obtain pure culture?
- Differentiate pour, spread & streak plate technique.
- What are the advantages & disadvantages of pour plate technique.
- What kind of experiments uses spread plate method?
- What are the purposes of performing streak plate?
- What is a bacterial colony?
- What is the purpose of using ethanol in the spread-plate technique?
- Describe the form of some common bacterial colonies.
- What is the purpose of the spread-plate technique?
- In the streak-plate technique, how are microorganisms diluted and spread out to form individual colonies?
- Which area of a streak plate will contain the greatest amount of growth? The least amount of growth? Explain your answers.
- Does each discrete colony represent the growth of one cell? Explain your answer. Why can a single colony on a plate be used to start a pure culture?
- In all routine laboratory work, petri plates are labeled on the bottom. Why?

- What is the main advantage of the pour-plate method over other methods of bacterial colony isolation? What are some problems?
- Why are the surface colonies on a pour plate larger than those within the medium?
- Why doesn't the 48° to 50°C temperature of the melted agar kill most of the bacteria?
- Explain how the pour-plate method can be used to isolate fungi.
- Why is it important to invert the petri plates during incubation?

Spotters: Pictures of pour plate, spread plate and streak plate techniques.

12. Cultural Variations of Bacteria

Aim

To study the cultural variations among microorganisms and use it as a tool for identification and classification through differentiation of character

Principle

The cultural charecteristics of bacteria refers to their macroscopic appearance in various media. The abundance of growth, size and colour of colonies provide certain useful clues, which are helpful in identification. Bacterial appearance can vary substantially depending on the organism, the medium and growth conditions. Some differentiation of bacteria can be well elucidated commonly. Agar plates, agar slants, gelatin stabs and broth media in tubes are used for such studies.

The macrocopically visible growth of microorganisms on agar plate commonly arrising from a single isolated cell and are called a colony. The main features of growth are summarized below. Diagrams also illustrated (Fig 12.1; 12.2; 12.3).

I.Growth on nutrient agar slants

Prepare Nutrient agar in tubes and sterilize at 121 ° C and made it as a slant. Streak Test organism on the surface of medium as straight single line streak. Incubate tubes at 37°C for 24 hours. After incubation observe tubes for various morphological features as described below. One organism has one type of morphology at any one condition.

a) Abundance of growth : Amount of growth is described as none, slightly, moderate or large.

b) Pigmentation: Chromogenic microorganisms may produce intracellular pigments, which are responsible for the colouration of the organism. Sometimes diffusible pigments may also produced, which may change colour of the medium.

c) Consistency: This may be evaluated based on the amount of light transmitted through growth. They may be opaque (no light transmission), translucent (partial transmission) or transparent (full transmission).

d) Form : The appearance of the single line streak growth on the agar surface maybe as follows.

i) Filiform : Uniform growth along the line of inoculation

ii) Echinulate : Margin of growth exhibit tooth like appearance

iii) Beaded : Separate or semiconfluent column is found along the line of inoculation

iv) Effuse : Growth is thin and vein like appearance

v) Arborescent : Branched tree like appearance

vi) Rhizoid : Root like appearance

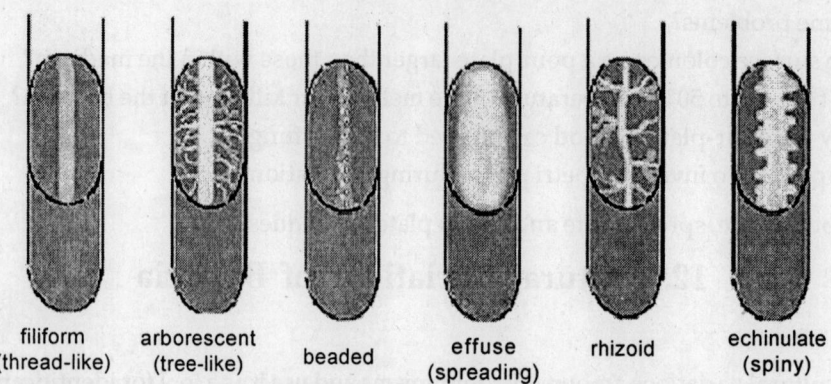

filiform (thread-like)   arborescent (tree-like)   beaded   effuse (spreading)   rhizoid   echinulate (spiny)

Fig 12.1: Growth on Slants

II. Growth on nutrient agar plates

Cultural character is evaluated in the following manner.

Nutrient agar plates are prepared and inoculated the plates by pour plate, spread plate or streak plate method

A) Size - Pinpoint, small, moderate, large.

B) Pigmentation - Pale yellow, colourless, brown, yellow, black, pink, red and green.

C) Form - This represents the shape of the colony

   a) Punctiform - Small circular pin headed colonies.

   b) Irregular - peripheral edged colonies.

   c) Circular - unbroken peripheral edge.

   d) Filamentous - threadlike spreading branch.

   e) Rhizoid - root like spreading growth with branches.

   f) Spindle - looks like a spindle with a central bulged area at both sides, tapering ends.

D) Margin - Here the appearance of outer edge is taken into consideration

   a) Entire - Shortly defined smooth even margin

   b) Undulate - Wavy indundations

   c) Lobate - Marked edge

   d) Rhizoid

   e) Filamentous - Thread like spreading edge

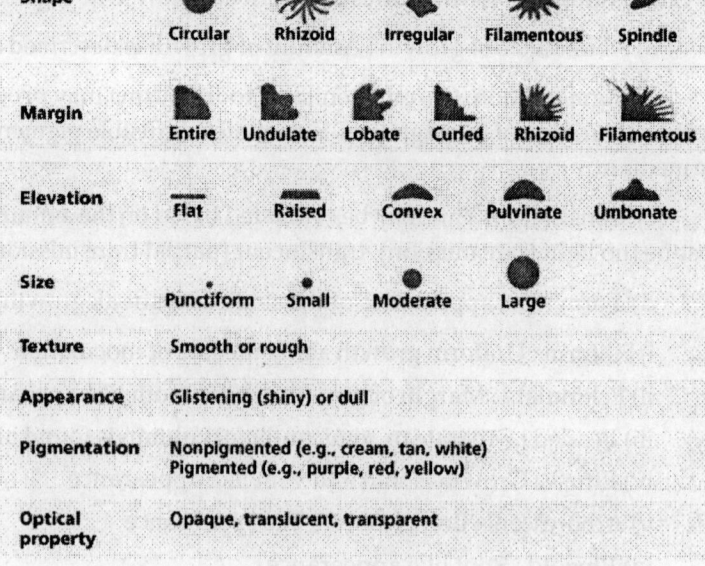

Shape	Circular	Rhizoid	Irregular	Filamentous	Spindle
Margin	Entire	Undulate	Lobate	Curled	Rhizoid	Filamentous
Elevation	Flat	Raised	Convex	Pulvinate	Umbonate
Size	Punctiform	Small	Moderate	Large
Texture	Smooth or rough
Appearance	Glistening (shiny) or dull
Pigmentation	Nonpigmented (e.g., cream, tan, white) Pigmented (e.g., purple, red, yellow)
Optical property	Opaque, translucent, transparent

Fig 12.2: Growth pattern on Agar plates

f) Curled - Intermediate between wavy and smooth resulting in concentric folding

E) Elevation

Degree to which the colony growth appears raised on the agar surface

a) Flat   -   Elevation not clear

b) Raised   -   With slight elevation

c) Convex   -   A slight dome shaped elevation

d) Pulvinate   -   A drop like deep convexed region

e) Umbonate   -   Raised convexed region with uplevel

f) Umblicate   -   A double convex region with a central depression

F) Opacity - Opaque, transleucent, transparent.

III. Growth on nutrient broth

These are evaluated based on turbidity and appearance of growth on the broth

GROWTH PATTERNS IN BROTHS

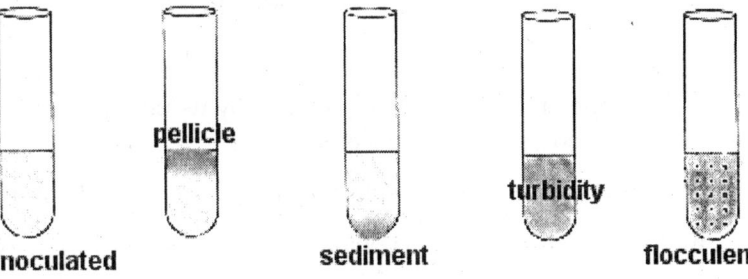

a) Uniform turbidity - Uniform growth through out the medium

b) Flocculent - Aggregates of growth dispersed in flocs throughout the medium

c) Pellicle - Thick pads like parallel growth on the surface.

d) Sediment - Concentration of growth in the bud region of the broth culture is high

Fig 12.3 : Growth pattern on Broth

e) Membranous - A thin membrane on the surface with evenly dispersed growth

f) Ring - A slightly thicker membrane with a central vacant hole

IV. Growth on nutrient gelatin

Liquefaction of the gelatin is taken into consideration

a) Crateriform - Liquefied surface in saucer form

b) Napiform - Bulbous liquefaction of the surface

c) Infundibuliform - Funnel shaped

d) Startiform - Complete liquefaction of the upper half of the medium

e) Scalate - Elongated tubular liquefaction

Observation

Test organisms colony morphology is noted with the help of above mentioned references carefully and carryout microscopic morphology, biochemical characterization serological and molecular analysis.

13. Morphological Variations of Bacteria

Aim

To study the morphological variation of Bacteria.

Introduction

Bacteria are one of the prokaryotic organisms, which exist in various sizes and shapes. They are unicellular and microscopic in nature. Bacterial cells are single, discrete, self-multiplying and physiologically complete organism. Morphological characters such as size, shape, and arrangements of cell are considered for the initial identification process.

Size

Bacteria show great variations in size. A spherical form is measures by its diameter. A rod or spiral form is measured by its length and width. Bacterial cell is measured by microns (μ). One micron is equal to 10^{-3} (1/1000mm). Spherical bacteria size ranges from 0.5-1.25μm in diameter. Rod shaped bacterial size ranges from 0.5 -1μm width and 2-5μm in diameter. Smaller size of the bacteria confers many advantages that are more nutrients can enter into the cell more wastes are removed easily, rate of growth is high and rate of metabolism also high.

Shape

The shape of the bacteria is governed by its rigid cellwall. Bacteria falls into four morphological shapes namely spheres, rods, spirals and pleomorphs.

Spheres: Bacteria showing spherical shapes are generally termed as cocci. E.g. *Staphylococcus aureus*

Rods: Rod shaped bacteria is generally termed as bacilli.e.g. *Bacillus subtilus*

Spirals: They are helically coiled or curved e.g. *Treponema pallidum*

Pleomorphic: Some bacteria exhibit varieties of shapes and they are said to be pleomorphic E.g. Mycoplasma.

Arrangements of Cells (Fig. 13.1)

Bacterial cells are usually arranged in a characteristic manner. These arrangements are useful for their identification. The bacteria arrange themselves in a definite pattern soon after cell division. The following patterns of arrangements were observed.

Spherical Bacteria

Diplococci : Here two coccus bacteria remain together in pairs e.g. Neisseria.

Streptococci : Many cocci are remaining together to give a chain like appearance. This is due to division in one plane e.g. *Streptococcus faecalis*

Tetrads: Four coccus bacteria attached together.

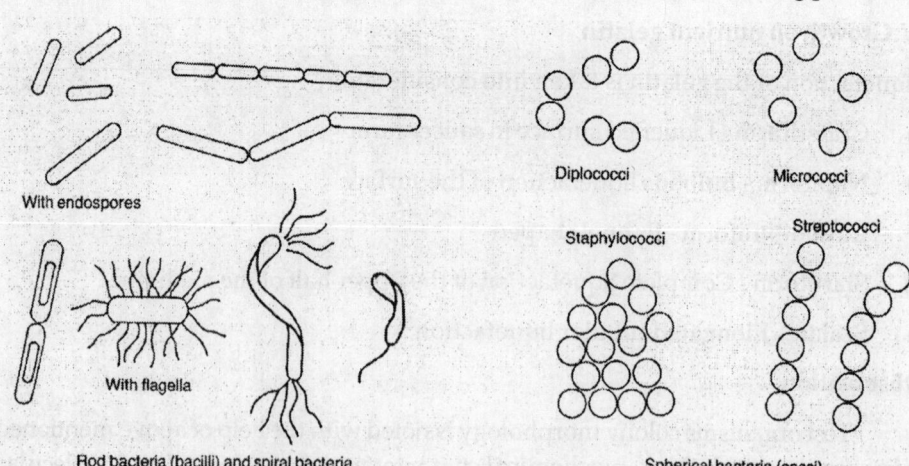

Fig 13.1 : Arrangements of Bacteria

Divisions in two planes produce tetrads e.g. Micrococci

Sarcina : Coccus bacteria arranged in a regular pattern. Here minimum number of bacteria will be 8. Three planes of division produce sarcina.

Staphylococci : Cocci are arranged in irregular forms, it looks like a bunch of grapes. This is due to division in many planes.

Rod Shaped Bacteria

Most of the rod shaped bacteria occurs in single. Few variations are observed through microscope, they are, two rods remain together are called **diplobacilli** e.g. *Klebsiella pneumoniae*. Some of the rods are arranged in chains be called **streptobacilli** e.g. *Bacillus subtilis*. Lactobacillus forms branching chains. The short rods with rounded ends are called coccobacilli. e.g. *Yersinia spp*. In *Corynebacterium diptheriae* cells remain attached at various angles resembling chineese letters. *Mycobacterium leprae* occurs as mass of rods. *Mycobacterium tuberculosis* appears like a tree. Vibrio shows *curved rods*. Stella occurs as *star shape*. Haloarcula occurs as *square shaped* one.

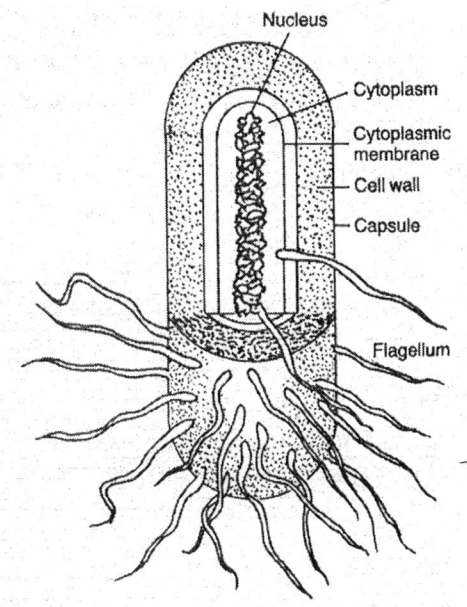

Fig 13.2: Morphology of Bacteria

Bacterial Cell Structure

It is prokaryotic one. It contains high concentration of inorganic ions and strong cell wall. The cell wall was strengthened by its peptidoglycon. On the basis of cellwall composition and staining properties, bacteria are classified into 2 types, gram positive and gram negative. In addition to cellwall, bacteria have capsule, slime, pili, flagella, cellmembrane, mesosomes, volutin granules, nucleoid, ribosome, PHB etc. Some bacteria produce spore during unfavorable condition. Bacteria multiply by single cell division by binary fission.

14. Staining Techniques
14a. Smear Preparation and Fixation

Aim

To preserve microorganisms.

To inactivate the microbial cells.

Introduction

Microscopical examination of stained preparations enables the morphology, relative sizing and arrangement of microorganism to be seen clearly. Better observation of microorganisms needs better smearing and fixation. Every slide should be labeled clearly with the date and the number.

Smearing

Smears should be spreaded evenly covering an area of about 15-20mm diameter on a slide. Purulent materials are smeared thinly using a sterile wire loop. The flame-sterilized loop must be allowed to cool before it is used.

Colonies should be emulsified in sterile distilled water before the preparation of thin smear. Non-purulent materials are centrifuged before smearing. A drop of well-mixed specimen is used for smearing. Swabs are smeared by rolling procedure. Sticks are used to smear sputum and faeces.

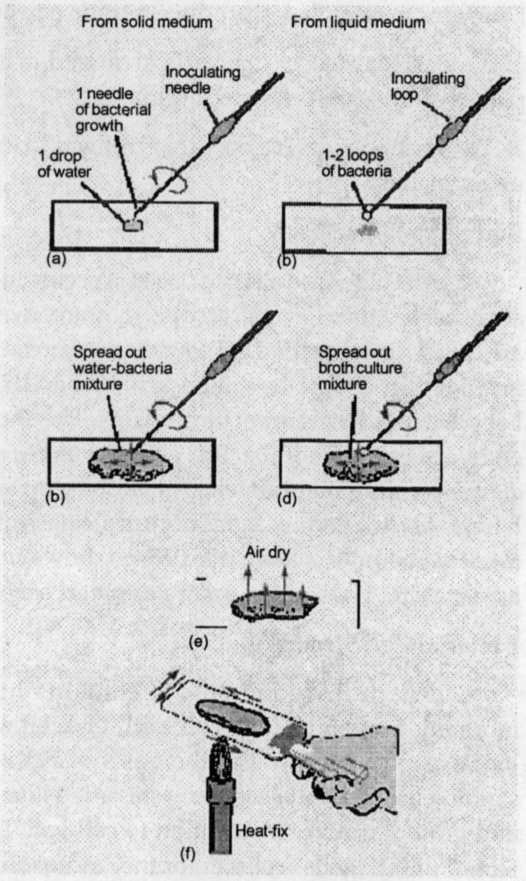

Drying

After the preparation of smears, the slides should be kept in a safe place to air dry, protected from flies and dust. If the smears cannot be stained immediately, they should be fixed and placed in a covered container.

Fixation

The purpose of fixation is to preserve microorganisms and to prevent the smear being washed from slides, during staining. Smears should be fixed by heat, alcohol or other chemicals before staining.

Heat fixation

It is a widely used method but can damage organisms. It may alter staining reactions especially if excessive heat is employed. Heat fixation is performed if the smear is prepared from solid media.

Procedure (Fig. 14.1)

- Prepare smear with the given culture or sample
- Allow smear to air dry.
- Hold the slide with smear facing upward.
- Rapidly pass the slide with smear 3 times through the flame of Bunsen burner.
- Allow the smear to cool before staining.

Fig. 14.1 : Smear preparation

Alcohol Fixation

This fixation is far less damaging to microorganisms than heat. Cells are well preserved. Alcohol is more bactericidal in nature. Alcohol fixation is performed when the smear is prepared from liquid culture or from direct samples (Clinical samples). Alcohol removes excess nutrients from the smear. Nutrients may interfere staining reactions.

Procedure

- Prepare the smear with the given culture or sample.
- Allow the smear to air dry.
- Hold the slide with smear facing upward.
- Add one or two drops of methanol or ethanol on the surface of the smear.
- Leave the solvent on the smear for minimum 2 minutes or until the alcohol dries on the smear.

Other Chemical Fixation

- Anthrax Bacilli containing smear is fixed with 4% potassium permanganate.

- Mycobacterium smear is sometimes fixed with Formaldehyde vapour.

Viva questions

- Why is smear needed for staining?
- What are the purposes of smearing and fixation?
- What are the methods available to fix the smear?

14b. Staining

Aim

To observe the minute cells under microscope

Types and Introduction

Visualization of microbial population in living state is more difficult because they are small transparent and colourless. If it is stained with any one of the dyes, it increases its visibility. Today various staining techniques are available to study the properties of various microorganisms and differentiation into specific groups / genera/ species. The chemical substances commonly used to stain bacteria are known as dyes. Dyes are classified as natural or synthetic. Chemically a dye is defined as organic compound containing a benzene ring plus a chromophore and auxochrome group. Such dyes are acidic, basic or neutral. The Acidic dyes are anionic and stains the cytoplasmic components which are more alkaline in nature. The basic dyes are cationic and combine with those cellular elements which are acidic in nature. Neutral dyes are prepared by mixing both basic and acidic components. Dyes are crude colouring agents whereas stains are prepared from purified dye. The stain is prepared by dissolving particular dye in distilled water or alcohol. There are two kinds of staining procedures, simple and differential.

Categories of staining

Simple staining - Methylene blue staining and Negative staining
Differential staining
    Separation into group - Gram staining and Acid - fast staining
    Visualization of structures - Capsule staining; Spore staining and Flagellar staining

Viva questions

- Name few acidic dyes
- Differentiate dye and stain
- How do you prepare neutral stain?
- What are the kind of dyes used to stain the cell wall of bacteria?

14ba. Simple Staining

Aim

To study the morphology of bacterial cells.
To observe the arrangements of bacterial cells.
To differentiate bacteria based on shape and arrangements.

Principle

The process of visualizing the morphology of microbial population by using single stain is called **simple staining**. In this staining, bacterial

---

Box: 14.1
Quality control for simple staining
Rod shaped bacterium
Escherichia coli, Bacillus sp.,
Lactobacillisp.,
Cooci Shaped - *Staphylococcus sp.*
Streptococcus sp.,

smear is stained with a single stain. Basic stains are usually preferred to determine the shapes and arrangements of bacteria. Since bacterial nucleic acids, cell wall components carry negative charge that strongly attracts cationic chromogen and imparts same colour to the bacteria. Most commonly used basic dyes are Methylene blue, Crystal violet and Carbol fuschin.

Materials required

24 hours bacterial cultures or sample, clean microscopic slides, Staining tray, Inoculating loop, Burner, Blotting paper, compound microscope etc.,

Staining reagents

Methylene blue or Carbol fuschin

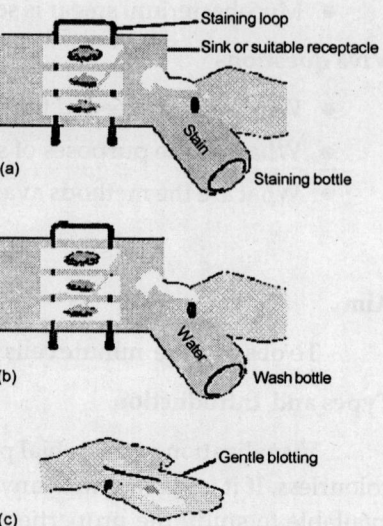

a. Staining
b. Destaining
c. Drying

Fig 14.2 : Simple staining

Procedure

- Prepare bacterial smear on a clean slide.
- Dry the smear with air and fix with heat prior to staining
- Flood the smear with methylene blue / carbol fuschin.
- Wash the stained smear with distilled water to remove excess stain
- Dry the smear using a blotting paper (do not wipe the slide).
- Examine the smear initially under 10X, then 40X and finally oil immersion field.

Observation

Rod or cocci shaped cells are seen as blue to purple in colour.

Viva questions

- Mention the uses of simple staining
- Name two simple stains other than methylene blue.
- Define basic dye, acidic dye, chromogen, auxochrome
- What is the purpose of simple staining?
- Why are basic dyes more successful in staining bacteria than acidic dyes?
- Name three basic stains.
- How would you define a properly prepared bacterial smear?

Spotters: methylene blue, carbol fuschin

14bb. Negative Staining Technique

Aim

To study the morphology of bacteria by negative staining technique.

Principle

Negative staining requires the use of an acidic stain such as Indian ink or nigrosin. The acidic stain with its negatively charged chromogen, will not penetrate the cell because of the negative charge on the surface of the bacteria. Stains that stain the background and not the bacteria are called negative staining. This technique is more advantageous than others are because, heat fixation is not required and the cells are not subjected to the distorting effect of chemicals and heat, their natural shape and size can be stained. Secondly, it is possible to observe bacteria that are difficult to stain e.g. Some spirilli.

Materials required

24-hour-old Culture, Smear slide, Spreader slide, Pasteur pipette, Microscope, laminar flow chamber, Nigrosin or India Ink etc.,

Nigrosin is prepared by adding 0.5g Nigrosin to 100 mL of distilled water.

Procedure

- Take two microscopic slide and cleaned properly.
- Place a drop of culture at one end of the slide.
- Add a drop of nigrosin on the culture.
- Place the spreader slide on the culture and hold at 45°
- Drag the spreader slide upto the next edge smoothly like blood smear preparation in differential count (Fig 14.3).
- Dry the smear in air
- Examine the dried smear microscopically

Observation

Organisms appear as hollow area and the background black.

Result

The given organism is found tobe rod or cocci Capsule nature also visualised

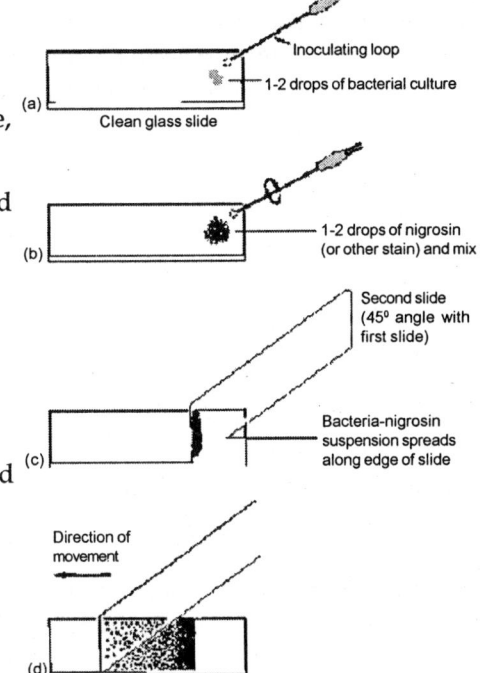

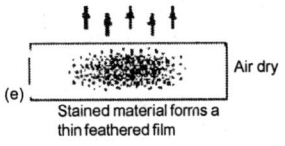

Fig 14.3: Negative Staining

Viva questions

- What are the significance of negative staining?
- What are the stains used in negative staining procedure?
- Is negative staining a differential staining?
- When is negative staining used?
- Why do the bacteria remain unstained in the negative staining procedure?
- What is an advantage of negative staining?
- Why is negative staining also called either indirect or background staining?

Spotters : Negatively stained bacterial picture, Nigrosin / India Ink

14 bc. Gram staining

Aim

- To understand the chemical and theoretical basics of differential staining procedure.

- To differentiate two important groups of bacteria.

Principle

The most important differential stain used in bacteriology is the Gram stain, named after Dr. Christian gram. It divides bacterial cells

> **Box: 14.2: Grams bacteria**
> Gram Positive cocci – *Staphylococci, Streptococci, Micrococci*
> Gram positive Rod – *Bacillus, Lactobacillus, Clostridium, Corynebacterium etc.,*
> Gram negative cocci – *Neisseria sp., Veillonella sp.,*
> Gram negative rod – *Escherichia coli, Salmonell., Pseudomonas, Rhizobium sp.,*

into two major groups, gram positive and gram negative, which makes it an essential tool for classification and differentiation of microorganisms. Those bacteria accepts and retain grams dye like grams crystal violet are called gram positive bacterium. If the bacteria losses grams dye are called as gram negative.

> Box: 14.3. Modifications of Gram staining
>
> Jensens modification
>
> Alcohol as decolourizer, weak neutral red as counter stain. Used for the examinations of *Neisseria* sp.,
>
> Kopeloff and Beermans modifications
>
> Uses acetone as decolourizer
>
> Preston and Morrells modifications
>
> Iodine acetone as decolourizer, gives goiod result, no need for carefull timing.

The gram stain uses four different reagents and their mechanism actions are as follows. Crystal violet (primary stain) is a cationic stain attracted by anionic cell wall and stains all the cells purple. Gram's Iodine (mordant) forms an insoluble complex by binding to the primary stain. The resultant CV – I complex serves to intensify the colour of the stain and all the cells will appear purple black. Only in gram positive cells, this CV – I complex binds to the magnesium-ribonucleic acid component of the cell wall. The resultant Mg-RNA-CV-I complex is more difficult to remove than the smaller CV-I complex. Ethyl alcohol 95% - It serves as a protein-dehydrating agent. Its action is determined by the lipid concentration of the microbial cell wall. In gram positive cells, the low lipid concentration is important for the retention of Mg-RNA-CV-I complex. Therefore small amount of lipid content is readily dissolved by the action of the alcohol, causing formation of minute cell wall pores. These are then closed by alcohol's dehydrating effect. As a consequence, the tightly bound primary stain is difficult to remove and the cells remain purple. In gram negative cells, the high lipid concentration found in the outer layers of the cell wall is dissolved by the alcohol, creating large pores in the cell wall that do not close appreciably on dehydration of cell wall proteins. This facilitates release of the unbound CV-I complex, leaving these cells colourless or unstained. Safranin is the final stain (Counter stain), which stains decolourized cells only. Gram negative cells appear pink in colour and Gram positive cells appear, purple in colour.

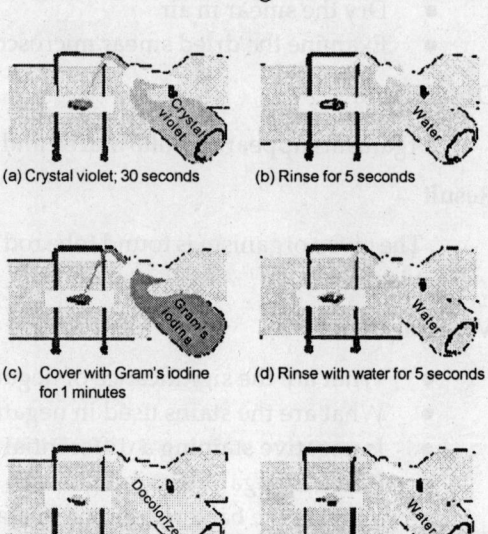

(a) Crystal violet; 30 seconds   (b) Rinse for 5 seconds

(c) Cover with Gram's iodine for 1 minutes   (d) Rinse with water for 5 seconds

Materials required

Bunsen flame, inoculation loop, microscopic slide, marker pen, crystal violet, grams iodine, grams decolourizer, safranin etc.,

Quality control

Gram positive – *Staphlococcus aureus, Bacillus sp.*,

Gram negative – *Escherichia coli*

Procedure

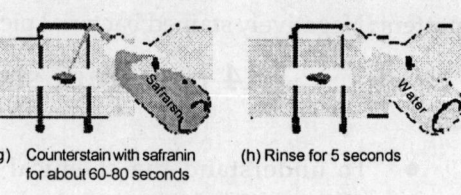

(e) Decolorize for 15-30 seconds   (f) Rinse with water for 5 seconds

(g) Counterstain with safranin for about 60-80 seconds   (h) Rinse for 5 seconds

- Prepare thin smear of given bacteria on a clean glass slide.
- Allow the smear to air dry and fixed with Heat.
- Place the slide on the slide rack for staining.
- Flood the smear with crystal violet and allow it for 30 seconds to one minute.
- Wash the smear with distilled water for few seconds, using running water.
- Stain the Smear with Iodine solution for one minute.

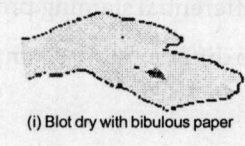

(i) Blot dry with bibulous paper

Fig 14.4 : Gram staining

- Wash Iodine solution with 95% ethylalcohol.
- Add Ethylalcohol dropwise, until no more colour flows from the smear.
- Wash the slide with distilled water and drained properly.
- Stain the smear finally with counter stain Safranin for 30 seconds.
- Wash the slide with distilled water and dried properly.
- Observe the slide under low and high power objectives of the compound microscope.

Observation and result

Pink colour or Purple colour cells are observed. Purple colour cells are called gram positive whereas pink colour cells are called gram-negative.

Viva questions

- Define gram stain and gram variable
- Differentiate gram positive and gram-negative cell wall.
- Why is gram stain called differential stain?
- List different counter stains used in gram staining
- What are the modified methods of gram staining?
- What is the difference between a simple and differential stain?
- Name the reagent used and state the purpose of each of the following in the Gram stain: a. mordant b. primary stain, c. decolourizer, d. counterstain
- Which is the most crucial step or most likely to cause poor results in the Gram stain? Why?
- When doing a Gram stain, What is the reason for using young cultures?
- Which part of the bacterial cell involved mostly with Gram staining, and why?

Spotters : Gram stained bacterial picture, Crystal violet, Grams iodine, Grams decolourizer, Safranin

14 bd. Capsule Staining

Aim

To demonstrate the capsule of bacteria.

To differentiate the capsule bearing bacteria from others.

Background information

Some bacteria secrete chemical substances that accumulate on the outer surface of the cell walls are called capsule. Capsule is water-soluble and non-ionic in nature. They have distinct chemical structure that can be clearly differentiated from the cell wall. There are two types of capsules, they are microcapsule and macro capsule. Macro capsules are 20 nm or more in size easily seen through light microscope. Microcapsule is less than 20 nm in diameter in size and seen under electron microscope. Capsules may be seen in stained or unstained preparations as a clear zone around the bacteria. Two types of staining procedures are employed to demonstrate capsules. In the positive staining procedures the capsule is stained and coloured whereas in the negative staining procedure the background is stained the capsule is seen as unstained hallow around the organisms. Two stains are used to distinguish capsule from cellwall. Cell wall of bacteria is initially stained with any positive dye and non ionic capsule is partially stained with neutral solutions like copper sulphate.

Materials required

24 hours old culture from slant or solid medium / direct sample (Should not use culture from broth because capsule is water soluble in nature), clean microscopic slide, Staining reagents

10% carbol fuchsin and 20% copper sulphate.

Quality control

Positive control – *Klebsiella sp.*

Negative control – *Escherichia coli*

Procedure

- Prepare a thin smear and air-dried (don't heat fix).
- Flood the Smear with Carbol Fuchsin and allowed to stain for 4-7 minutes.
- Rinse the smear with Copper Sulphate several times.
- Pour off excess solution and dry the smear (Don't wash the smear with water).
- Examine the smear under oil immersion objective

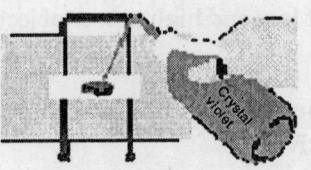 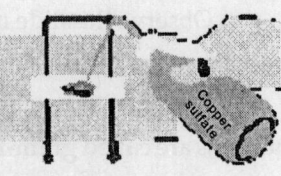

(a) Flood the slide with crystal violet; let stand 4-7 minutes

(b) Rinse thoroughly with copper sulfate

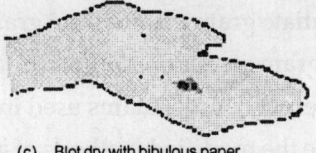

(c) Blot dry with bibulous paper

Fig 14.5: Capsule staining

Observation

Bacteria are observed as purple/pink and capsule is blue in colour.

Viva questions

- Explain the nature of capsule
- Differentiate capsule from slime
- Why are broth cultures are not used in capsule staining?
- What three chemical substances have been identified in bacterial capsules?
- What is the relationship between the presence of capsules and bacterial pathogenicity?
- What is the dual function of copper sulfate in capsule staining?
- In staining bacterial capsules, why is heat-fixing omitted?
- How is the capsule stain used in clinical microbiology?

Spotters - Copper sulphate, Picture of capsulated organism.

14be. Spore Staining

Aim

To differentiate normal vegetative cells from spore formers.

To find out endospore producing ability of the test organism.

Background informations

Bacteria belonging to the genera Bacillus and Clostridium possess resting and resisting structures called endospores. They are present intracellularly or as free spores. The position of the spore may be central, sub terminal or terminal. It has the capacity to resist heat, radiation and chemicals. The heat resistant of spores has been linked to their high content of calcium and dipicolinic acid. Spore is formed by a process called sporulation (Fig. 14.6). Endospore is surrounded by impermeable layers called spore coats. Endospores are completely resistant to heat, radiation, chemicals and agents that are lethal to microbial growth.

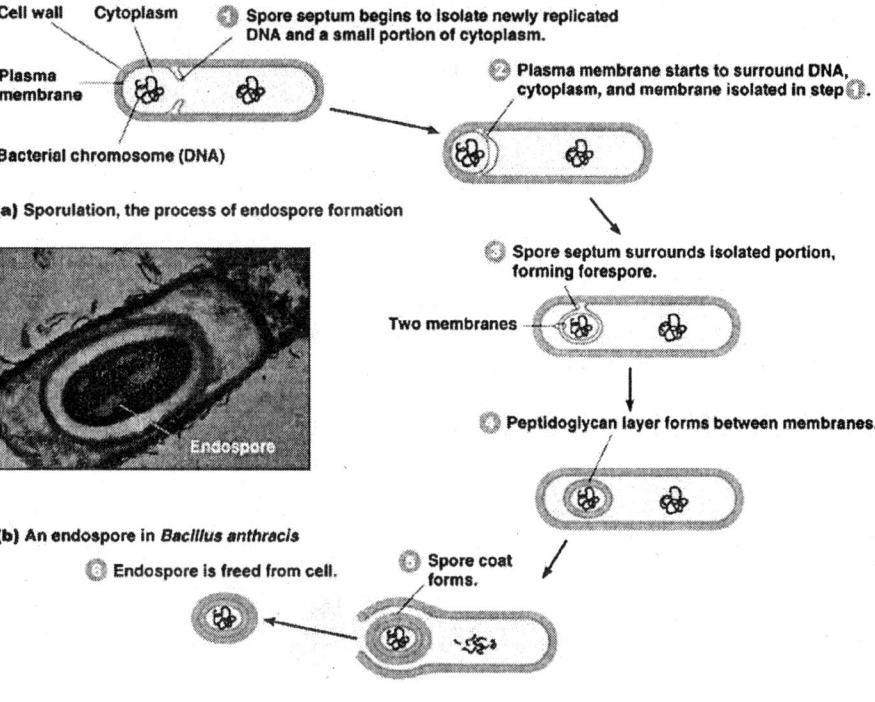

(a) Sporulation, the process of endospore formation

(b) An endospore in *Bacillus anthracis*

Principle

Endospores strongly resist the application of simple dyes but once stained, are quite resistant to decolourization. Unlike other cells, the spore will not accept the primary stain easily. Heat is applied to increase penetration.

Fig 14.6: Sporulation

After heating vegetative cells and spores appear greenish. Once the spore accepts the stain, it cannot be decolourized by tap water, which removes only excess stain. The spore will remain green. On the other hand, the vegetative cells do not have strong affinity for stain. Hence, water removes it and vegetative cells look colourless. To make the distinction between the spore and vegetative portion of the cell, a contrasting counter stain is usually applied in the ordinary fashion the resulting picture shows the initial stain taken up by the spore and stain appear in the cytoplasm.

Materials required

Nutrient agar slant cultures (more than 72 hours old), slides, glass rods, pasteur pipettes, blotting paper, Microscope with oil immersion lens, Malachite green, safranine etc.

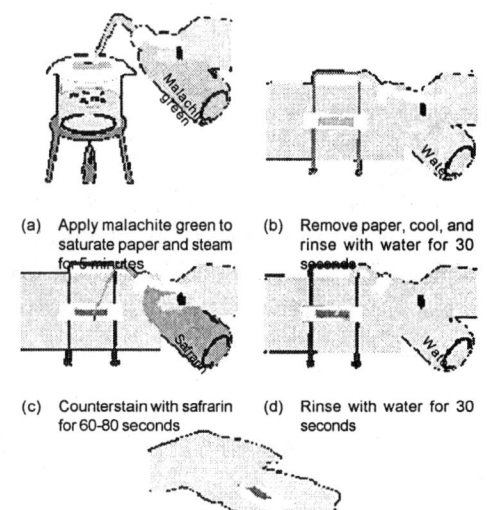

(a) Apply malachite green to saturate paper and steam for 5 minutes

(b) Remove paper, cool, and rinse with water for 30 seconds

(c) Counterstain with safrarin for 60-80 seconds

(d) Rinse with water for 30 seconds

Procedure

- Prepare the smear, air dry and fix with heat.
- Place a piece of blotting paper on the smear.

(e) Blot dry with bibulous paper

Fig 14.7: Spore staining

- Saturate the paper with malachite green allowed it to act for 2 minutes then heat the stain till it steams. It is allowed to act for another 3 minutes (Do not allow the stain to dry on the slide)
- Wash the smear with tap water for 1 minute.
- Counter stain the smear with safranine for 1 minute.
- Wash the stained smear with tap water and dry properly.
- Use Oil immersion objective to examine the smear.

Observation

Bacterial endospores are green in colour . Bacterial cytoplasm light blue and Vegetative cells are pink in colour.

Viva questions

- Give examples for endospore forming bacteria
- Explain about spore formation
- Name the chemical which is formed during spore formation
- How spore forming bacteria withstand an extreme environment?
- Why is heat necessary in order to stain endospores?
- Where are endospores located within vegetative cells?
- In the Schaeffer–Fulton endospore stain, what is the primary stain and the counterstain?
- Name two disease-causing bacteria that produce endospores.
- What is the function of an endospore?
- Why are endospores so difficult to stain?
- What do endospore stains have in common with the acid-fast (Ziehl–Neelsen) stain?

Spotters – Sprorulation, Malachite green, Spore structure, Picture of *Clostridium sp.*

14 bf. Acid Fast Staining

Aim

To differentiate bacteria based on mycolic acid content in cellwall.

To become familiar with theoretical and practical basics of acid fast staining.

To diagnose tuberculosis and leprosy quickly.

Introduction

It is a differential staining. Paul Ehrlich developed it in 1882, which was later on modified by Ziehl-Neelsen and is being used by present day microbiologists. Certain species of bacteria, particularly the organisms of the genus Mycobacterium and some strains of Nocardia, once stained with dyes like carbol fuchsin, resist decolourization by strong mineral acid solution. This feature of acid fastness is associated with intact cellwall and the presence of large quantities of unsaponifiable wax fraction (mycolic acid), which makes penetration by stains extremely difficult.

Principle

Bacteria are classified as acid-fast if they retain the primary stain after washing with strong acid and appear red or as non acid-fast if they lose their colour on washing with acid. Heat is applied to increase the penetration of dye during primary staining. Once stained, the stain cannot be removed when it is treated with strong acid. Mycolic acid content of bacterium confers acid fastness to the bacterium. Non acid fast bacterium decolourizes easily and readily accepts counter stain. Acid fast bacteria appears as red colour. Degree of acid fastness vary depends on the species.

> **Box :14.4 Modified versions of Acid fast staining**
> Kinyouns modification
> 5% Sulphuric acid is used as a decolourizing agent for *Mycobacterium leprae* staining
> 1% Sulphuric acid is used as a decolourizing agent for *Nocardia* staining

Materials Required

Sputum or Mycobacterium culture, Staining rack, Hot plate, Glass slides, Blotting paper, Inoculation loop, Microscope, Carbol fuschin, 3% Sulphuric Acid and methylene blue.

Procedure

- Transfer purulent part of the sputum (especially that containing any piece of yellow caseous material) or Mycobacturium culture to clean microscopic slide using a piece of stick or inoculation loop.

- Prepare thin smear using a circular movement to spread the specimen.

- Allow the smear to air dry in a safe place and fixed the smear with alcohol by covering it with one or two drops of ethanol or methanol for 2-3 minutes.

- Place a piece of filter paper and saturate the paper with the filtered carbol fuchsin stain and heats the stain until vapour begins to rise (Do not over heat).

- Allow the heated stain to remain on the slide for 5 minutes.

- Wash off the stain with clean water.

- Decolorize the smear with 3% v/v acid for 5 minutes or up to sufficient decolourization i.e. pale pink.

- Wash the smear with clean tap water.

- Again flood the smear with methylene blue for 1-2 min and wash properly with clean tap water.

- Wipe back of the slide and allow air dry.

- Examine the smear microscopically.

> **Box : 14.5 Other structures stained with acid fast staining**
> Cryptosporium sp.
> Isospora
> Fungal spores
> Spermatozoa head

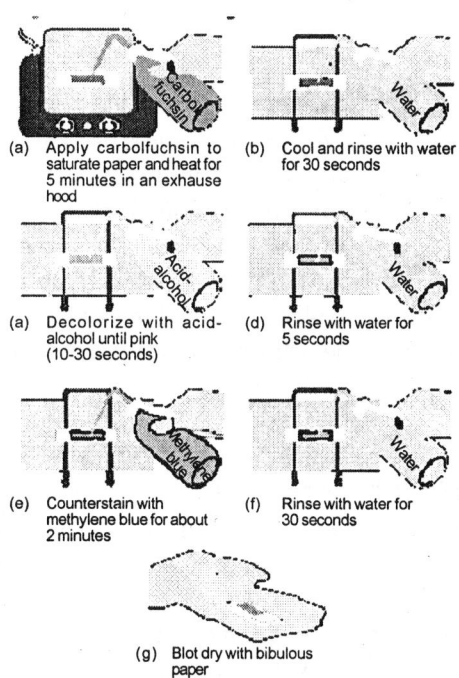

(a) Apply carbolfuchsin to saturate paper and heat for 5 minutes in an exhause hood

(b) Cool and rinse with water for 30 seconds

(a) Decolorize with acid-alcohol until pink (10-30 seconds)

(d) Rinse with water for 5 seconds

(e) Counterstain with methylene blue for about 2 minutes

(f) Rinse with water for 30 seconds

(g) Blot dry with bibulous paper

Reporting

More than10 AFB/field	-	+++
1-10 AFB/field	-	++
10-100AFB/100field	-	+
1-9AFB/100field	-	report the exact number

Fig 14.8: Acid Fast staining

Observation

AFB cells are observed as red colour and Non AF Bacilli are seen as blue coloured cells.

Viva questions

- What are the principles of acid fast staining?
- List out various reagents used in acid fast staining.
- Why is staining technique called acid fast?
- Why is acid fast staing also called Ziehl Neelson technique?
- What are the modifications of Acid fast staining?
- Name the type of cells which are stained with acid fast staining?
- What is the purpose of the heat during the acid-fast staining procedure?
- What is the function of the counterstain in the acid-fast staining procedure?
- For what diseases would you use an acid-fast stain?

- What makes a microorganism non-acid-fast?
- Name the chemical which is responsible for the acid-fast property of Mycobacteria?
- Is a Gram stain an adequate substitute for an acid-fast stain? Why or why not?

Spotters: Acid fast bacilli photo / structure, carbol fuschin, Methylene blue, acid alcohol.

14 bg. Alberts Staining

Aim

To stain the metachromatic granules and differentiate bacteria.

Principle

The Albert technique is used to stain the volutin or metachromatic granules of *Corynebacterium diphtheriae*. The granules are most numerous after the organism has been cultured on a protein rich medium such as Dorset egg or loeffler serum. Metachromatic granules can also be found in other Corynebacterium species and occasionally in some Bacillus species. These granules are madeup of poly meta phosphate and are seen in unstained preparations as round, refractile bodies within cytoplasm. With basic dyes granules tend to stain more strongly than the rest of the bacterium. Neisser stain, Pouch stain, alberts stains are used to stain these granules. Granules of Diphtheria bacilli exhibits metachromasia when it is stained with alberts staining.

Material Required

Young culture of *Corynebacterium diphtheriae* in Dorset egg or loeffler serum, microscopic slide, cover slip, distilled water, water bath, blotting paper, microscopie with oil immersion lens, wash bottle etc.

Toludine blue- malachite green (Alberts stain I), Albert's iodine

Procedure

1. Prepare thin smear and air-dried.
2. Fix air dried smear using alcohol
3. Cover the smear with toludine blue -malachite green stain for 3-5 minutes.
4. Wash excess stain with the clean water.
5. Cover the smear again with Albert's iodine for 1 minute and washed off with water.
6. Wipe slide back and allow the slide to dry.
7. Examine the smear microscopically, first with the 40x objective to check the staining and to see the distribution of the material and then with the oil immersion lens to look for bacteria containing metachromatic granules

Observation

Bacterial cells are seen as green and Metachromatic granules are observes as green black dot on the cell.

Viva questions

- What are the significance of granules in bacteria?
- Define metachromacia.
- What are the other stains used to stain metachromatic granules?
- Give the other names for metachromatic granules.

Spotters: Alberts iodine, metochromatic granule stained cells

14 bh. Silver Staining For Flagella

Aim

To demonstrate nature of flagella.

Background information

Some bacteria possess organelles of locomotion, a thread like structure called flagella with which they move from place to place and exhibit motility. Flagella maybe classified into following types

Monotrichous   -flagella at one end e.g., *Vibrio cholerae* (Fig. 14.9a)

Amphitrichous   -flagella at both ends e.g., Pseudomonas (Fig. 14.9c)

Lopohtrichous   - tuft of flagella present at one or both ends e.g., Spirillum (Fig. 14.9 b)

Peritrichous   -flagella found around the surface the cell e.g., *Salmonella typhi* (Fig. 14.9 d)

These are very small structures and are not visible under light microscope using ordinary staining procedures. To see them under light microscope special staining techniques are used, in which the thickness of the flagella are increased by special staining.

Materials required

4 hours broth culture of *Proteus vulgaris/ Escherichia coli*, microscopic slide, cover slip, distilled water, water bath, blotting paper, microscope with oil immersion lens, DPX mount, wash bottle etc.

Mordant solution and Silver nitrate

Procedure

- Prepare the smear and air-dried
- Add mordent solution to cover the smear and allowed it to act for 3-5 minutes.
- Rinse smear with distilled water and air dry
- Add several drops of silver nitrate solution to cover the smear.
- Heat the slide to 45-50°C for 1-3 minutes.
- Rinse the smear with water and air dry.
- Add drop of DPX moundant to the smear and cover it with a cover glass.
- Observe the smear microscopically and look for flagella.

Observation

Flagella and bacteria stains dark.

Viva questions

- What is the principle of silver staining?
- Name the bacterium that shows monotrichous flagella.
- How do you observe flagella under microscopy after staining?

Spotters: Silver nitrate solution, Pictures of bacteria with flagella.

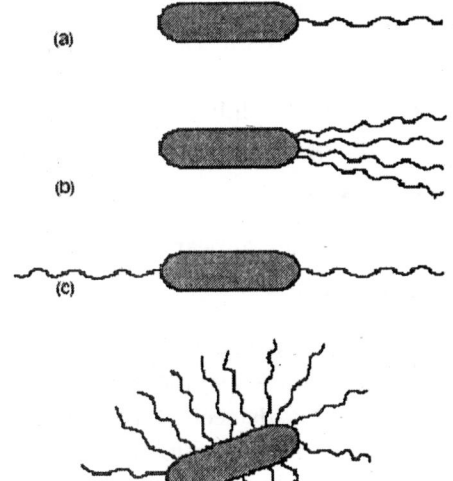

Fig 14.9 : Types of Flagella

14 bi. Fontana Stain

Aim

To stain the spirochaetes by fontana staining method

Principle

Spirochaetes are delicate organisms and are not resolved by ordinary light microscope. Depositing silver salts over them so that they can be resolved by light microscope. Silver nitrate increases the thickness of the organisms.

Materials required

Clinical sample, microscopic slide, cover slip, distilled water, water bath, blotting paper, microscope with oil immersion lens, wash bottle alcohol etc.

Fixative is prepared by adding 1 mL of Acetic acid, 2mL of Formalin to 100mL of distilled water.

Mordant is prepared by dissolving 1g Phenol and 5g Tannic acid in 100mL of distilled water.

Ammoniacal silver nitrate solution is prepared by mixing 35 mL of ammonia solution (5mL of concentrated ammonia in 45mL of distilled water) in 90 mL of silver Sitrate (Silver nitrate 0.5g in 100mL distilled water) as dropwise till the white precipitate formed and redissolves to give a faint opalescent solution.

Procedure

- Prepare thin smear.
- Treat the smear with fixative 3 times for 30 seconds, wash with obsolute alcohol and allow to act for 3 minutes.
- Drain the alcohol and the slide is passed over the flame and dried.
- Add Ammoniacal silver nitrate solution and heated till steam rises from the smear and allowed to act for 5 minutes.
- Wash the slide with distilled water, dried and examined under oil immersion objective preferably after fixing a coverslip over the smear.

Observation

Spirochaetes appears as brownish black with backround brownisn yellow.

Viva questions

- Why is there a difficulty on the observation of spirochaetes on ordinary staining?
- Mention few spirochaetes of medical importance.
- What is the need of fixation in staining?
- Name special staining techniques used for the identification of Treponema.
- What is the purpose of performing Fontana staining?
- What are the principles of Fontana staining?
- How do you look microbes under microscope after Fontana staining?

Spotters – Silver nitrate, Phenol, Tannic acid, Acetic acid, Formaldehyde

14 bj. Wayson Staining

Aim

To see and differentiate *Yersinia pestis* from other bacteria.

Principle

It is also called as bipolar staining technique. Bipolar stainging provides clue for the presumptive diagnosis of *Yersinia pestis* in pure form as well as in clinical samples. Organisms appears as like safety pin.

Materials required

Bacterial culture *Yersinia pestis*, microscopic slide, cover slip, distilled water, water bath, blotting paper, microscope with oil immersion lens, wash bottle etc.

Wayson's stain is prepared by adding 200mG Basic fuschin, 75mG Methylene blue, 20mL 95% Ethanol and 10g Phenol in 100mL of distilled water. Make the volume of the stain to 200mL using standard measured flask.

Procedure

- Prepare smear and air dried.
- Fix smear with the help of alcohol.
- Flood smear with Wayson's stain for 10-20 seconds.
- Wash stain with clean water.
- Wipe back of the slide and placed in a draining rack for the smear to air-dry.
- Examine smear microscopically, first with the 40x objective to see the distribution of material and then with the oil immersion objective to look for bipolar stained bacteria.

Observations

Bacteria are seen as Blue with pink ends.

Viva questions

1. What are the ingredients of wayson stain?
2. Why is phenol added in this stain?
3. What is the purpose of doing this staining technique?

Spotters – Yersinia Picture or Stained Yersinia preparations

15. Motility Test

Aim

- To perform the hanging-drop procedure for microscopic observation of living bacteria.
- To study motility of Bacteria.
- To observe cell activities such as motility and binary fission.
- To Observe the natural size and shape of the cells, since heat fixation and exposure to chemicals during staining cause some degree of distortion.

Principle

Bacteria, because of their small size and a refractive index that closely approximates that of water, do not lend themselves readily to microscopic examination in a living, unstained state. Examination of living microorganisms is useful because motility is one of the important parameter for the identification of bacteria.

Bacteria uses flagella to move towards food sources (Chemotaxis), move towards light (Phototaxis) and to move away from toxic chemicals. Some organisms motile at room temperature (30⁰C) but non motile at body temperature

(37⁰C) e.g., *Yersinia enterocolitica, Listeria monocytogens*. There are different methods are available to detect motility of bacteria. They are hanging drop method, dark field microscopy, flagella staining and semisolid media. Motility of anaerobic bacteria are detected by capillary tube method. Here culture is growing in Robertson cooked meat media or fluid thioglycollate medium. Then the culture is filled in capillary tube and sealed properly. Sealed capillary tube is directly observed under bright field microscopy.

Hanging drop method is a direct and best method to detect motility of bacteria. The name hanging drop is because a drop of culture is hanged in a concavity of slide on coverslip. In liquid suspension false motility (Brownian movement) is also observed. It is essential to differentiate between actual motility and Brownian movement, a vibratory movement of the cells because of their bombardment by water molecules in the suspension. Bacteria exhibits different types of Motility (Box 15.1) with Monotrichous, Amphitrichous, Lopohtrichous and Peritrichous flagella (Fig. 14.9).

Materials required

24 hour broth culture of *Pseudomonas aeruginosa, Bacillus cereus* and *Staphylococcus aureus*, Bunsen burner, Inoculation loop, Depression slide, Cover slip, Microscope, Petroleum jelly, tooth pick etc.,

Quality Control (Table 15.1)

Positive control-*Escherichia coli*

Negative control- *Shigella sonnei*

Procedure

- Apply Petroleum jelly / Vaseline around the concavity of the depression slide as ring.

- Place loopful of the culture in the centre of a clean coverslip using aseptic technique.

- Place depression slide with the concave surface facing down, over the coverslip so that the depression covers the drop of culture. Press the slide gently to form a seal between the slide and the coverslip. (Fig. 15.1)

- Quickly turn slide right side up so that the drop continues to adhere to the inner surface of the coverslip.

Box: 15.1 -Different kinds motility
Dartling motility by Vibrio & Campylobacter
Cork screw motility by Spirochaetes
Flexion & Extension motility by Capnocytophaga (Gliding Bacteria).
Tumpling motility by Listeria monocytogens
Swarming motility by Proteus sp.
Active serpendine, wrigging motility by Salmonella sp.

Table :15.1 Motility nature of Bacteria	
Motile	Nonmotile
Aeromonas sp.	*Staphylococcus sp.*
Alkaligens sp.	*Streptococcus sp.*
E. coli	*Enterococcuus sp.*
Serratia sp.	*Micrococcus sp.*
Salmonella typhi	*Neisseria sp.*
Vibrio cholerae	*Lactobacilli sp.*
Plesiomonas sp.	*Bacillus anthracis*
Rhizobium sp.	*Fusobacterium*
Y. enterocolitica	*Yersinia pestis*
Pseudomonas sp.	*Rickettsia*
Citrobacter sp.	*Chlamydia*
Proteus sp.	*Brucella*
Bacillus sp. except B. anthracis	*Mycoplasma*
	Corynebacterium

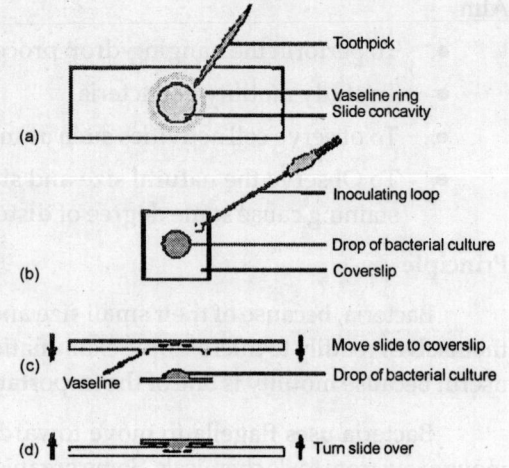

Fig. 15.1- Hanging drop technique

- For microscopic examination, Focus edge of the drop under the low-power objective with reduced light, then observe the drop with high powed objective. Use oil- immersion objective for detailed observation.

Observation

Active motility of motile cells or non motile stable cells are observed.

Viva questions

- Name the locomotary organ of bacteria?
- What are the methods are available to demonstrate motility.
- What is the purpose of performing motility test?
- Mention different types of motility.
- Define Monotrichous, Amphitrichous, Lophotrichous and Peritrichous flagella.

Spotters – Different types of flagella picture, SIM medium.

16. Calibration of the ocular micrometer

Aim

To measure the size of the microorganisms.

To know the principles and applications of stage and ocular micrometer.

Principle

Accurate measurement of the size of bacteria, trophozoites, eggs or other parasitic forms is often necessary in making a species identification. The measurement can be made with a calibrated scale called a micrometer. The ocular micrometer, a small, round glass disk etched with fixed scale, is in-expensive and easy to use, and is recommended for laboratory use. Ocular micrometers are etched with a fixed scale, usually consisting of 50 parallel lines. Depending on the magnifying power of the set of objectives used in the compound microscope, each division in the ocular micrometer represents different measurements. Therefore each set of oculars and objectives used. The ocular micrometers are usually calibrated by using stage micrometer etched with a scale (0.1 mm and 0.01mm divisions)

Materials Required

Ocular micrometer, Stage micrometer, Standard compound microscope, bacterial stained smear etc.,

Procedure

- Remove ocular lens of the microscope from the microscope (If a binocular microscope is used, it is customary to remove the right ocular).
- Unscrew top of the ocular lens and insert the micrometer wafer so that it rests on the diaphragm ring inside the ocular (Ocular micrometer is inserted with the engraved side down. The micrometer should be handled with lens paper and every effort made to prevent lint from, adhering to the surface).
- Replace ocular lens in its house. When it is viewed through the ocular the mircometer scale appears as a series of lined divisions, illustrated in figure 16.1.
- Place stage micrometer under the objective of the microscope that is to be calibrated. Bring into view the stage micrometer scale, which appears as a series of lines divided into 0.1mm and 0.01mm divisions as shown in the simulated view through the microscope in Fig 16.2.

- Adjust stage micrometer so that the 0 line on the ocular micrometer. Superimposed with the 0.0 line on the stage micrometer scale. When it is viewed under high magnification (X 450), the superimposition of the two scales appears as in the simulated view through the microscope, illustrated in Figure 16.3.

- Without further manipulation, look across the two scales and find the next pair of lines that exactly coincide. For Example, the coinciding lines are the 40 mark on the ocular scale and 9th mark on the stage micrometer scale.

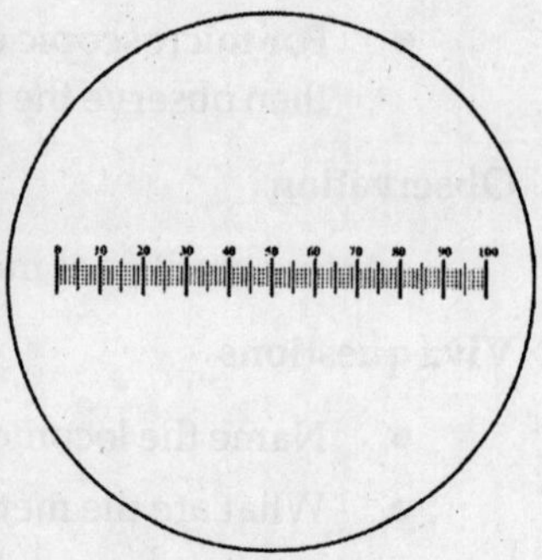

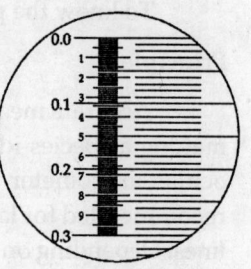

Fig. 16.1 : Ocular Micro meter

Calculation

The object of the calibration is to determine the width in micrometers of each ocular scale division, when calibrated against the stage micrometer scale.

40 units on the ocular scale are equal to 9 divisions on the stage micrometer scale.

1 stage division = 1μm

ie one ocular division =9/40X1

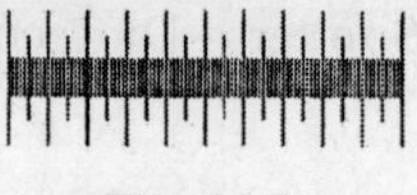

each ocular micrometer division in the calibration is equal to 0.23μm.

Thus if an object that is viewed under the microscope occupies 3 occular scale divisions, it would measure 0.23 x 3 = 0.69μm.

Size of the given bacterium is 0.69μm.

This same calculation can be used for the calibration of any set of oculars and objectives substituting the appropriate numbers.

Fig. 16.2 : StageMicrometer

Viva questions

What is the need of microbial size measurement?

Is any other method available to measure the size of microorganisms

Fig. 16.3
Super imposed view

Spotters – Stage micrometer, ocular micrometer

17. Cultivation of anaerobes

Aim

To cultivate anaerobic bacteria.

Introduction

Microbes exhibit great diversity as to their ability to use free oxygen for growth. These variations in oxygen requirements reflect the differences in the bio oxidative enzyme system present in the various species. The microbes can be classified in to various types based on its oxygen requirements.

- Aerobes - require oxygen as a terminal electron acceptor and will not grow in the absence of oxygen.

- Anaerobes - do not use oxygen for growth and metabolism but rather obtain their energy from fermentative process.

- Microaerophilic - require oxygen as a terminal electron acceptor but fail to grow on the surface and no growth under anaerobic condition.

- Facultative anaerobes - can grow either oxidatively or anaerobically.

● Capnophilic - requires carbondioxide for growth.

Anaerobic metabolism is essentially fermentative and may include an electron transport system with an organic final electron acceptor. Products of anaerobic metabolism include short chain fatty acids, alcohols and amines. Oxygen toxicity is due to alteration of redox potential in the presence of oxygen rendering enzymes inactive and to the ability of anaerobes to deal with the toxic products of oxygen metabolism (hydrogen peroxide, superoxide, hydroxy free radicles, singlet oxygen).

Anaerobes can be grown on agar plates in an atmosphere without oxygen usually nitrogen 80%, carbondioxide 10% and hydrogen 10 %. The carbondioxide stimulates growth and the hydrogen combines with oxygen and that may be used to maintain anaerobic condition. This is achieved in anaerobic jars with sealed and clamped lids from which air is evacuated and replaced by the anaerobic gas mixtures. In all cases oxygen and hydrogen reaction is promoted by the presence of catalyst. Anaerobes may also be grown in liquid cultures in an anaerobic jar / chambers or even in deep broth with reducing agents.

All facultative anaerobes and aerobes have the following pathways for handling oxygen but most anaerobes do not have it.

Cytochrome metabolic pathways for oxygen

Superoxide dismutase , which catalyses the reaction

$$H_2 + 2O_2 ----> H_2O_2 + O_2$$

Catalase , which catalyses the reaction

$$2H_2O_2 -------> 2H_2O + O_2$$

Anaerobes cannot be cultivated in the presence of oxygen. An anaerobic environment is essential for the growth of strict anaerobes. Anaerobic bacteria cause a variety of infections in humans. Anaerobic infections are generally endogenous. According to various reports 50-60% of important infections are caused by anaerobic bacteria. Anaerobes are very important because they can resist many anti microbial agents.

Anaerobic Bacteria

Gram Positive bacilli – *Clostridium, Desulfotomaculum , Acetobacterium, Lactobacillus, Propionebacterium acnes,* *Eubacterium lentum,* Bibidobacterium, *Actinomycetes*

Gram Positive cocci - *Peptococcus , Peptostreptococcus, Ruminococcus, Sarcina.*

Gram Negative bacilli – *Anaerobacter, Bilophila, Desulpholobus , Bacteroides , Prevotella, Porphyromonas ,* *Fusobacterium*

Gram Negative cocci – *Veillonella,* Acidaminococcus

Anaerobic Infections

Appendicitis, Cholecystitis, Otitis media, Dental and oral infections., Endocarditis, Endometritis, Myocarditis, Osteomyeletis, Peritonitis, Empyema, Salpingitis, Septic arthritis, Sinusitis, Trauma, Bacteremia

Materials required

Specimen

Anaerobes are often missed unless the specimen is properly collected, transported to the laboratory and then isolated properly.

Head and neck   - Abscess and Biopsy

Lungs	-	Transtracheal aspirate, lung puncture and biopsy
CNS	-	Abscess, Biopsy ,lumbar puncture
Abdomen	-	Peritoneal Fluid and Biopsy
Urinary tract	-	Suprapubic Aspirate
Female genital tract	-	culdoscopy specimen, endometrial aspirate
Bone & joint	-	aspirate
Soft tissue	-	aspirate

Aspirates are transported with vials with anaerobic atmosphere

All specimens should be transported within 30 minutes.

Media

Successful isolation of anaerobes depends on choosing the correct primary growth media and environmental condition. Most anaerobes require hemin and vitamin K for growth.

Brucella blood agar	-	Brucella
Phenylethyl alcohol agar	-	inhibit facultative gram-negative rod.
Bacteroides bile esculin agar.	-	Bacteroides
Cycloserine cefoxtin	-	*C.difficile*
Egg yolk agar	-	*Clostridium perfringens*
Robertson cooked meat medium	-	Clostridium
Chopped meat broth	-	Clostridium
Columbia blood agar	-	Prevotella
CDC anaerobic agar (TSA+YE+hemin+VitK,L-Cystine)	-	Prevotella, Fusobacterium
Anaerobic kanamycin vancomycin blood agar	-	Fusobacterium
LKV medium	-	Fusobacterium, Bacteroides, Prevotella

Procedure

Both microscopic and culturing techniques are performed.

Microscopy

Modified Gram staining is a common microscopic technique (Kopeloff's modification)

- Prepare Smear
- Fix by using Methanol
- Flood alkaline crystal violet and add 5 drops of sodium bicarbonate. Wait for 2-3 minutes
- Wash with water
- Add kopeloff's iodine for 2 minutes
- Decolourize with 3:7 acetone alcohol.
- Flood safranin for 10 –30 seconds.

Culturing

- Streak the specimen on selective and differential medium.
- Use capillary pipettes for the inoculation on primary inoculation media with liquid specimen.
- Inoculate liquid media near the bottom with 1 or 2 drops of inoculum.
- For streaking place one drop of sample on each medium and then streak the drop with platinum or nichrome loop, using a quadrant streak technique.
- Mince the solid tissue specimens with sterile scissors. Add one part of enriched thioglycolate medium per volume of tissue and grind the mixture with sterile tissue grinder.
- All the plates should be incubated under anaerobic condition.

Available methods of anaerobiosis are

- Pyrogallol method or rolling tube or wrights tube method
- Agar shake method
- Jar technique
- Evacuation and replacement method
- Gas pak method
- Anaerobic glove box technique.
- Anaerobic holding jar method
- Pre Reduced Anaerobically Sterilized Media (PRAS)

Rolling Tube Method

- It was developed by Hungate in 1950 to isolate strict anaerobes.
- Prepare medium and sterilize at 121^{0}C for 15 minutes and make a slant.
- Inoculate the slant with the test specimen.
- Burn the cotton and Insert a plug of burned cotton into the middle region of the tube.
- Add few pellets of pyrogallol and pour 0.5mL of 1M Sodium Hydroxide.
- Seal the tube with rubber bunk.
- Incubate the tubes at 37°C for 72 hours.

Agar Shake Method

It is a simple method requiring simple equipment and yet it is extremely effective for the isolation of anaerobes. Van Niel pioneered this method in 1931.

Procedure

- Prepare 9mL of 1% agar containing media in a series of test tubes.
- Keep the media in test tube at 42-44°C
- Inoculate the first tube in the dilution series with preferable amount of soil or water or sediment and shake well.
- Perform dilution from first tube to the end.
- Cool the tubes after dilution and sealed with a film of liquid paraffin.

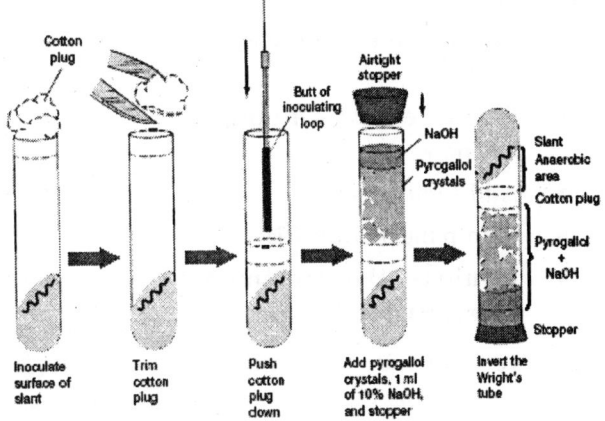

Fig. 17.1 : Rolling tube

- Insert absorbent cotton into the tubes and add few pellets of pyrogallol and 0.5mL of 1M calcium carbonate prior to sealing.
- Seal the tubes with a rubber bunk, an additional safe guard to prevent the entering of oxygen.
- Incubate all tubes at room temperature for 72 hours.
- Isolate the colonies from the tube by using sterile pasture pipette and purify the isolates.

Anaerobic Jar Technique

An anaerobic jar is a cylindrical container made up of plastic, glass or metal. A metal or plastic lid is clamped to a flange at the top of the jar to create an airtight seal. Some jar lids have vents or valves through which air can be evacuated and an anaerobic gas mixture can be added.

Evacuation-Replacement Jar Procedure (ER)

A suitable gas mixture for the ER procedure is 10% hydrogen, 5% carbon di oxide and 85% nitrogen. Eliminating the need for a vaccum pump can use this device with an in-house vaccum pump, there. To perform the procedure, replace the used catalyst in the lid of the jar with fresh one. Put the material to be incubated inside the jar. Place methylene blue indicator in the jar. After closing the jar with lid, connect the vent on the lid and evacuate the jar to 20-24in. of mercury and fill the jar with commercial grade nitrogen. Repeat the cycle. After the 3rd evacuation, fill the jar with anaerobic gas mixture. Clamp the rubber tubing attached to the vented jar, disconnect the jar from the vaccum and gas line. Then place the jar in an incubator.

Anaerobic Gas-Pak Jar Method

It uses the cold catalyst consisting of palladium coated alumina pellets, which is active at room temperature. The disposable gas pak H_2-CO_2 generator consists of a sealed foiled envelope containing two tablets. One contains citric acid and sodium bicarbonate and the other containing sodiumborohydride. When water is introduced in to envelope, the former tablet releases CO_2, while the other releases H_2. Hydrogen combines with oxygen forms water through condensation process.

Procedure

- Replace the used catalyst with fresh one.
- Put the material to be incubated inside the jar.
- Place methylene blue indicator in the jar.
- Cut the corner of the gas pak envelope.
- Place the envelope in upright position.
- Add 10mL of water.
- Clamp the lid on the jar.
- Incubate the jar under appropriate environment.

Anaerobic Glove Box Technique (Fig. 17.2)

Anaerobic glove box is a self-contained anaerobic system. It consists

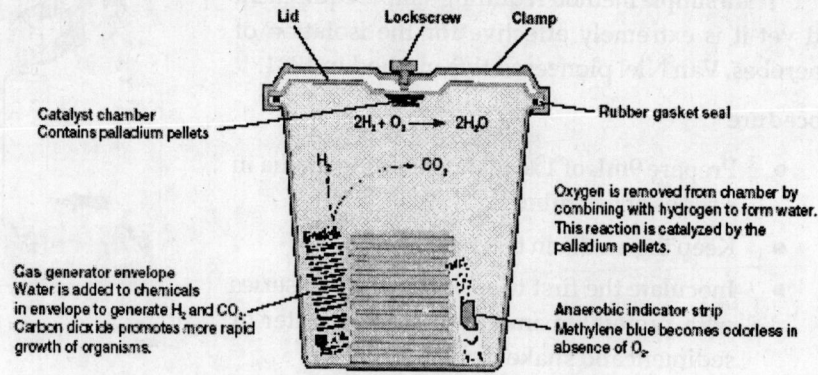

Fig. 17.2 : Evacuation - Replacement Jar

of a gas tight chamber with glove portals and an entry lock for the transfer of materials in or out of the chamber. The operator of the chamber places his or her hands and arms in gloves to handle the culture. A H_2 containing atmosphere is recirculated through palladium catalyst to remove O_2 from inside chamber. R.G.Freter and colleagues at the university of Michigan develop flexible-vinyl plastic glove box. Media are incubated in an incubator placed inside the chamber. Accessories of glove box are a rigid metal entry lock, vaccum pump, a gas mixture tank (85% N_2, 10% H_2 and 5% CO_2) and a tank of commercial grade N_2. Relative humidity within glove box should be maintained at 70 - 85% moisture.

PRAS and the Roll Streak Tube Method (Pre Reduced Anaerobic System)

W.E.C. Moore and associates developed it. Their system is based on R.E. Hungate method. During preparation PRAS media, media components are combined, boiled to remove dissolved O_2 and then autoclaved and stored in butyl rubber stopper tubes under O_2 free environment. Commonly Three types of commercially available CO_2 can be used for gassing roll tubes and liquid media.

1. Anaerobic grade CO_2 – Does not pass thorough catalyst.

2. Commercial grade CO_2 – Pass through copper catalyst

3. 97% CO_2 and 3% H_2 are used.

Anareboic Disposable Plastic Bag

The anaerobic bio-bag consists of a clear plastic bag, an H_2-CO_2 generator, palladium catalyst pellets, and a resazurin indicator, the generator is activated, and then the bag is sealed.

Anareboic Holding Jar

Three holding jars are used, the first to hold an inoculated media, the 2nd for plates that are growing colonies to be subculture, and the 3rd to receive freshly inoculated plates. Commercial grade N_2 can be used in the holding jar system. Flow rate of N_2 to each jar is regulated by the needle valves on the many fold, and adjust the gas tank regulator to 416/in^2 for 1 to 2 minutes to purge the jar of air. Then decrease the flow rate to 1or 2 bubbles per seconds.

Anaerobic Jar With Hydrogen

Removing most of the air from the anaerobic jar and replacing it with hydrogen or preferably hydrogen mixed with carbon di oxide and nitrogen obtained anaerobic condition. In the presence of catalyst hydrogen reacts with oxygen to form water. A common catalyst used is palladium.

Observations

Anaerobic bacteria can be cultivated any one of the method mentioned. Agar shake and rolling tube methods are very simple methods easily performed in ordinary laboratory also. Growth of bacteria is noted

Viva Questions

- Explain how an anaerobic atmosphere can be created in a jar.

- Explain what happens in a Wright's tube.

- Differentiate between the following: a. an obligate anaerobe, b. an obligate aerobe, c. a facultative anaerobe d. an aerotolerant anaerobe, e. a microaerophile

- What are the ingredients in Brewer's anaerobic agar that remove O2 from the medium?

- Of the methods used in this exercise to create an anaerobic environment, which works the best, and why?

Spotters: Pyrogallol, anaerobic Jar, Anaerobic Gas Pak.

6

18. Preservation of Microorganisms

Aim

To preserve bacteria and other microorganisms.

Background information

Pure cultures of microorganisms are required for research as well as for other teaching purposes. The methods used for maintenance and preservation should conserve all the characteristics of the organisms. Some of the simple methods of culture maintenance and preservation are explained in this experiment. Long-term use of microorganisms needs to be stored in proper environmental conditions. Most of the cultures are preserved by culture collection centers. Main objectives of culture collection centers are depositing cultures from different sources, supplying authentic cultures to researchers and also for teaching. Authentic cultures are helpful in identification of unknown cultures, production of industrially economically viable compounds. Different methods are available to preserve microorganisms.

Method I

Maintanence in Fresh Media

Microbial cultures can be maintained by periodic transfer on fresh, sterile media in tubes. The frequency of transfer however varies with the organisms. To keep the cultures viable, it is necessary to use an appropriate growth medium and a proper storage temperature. Many heterotrophic bacteria can be maintained on a medium such as nutrient agar with transfers to fresh medium after every 20-30 days.

Materials required

Nutrient agar for heterotrophic bacteria, PDA for yeast and fungi, any suitable medium for specific bacteria, Test tubes, conical flask, refrigerator, incubator etc.,

Procedure

- Prepare nutrient agar / PDA/ any other appropriate medium.
- Pour 2 – 3mL quantities of medium into 7mL test tubes or culture tubes.
- Sterilize the medium appropriately.
- Make one agar slant and one deep for each culture to be stored.
- Inoculate the slant / deep with suitable culture using inoculation loop / needle.
- Incubate the cultures at appropriate temperature (37°C for mesophilic bacteria; 25°C for yeast and fungi).
- Store grown bacterial / fungal culture in refrigerator after proper labeling.
- Review the culture after 15 – 30 days.

Method II

Storage in Sterile Soil

This method is widely used for preserving spore forming bacteria and fungi. Bacterial cultures maintained by this procedure have been remained for 70-80 years.

Materials required

Sterile Soil, sterile screw cap tubes, refrigerator, agar plate with cultures, tube with sterile water, hot air oven etc.,

Procedure

- Grow bacteria / fungi on appropriate plate medium up to the level of spore formation.
- Suspend the spore of pure culture in sterile water .
- Take garden soil in a screw cap bottle.
- Sterilize the soil 2 – 3 hours at 110°C for 3 days.
- Add spore suspension to sterile soil and allowed to dry at room temperature.
- Store dried screw cap tube containing culture in a refrigerator.
- Review the culture after 50 days.

Method III

Storage in Mineral Oil

This method also recommended for the preservation of bacteria and fungi. Mineral oil / liquid paraffin of Specific gravity 0.83 – 0.89 are used. It prevents dehydration, maintain slow metabolic rate and also reduce oxygen tension. Mineral oil covered cultures are stored at 0-5°C. Some microorganisms have been preserved satisfactorily for more than 15-20 years by this method.

Materials required

Mineral oil / liquid paraffin, agar slant, pure culture, inoculation loop, incubator, refrigerator etc.,

Procedure

- Prepare suitable agar medium in test tubes.
- Sterilize the tubes properly.
- Make agar slant.
- Inoculate test organism as zig zag streak.
- Incubate at appropriate temperature for 24-48 hours.
- Sterilize liquid paraffin / mineral oil at 120°C for 40 minutes twice.
- Pour sterile mineral oil on the surface of the growth to a level of 1cm above the highest point of agar slant.
- Store cultures at 0-5°C.
- Review cultures after 90 – 100 days.

Method IV

Storage at Low Temperature / liquid nitrogen

In this method, cultures are frozen in the presence of a protective agent such as glycerol or dimethylsulfoxide in liquid nitrogen (-196°C). This procedure has been successful with many organisms which cannot be preserved by lyophilization.

Materials required

Ultra low temperature cabinet (Deep Freezer), liquid nitrogen, glycerol or dimethyl sulfoxide, agar slant, microbial culture etc.,

Procedure

- Grow bacteria / fungus in a slant medium.
- Add 4mL of glycerol / DMSO on the surface of growth.
- Scrap the culture using needle or inoculation loop.
- Collect 0.5mL of cell suspension.
- Transfer the cell suspension in storage based cryo tube.
- Store the culture in liquid nitrogen containing ultra low temperature cabinet after proper labeling.

Method V

Lyophilization

Lyophilization is a process in which the cell suspensions are placed in small vials, which are then frozen by immersing in a mixture of dry ice and acetone or liquid nitrogen. The vials are then evacuated and dried under vacuum, sealed and stored at a low temperature. This method provides long-term culture survival without a change in any characteristic. Also, lyophilized cultures take little space for storing. Although cultures can be stored for long periods by this method, viability depends on the quality of glass vials used. It has been found that loss of vacuum during storage leads to inactivation of cultures. Lyophilization needs high cost equipment.

Method VI

Storage in Silica Gel

Both bacteria and yeast can be stored in silica gel powder at low temperature for a period of 1-2 years. In this method, finely powdered, heat sterilized and cooled silica powder is mixed with a thick suspension (paste) of cells, mixed and stored at a low temperature. The basic principle in this technique is quick desiccation at low temperature, which allows the cells to remain viable for a long period.

Spotters

Lyophilized vial, agar deep with culture, agar slant with culture.

Viva questions

What are the methods available to preserve microorganisms?
Which method is suitable for ordinary microbiology laboratory?
Define lyophilization
How fungal cultures are preserved?

• • •

Microbial Physiology

CHAPTER 2

19. Measurement of Growth and Growth Curve

Aim

To study the population growth of microorganisms.

To measure the growth of microorganisms.

Background information

Growth is defined as an increase in cellular constituents and may results in an increase in a microorganism's size, population number or both. Population growth is studied by analyzing the growth curve of a microbial culture. In liquid medium, microbes are usually grown as batch culture. In a closed system, population growth remains exponential for only a few generations then enters a stationary phase due to factors such as nutrient limitations and waste accumulation. The microorganisms are reproduced by binary fission. Growth of microbes can be plotted as the logarithm of cell number versus the incubation time. The resulting curve exhibits four distinct phases. Growth can be determined by various methods. The methods are as follows 1) Direct microscopic examination, 2)Viable count by standard plate count method and 3) Population measurement by turbidity method.

Growth phases

Four types of phases are observed during cell growth. They are Lag phase, Log phase, Stationary phase and Decline phase

Lag phase

When microorganisms are introduced into fresh culture medium, usually no immediate increase in cell numbers or mass occurs therefore this period is called as lag phase. In this phase, all the microbes adopt themselves and ready to prepare ATP, essential cofactors and ribosomes. Lag phase varies considerably in length with the condition of the microorganisms and nature of the medium. Inoculation of culture into chemically different medium results in long lag phase. When young cultures are inoculated to the same sterile medium, the lag phase will be short or absent.

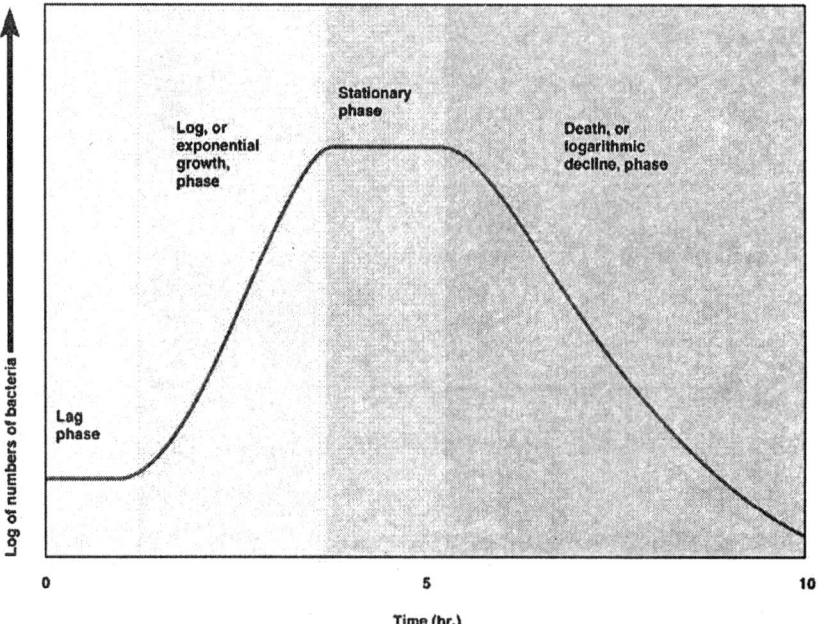

Fig 19.1: Growth Curve

Log phase

It is also called Exponential phase. In this phase microbes grow and divide at higher rate. The rate of growth is constant. The population is most uniform in terms of chemical and physiological properties.

Stationary phase

In this phase, growth is attained by bacteria at a population level of around 10^9 cells/mL. Final population depends on nutrient availability. The total number of viable microorganisms remains constant. This may results from a balance between cell division and cell death. Microbes enter into a stationary phase for several reasons. They are nutrient limitation, oxygen availability and accumulation of toxic material.

Death phase

During this phase cells stepup the death line and reduce the number of viable cells. Dead cells are settled in the bottom of the culture vessel.

Time required for a microbial population to double in number is called generation time. Generation time vary with the species of microorganisms. Eg. Generation time for *E.coli* is 20 minutes (Box 19.1).

Box: 19.1 Generation time	
Beneckea natriengens	- 16 min
B.subtilis	- 43 min
C. botulinum	- 58 min
M.tuberculosis	-12 hours
Saccharomyces	- 2 hours

Measurement of cell mass

Increase in the total cell mass as wells as in cell numbers accompany population growth. Some people performed measurement of cell mass by measuring dry weight. It is a time consuming and not a very sensitive method. Spectrophotometric method is the more rapid and sensitive technique depends upon the fact that microbial cells scatter light striking them. Because microbial cells in a population are of roughly constant size, the amount of scattering is proportional to the concentration of cells present. This type of measurement is also called Turbidity measurement. It is performed with the help of calorimeter or spectrophotometer. Spectrophotometer works under the principle of Beer Lamberts law.

Materials required

Overnight culture of *Escherichia coli*, Calorimeter / Spectrophotometer, Glass cuvette, Conical flask, Test tubes, Pipettes, Inoculation loop etc.

Procedure

1st day

- Prepare 50mL of nutrient broth and sterilize at 121 °C for 15 minutes.
- Inoculate loopfull of *Escherichia coli* and incubate at 37°C for overnight.

2nd day

- Prepare 100 mL nutrient booth and sterilize at 21 °C for 15 minutes.
- Inoculate 1mL of overnight culture into the culture medium
- Incubate the culture flask with medium at 37°C with shaking
- Measure the growth pattern at 600nm using spectrophotometer / calorimeter (every ½ to 1 hour intervals.)

Measurement of Cell Number

Both viable and dead cells are measured using turbidity method. *Neubauer* counting chamber and ordinary measured microscopic slide are the most obvious way to determine microbial numbers. The use of a counting chamber is easy, inexpensive and relatively quick. It also gives information about the size and morphology of the microorganisms.

Count by Neubauer counting chamber

Materials Required

Neubauer counting chamber, RBC pipette, Formaldehyde, Nutrient broth, Bacterial culture

Procedure

- Prepare 100 mL nutrient broth and inoculate one mL of culture

- Incubate the culture at 37°C.

- Count the cells at 30 minutes intervals.

- Wash, drain and dry the counting chamber and cover slip.

- Fix the bacterial suspension to be counted by adding 2-3 drops of 40% formaldehyde per 10 mL of culture and mix thoroughly.

- Place the drop of bacterial suspension on the center of the platform using RBC pipette (the suspension should fill only the space between platform and cover slip.)

- Count the cells in RBC counting areas of the haemocytometer platform and calculate number of cells per mL by the following calculations

Calculation

25 squares cover an area of 1mm x 1mm area.

Chamber depth is about 0.02mm

Volume of the chamber $= 1mm \times 1mm \times 0.02mm$

$= 1/10cm \times 1/10 cm \times 1/200 cm^3$

$= 0.00005 cm^3$

0.00005 cm^3 area hold 0.00005 mL of fluid

That is 5 $\times 10^{-4}$

5$\times 10^{-4}$ holds 5 $\times 10^{-4}$ mL fluid

Bacteria per cm^3 is = number of bacteria/ square $\times 25$

Number of bacteria per mL is

= Number of cells / square $\times 25 \times 5 \times 10^{-4}$

Microscopic Slide Counting

Procedure

- Mark 1 cm^2 area on a clean glass slide.

- Spread 0.01mL of culture uniformly over this area.

- Air dry the smear

- Stain the smear with methylene blue for 1-2 minutes.

- Examine the slide under oil immersion microscope and count the number of microorganisms / field.

Calculations

Diameter of one oil immersion field	=0.6mm
Area of microscopic field	$=\pi r^2$
π	=3.14
r^2	=0.3mm^2
	=3.14 x 0.09
	=2.83mm
1cm^2	=10mm^2
That is 100/2.83	=35 fields/cm^2

1/100mL was spreaded over 1cm^2 area

Each microscopic field has $\dfrac{1}{100} \times \dfrac{1}{35} = \dfrac{1}{3500}$

Total number of cells in mL of sample

=Number of cells in one field x 3500

=— — — — — — — —Cells / mL of sample

Viable Count

It is performed by serial dilution and pour plate method. Cells are counted in the form of colonies. Each colony represents one viable cell.

Materials required

Procedure

- Prepare 100 mL culture media and sterilize it properly.
- Inoculate 1mL of overnight culture.
- Incubate culture flask at 37 ° C with shaking.
- Perform pour plating every one-hour by counting the cells by pour plate method.
- Take 1-mL culture from the flask.
- Dilute the culture up to 10^{-8}.
- Add 1 mL culture from 10^{-5}, 10^{-6}, 10^{-7} and 10^{-8} dilution to appropriately labelled petriplates
- Pour 20 mL of sterile molten medium to petriplates and mix properly.
- Allow plates to solidify.
- Incubate all plates at 37 ° C.

Advantage of viable count technique

In this technique only viable cells are counted because only viable cells are emerged as a colony but all other techniques allows to measure all viable and dead cells.

Observations

Various types of observations are made with different techniques.

All the results were tabulated and draw the growth curve of the particular microorganisms.

Table 19.1: observation report table (For All Methods)

S.No	Time	Indirect method			Viable count CFU/mL
		Turbidity(OD)	Neubauer Cells/mL	Microscopic CountCells /mL	
1					
2					
3					
4					
5					
6					
7					
8					
9					
10					

Viva questions

What is the difference between % T and absorbance?

Why is absorbance used in constructing a calibration curve instead of percent transmittance?

What is the purpose of constructing a calibration curve?

What is a CFU?

How would you prepare a series of dilutions to get a final dilution of 10^{-10}? Outline each step.

Why was 550 to 600 nm used in the spectroscopy portion of this experiment?

How would you define biomass?

What are several advantages to spectrophotometric determination of bacterial numbers? and the Disadvantages?

Spotters : Spectrophotometer, Growth curve

20. Effect of pH on Growth

Aim

To analyze the effect of pH on growth.

Background information

pH is a measure of the hydrogen ion activity of a solution and is defined as the negative logarithm of the hydrogen ion concentration. pH scale extends from pH 0.0 to pH 14. Each pH unit represents a tenfold change in hydrogen ion concentration. pH dramatically affects microbial growth. Each species has a definite pH growth range and pH growth optimum.

Acidophiles have their growth optimum between 0 and 5.5, neutrophiles between pH 5.5 and 8 and alkalophiles prefer the pH range of 8.5 to 11.5. Microorganisms frequently change the pH of their own habitat by producing acidic or basic metabolic products.

Box : 20.1.pH Scale
0 – Concentrated Nitric acid
1 – gastric content
2 – lemon juice
3 – vinegar
4 – orange juice
5 – cheese
6 – beef, rainwater
7 – saliva, pure water and blood
8 – Seawater
9 – alkaline lakes
10 – soap
11 – Household ammonia
12– Saturated calcium hydroxide solution
13 – Bleaching powder

Materials Required

Nutrient broth with various pH (3, 4. 5, 6, 7, 8, 9), Test organism, petriplates, conical flask, spectrophotometer, pH meter etc.,

Procedure

- Prepare nutrient broth tubes of various pH like 3,4, 5, 6, 7,8 and 9.

- Inoculate all tubes with a loopful of culture (test organism).

- Incubate all tubes at 37 ° C for 24 hours.

- Measure turbidity with the help of spectrophotometer at 600nm.

- Plot the values in the graph paper and draw line graph.

- Interpretate the results based on the graph.

Table 20.1 Observation record

S. No	pH	Optical density
1	3	
2	4	
3	5	
4	6	
5	7	
6	8	
7	9	

Viva questions

Which microorganism grew best in the acid pH range?

Which microorganism grew best in the neutral pH range?

Which microorganism grew best in the alkaline pH range?

Which microorganism has the widest pH growth range?

Which microorganism has the narrowest pH growth range?

Why are buffers added to culture media?

Why do microorganisms differ in their pH requirements for growth?

List and describe the chemistry of several common buffers used in microbiological media.

How would you define a buffer?

How do microorganisms change the pH of their own environment?

21. Effect of Temperature on Growth

Aim

To analyze the effect of temperature on growth.

Background information

A most important factor influencing the effect of growth is the temperature. High temperatures damage microorganisms by denaturing enzymes, transport carriers and other proteins. Microbial membranes are also disrupted by temperature extremes. At very low temperatures, membranes modified and enzymes do not work rapidly. Microbial growth can be classified into three based on the temperature. They are Minimum, optimum & maximum. Psychrophiles grow well at 0^0C and have an optimum of 15^0C or lower (*Pseudomonas fluorescence*). Mesophiles are microorganisms with growth optimum around 20 – 45^0C, optimum temperature 37 ^{0}C. Some microbes are thermophiles, they can grow at temperatures of 55 ^{0}C or higher. Their minimum growth is usually around 45 ^{0}C and they often have optimum between 55 and 65^0C.

Materials Required

Nutrient broth, spectrophotometer / calorimeter, Nutrient agar, test organisms, pipettes, test tubes, incubator, hot air oven, cooker etc.,

Procedure

- Prepare one nutrient broth tube for each test organism. Maintain one tube as control.

- Sterilize all tubes at 121 ° C for 15 minutes.

- Label tubes as 30, 40, 50, 60 and 70 individually.

- Inoculate all tubes with test organism as per label.

- Incubate all tubes at various temperatures (30, 40, 50, 60 and 70^0C) for 24 hours.

- Observe growth and measure optical density at 600nm.

- Plot the values in the graph paper and draw line graph.

- Based on the graph observation interpretate the results.

Table 21.1 :Observation record

S. No	Temperature	Optical density
1	30^0C	
2	40^0C	
3	50^0C	
4	60^0C	
5	70^0C	
6	Control	

Viva questions

How does temperature inhibit the growth of microorganisms?

Define thermophile, psychrophils?

How does thermopiles withstand high temperature?

What are extremophiles and mesophiles?

How can you be sure that the turbidity produced in the broth tubes was caused by the bacteria?

How can you determine experimentally whether a bacterium is a psychrophile or a mesophile?

What are the limitations for using boiling water as a means of sterilizing materials?

Is *S. aureus* a mesophile? Explain your answer.

Spotters : Hot air oven, incubator

22. Effect of Salinity (High Salt Concentration) on Growth

Aim

To analyze the effect of sodium chloride concentration on growth

To assess the effect of osmotic pressure of the environment.

Background Information

Growth of bacteria can be profoundly affected by the amount of water entering or leaving the cell. Solution is composed of two parts, that which is dissolved (the solute) and the fluid in which the solute is dissolved (the solvent). The solute concentration is related to a phenomenon known as osmotic pressure. On the basis of solute concentration the medium is divided into three types, hypotonic (low solute content), isotonic and hypertonic (high solute content). In hypotonic solution the solute concentration of the protoplasm is higher than outer side, there fore the osmotic pressure inside of the cell is higher than outside. This internal pressure pushes the cells plasma membrane against the cell wall. As a result ,Water enters inside of the cell. In hypertonic solution, protoplasm concentration is lower than outer environment concentration, so fluid is effluxed from the cell.

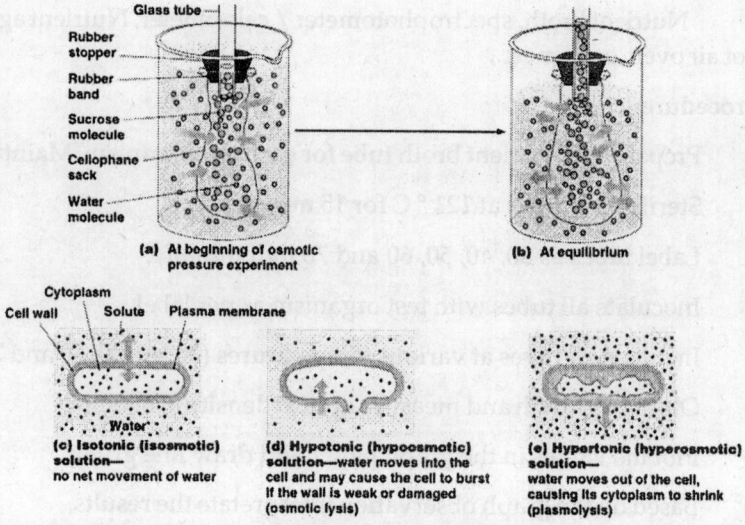

Fig 22.1: Osmo lysis

In isotonic solution, both cell and outer environment solute concentration are same. Physiological saline is an example for isotonic solution. Blood also act as a isotonic solution. Generally the bacterial cellwall has sufficient strength to withstand the difference in solute concentration. During the differentiation of osmotic pressure cell will burst or shrinked. This phenomenon is known as Plasmolysis. It does not occur in all bacteria. Those bacteria that withstands higher sodium chloride concentration are called halophills or halotolerent. In this experiment we will test the degree of inhibition of organisms that results with media containing different concentration of sodium chloride.

Material Required

Bacterial cultures (*Escherichia coli, Staphylococcus aureus, Enterococcus sp.*) , 0.5%,1%,2%,5%,10% and 15% sodium chloride containing nutrient agar medium, Petriplates, Pipettes, Inoculation loop,

Procedure

- Prepare nutrient broth and inoculate with test organism and incubate for 24 hours at 37°C.

- Prepare nutrient agar with different concentrations of sodium chloride (0.5%,1%,2%,5%,10% and 15%).

- Streak test organism on various concentration of sodium chloride containing nutrient agar plates as single line streak.

- Streak at least four organism in a single plate.

- Incubate all plates at 37° C for 24 hours

- Observe the plates and record the results

Table 22.1: Observation record table

S. No	Test organism	Salt concentration					
		0.5%	1%	2%	5%	10%	15%
1							
2							
3							
4							

Result

The given bacteria tolerates up to — — — % Sodium chloride concentrations

Viva questions

How does high salt concentration disturb microbial cells?

What are barophiles, halophiles?

Define osmophils, hypertonic, hypotonic, isotonic.

Name bacteria which tolerates the most salt, least salt and tolerates a broad range of salt?

Define: a.osmosis, b.osmotic pressure, c.plasmolysis, d.halophilic

How is it possible for a bacterium to grow in a hypertonic environment?

What are the optimal concentrations of NaCl for most bacteria?

What kinds of food do you think of that are protected from microbial destruction by salting?

Why don't bacteria lyse when it is placed in a hypotonic solution?

Spotters : diagram of cell lyses and cell shrinkage

23. Effect of Sunlight Radiation on Growth

Aim

To analyze the effect of sunlight radiation on the growth of bacteria.

Background Information

Our globe is bombarded by electromagnetic radiation. Sunlight is the major source of radiation on the earth. It includes visible light, ultraviolet rays, infrared rays and radio waves. UV radiation, kills all kinds of microbes due to its shorter wavelength and high energy. The most leathel UV radiation has a wavelength of 260nm; DNA most effectively absorbs the wavelength. The primary mechanism of the UV radiation is the formation of thymine dimer. When UV exposure is too high, the damage is so extensive. Visible light also kills microbes if its intensity is too high for a longer period.

Materials Required

Nutrient agar, Test tubes, Petriplates, L rod, Conical flask, Black cloth, Pipettes, overnight culture of *Escherichia coli* etc…

Procedure

- Prepare five nutrient agar plates.

- Spread 0.1 mL of overnight culture.

- Allow drying for 5 minutes.

- Expose all plates to UV light for different time (2, 5, 10, 15 and 20 minutes)

- Cover the plates with dark cloth; to prevent the entry of visible light, it may repair the damage through photo reactivation.

- Incubate all plates at 37°C for 24-48 hours.

- Observe and record the results.

Table 23.1 Observation Record table

S. No	Culture	Time of UV exposure				
		2 min	5min	10 min	15 min	20 min

Observation and result

The bacterial growth is observed up to 5 minutes of UV exposed plates. This indicates long term UV exposure is lethal to the life.

Viva questions

Thymine dimer, Wavelength of UV radiation, photo reactivation, photolyase

Mutation, repair mechanisms

Spotters : Picture of TT dimer, UV lamp

24. Effect of disinfectant - Phenol coefficient test

Aim

To measure the efficiency of disinfectants and antiseptics.

To evaluate the effectiveness of given disinfectant.

To compare the effect of commercial disinfectant with phenol.

Background information

Disinfectants used in hospitals and laboratories must be tested periodically to ascertain its potency and efficacy. As certain disinfectants lose potency on standing and addition of organic matter, their efficacy must be tested. Some methods compare the performance with that of phenol whereas other methods simply state the effectiveness of disinfectants. Disinfection process validation is defined as "establishing documented evidence that a disinfection process will consistently remove or inactivate known or possible pathogens from inanimate objects." **Phenol coefficient** is a measure of the bactericidal activity of a chemical compound in relation to phenol. To calculate phenol coefficient, the concentration of the test compound at which the compound kills the test organism in 10 minutes, but not in 5 minutes, is divided by the concentration of phenol that kills the organism under the same conditions. A method for evaluating water-miscible disinfectants in which a test organism is added to a series of dilutions of the disinfectant; the phenol coefficient is the number obtained by dividing the greatest dilution of the disinfectant killing the test organism by the greatest dilution of phenol showing the same result.

Materials required

Test tubes, Phenol, Lysol or any other commercial disinfectant, petri plates, Incubator, Inoculation loop, Nutrient agar.

Procedure

- Prepare a series tubes (10nos) with 2mL-distilled water.

- Add 1mL of phenol to the first tube and dilute by transferring 1mL to next tube (Up to 5 dilutions).

- Similarly dilute commercial disinfectant (Phenol is diluted from 1:200 to 1:800 and the test disinfectant is diluted from 1:75 to 1:125)

- Inoculate test disinfectant tube and phenol diluents with a drop *Salmonella typhi* and incubated at 37°C

- Remove samples from commercial and phenol disinfectant tubes at 2.5 min intervals and inoculated into fresh petri plates containing nutrient agar medium

- The cultures are incubated at 37°C for 2 days

- The highest dilution that kills the bacteria after a 10 min exposure, but not after 5 min, is used to calculate the phenol coefficient

Calculation

Phenol coefficient　　　=　　　concentration of disinfectant that kills the test organism
　　　　　　　　　　　　　　　Concentration of phenol that kills the test organism

For example, after 10 minutes, the test organism was killed by the test disinfectant at a dilution of 1:600. In the same period the test organism was killed by phenol at a dilution of 1:100.

　　　　　　　　=　　　600/100 = 6

This result indicates that the test disinfectant can be diluted six times as much as phenol and still possess equivalent killing power for the test organism.

Spotters

Phenol, dettol, lysol

Viva questions

Define disinfectants and antiseptics.

What are the needs of testing disinfectants?

What is phenol coefficient?

How do you perform phenol coefficient tests?

25. Biochemical Reactions of Bacteria
25a. Indole Test

Aim

To determine the ability of microorganisms to degrade the aminoacid tryptophan.

To determine the ability of microorganisms to produce indole.

Principle

Tryptophan is an essential aminoacid that can undergo oxidation by the enzymatic activities of some bacteria. Conversion of tryptophan into metabolic end product is mediated by the enzyme tryptophanase.

The presence of indole is detectable by adding Kovac's reagent, which produces a cherry red reagent layer. The colour is produced by the reagent, which is composed of P- dimethylaminobenzaldehyde, butanol and hydrochloric acid. Indole is extracted from a medium into the reagent layer by the acidified butanal component and forms a complex with the P- dimethyl amino benzoldehyde, yielding a cherry red colour (Rosindole dye).

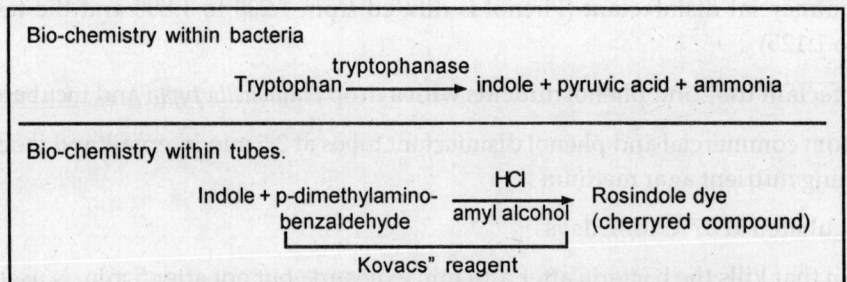

Fig 25.1: Principle and reactions of Indole Test

Cultures producing a red reagent layer following the addition of kovacs reagent are indole positive. The absence of red colouration demonstrates that the substrate tryptophan is not hydrolysed and indicates an indole negative reaction.

Materials required

SIM agar or Peptone water., Kovacs indole reagent, Test tubes, cotton, conical flask, pH paper/ pH meter etc.,

Quality Control

Positive control: *Escherichia coli*

Negative control: *Klebsiella pneumoniae*

Procedure

- Prepare SIM agar or peptone water medium and sterilize at 121^0C for 15 minutes.
- Inoculate the medium with test organism by using suitable technique.
- Incubate the medium at 37^0C for 24 hours.
- Look for growth after 24 hours and add one mL of kovacs indole reagent.
- Observe colour change and record the results.

Observation

Cherry red colour formation indicates positive result. Yellow or other colour change indicates negative results.

Viva questions

Is there any relationship between root nodule formation and indole test?

What is the reason behind cherry red colour formation in indole test?

What is the principle of indole test?

Which is the major ingredient in indole test medium?

What are the major end product of Tryptophan metabolism?

Spotters-SIM agar, peptone, Kovac's indole reagent, Indole acetic acid, Indole test positive or negative test result.

25b. Methyl Red Test

Aim

To determine the ability of micro organisms to oxidize glucose with the production of high concentration of acid end products.

Principle

Methyl red is a pH indicator with a range between 6 (yellow) and 4.4 (red). The pH at which methyl red detects acid is considerably lower than the pH of other indicators used in bacteriological culture media. Thus to produce a colour change, the test organism must produce large quantities of acid from the carbohydrate substrate being used. Methyl red test is a quantitative test for the detection of mixed acid production (lactic, formic, acetic and pyruvic acids) from glucose through mixed acid fermentation pathway.

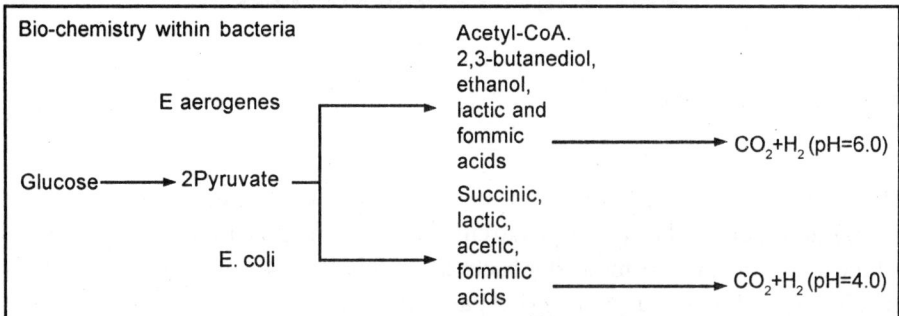

Fig 25.2: Principle and reactions of MR test

Materials required

MR-VP broth, Methyl red pH indicator, Test tubes, Inoculation loop, Cotton etc.

Quality Control

Positive control: *Escherichia coli*

Negativecontrol: *Klebsiella pnemoniae*

Procedure

- Prepare MR-VP broth in test tubes and sterilize at appropriate temperature.
- Inoculate the test organisms using sterile technique.
- Incubate tubes at 37⁰C for 24- 48 hours.
- At the end of incubation, add 5 drops of methyl red indicator directly to the medium.
- Gently shake the medium
- Observe for colour change.

Observation

Colour change is observed

Result

Positive -red or pink colour

Negative -yellow colour

Viva questions

Why is methyl red test used methyl red indicator?

Why is mixed acid fermentation test is called methyl red test?

Why is phenol red or phenolphthalein not used in methyl red test?

What are the principles of MR test?

How is mixed acid fermentation of bacteria detected?

List any 5 MR positive bacteria

Which is the major component in MR test medium

Spotters – MR-VP medium, MR test result.

25c. Voges Proskauer Test

Aim

To differentiate enteric organisms.

Principle

Voges and Proskauer are the two microbiologists working at the beginning of the 20th century. They first observed red colour reaction produced by appropriate culture media after treatment of potassium hydroxide. It was later discovered that the active product formed after bacterial metabolism is acetyl methyl carbinol (acetoin) a neutral reacting end product. It is a product of butylene glycol pathway.

Pyruvate is formed during the fermentative degradation of glucose, which is further metabolized by bacterial enzymes through butylene glycol path way and produce acetoin. In the presence of atmospheric oxygen and 40% KOH, acetoin is converted in to diacetyl and creatine. Alpha naphtol serve as a catalyst to bring out a red complex.

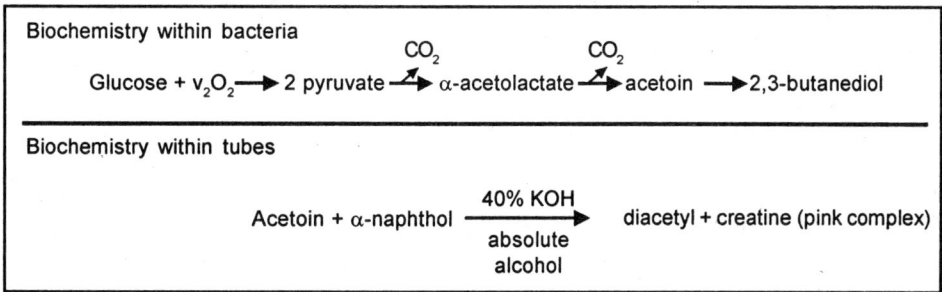

Fig 25.3: Principle and reactions of VP test

Materials required

MR-VP broth, α napthol, Potassium hydroxide, Test tubes, Inoculation loop, Cotton etc.

Quality Control

Negative control: *Escherichia coli*

Positive control: *Klebsiella pnemoniae*

Procedure

- Prepare MR-VP broth in test tubes and sterilize at 121^0C for 10 minutes.
- Inoculate the test organisms using sterile technique.
- Incubate tubes at 37^0C for 24- 48 hours
- At the end of incubation, add 0.5 mL of α napthol, followed by 0.2mL of KOH.
- Shake the tube gently to expose the medium to atmospheric oxygen and allow the medium to stand for 10-15 minutes.
- Observe colour change and record the results.

Observation

Colour change was observed

Result

Positive -red or brown colour

Negative -black or pale yellow colour

Viva questions

Give other name of acetoein

How do you detect acetyl methyl carbinol in VP test medium?

Name the end product of butanediol fermentation.

Reason for namology in VP test

What are the reagents used in VP test?

Spotters – MR VP medium, VP positive or negative results

25d. Citrate Utilization Test

Aim

To differentiate bacteria

To detect the ability of bacteria to utilize citrate as a carbon source.

Principle

Sodium citrate is a salt of citric acid, a simple organic compound found as one of the metabolites in the TCA cycle. Some bacteria can obtain energy in a manner other than by the fermentation of carbohydrates by using citrate as the sole source of carbon. The measurement of this characteristic is important in the identification of many members of the Enterobacteriaceae. Any medium used to detect citrate utilization by test bacteria must be devoid of protein and carbohydrate as source of carbon. The utilization of citrate by a test bacterium is detected by the production of alkaline by products. The medium includes sodium citrate, an anion, as the sole source of carbon and ammonium phosphate as a sole source of nitrogen. Bacteria that use citrate also extract nitrogen from the ammonium salt, with the production of ammonia, leading to alkalization of the medium from conversion of the NH_3^{2+} to NH_4OH

> **Box:25.1 Media for citrate test differentiation**
> Simmons citrate and Kosers citrate medium are used to study citrate utilization. Kosers medium is a liquid medium without any indicator. Citrate utilization is detected with turbidity observation. Simmons medium is a solid and indicator medium. Growth and colour change indicates citrate utilization.

Table :25.1 Quality control

Citrate Positive	Citrate Negative
Klebsiella pneumoniae	*E. coli*
Citrobacter sp.	*Salmonella sp.*
Enterobacter sp.	*Shigella sp.*
Serratia sp.	*Yersinia sp.*

Materials required

Test tubes, Conical flask, inoculation loop, cotton plug, Simmons citrate agar, test organisms etc.,

Procedure

- Prepare simmons citrate medium and poured in test tubes.

- Sterilize the medium at 121^0C for 15 minutes.

- Pick a well-isolated colony from the surface of a primary isolation medium and inoculated as a single streak on the slant surface of the citrate agar tube.

- Incubate the medium at 37^0C for 24 hours.

- Observe colour change after incubation period.

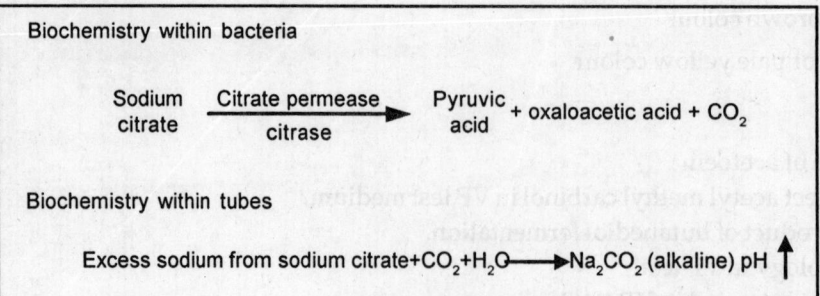

Fig 25.4: Principles and reactions of Citrate test

Result

A positive test is represented by the development of a deep blue colour within 24-48 hours, indicating that the test organism has been able to utilize the citrate contained in the medium, with the production of alkaline products. A positive test may also be read without a blue colour if there is visible colonial growth along the inoculation streak line.

Viva questions

Name the triple indicator used in citrate utilization test

What is the principal component in citrate medium?

Name any two citrate utilizing medium'

How do you detect citrate utilization in medium?

Spotters – Simmons citrate medium, Citrate test result tube or picture

25e. Triple Sugar Iron agar test (H₂S production)

Aim

To detect fermentative nature of bacteria

To determine the ability of microorganisms to produce hydrogen sulphide from specific substrate.

Principle

Some bacteria liberate sulphur from sulphur containing aminoacids or other sulphur containing compounds. The sulphur is used as final hydrogen acceptor during anaerobic respiration leading to the formation of hydrogen sulphide. When the following conditions are present, hydrogen sulphide can be detected by the test system.

Table : 25.2 - H₂S production	
Sulphur source	**H₂S indicator**
Sodium thio sulphate	Ferrous sulphate
Peptone	Ferrous ammonium
Sulphate	sulphate
Tryptophan	Lead acetate
	Iron metal
Common media for H₂S detection Haektoein enteric agar, XLD agar, SIM agar, Bismuth sulphite agar, SS agar, Deoxycholate citrate agar.	

Medium must contain a sulphur source either in the form of organic compounds or in the form of inorganic compounds.

Presence of hydrogen sulphide indicator. Indicator maybe heavy metals ions (Fe^{2+} or Fe^{3+})

The test organism must possess the enzyme system to produce hydrogen sulphide.

The medium must support the growth of microorganisms.

The following are the series of steps involved in the production and detection of hydrogen sulphide.

Bacterial enzyme system release sulphide from sulphur source.

Cysteine Desulphurase

Cysteine – – – – – –> pyruvic acid+ hydrogen sulphide -+ammonia

Thiosulphate Reductase

Thiosulphate+4H+4e⁻ – – – – – – – –> 2sulphite+ 2hydrogen sulphide

Positive control

Citrobacter fruendi, Salmonella typhi, Salmonella typhimurium, Proteus sp., Edwardsiella sp. are the common hydrogen sulphide producing organisms.

Materials required

Test tubes, Conical flask, inoculation loop, cotton plug, TSI agar, etc.,

Procedure

- Prepare and sterilize TSI agar medium and make it as a slant with enough amount of butt (Slant and butt must be in equal length)

- Pick Single colony from primary isolation plate and inoculated by stabbing down the centre of agar butt carefully. Withdraw the inoculating needle carefully and then streaked the surface of the slant.

- Incubate the tube at 37°C

- Note the result only after 18- 24 hours.

Result and interpretation

Hydrogen sulphide production was indicated by the development of black colour. Yellow colour of the butt is due to glucose fermentation. Yellow colour of the slant indicates acid production due to lactose or sucrose fermentation.

Precaution

Stap inoculation must be done. Butt and slant must be same length. Black colouration of the butt or slant is read as acid slant acid butt because hydrogen sulphide production requires hydrogen ions. Hydrogen ions are acid. TSI contain ten times less glucose than lactose and sucrose. During metabolism glucose is utilized first. In the butt glucose is converted into pyruvic acid anaerobically. In the slant pyruvate is further metabolized aerobically to acid end products. Thus acid products cause the colour of the indicator to yellow. This occurs within 6-8 hours. After depletion of glucose, lactose fermentors will utilize lactose and the same reaction persists upto 18- 24 hours. But in the case of nonlactose and non sucrose Fermentors, after the depletion of glucose, the organisms metabolize peptone aerobically for their energy and produce alkaline end products. These results in the formation of pink colour in the slant. Thus the colour of slant changed yellow to pink after 8 hours. That is why the result must read after 24 hours.

Viva questions

Name sulphur source used in TSI agar.

What are the kinds of respirations detected in TSI test?

How is H_2S detected in TSI medium

Why butt and slant length must be in same length in TSI medium?

List any 5 medium used to detect H_2S production.

Name the indicator used in TSI medium.

Explain the role of Ferrous ammonium sulphate in TSI medium.

Why must TSI test observations be made between 18 to 24 hours after inoculation?

Distinguish between an acid and alkaline slant.

What is the purpose of thiosulfate in the TSI agar?

What is meant by a saccharolytic bacterium? What reaction would it give in a TSI tube?

Why is there more lactose and sucrose in TSI agar than glucose?

What is the pH indicator in TSI agar?

Spotters – TSI medium, Results of TSI test

25f. Catalase Test

Aim

To demonstrate the availability of catalase in test organisms.

To demonstrate the role of catalase.

Principle

Catalase is an enzyme that decomposes H_2O_2 into water and oxygen. Chemically, catalase is a haemoprotein, similar in structure to haemoglobin, except that the four iron atoms in the molecule are in the oxidized, rather than the reduced (Fe^{2+}) state. Excluding Streptococci, most aerobic and facultative bacteria possess catalase activity. Hydrogen peroxide forms as one of the oxidative product of aerobic carbohydrate metabolism. If allowed to accumulate, it is lethal to bacterial cell. Catalase converts H_2O_2 into H_2O and O_2. Maxiumum number of intracellular pathogens possesses catalase enzyme as one of the defense mechanism.

$$2O_2^- + 2H^+ \xrightarrow{\text{superoxide dismutate}} O_2 + H_2O_2$$

Oxygen   Hydrogen peroxide

$$2H_2O_2 \xrightarrow{\text{catalase of peroxidase}} 2H_2O + O_2$$

Water   Free oxygen

Fig 25.5: Principle of Catalase test

Materials required

Test organism in nutrient broth or agar, Glass Slide, wooden stick, cotton plug, 3% H_2O_2 etc.,

Quality control

Positive control: *Staphylococcus aureus*

Negative control: Streptococcus species

Procedure

Method 1

- Transfer small quantity of culture from the plate or slant to the surface of a glass slide with a wooden applicator stick.

- Add 1 drop of 3% H_2O_2 on the culture with the help of Pasteur pipette and observed for bubble formation.

Method 2

- Take one mL of 3% H_2O_2 in a test tube.

- Add one drop of culture from nutrient broth to the tube with the help of Pasteur pipette.

- Observe the tube for bubble formation.

Result

The rapid and sustained appearance of bubbles or effervescence constitutes a positive test. Catalase is present in RBC, so care must be taken to avoid carryover of RBC with the colony material (If the medium is Blood agar).

Viva questions

How do you interpretate catalse test result?

What are the principles of catalase test?

Why is inoculation loop not used in transferring culture in catalase test?

What are the clinical / medical significance of catalase test?

What is the importance of catalase to certain bacteria?

Do anaerobic bacteria require catalase? Explain your answer.

Write a balanced equation for the degradation of H_2O_2 in the presence of catalase.

What two groups of bacteria can be differentiated with the catalase test?

What are several bacteria that produce catalase?

What is the substrate of the catalase reaction?

Spotters - H_2O_2 Catalase test result.

25g. Oxidase test

Aim

To determine the oxygen requirement of the bacteria

To demonstrate the presence of oxidase enzyme

To demonstrate metabolic nature of bacteria.

Principle

The cytochromes are iron containing haemoproteins that act as the last link in the chain of aerobic respiration by transferring electrons to oxygen, with the formation of water. The cytochrome system is found in aerobic or micro aerphilic and facultative anaerobic organisms. Oxidase test is important in identifying organisms based on oxygen utilization. This test is most helpful for the identification of *Aeromonas, Pseudomonas, Neisseria, Camphylobacter, Pastuerella* and enterobacteriaceae members. The cytochrome oxidase test uses certain reagent dyes, such as p-phenylenediamine dihydrochloride, that substitute for oxygen as artificial electron acceptor. In the reduced state the dye is colourless; however, in the presence of cytochrome oxidase and atmospheric oxygen, p-phenylenediamine is oxidised, forming indophenol blue.

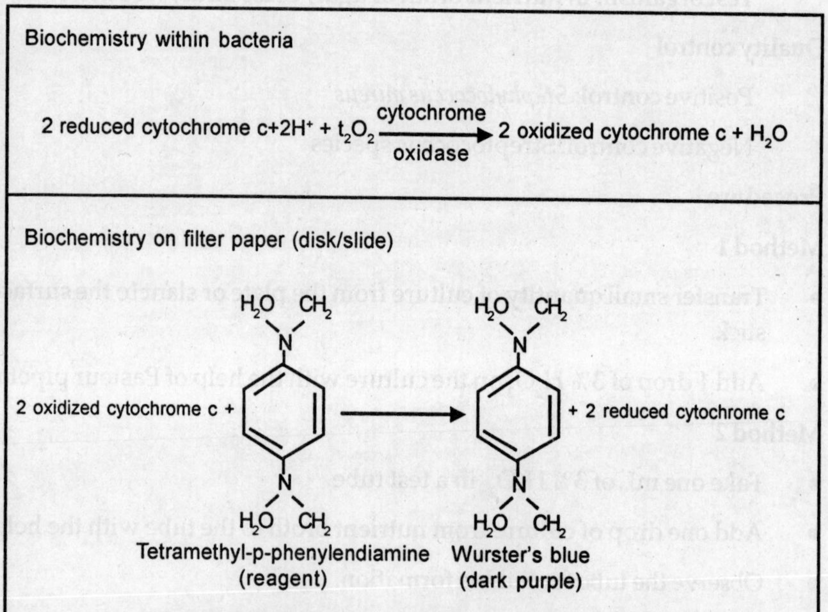

Biochemistry within bacteria

$$2 \text{ reduced cytochrome } c + 2H^+ + t_2O_2 \xrightarrow[\text{oxidase}]{\text{cytochrome}} 2 \text{ oxidized cytochrome } c + H_2O$$

Biochemistry on filter paper (disk/slide)

2 oxidized cytochrome c +

Tetramethyl-p-phenylendiamine (reagent)

→

+ 2 reduced cytochrome c

Wurster's blue (dark purple)

Fig 25.6: Principle and reactions of Oxidase test

Tetra methyl paraphenylene diamine is recommended because the reagent is more stable in storage and is more sensitive to detection of cytochrome oxidase and is less toxic than the dimethyl derivative.

Precautions

Iron wire, nichrome loop should not be used to transfer culture. Should not use colony from selective media and result should be observed within 10 seconds.

Materials required

Test organism, Tooth pick, Slide, Oxidase disc.

Quality control

Positive control: *Pseudomonas aeruginosa*

Negative control: *Escherichia coli*

Procedure

Method 1

- Take a pure culture.
- Inoculate in a tube containing 5-10mL of nutrient broth.
- Incubated at 37^0C for 12 – 24 hours.
- Take Oxidase disc in a clean microscopic slide.
- Place One or two drops of culture on the disc.
- Observe for colour change within 10 seconds.

Method 2

- Take a pure culture and grow in nutrient agar plate.
- Take oxidase disc in a clean microscopic slide.
- Take small quantity of bacterial culture in a wooden stick.
- Paste the culture on oxidase disc
- Observe for colour change within 10 seconds.

Observation and results

Bacterial colonies having cytochrome oxidase activity develop a deep blue colour at the inoculation site within 10 seconds. Any organism producing a blue colour in the 10-60 second period must be tested further because it probably doesn't belong to the enterobacteriaceae. Stainless steel or nichrome inoculating loops or wires should not be used for this test because surface oxidation products formed when flame sterilizing may result in false positive reaction

Viva questions

What are the precautions to be observed while doing oxidase test?

What are the principle of oxidase test?

What are the kinds of organisms possess oxidase in large quantities?

What metabolic property characterizes bacteria that possess oxidase activity?

What is the importance of cytochrome oxidase to bacteria that possess it?

What is the function of the test reagent in the oxidase test?

The oxidase test is used to differentiate among which groups of bacteria?

Why should nichrome or other iron-containing inoculating devices not be used in the oxidase test?

Spotters – oxidase disc, positive result of oxidase, oxidase reagent.

25h. Urease test

Aim

To demonstrate the presence of urease, an intracellular enzyme in the bacteria.

To distinguish the bacteria / fungi based on the urease activity.

Introduction

Certain bacteria and fungi possess the enzyme urease that hydrolyzes urea, releasing ammonia into the medium. This produces a change in the pH that can be detected by the colour change. This test can be used to differentiate different groups of bacteria and fungi especially *Cryptococcus neoformance*. *Helicobacter pylori* produces strong strong urease in human stomach.

Principle

Urea is a diamide of carbonic acid. Urease, the enzyme produced by the bacteria and fungi, hydrolyses urea and releases ammonia and carbon dioxide. Ammonia reacts in solution to form ammonium carbonate, which is alkaline leading to an increase in pH of the medium. Phenol red is incorporated in the medium changes its colour from yellow to red, thus indicating the presence of urease activity.

Materials required

Test tube, conical flask, Autoclave, Balance, Inoculation loop, hot air oven, test cultures like *Escherichia coli* and *Citrobacter sp.*, Christension urea agar etc.,

Procedure

● Prepare Christensen's urea agar and sterilize properly.

● Prepare agar slant by placing the tube of medium in slanting position (Refer slant preparation)

● Inoculate test organism on the medium as zig zag streak.

● Incubate the medium at 37⁰C for 18 hours.

● Observe the medium for change of colour.

Observation

Pale yellow – Negative

Pink – Positive

Viva questions

Describe the principles of urease test.

Name the organism used in urease test as control.

What are the medium used to find out urease activity?

List urease Negative microorganism.

What are the important uses of urease test in mycology?

Which pH is mentioned to perform urease test?

Name the indicator used in urease test.

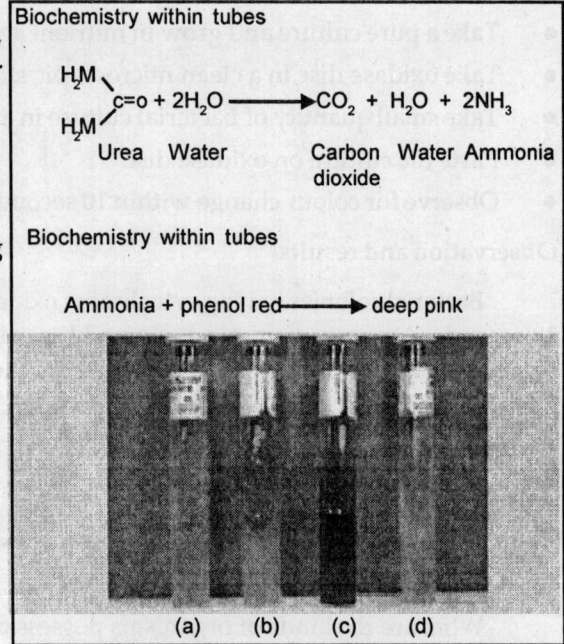

Biochemistry within tubes

$$\begin{matrix} H_2M \\ \quad \\ H_2M \end{matrix} c=o + 2H_2O \longrightarrow CO_2 + H_2O + 2NH_3$$

Urea Water   Carbon Water Ammonia
                    dioxide

Biochemistry within tubes

Ammonia + phenol red ⟶ deep pink

(a)   (b)   (c)   (d)

Fig 25.7: Principle and reactions of Urease test

What is the purpose of using indicator in urease test?

Which organisms produce strong urease activity in human?

Explain the biochemistry of the urease reaction.

What is the purpose of using phenol red in the urea broth medium?

When would you use the urease test?

What is in urea broth?

Spotters : urea agar, urease positive tube, urea.

25i. Nitrate Test

Aim

To identify the organisms on the basis of nitrate reduction.

To study the organisms ability to reduce nitrate to nitrite

Principle

Nitrate is one of the nitrogen sources. Nitrate acts as a electron acceptor in anaerobic respiration. Nitrate reduction ability of the microorganisms maintains Nitrogen cycle in ecosystem. The capability of organism to reduce nitrates to nitrites is an important characteristic used in the identification and species differentiation of many groups of microorganisms. Organisms demonstrating nitrate reduction have the capability to extracting oxygen from nitrates to form nitrites and other reduction products.

The presence of nitrites in the test medium is detected by the addition of alpha naphthylamine and sulfanilic acid, with the formation of a red diazonium dye, P sulfo benzene-azo-alpha-napthylamine. This gives red colour to the positive reaction.

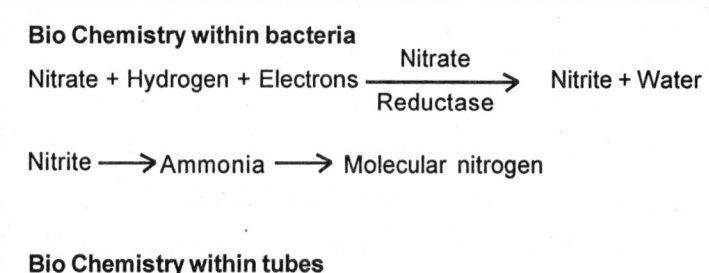

Bio Chemistry within bacteria

$$Nitrate + Hydrogen + Electrons \xrightarrow[\text{Reductase}]{\text{Nitrate}} Nitrite + Water$$

Nitrite ⟶ Ammonia ⟶ Molecular nitrogen

Bio Chemistry within tubes

Sulphanilic Acid + Alpha napthylamine

⟶ coloured compound

Materials required

Nitrate Broth, Alpha naphthylamine reagent and Sulfanilic acid reagent.

Test tube, Cotton, Inoculation loop, conical flask, Incubator etc.,

Quality control

Positive control: *Escherichia coli*

Negative control: *Acinetobacter baumannii*

Procedure

- Prepare nitrate broth and sterilize properly.
- Inoculate the medium with test organism Incubate at 37⁰C for 24-48hrs.

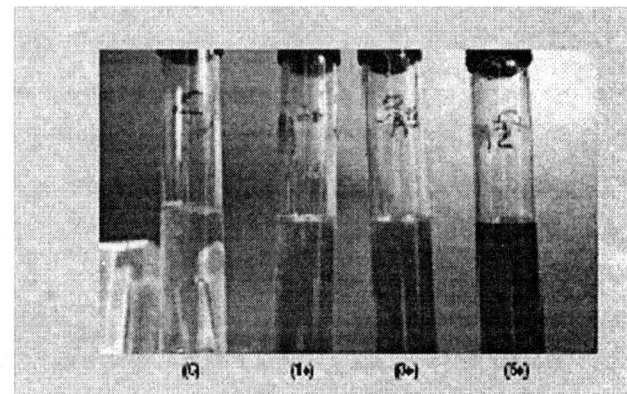

Fig 25.8: Principle and reactions of nitrate test

- At the end of incubation, add 1mL each of Alpha naphthylamine reagent and Sulfanilic acid reagent to the test medium, in that order.

- If the test showed negative result, sprinkle little Zinc metal dust and observed colour change.

Observation and result

Red colour within 10 seconds-Positive

Red colour after the addition of zinc-Negative

No colour change-Negative

No colour change after the addition of zinc- positive

Interpretation

The development of a red colour within 30 seconds after adding the test reagents indicates the presence of nitrites and represents a positive reaction for nitrate reduction. If no colour develops after adding the test reagents, this may indicates either that nitrates have not been reduced or that they have been reduced to products other than nitrites such as ammonia, molecular nitrogen, nitric oxide (NO) or nitrous oxide (N_2O) and hydroxylamine. Because the test reagents detect only nitrites, the latter process would lead to a false negative reading. Thus it is necessary to add a small quantity of Zinc dust to all negative reaction. Zinc ions reduce nitrates to nitrites, and the development of a red colour after adding Zinc dust indicates the presence of residual nitrates and confirms a true negative reaction.

Viva questions

What are the principles behind the nitrate test?

Name the reagents used to detect nitrite

Name major ingredients available in nitrate broth

Mention the role of zinc in nitrate test

Importance of nitrate reduction in bacteria

From your results, which bacteria are negative for nitrate reduction? Which are positive?

Why is the development of a red colour a negative test when zinc is added?

What are the end products that may result from the action of bacteria with nitrate-reducing enzymes?

Spotters : Sodium nitrate, zinc, Nitrate positive tube.

25j. Oxidative Fermentative Test (OF)

Aim

To differentiate the bacteria based on oxidation and fermentation of carbohydrates.

To identify the bacteria.

To identify the saccharolytic and fermentative reactions of bacteria

Principle

Saccharolytic microorganisms degrade glucose either fermentatively or oxidatively. The end products of fermentation are relatively strong mixed acids that can be detected in conventional fermentation test medium. The acids formed in oxidative degradation of glucose are extremely weak and are not detected in ordinary fermentation medium. Hence to differentiate oxidation from fermentation more sensitive oxidative-fermentation medium of Hugh and Leifson is used. The OF medium of Hugh and Leifson differs from carbohydrate fermentation media as follows.

The concentration of peptone is decreased from 1% to 0.2%.

The concentration of carbohydrate is increased from 0.5% to 1%.

The concentration of agar is decreased from 1.5 to 0.3%.

The lower protein/higher carbohydrate ratio reduces the formation of alkaline amines that can neutralize the small quantities of weak acids that may formed from oxidative metabolism. The relatively large amount of carbohydrate serves to increase the amount of acid that can potentially be formed. The semisolid agar consistency permits acid that form on the surface of the agar to penetrate throughout the medium, making interpretation of the pH shift of the indicator easier to visualize. Motility can also be observed in this medium.

Materials required

OF Basal Medium, Test tubes, conical flask, membrane filter & apparatus, sterile mineral oil or liquid paraffin, carbohydrate to be tested (Glucose, Lactose, Sucrose etc.,)

Quality Control

Glucose oxidative – *Pseudomonas aeruginosa*

Glucose fermentative- *Escherichia coli.*

Non saccharolytic – *Moraxella sp.*

Procedure

- Prepare two tubes of OF basal medium for each carbohydrate.
- Sterilize at 120 ^{0} C for 10 minutes.
- Inoculate test organism using needle.
- Add one mL of sterile liquid paraffin / mineral oil to one tube of each pair.
- Incubate each tubes at 35 ^{0} C.
- Observe colour change at an regular interval for several days.
- Record the results and interpretate it.

Result

Acid production is detected in the medium by the appearance of yellow colour. In the case of oxidative organisms, colour production maybe first noted near the surface of the medium.

Open tube	Covered tube	Metabolism
Acid	Alkaline	Oxidative
Acid	Acid	Fermentative
Alkaline	Alkaline	Nonsaccharolytic

Viva questions

OF basal medium is also called as_____

Why are we adding mineral oil /liquid in OF test?

Why is low quantity of peptone added in OF basal medium.

What is the need of filter sterilization of sugars?

Why is 0.3% agar agars added in OF medium?

What are the purposes OF test?

What are the principles OF test?

How do you differentiate oxidation & fermentation in OF test?

Spotters: OF medium, mineral oil, positive & negative reactions.

25k. Carbohydrate Fermentation Test

Aim

To determine the ability of microorganisms to ferment carbohydrates with the production of an acid or acid and gas.

Principle

In fermentation, substrates such as carbohydrates and alcohols undergo anaerobic dissimilation and produce an organic acid (for example, lactic, formic, or acetic acid) that may be accompanied by gases such as hydrogen or carbon dioxide. Facultative anaerobes are usually the so called fermenters of carbohydrates. Fermentation is best described by considering the degradation of glucose by way of the **Embden-Meyerhof pathway,** also known as the **glycolytic** pathway.

Fermentative degradation under anaerobic conditions is carried out in a fermentation tube containing a Durhams tube, an inverted inner vial for the detection of gas production. Nutrient broth ingredients are added to the medium for the support of the growth of all organisms. A specific carbohydrate that serves as the substrate for determining the organism's fermentative capabilities.

The pH indicator phenol red, which is red at a neutral pH (7) and changes to yellow at a slightly acidic pH of 6.8, suggesting that slight amounts of acid will cause a colour change. Following incubation, carbohydrates that have been fermented with the production of acidic wastes will cause the phenol red to turn yellow, thereby indicating a positive reaction. In some cases, acid production is accompanied by the evolution of a gas (CO_2) that will be visible as a bubble in the inverted tube. Cultures that are not capable of fermenting a carbohydrate substrate will not change the indicator and the tubes will appear red. This is a negative reaction.

Materials Required

Test Tubes, Durham's Tube, Cotton, test organisms, conical flask, carbohydrate fermentation medium.

Quality Control

Glucose fermentative- *Escherichia coli*

Glucose non fermenter – *Pseudomonas aeruginosa*

Procedure

- Prepare carbohydrate fermentation medium with specific carbohydrate and pour in to test tube.
- Insert Durham's tube and filled with medium without any air bubble (used to detect gas production during fermentation).
- Sterilize the medium at 120°C for 5 minutes. Excess heat may denature carbohydrate.

- Inoculate the medium with test organism.
- Incubate tubes at 37°C for 24 hours.
- Look for colour change and gas bubbles in Durham's tube.
- Record the results and interpretate the results.

Result

Colour change and air bubble in durham's tube interpretates carbohydrate fermentation

Viva questions

Define fermentation

Mention different types of fermentation.

Is fermentation different from anaerobic respiration?

Which component acts as a final electron acceptor in anaerobic respiration?

Name the indicator used in carbohydrate fermentation test.

Name the organism responsible for glucose & lactose fermentation.

What are the roles of Durham's tube in carbohydrate fermentation?

Spotters: Carbohydrate fermentation medium, Positive & Negative reactions of carbohydrate fermentation test, Durham's tube

25l. Phenylalanine Deaminase Test

Aim

To understand the biochemical process of phenylalanine deamination.

To describe how to perform the phenylalanine deamination test

Principle

Phenylalnine is an aminoacid. Upon deamination, it forms ketoacid, phenyl pyruvic acid. Among enterobacteriaceae, only members of the Proteus, Moraxella and Providencia possess the deaminase enzyme necessary for the conversion. The phenylalanine test depends on the detection of phenylpyruvic acid in the test medium after growth of the test organism. Test is positive if a viable green colour develops on addition of a solution of 10% Ferric chloride.

Materials required

Phenylalanine medium, Ferric chloride reagent, test tubes, Conical flask, inoculatation loop, test organisms, incubator etc.,

Quality control

Positive control: Proteus species.

Negative:*Escherichia coli*

Procedure

- Prepare phenylalanine medium.
- Pour the medium into test tubes and sterilize at 121°C for 15 minutes and make it as slant.

- Inoculate the medium with a single colony of the test organism
- Incubate at 37⁰C for 18 to 24 hours
- Add 4 or 5drops of the ferric chloride reagent to the surface of the agar.
- Rotate the tube to dislodge the surface colonies.
- Observe for colour change.

Result

The immediate appearance of green colour indicates the presence of phenyl pyruvic acid and said to be positive test.

Viva questions

What are the principles of deaminase test?

What is the main purpose of deaminase?

Is deaminase is an aerobic reaction or anaerobic reaction.

What happened if deaminase medium is over laid with oil?

Name deaminase positive organism

How do you prepare ferric chloride reagent.

What is the purpose of the ferric chloride in the phenylalanine deamination test?

When would you use the phenylalanine deamination test?

Name some bacteria that can deaminate phenylalanine.

Describe the process of deamination.

Describe the colour of an uninoculated tube of phenylalanine agar.

Spotters : Phenylalanine, Positive reactions of deaminase.

25m. Decarboxylase Test

Aim

To understand the biochemical process of decarboxylation.

To explain how the decarboxylation of lysine can be detected in culture.

To perform lysine and ornithine decarboxylase tests.

Principle

Decarboxylases are a group of substrate specific enzymes that are capable of reacting with carboxyl portion of aminoacids, forming alkaline-reacting amines. This reaction is known as decarboxylation, forms Co_2 as the second product. Each decarboxylase enzyme is specific for an aminoacid. Lysine, ornithine and arginine are the three aminoacids routinely tested in the identification of Enterobacteriaceae. The specific amine products are as folows.

Lysine — — → cadaverine; Ornithine-→ putrescine; Arginine — →citruline.

The conversion of arginine to citruline is a dihydrolase, rather than a decarboxylase reaction, in which an NH_2 group is removed from arginine as the first step. Ornithine undergoes decarboxylation to form putrescine. Moellar decarboxylase medium base is most commonly used for determining the decarboxylase capabilities of the organism. The aminoacid to be tested is added to the decarboxylase base before inoculation with the test organism. A control tube, consisting of only the base without the aminoacid, must also be setup in parellal. Both tubes are incubated anaerobically by overlaying with mineral oil. During the initial stages of incubation, both tubes turn yellow, owing to the fermentation of the small amount of glucose in the medium. If the aminoacids is decarboxylated, alkaline amines are formed and the medium recovers its original purple colour.

Materials required

Moellar Decarboxylase broth base, test tubes, Conical flask, inoculatation loop, test organisms, , incubator, L Lysine, L Ornithine, L Arginine.

Quality control

Aminoacid	Positive control	Negative control
Lysine	Enterobacter aerogens	Enterobacter cloacae
Ornithine	Enterobacter cloacae	Klebsiella pneumoniae
Arginine	Enterobacter cloacae	Enterobacter aerogens

Procedure

- Prepare moeller decarboxylase medium base in two conical flasks.

- Divide one flask containing medium into 3 portions.

- Add 1% of any one L aminoacids (L Lysine/ L Ornithine/ L Arginine) to each of the portion of medium.

- Pour L aminoacid medium into one test tube and medium without aminoacid (Control) in to one tube.

- Sterilize at 121°C for 15 minutes.

- Inoculate test organism into both tubes.

- Overlay both tubes (one with aminoacid and one without aminoacid) with sterile mineral oil to cover about 1cm of the surface

- Incubate at 35°C for 18-24 hours.

- Observe for growth and colour change.

Result

Coversion of the control tube to a yellow colour indicates that the pH of the medium has been lowered sufficiently to activate the decarboxylase enzymes. Reversion of the tube containing the aminoacid to a blue purple colour indicates a positive test owing to the formation of amines from the decarbozylation reaction.

Viva questions

Define decarboxylation.

Name the medium used to detect decarboxylase activity.

Name the amino acids used to perform decarboxylase activities.

Name end product of lysine decarboxylation.

Mention the role of glucose in decarboxylase medium.

Why pyridoxol is incorporated in decarboxylase medium?

Why mineral oil is over laid in decarboxylase medium?

Name the indicator used in decarboxylase test.

Explain what occurs during decarboxylation?

How does the pH indicator bromo cresol purple indicate a change in pH?

Spotters: Lysine , Arginine, ornithine, Moeller decarboxylase medium , reaction of decarboxylase test/ photo.

25n. O-NitroPhenyl β-D-Galacto Pyranoside (ONPG)

Aim

To differentiate non lactose Fermentors from late lactose fermenting microorganisms.

Principle

ONPG is structurally similar to lactose, except that orthonitrophenyl has been substituted for glucose. On hydrolysis, through the action of the enzyme β galactosidase, ONPG cleaves into galactose and ortho nitro phenol. ONPG is a colourless compound, ortho nitrophenol is yellow, providing visual evidence of hydrolysis. Lactose fermenting bacteria possess both lactose permease and galactosidase, two enzymes required for the production of acid in the lactose fermentation test. The permease is required for the lactose molecule to penetrate the bacterial cell where the galactosidase can cleave the galactoside bond, producing glucose and galactose. Non lactose Fermentors are devoid of these two enzymes and are incapable of producing acid from lactose. Some bacterial species are appear to be non lactose fermentor because they lack permease, but do possess β galactosidase and give a positive ONPG test. So-called late lactose Fermentors may be delayed in their production of acid from lactose because of sluggish permease activity. In these instances, a positive ONPG test may provide a rapid identification of delayed lactose fermentation.

$$\text{ONPG} \xrightarrow[\beta \text{ galactosidase}]{H_2O} \text{galactose+ortho nitrophenol (yellow)}$$

Materials Required

1M Phosphate buffer(pH-7), ONPG, Physiological saline, Toluene, test tubes, Conical flask, inoculatation loop, test organisms, incubator.

Quality control

Positive control: *Escherichia coli*

Negative control: *Proteus sp,*

Procedure

- Bacteria grown in media containing lactose, such as Mac Conkey, KIA or TSI agar produce optimal results in the ONPG test.

- Emulsify a loopful of bacterial growth in 0.5mL of physiological saline to produce heavy suspension.

- Add one drop of toluene to the suspension and mix for a few seconds to release the enzyme from the bacterial cell.

- Add an equal quantity of buffered ONPG solution to the suspension.

- Place the mixture in a 37⁰C water bath for 24 hours.

- Observe for colour change.

Result

The rate of hydrolysis of ONPG to ortho-nitrophenol may be rapid for some organisms, producing a visible yellow colour reaction within 5-10 minutes. Most tests are positive within 1 hour; however, reactions shouldn't interpret as negative before 24 hours of incubation. The yellow colour is usually distinct and indicates that organism has produced ortho-nitrophenol from the ONPG substrate through the action of β galactosidase.

Viva questions

Expand ONPG.

What is the purpose of performing ONPG?

How do you prepare ONPG?

Why toluene is added in test culture when performing ONPG?

What kinds of lactose fermenting bacteria are subjected to ONPG test?

Name the Positive organisms of ONPG test.

Spotters: ONPG, Positive reaction of ONPG/photo.

25 o. Malonate Utilization Test

Aim

To demonstrate the effect of malonate.

To differentiate bacteria based on malonate utilization.

Principle

Malonate is an enzyme inhibitor. It interferes with oxidation of succinic acid to fumaric acid. It binds to enzyme succinate dehydrogenase and prevent conversion of succinic acid. This results in accumulation of succinic acid in cell leads to cell death. To overcome this problem, microbes should use melonate as sole carbon source. Malanoate utilization leads to accumulation of alkaline end products, which is indicted as colour change from green to blue.

Materials required

Test tube, conical flask, Autoclave, Balance, hot air oven, test cultures like *Escherichia coli* and *Citrobacter sp.*, **Malonate Medium**.

Quality control

Positive control: Escherichia, Klebsiella, Alkaligens, Enterobacter

Procedure

- Prepare malonate medium and sterilize at 121 ° C for 15 minutes.
- Inoculate the broth from young culture to be tested.
- Incubate at 37°C for 24 hours
- Observe for colour change

Observation

Positive result is indicated by change of colour from green to blue, due to the utilization of sodium malonate.

Viva questions

How do you perform malonate utilization test?

What is the nature of melonate?

What happened if there is an accumulation of succinate in cell?

How do you find out the positive reaction of melanoate utilization test?

Spotters : Sodium malanoate, Malonate medium

25 p. Esculin hydrolysis (bile esculin test)

Aim

To check whether the bacteria hydrolyse esculin or not.

To differentiate gram positive bacteria.

Principle

The bile esculin test is based on the ability of certain bacteria, notably the gp D Streptococci and Enterococcus sps., to hydrolyze esculin in the presence of bile(4% bile salt or 40% bile). Esculin is a glycosidic coumarin derivative (6-beta-glucoside-7-hydroxy coumarin) are linked together by an ester bond through oxygen. For this test, esculin is incorporated into a medium containing 4% bile salt. Bacteria that are bile esculin positive are first of all, able to grow in the presence of bile salts. Hydrolysis of the esculin in the medium results in the formation of glucose and a compound called esculatin. Esculatin, inturn, reacts with ferric ions to form a black diffusable complex.

$$\text{Esculin} \xrightarrow{\text{Fe 3+}} \text{glucose+esculetin} \longrightarrow \text{black complex.}$$

Animal tissue peptones and infusions from heart muscle provide amino acids or other nitrogenous substances that support bacterial growth. Sodium chloride maintains osmotic equilibrium. Esculin is a glycoside incorporated as a differential agent to facilitate the identification of various organisms, including *Enterobacteriaceae*, enterococci and anaerobes. Hydrolysis of esculin yields esculetin and dextrose. In the presence of an iron salt, esculetin forms a brown-black complex that diffuses into the surrounding medium

Materials required

Bile esculin agar medium, inoculation loop, petriplates, test tubes, incubator

Quality control

Positive control: *Enterococcus faecalis*

Negative control: viridans streptococci.

Procedure

- Prepare sterile Bile esculin agar slant or plate.
- Inoculate 2 or 3 morphologically similar colonies using zig zag motion on slant & Quadrant streak on plate.
- Incubate the tubes / plates at 35°C for 24-48 hours in an ambient air incubator.
- Observe for colour change.

Result

Diffuse blackening of more than half of the slant within 24-48 hours indicates esculin hydrolysis. On plates, halos will be observed around isolated colonies and any blackening is considered as positive. All gp D streptococci will be bile esculin positive within 48 hours.

Limitation

Some viridence streptococci may also hydrolyze esculin in the presence of bile.

Viva questions

What is the principle of Esculin hydrolysis ?

What is the purpose of esculin hydrolysis test?

Spotters: Esculin, bile salt, Positive reaction of esculin test/ photo.

25 q. Coagulase test

Aim

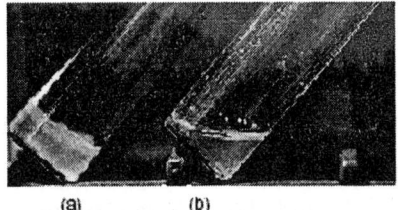

To demonstrate the presence of coagulase.

To distinguish the bacteria based on the coagulase activity.

(a)   (b)

Fig 25.9: Tube coagulase test

Background Information

The enzyme, coagulase, produced by a few Staphylococcus species, is a key feature of pathogenic Staphylococcus. The enzyme causes coagulation of blood, allowing the organism to produce more severe infection.

Coagulase is a protein having a prothrombin – like activity capable of converting fibrinogen into fibrin, which results in the formation of visible clot. In the laboratory, the coagulase test is used to identify S. aureus and differentiate it from the other species of coagulase negative Staphylococcus.

Principle

S.aureus produces the enzyme coagulase in 2 forms; they are bound coagulase and free coagulase.

Bound coagulase

Bound coagulase is also known as clumping factor. It is bound to the bacterial cell wall and is not present in culture filtrates. Presence of this enzyme is tested by slide coagulase test. Fibrin strands are formed between the bacterial cell when suspended in plasma (fibrinogen) , causing them to clump into visible aggregates.

Free coagulase

Free coagulase is a thrombin – like substance present in S. aureus culture filtrates. Presence of free coagulase is tested by tube coagulase test. In this method, a suspension of coagulase producing Staphylococci is prepared in plasma in a test tube, and incubated at 37^0 C for 3-6 hours. In a positive test, the enzyme coagulase secreted by S.aureus is liberated to the medium, which reacts with fibrinogen to produce a visible fibrin clot.

Materials Required

Rabbit plasma with EDTA anticoagulant, saline, glass slides, test tubes, glass rod/platinum loop/plastic loop etc.,

Specimen

Pure growth of *S.aureus* from solid media preferably from non-blood agar plates.

Procedure

Slide test

- Take a clean glass slide.

- Mark it into two halves by a glass marking pencil.

- Add two drops of sterile saline on two halves of the glass slides.

- Pick up the colonies of *S.aureus* to be tested from agar culture and gently emulsify with drops of saline.

- Add a drop of undiluted plasma to the bacterial suspension and mix with a wooden applicator stick.

- Place another drop of saline in other half of the slide as a control.

- Rock the slide, back and froth and observed for the prompt clumping of the bacterial suspension within 10-15 seconds.

Tube test

- Take 0.5 mL of rabbit plasma (diluted 1 in 5 with saline) in a test tube.

- Add approximately 5 drops (250 µL) of overnight broth culture or small amount of the colony growth of *S. aureus* to the diluted plasma in the test tube.

- Incubate the tube at 37^0C for 4 hours.

- Observe for clot formation by gently tilting the tube.

- If no clot is observed at that time, re incubate the tube at room temperature and read again after 18 hours.

Quality control

Positive control : *S. aureus* (Coagulase Positive bacteria)

Negative control : *S.epidermidis* (Coagulase negative bacteria)

Observations

In a positive slide test, prompt clumping of the organism shows the presence of the bound coagulase.

In a positive tube test, the plasma in the tube clots and does not flow when the tube is inverted.

Note : on continued incubation, the clot may be lysed by fibrinolysin secreted by some strains.

Box 25.2 List of coagulase positive bacteria
Staphylococcus aureus.
Staphylococcus schleiferi
Staphylococcus felis
Staphylococcus lutrae
Staphylococcus intermedius
Staphylococcus hyicus
Staphylococcus hydrogenalis

Results and interpretation

In slide test, positive reaction will be detected within 10-15 seconds of mixing the plasma with the suspension by the formation of a white precipitate and agglutination of the organisms. The test is considered negative if no agglutination is observed after 2 minutes. All strains that are coagulase positive can be reported as *S. aureus*. All strains producing negative slide tests must be tested with the tube coagulase test.

The tube coagulase test is considered positive if any degree of clotting is noted.

Viva question

Mention different methods of coagulase test.

Give examples for coagulase positive bacteria.

Describe mode of action of coagulase.

What is clumping factor?

What are the difference between clumping factor and coagulase?

Mention other name of clumping factor.

What are the purposes in performing coagulase test?

What is that method is performed to detect clumping factor?

What are the role of coagulase in bacteria?

Spotters: Positive result pictures of coagulase test.

25 r. Optochin Susceptibility Test

Aim

To detect susceptibility pattern of bacteria on Optochin.

To conform *Streptococcus pneumoniae*.

Principle

Ethyl hydrocuprene hydrochloride(Optochin), a quinine derivative, selectively inhibits the growth of *Streptococcus pneumoniae* at very low concentrations(5µG/mL or less). Optochin may also inhibit other viridans streptococci, but only at much high concentrations. The test has sensitivity of more than 95% and is simple to perform, and is inexpensive. Optochin is water soluble and diffuses readily into agar medium. Therefore, fillter paper disks impregnated with optochin can be used to determine susceptibility of suspected pneumococci. This test is used to confirm *S. pneumoniae*.

Materials required

Test Organisms, Blood agar Plate, Optochin disc, forceps, needle etc.,

Quality control

Positive control : *Streptococcus pneumoniae*

Negative control : *Streptococcus pyogenes*

Procedure

- Using an inoculating loop, select three to four well isolated colonies to be tested and streak on blood agar plate. The inoculated area should be about 3 cm².

- Place an optochin disc in the upper third of the streaked area. Tamp down the disk with flamed forceps so that the disk adheres firmly to the agar surface.

- Incubate the plate at 37°C for 18-24hours in a candle jar or in 5% to 7% CO_2 containing environment.

Result

Streptococcus can be presumptively identified as *S. pneumoniae* if it shows a zone of inhibition of 14mm or more around a 6mm disc, or a zone of 16mm or more around a 10mm disk. Organisms showing zones smaller than these should be tested for bile solubility.

Viva questions

What are the principles of optochin test?

Name the chemical nature of optochin

How do you perform optochin test?

Spotters : Blood agar plate, Optochin disc.

25 s. Bacitracin and SXT Susceptibility Test

Aim

To test susceptibility of bacteria to bacitracin.

To differentiate Gp A & GpB β haemolytic Streptococci.

Principle

Susceptibility to low concentrations of the polypeptide antibiotic bacitracin and to the combination sulfonamide trimethoprim-sulfamethaxazole(SXT) provides an easy and inexpensive method for the presumptive identification of both group A and group B β haemolytic Streptococci.

Group A Streptococci are susceptible to relatively low concentrations of bacitracin and are resistant to SXT. Group B Streptococcus are resistant to both antibiotic. Other beta haemolytic Streptococci show varying susceptibility to bacitracin, but these organisms are usually susceptible to SXT test along with the bacitracin test increases the sensitivity and predictive value of the bacitracin test.

Material required

β haemolytic bacteria , blood agar plate , inoculation loop , L- rod

Bacitracin disc , SXT disc , incubator, etc;

Procedure

- Pick 3-4 isolated colonies of the β haemolytic streptococcus and streak the inoculum down the center half of a blood agar plate.

- Using a sterile swab or a bacteriological loop spread the inoculam as a lawn over the entire half of the plate.

- Aseptically place a bacitracin disk and SXT disk on the inoculated area. Make sure that the discs are spread evenly. Using flamed forceps, gently tamp down the discs so that they adhere to the agar surface.

- Incubate the plate in ambient air at 35°C.

Result

Susceptible (S): Any zone around either of the disc.

Resistant(R) : Growth upto the edge of the disc.

Bacitracin	SXT	Identification
S	R	GpA
R	R	Gp B
S/R	S	Not Gps A or B

This test is generally performed on throat isolates, for which gpA Streptococci are being sought, the gp B is generally not reported.

Limitations: Only gpB Streptococci should be tested, because many alpha haemolytes are susceptible to low concentrations of bacitracin.

No data are available to indicate that zones of inhibition should be measured.

The lawn of bacterial inoculum should be confluent.

Viva questions

What are the purposes of SXT & bacitracin test?

How do you differentiate GpA& GpB streptococci.

Spotters: Bacitracin , SXT, blood agar, chain of cocci.

25 t. Novobiocin Sensitivity Test

Aim

To differentiate coagulase positive and negative Staphylococcus based on Novobiocin susceptibility

Principle

Coagulase negative Staphylococci can be divided into novobiocin susceptible and novobiocin resistant species. Among the novobiocin-resistant species *S. saprophyticus* is the one commonly recovered from humans as a cause of urinary tract infections. Therefore, screening coagulase negative Staphylococci isolated from quantitative urine cultures are susceptible to novobiocin provides a reliable presumptive identification of this species.

Materials Required

Novobiocin disc (5μG), Sheep blood agar plate, Test tubes, forceps, cotton plug, inoculation loop etc.

Quality control

Positive control: *Staphylococcus saprophyticus* (Resistant)

Negative control: *Staphylococcus aureus* (Sensitive)

Procedure

- Prepare a suspension of the organism to be identified in sterile distilled water or broth.
- The suspension should be equivalent in turbidity to a 0.5 Mcfarland standard. (Refer Annexure)
- Spread 0.1mL of the suspension over half of the blood agar plate.
- Aseptically place a novobiocin disc on the inoculated area.
- Susceptibility to furazolidone may be assessed on the same plate by placing a discs about 4mm apart on the Novobiocin disc. Gently tamp the disc with sterile forceps to ensure contact with agar surface. Incubate the plates aerobically for 18-24 hours at 35°C.

Result

Staphylococcus saprophyticus is novobiocin resistant. Other coagulase negative Staphylococci and *Staphylococcus aureus* are novobiocin susceptible and will show zones of 16mm are larger.

Viva questions

What is the purpose of novobiocin test?

Is coagulase positive Staphylococcus is sensitive to novobiocin?

Spotters : Blood agar plate, Novobiocin disc

25 u. Bile Solubility Test

Aim

To differentiate Streptococcus sp.

To understand the principles of bile solubility test

Principle

Bile salt, specifically sodium deoxycholate and sodium taurocholate, have the capability to selectively lyse *Streptococcus pneumoniae* when added to actively growing bacteria in agar medium. *Streptococcus pneumoniae* produce autolytic enzymes(autolysins) that account for the central depression or umplication characteristic of older pneumococcal colonies on agar media. The addition of bile salt activates the autolysins and accelerates the natural lytic reaction observed with cultures. The bile solubility test can be performed either with a broth culture of the organism or with colonies grown on agar medium. The turbidity of the broth suspension visibly clears on addition of bilesalts if the organism is soluble.

Materials required

Sheep blood agar plates, 10% sodium deoxycholate (bile salt), Phenol red solution, 0.1N sodium hydroxide solution.

Procedure

- Transfer approximately 0.5 mL of 18- 24 hour broth culture to two clean test tubes. Containing 0.5 mL of phosphate buffered saline (pH-7).

- Add one drop of phenol red indicator to each tube.

- Add 0.1 N NaOH to adjust the pH to 7.

- Add0.5 mL of 10% sodium deoxycholate to one of the tube.

- Add 0.5mL of sterile normal saline to other tube.

- Gently agitate both tubes and place them in an incubator or water bath at 35°C for three hours and check hourly.

Result

There is visible clearing of the suspension in the tube containing the sodium deoxycholate, with no colour change in the saline control suspension.

Viva questions

List out other names of bile salt.

How *Streptococcus pneumoniae* solublizing bile salt.

How do you perform bile solubility test

Give reason for adding sodium hydroxide in bile solubility test

Spotters: Bile salt.

25 v. The CAMP Test

Aim

To check CAMP activity.

To assess synergistic haemolysis.

Principle

The presumptive identification of gpB beta Haemolytic Streptococci can be done with the CAMP test, which is reliable and easy to perform. Christie, Atkins and Munch-Petersen first described the haemolytic phenomenon in 1944 and it is their names that provide the acronym for the test. The beta haemolysis produced by most of the strains of *Staphylococcus aureus* is enhanced by an extra cellular protein produced by gpB beta haemolytic *Streptococci*. Interaction of the beta haemolysin with this factor cause "synergistic haemolysis", which is easily observed on a blood agar plate. This phenomenon is seen with both haemolytic and nonhaemolytic isolates of Streptococci.

Materials Required

Beta haemolysis producing strain of *Staphylococcus aureus and Streptacoccus*, Sheep blood agar plate.

Quality control

Positive control: gpB Strepococci

Negative control: gpA Strepococci

Procedure

- Down the center of a blood agar plate, make a single straight-line streak of beta haemolysin producing *Staphylococcus aureus*.

- Taking care not to intersect the *Staphylococcus aureus* streak, inoculate a streak of the beta haemolytic Streptococcus to be identified perpendicular to the *Staphylococcus aureus* streak. Make these streaks so that, after incubation, the growth of the organism will not be touching. The Streptococcus should be 3-4 cm long. Known gpA and gpB Streptococci strain should be similarly inoculated on the same plate as positive and negative controls, respectively.

- Incubate the plates at 35 ° C for 18-24 hours.

Result

An increased area of haemolysis occurs where the beta hemolysin secreted by the Staphylococci and CAMP factor secreted by the gpB streptococci intersects.

Viva questions

Expand CAMP

Why is the test called CAMP?

What is synergistic haemolysis?

Name the test organisms used in CAMP test

Spotters : Picture of CAMP test

25 w. Litmus milk reaction

Aim

To differentiate bacteria based on milk substrate utilization.

To check the organisms ability to utilize and metabolize different components of milk.

Principle

Milk is an excellent medium for the growth of microorganisms because it contains the milk protein casein, the milk sugar lactose, vitamins, minerals and water. Litmus, a pH indicator is incorporated in the medium for the detection of production of acid or alkali and oxidation-reduction activities. A variety of different chemical changes occur in milk, depending upon which milk ingredients are utilized by the bacteria. Once again, this is depend upon the type of enzymes that the organism is able to produce enzymes. Litmus milk medium consists of 10% powdered skim milk and the dye litmus. Litmus, upon addition to rehydrated skim milk, changes the colloidal milk suspension from white to lavender (pale bluish purple). Characteristic reactions observed with litmus milk are lactose fermentation (lactic acid production), Alkali reaction, Curd formation (acid curd and rennin curd), Litmus reduction, Proteolysis (peptonization), Gas formation, Production of acid.

Some bacteria ferment the lactose of milk with the production of lactic acid which is detected when litmus medium changes from blue (or purple) (neutral pH) to red (or pink) (pH 4). The accumulation of acid acts on the milk protein, casein, resulting in the formation of **curd** (clot) due to the precipitation of casein as **calcium caseinate** which is very firm. As the acidity increases, the curd becomes so solid that there is a squeezing out of a clear liquid (**whey**) from the curd. Acid curd is identified by the clot, which remains immobile when the tube is inverted.

Some bacteria produce an enzyme, **rennin**, which acts on casein and in the presence of calcium ions forms **calcium paracaseinate** that is insoluble and is called **rennet curd**. Unlike acid curd it is a soft semisolid clot that will flow slowly on tilting the tube. Acid or rennet curds are quite palatable dairy products known as **cottage cheese**. Some bacteria possess proteolytic enzymes (e.g.**caseinase**) and hydrolyze casein (called **proteolysis, peptonization**) resulting in the release of large quantities of ammonia that makes the medium alkaline with foul smell, the litmus, turns a **purplish-blue**. With further incubation of the medium, an opaque clearing of the milk occurs as the casein is hydrolyzed to peptides and aminoacids. The opaque (turbid) liquid supernatant (whey like appearance) turns **brown** in colour.

Reduction of the litmus by oxidation-reduction activities of bacteria can be shown by loss of litmus colour. In the litmus milk test, litmus (purple in the oxidized state) acts as such an acceptor of hydrogen from the substrate and becomes reduced and turns **white** or milk coloured. An **alkaline reaction** due to partial degradation of casein into shorter polypeptide chains with the simultaneous release of alkaline end products is evident when the colour of the medium either **does not change** or **changes to a deeper blue**.

Materials required

Streptococcus lactis, Escherichia coli, Proteus vulgaris, Alcaligenes faecalis and *Pseudomonas aeruginosa,* Sterile tubes of litmus milk medium (10mL/tube) Bunsen burner, Inoculation loop , Wax marking pencil.

Procedure

- Prepare Litmus milk medium and sterilize at 120°C for 5 minutes.

- Label each of the litmus milk medium tubes with the bacterium to be inoculated.

- Inoculate tubes of litmus milk, using loop inoculation, with each of the appropriate bacterial species and keep one tube as an uninoculated comparative control. Two tubes are used to each organism to be inoculated.

- Incubate the tubes at 37°C for 24-48 hours.

- Refrigerate the uninoculated control tube of litmus milk.

Observations and results:

Make frequent observations of the incubated tubes for the colour and consistency of the medium and present the results in a tabular form.

Table 25.5 : Litmus milk reactions

Bacterial species	Acid	Alkaline	Litmus milk reactions			
			Curd	Pep	Red	Gas
Streptococcus lactis	+	-	+	-	+	-
Escherichia coli	+	-	+/-	-	+/-	+/-
Proteus vulgaris	-	+	-	-	-	-
Alcaligenes faecalis	-	+	-	-	-	-
Pseudomonas aeruginosa	-	-	-	+	-	-

Viva questions

What are the principles of litmus milk reactions?

Define curd, rennin, rennet curd and whey.

What is peptonization?

How is litmus milk reaction helpful in microbial identification?

Spotters : Litmus milk

25 x. Starch Hydrolysis

Aim

To determine the ability of microorganisms to excrete hydrolytic extracellular enzymes capable of degrading starch.

Principle

Carbohydrates are characterized by the glycosidic bond. The type of the glycosidic bond to a large extent determines the specificity of the carbohydrates splitting digestive enzymes. Starch, a highly polymerized structure, consists of amylase, a straight chain α 1,4 glycosidic links and half amylopectin, a branched component with 1,6 bonds. Amylase, one of the enzyme acts on starch, hydrolyzing 1-4 linkages, producing limit dextrin, maltose, triose and maltose at an optimum pH of 7. Bacteria are known to produce amylases abundantly. The cell into the medium secretes these enzymes. These enzymes hydrolyze starch into carbohydrate of low molecular weight units. They are now able to pass through the membrane into the cell and get used for energy production through the process of glycolysis. In this experiment, starch agar is used to demonstrate the hydrolytic activity of starch.

Materials required

Bunsen burner, Inoculation loop, 24-48 hours cultures of *Bacillus subtilis*, *Escherichia coli*, *Enterobacter* sp., *Pseudomonas* sp., Gram's iodine solution, starch agar etc.,

Procedure

- Prepare and sterilize Starch agar medium and poured into sterile petriplates.

- Streak the plates individually with the given bacterial cultures (Extensive streaking on the plate should be avoided).

- Incubate the inoculated plates at 37°C for 24 hours.

- Following incubation period, flood iodine solution over the entire starch agar surface.

- Examine the plates for the presence or absence of the blue-black colour surrounding each test organism.

- Record the results.

Observation

The zone of hydrolysis is seen in *Bacillus cereus* and *Bacillus subtilis* and not seen in *E. coli*.

Result

The *Bacillus cereus and Bacillus subtilis* have the ability to produce amylase and utilizes starch as carbon source. So, when iodine is poured, due to the absence of starch, zone is formed around the organism showing positive result. The *E. coli* doesn't have the ability to produce amylase so starch is not utilized and zone is not formed around the organism.

Viva questions

What is the chemical nature of starch?

Name enzyme responsible for starch hydrolysis.

What is the nature of amylolytic enzyme.

How do you perform starch hydrolysis?

How do you detect starch hydrolysis?

Name the bacteria responsible for starch hydrolysis.

Describe the function of hydrolases.

Describe the chemistry of starch hydrolysis.

The chemical used to detect microbial starch hydrolysis on starch plates is — — — — —

The smallest product of this hydrolysis is called — — — — — — — — —

How is it possible that bacteria may grow heavily on starch agar but not necessarily produce α-amylase?

What are the ingredients of starch agar?

Spotters : Starch, Iodine.

25 y. Gelatin Hydrolysis

Aim

To determine the ability of some microbes to produce gelatinase, proteolytic exoenzyme capable of liquefying gelatin.

Principle

Gelatin is of great value in identifying bacterial species although its nutrient value is questionable. Since it lacks the essential aminoacid tryptophan produced by the hydrolysis of collagen, which is a major compound of gelatin. It is a protein of connective tissues in man and animal. Below 25°C gelatin will maintain its gel properties and exists as a solid. At temperatures above 25°C gelatin is in a liquefied state. Some microorganisms are capable of hydrolyzing gelatin and they have the enzyme gelatinase, which is a proteolytic enzyme. In this experiment, nutrient gelatin agar plates are used. The medium consists of nutrient agar supplemented with 1% of gelatin. Gelatin though a protein, many microbes can't digest it as it is because of its molecular size. Gelatinase is secreted extraordinarily which hydrolyze gelatin to digestible product and are then consumed. In some microbes the ability to hydrolyze gelatin is absent and they do not produce gelatinase in the medium and gelatin remains unhydrolysed.

Materials Required

24-48 hours cultures of *Escherichia coli* and *Bacillus spp.*, Mercuric chloride solution, Nutrient gelatin agar plate, Petriplates, Inoculation loop

Procedure

- Prepare Nutrient gelatin medium and sterilized at 121° C for 15 minutes.
- Streak the given bacterial culture on the surface of the medium as single line streak.
- Incubate plates at 37 ° C for 24 hours
- Following incubation ,flood the gelatin precipitating reagent(Mercuric chloride)
- A clear zone around the bacterial colony indicates positive result

Observation

A clear zone is formed aroud colony after the addition of mercuric chloride solution.

Result

The given organism possess an enzyme which degrade gelatin.

Viva questions

How can gelatin hydrolysis be beneficial to certain bacteria?

What is gelatin?

Spotters : Gelatin, Mercuric chloride

25 z. Casein Hydrolysis

Aim

To determine the ability of microbes to elaborate proteolytic enzyme capable of degrading casein

Principle

Casein, milk protein is a macromolecule composed of aminoacid subunits linked together by peptide bond (CO-NH) molecule. Some microorganisms have the ability to degrade the protein casein by producing proteolytic exo enzyme called proteinases which breaks the peptide bond by introducing water into the molecule, liberating smaller chains of aminoacids called peptides, which are later break down into free amino acids by extra cellular or intracellular peptidases, which are transported through cell membrane into the intracellular aminoacid pools for use in the synthesis of proteins. Casein hydrolysis was demonstrated by supplementing nutrient agar with milk. The medium is opaque due to casein in colloidal suspension. The positive result is indicated by the formation of clear zone around the colonies.

Materials required

Bacterial test organisms, Skim agar medium, petriplates, Conical flask, Inoculation loop, Autoclave etc.

Procedure

- Prepare skim milk medium or casein medium
- Sterilize at 110°C for 10 minutes
- Inoculate test organism in to the plate as single line streak.
- Incubate at 37 ° C for 24 hours
- Observe for zone around the colonies.

Observation

Observe all the inoculated plates for any clearance around the line of streak.

Result

The given organism is found to be positve to casein hydrolysis

Viva questions

Define the following terms: a. protein, b. hydrolysis, c. casein, d. protease, e. amino acid, f. peptide bond g. proteolysis

Why sterile skim milk used in this experiment?

Spotters : Casein.

25 aa. Lipid Hydrolysis

Aim

To Understand the biochemical process of lipid hydrolysis.

To determine the ability of bacteria to hydrolyze lipids by producing specific lipases.

To Perform a lipid hydrolysis test.

Principles

Lipids are high molecular weight compounds possessing large amounts of stored energy. The two common lipids catabolized by bacteria are the **triglycerides (triacylglycerols)** and **phospholipids.** Triglycerides are hydrolyzed by the enzymes called **lipases** into glycerol and free fatty acid molecules. Glycerol and free fatty acid molecules can then be taken up by the bacterial cell and further metabolized through reactions of glycolysis, oxidation pathway and the citric acid cycle. These lipids can also enter other metabolic pathways where they are used for the synthesis of cell membrane phospholipids. Since phospholipids are functional components of all cells, the ability of bacteria to hydrolyze host-cell phospholipids is an important factor in the spread of pathogenic bacteria. When lipase-producing bacteria contaminate food products, the lipolytic bacteria hydrolyze the lipids, causing spoilage termed **rancidity.** When these same lipids are added to an agar solidified culture medium and are cultured with lipolytic bacteria, the surrounding medium becomes clear and transparent.

Materials Required

Tributrin agar, Broth cultures of *Proteus mirabilis* and *Staphylococcus epidermidis*, Petri plate, inoculation loop, incubator, wax pencil, Bunsen burner

Procedure

- Prepare Tributrin agar and sterilize at 121°C for 15 minutes.
- Pour the medium on Petriplate & allowed to solidify
- Inoculate test organism as spot.
- Incubate the plate in an inverted position for 24 to 48 hours at 35°C.
- Examine the plate for evidence of lipid hydrolysis .
- Observe for any change. Lipid hydrolysis is evidenced by appearance of oil droplets and halo (clearence) around colony.

Observation and result

Oil dropets / clearence around colony indicated that the given organism posses s lipase enzyme.

Viva Questions

What is the function of lipases?

How can one determine whether a bacterium is lipolytic?

What are two functions of lipids in bacterial cells?

Give some examples of foods that might be spoiled by lipolytic bacteria.

How is the ability of certain bacteria to attack phospholipids related to pathogenicity?

What is the difference between a triglyceride (triacylglycerol) and a phospholipid?

What are several pathways that bacteria use to metabolize lipids?

25 ab. Salt Tolerance Test

Aim

To check the organisms ability to tolerate high salt concentrations.

To differentiate Enterococci and gpD Streptococci.

Principle

Ability to grow in the presence of variable amount of sodium chloride is a test that has been used to characterize several bacteria, including viridence streptococci. It is particularly useful, however, for presumptive identification of the enterococcal group D organisms, which have the specific ability to grow in the presence of 6.5% of sodium chloride incorporated into either a broth or an agar medium. This test along with bile esculin test, is used in many laboratories to distinguish *Enterococcus* from the group D *Streptococci, S. bovis* and *S.equinus*.

Heart infusion broth is a general purpose nutritional medium that is used for the cultivation of many bacteria. It normally contain 0.5% sodium chloride. By increasing the salt concentration to 6.5%, the medium becomes semi selective for the growth of *Enterococci*.

Materials required

6.5% Sodium Chloride agar, (Nutrient agar with 6.5% Sodium Chloride) Petriplates, Conical flasks, inoculation loop, incubator etc.

Quality Control

Positive control : *Enterococcus faecalis*
Negative control: *Streptococcus bovis*.

Procedure

- Prepare medium with 6.5% sodium chloride concentration and sterilize at 121°C for 15 minutes
- Pour it into sterile petriplate and allow to solidify.
- Inoculate three or four colonies.
- Incubate at 37°C in air incubator.
- Observe for growth.

Result

A positive test is the presence of obvious growth in the medium, with or without colour change in the indicator. If the organism is bile esculin positive and grows in the 6.5% sodium chloride broth, the organism is an enterococcus species. If the organism is bile esculin positive and fails to grow in the 6.5% sodium chloride broth, the organism is a group D streptococci.

Viva questions

What is the purpose & principle of salt tolerance test?

How does sodium chloride inhibit the growth of bacteria?

How do you confirm group D streptococci?

How do you differentiate enterococci & gp D streptococci?

Spotters : Sodium chloride

Immunology

CHAPTER 3

26. ABO Blood Grouping

Aim

To find out the blood group (ABO) of an individual.

To know the type of antigen and antibody present in the blood RBC.

Background Information

Blood grouping was discovered by **Landsteiner's** in 1900. A vast number of antigens have been detected in human blood cells, of which about 10-15 % form well defined systems and only 1-2% play a significant role in blood transfusion. At least 100 antigens have been recognized on R.B.C. surface. However out of all, only ABO & Rh are important and others are less important because the antigens are weak and there is no corresponding antibodies in the serum. ABO blood system consists of four main groups. They are A, B, AB and O. Blood group of an individual are determined by A and B antigens on the RBC. Therefore the blood group of the individual may be Group A (presence of A antigen), Group B (presence of B antigen), Group AB (presence of both A&B antigen), Group O (absence of both A&B antigens). Now a day the group A having another sub groups A1 and A2 (Fig 26.1 and table 26.1).

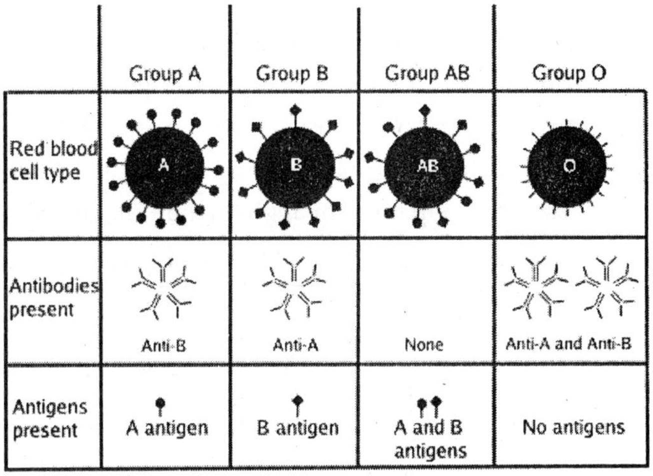

Fig 26.1: Blood group antigen and Antibodies

Specific antibodies are available in individuals blood. These antibodies had no effect on the red blood cells of the same individual but when mixed with the RBC antigen of a different blood type, a violent, incompatible reaction may result and may be fatal. Type O blood group could be used in any transfusion because it lacks both the antigens, as the person of this group is called **universal donor**. A person with blood group AB called a **universal recipient**, can receive any type of blood because it lacks both antibodies a and b

Table 26.1 : ABO blood group classification system

Blood group	Antigen	Antibody	Genotype
A	A	Anti b	AA, AO
B	B	Anti a	BB, BO
AB	AB	None	AB
O	None	Anti a&b	OO

ABO blood grouping is based on agglutination reaction, type of reaction that occurs between particulate antigen and specific antibodies that leads to clumping or agglutination of cells. When the cells involved are red blood cells, the reaction is termed as haemagglutination.

Material Required

Human blood, Antisera A, Antisera B, Microscopic slides, Spirit, Lancet, Cotton, AntiseraA1, Mixing sticks etc... Blood sample is collected by finger puncture method, Antiseras are available commercially.

Procedure

- Rapid slide method is adopted to perform ABO blood grouping.
- Take two microscopic slides or one rectangular slide.
- Divide the slide in to two portions by drawing a line in the middle transversely.
- Mark the slide as A and B.
- Wipe the middle finger with cotton moistened with 70 % alcohol and allowed to dry.
- Prick disinfected area with a sterile lancet.
- Squeeze a finger and allows a drop of blood to fall on each division of the slide.
- Add one drop of antiserum in to appropriately labeled drop of blood on the slide
- Mix serum and blood drops with an applicator stick.
- Rock the slide back and forth for two minutes between fingers.
- Observe the mixtures for agglutination and record the blood groups (Table 26.2).

Table 26.2: Serological Reactions In ABO blood group system

Agglutination with			Blood group
Anti A	Anti A1	Anti B	
+	+	0	A 1
+	0	0	A2
+	+	+	A1B
+	0	+	A2B
0	0	+	B
0	0	0	O
+ -Agglutination		0-No agglutination	

Observation and Result

Agglutination is noted in specific blood group slide. The given blood is found to be $-----$ group

Viva Questions

Why blood group O is considered as universal donor &AB as recipient?

Who discovered blood grouping?

Define agglutination & haemagglutination.

What is the role of antigens in blood grouping?

What happens if A blood group individual receives B blood?

Could a type AB type blood group individual receive blood from a type B individual? Who would receive type O blood? Explain your answers.

Could a person with blood type AB receive blood from a primate with the same blood type? Explain your answer.

Why would a person with blood type A exhibit a transfusion reaction if given type B blood?

What causes clumping to occur?

Spotters: Anti A, Anti B, Lancet, Picture of blood grouping reactions.

27. Rh factor typing

Aim

To determine D antigen of an individual.

Background Information

Landsteiner and **Weiner** are the first persons to report in 1940 that the rabbit serum contained the Rh factor. This factor is later designated as D antigen. The Rh factor is a complex of many antigens. Rhesus (Rh) factor is so named because injecting RBCs of rhesus monkey into rabbits and guinea pigs raised the original antibody. For the clinical purpose, the detection of Rh factor is highly essential. If the fetus developed from Rh negative mother and Rh positive father genetically can have Rh positive RBCs. These Rh-positive fetal antibodies may pass through placenta into the maternal circulation and stimulating the formation of Rh antibodies by the mother. These Rh antibodies can re-cross the placenta into the fetus.

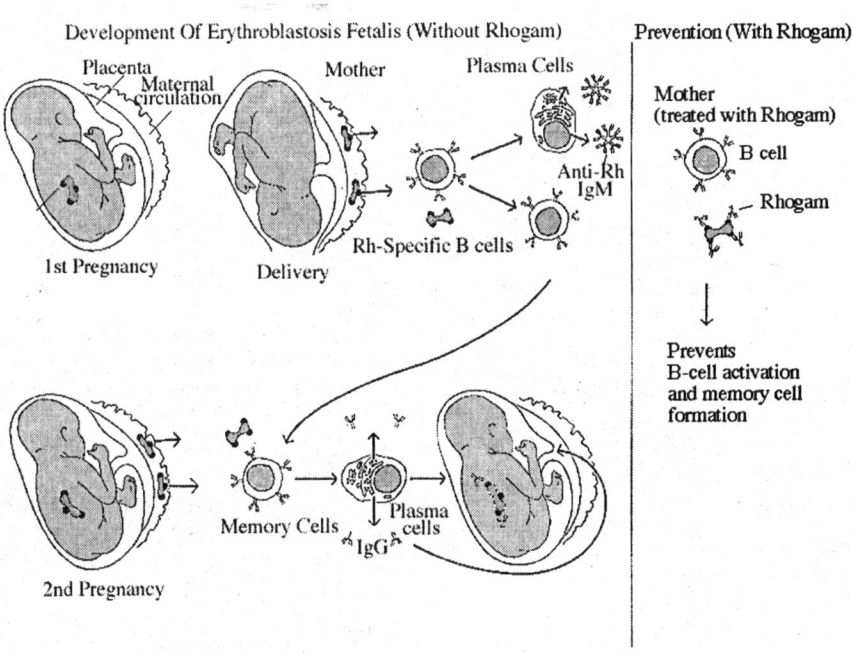

Fig 27.1: Developments of Erythroblastosis fetalis

Resulting antigen antibody reaction may produce anaemia, jaundice and sometimes death in the newborn. This disease is often called hemolytic disease of the newborn (HDN) or Erythroplastosis fetalis (Fig. 27.1). Prevention of this disease in newborn is with the therapy Rh immuno globulin. The presence of Rh factor in human blood is determined by agglutination reaction between Anti D typing serum and red blood cells.

Materials Required

Anti D, Blood, Microscopic slide, Spirit, Lancet, Cotton, Tooth picks etc… Blood sample is collected by finger puncture method, Antisera are available commercially.

Procedure

- Take one microscopic slide and mark as D.

- Wipe middle finger with cotton moistened with 70 % alcohol and allow to dry.

- Prick disinfected area with a sterile lancet.

- Squeeze a finger and allows a drop of blood to fall on the slide.

- Add one drop of anti D in to the drop of blood on the slide.

- Mix serum and blood drops with an applicator stick.

- Rock the slide back and forth for two minutes between your fingers.

- Observe the mixtures for agglutination and record the findings.

- Agglutination indicates Rh positive.

Observation

Agglutination was noted in Anti D added circle

Result:

The given blood is Rh positive

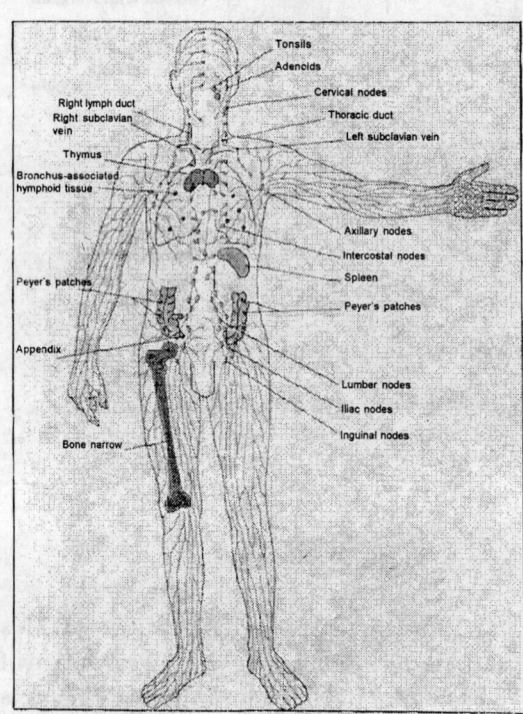

Fig. 28.1 : Lymphoid organs of Human

Viva Questions

What is Rh?
Why the name Rh given to blood group system?
Define erythroplastosis faetalis and HDN
What are D antigens?
What is the significance of Rh typing in blood transfusion?
Who discovered Rh antigen?
How do you perform Rh typing?

Spotters : Anti D, Lancet, Picture of Rh Positive blood .

28. Demonstration of Lymphoid Organs in Laboratory Animal

Aim

To know various lymphoid organs of mammals

Background Information

Immune organs are morphologically and functionally diverse organs and tissues. They have various functions in the development of immune responses. These can be distinguishes by function as primary lymphoid organs and secondary lymphoid organs. Thymus and bone marrow are the primary lymphoid organs. Lymph nodes, spleen, MALT and GALT are the secondary lymphoid organs. Primary lymphoid organ helps the maturation of lymphoid cells. Secondary lymphoid organ traps the antigen and provides the site for lymphocyte maturation. Primary lymphoid organs are also called central lymphoid organs. Secondary lymphoid organs are also called peripheral lymphoid organs. Primary lymphoid organs are the generative organs. Secondary lymphoid organs are the differentiate organs. Cutaneous associated lymphoid organs are called tertiary lymphoid tissues, which normally contain fewer lymphoid cells than secondary lymphoid organs (Fig : 28.1)

Thymus

Thymus is a flat, bilobed organ situated above the heart. Each lobe is surrounded by a capsule and is divided into lobules, which are separated from each other by strands of connective tissue called trabeculae. Lobules are organized into two compartments, outer compartment or cortex, is densely packed with immature T cells. The inner compartment is called medulla. Thymic epithelial cells in the outer cortex, called nurse cells. Cortex and medulla of the thymus are criss-crossed by a three dimensional stromal-cell network composed of epithelial cells, dentritic cells and macrophages, which made

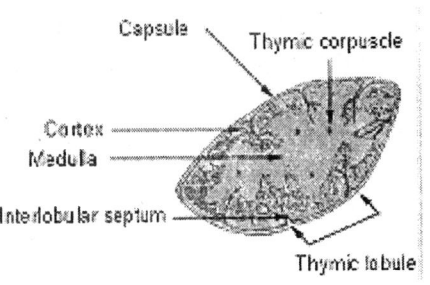

Fig. 28.2 - Thymus

> **Box 28.1: Di George Syndrome** is a disorder caused by the deletion of a small piece of chromosome 22. It is an immunodeficiency syndrome in humans and mice, associated with thymic hypoplasia or aplasia and absence of T lymphocytes, resulting from a congenital absence of the third and fourth branchial pouches
>
> DiGeorge syndrome causes migration defects of neural crest-derived tissues, particularly affecting development of the third and fourth Branchial pouches.

up the organ and contribute to the growth and maturation of thymocytes. Nurse cells have long membrane extensions that surround as many as 50 thymocytes forming multicellular complexes. Each and every thymocytes that developed in thymus expresses high level of MHC molecule. Any developing thymocytes that are unable to recognize self-MHC are eliminated by programmed cell death. About 95-99% of the thymocytes undergo programmed cell death. *DiGeorge syndrome* (Box 28.1) is related to thymus. Thymulin and thymostimulin are the enzymes responsible for the development of thymocytes (Fig – 28.2).

Bonemarrow

Red marrow is found in bones consists of a sponge- like reticular framework located between long trabaculae. The proliferation and maturation of precursor cells in the bone marrow are stimulated by cytokines. Many of these cytokines are called colony-stimulating factors. The marrow contains mature lymphocytes, which have developed from progenitor cells (Fig 28.3).

Lymphnodes

Lymphnodes are encapsulated bean shaped structures containing reticular network packed with lymphocytes, macrophages and dentritic cells. Morphologically a lymphnode can be divided into

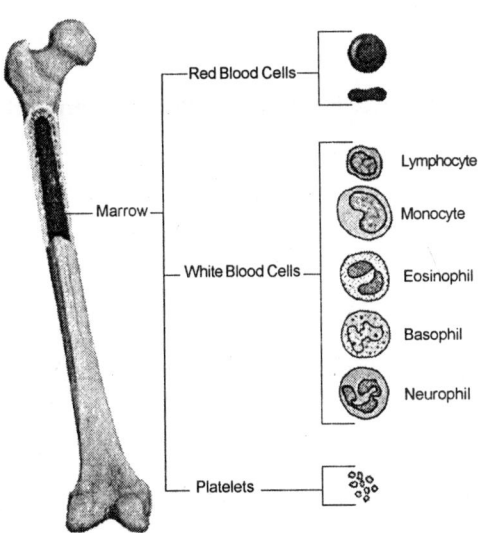

Fig. 28.3 : Bone Marrow

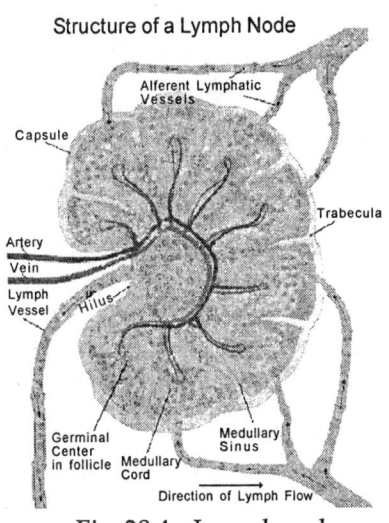

Fig. 28.4 – Lymph node

three roughly concentric regions (Cortex, paracortex and the medulla). Cortex contain lymphocytes (mostly B cells), macrophages and follicular dentritic cells arranged in primary follicles. After antigenic challenge the primary follicle enlarge in to secondary follicles, each containing germinal center. Para cortex is populated largely by T lymphocytes and dentric cells. It sometimes referred as thymus dependent area. Cortex is a thymus independent area. Medulla is populated with plasma cells (Fig. 28.4).

Spleen

It is a large ovoid organ situated high in the left abdominal cavity. A capsule that extends a number of projections (trabeculae) into the interior to form a compartmentalized structure. Compartments are of two types, the red pulp and white pulp, which are separated by a diffuse marginal zone. Red pulp is populated by macrophages and RBC. White pulp is populated with T lymphocytes (Fig: 28.5).

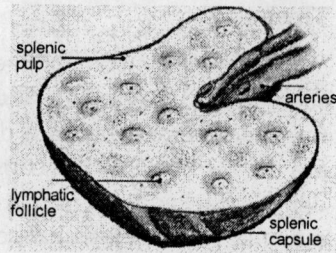

Fig. 28.5 - Spleen

MALT

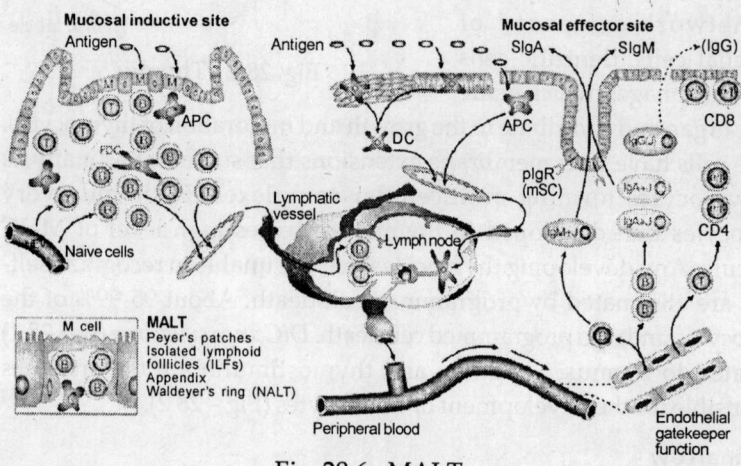

Fig. 28.6 - MALT

Mucous membrane lining the digestive, respiratory and urogenital systems have a combined surface area about 400^{m2} and are the major sites of entry for most pathogens. These areas are protected by a group of organized lymphoid tissue known as MALT. The outer mucosal epithelial layer contains so called intraepithelial lymphocytes. Lamina propia, which lies under the epithelial layer, contains large number of B cells, plasma cells, activated T cells and macrophages in loose clusters. About 15,000 lymphoid follicles are available within lamina propia. The subcutaneous layer beneath the lamina propia contains payer's patches, nodules of 30-40 lymphoid follicles (Fig. 28.6).

Materials Required

Healthy laboratory animal, Dissection set, Dissection board, Pins, Hammer, Scissors, Chloroform, Clean cloths, Sponge, Cotton etc.,

Procedure

- Hold animal in a dissection board with the help of pins.
- Cut the outer layer of the skin from the abdominal region upto the mouth.
- Cut open the body and expose major lymphoid organs.
- Label all lymphoid tissues clearly and visually.
- Observe the morphology of lymphoid organs and record the observations.

Observations: Different lymphoid organs are observed and differentiated.

Viva question

List out different lymphoid organs of human.

What are primary lymphoid organ?

Distinguish primary lymphoid organ from secondary lymphoid organ.

What are the purpose of this experiment?

What is *DiGeorges syndrome*?

What are the significance of spleen?

Define MALT and GALT.

29. Antigen Preparation

Aim

To prepare antigens from bacteria
To inactivate prepared bacterial antigens
To check quality of prepared antigens

Principle

Antigens that used for antibody production / detection can be prepared in laboratory by various processes. It may be chemical process, physical process or mechanical means. Various types of antigens are available in microorganisms. For example the *Salmonella* having more than 2000 serotypes. This is because of antigenic variations. The antigens detected from the microorganisms are somatic (O) antigen, flagellar (H) antigen, surface (Vi) antigen, fimbrial (F) antigen, M and N antigens

Materials Required

Bacterial cultures, Formaldehyde, Nutrient agar, Nutrient broth, Barium chloride, Sulphuric acid etc.,

Procedure

Preparation of antigen by heat treatment

1. Cultivate the bacteria in a nutrient broth and incubated for 24 hours at 37°C.
2. Heat the bacterial suspension in a boiling water bath at 100° C for 30 minutes.
3. Centrifuge the culture suspension at 10000 rpm for 10 minutes
4. Discard Supernatant.
5. Suspend pellet in saline.
6. Repeat the centrifugation for three or four times.
7. Suspend the pellet after final wash in sterile saline.
8. Adjust the turbidity to Mcfarland Standard 3 and Mcfarland Standard 4.
9. Use this final antigen for immunization or antigen antibody reactions.

Preparation of antigen by chemical treatment

1. Cultivate bacteria in a nutrient broth and incubate for 24 hours at 37°C.
2. Add formaldehyde to a final concentration of 0.2%.
3. Keep the formalized culture at 37 ° C overnight in incubator.

Perform experiment by following 3 –9 points of **preparation of antigen by heat treatment (previous section)**

Preparation of antigen by sonication method

1. Cultivate the bacteria in a nutrient broth and incubated for 24 hours at 37°C.
Perform experiment by following 3 –8 points of **preparation of antigen by heat treatment (previous section)**
Suject the cell suspension to high vibration in sonictor (During this time all viable cells were broken and considered as antigen).
Use this final antigen for immunization or antigen antibody reactions.

Quality control of the antigen

Viability checking is one of the quality control procedure in the antigen preparation procedure.

After antigen preparation the antigen suspension should not be grown on any of the artificial or natural medium. Quality control of antigen is performed by viable plate count method

Streak antigen suspension on nutrient agar plate.

Incubate nutrient agar plate at 37°C for 24 hours.

Observe plates for growth.

Observation

If there is no growth the antigen is subjected to immunization or antigen antibody reactions. If there is any growth the suspension may be discarded.

Viva questions

Define the following: Antigen, H antigen, Vi antigen, O antigen and K antigen.
What is Mcfarland standard?
How do you check viability of antigen?
Mention about quality control of antigen.

Spotters: Different types of antigen, $BaCl_2$, H_2SO_4

30. PolyClonal Antibody Production

Aim

To immunize the laboratory animal and the production of polyclonal antibodies

Principle

Antigen is a substance that when injected into a suitable animal gives rise to an immune response. During the immune response animals produce antibodies against the particular antigen. Antigens may be a parasite or any protein substance. The antibodies are available in the serum of the animal blood. The immunized animals can produce specific antibodies naturally. When purified antigen is injected into the host, the host immune system recognises and responds to the antigen. B cells of the host then proliferate and differentiate to produce specific antibodies. Adjuvants are mixed with antigen to promote the efficiency of antigen stimulation.

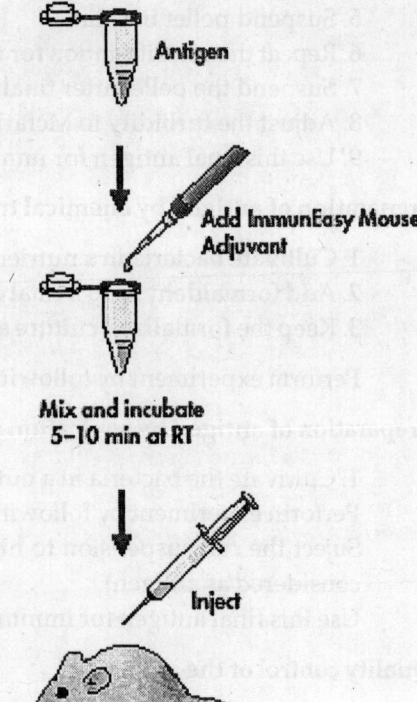

Fig. 30.1 – Process of antigen inoculation

Materials Required

Rabbit, Bovine serum albumin (BSA) or any one antigen, 21 gauge needle for injecting antigen, Scissors, Xylene, Spirit, cotton, 1 mL syringe, 5 mL syringe, 24 gauge butterfly needle, Adjuvants.

Procedure

● Accommodate rabbit to the laboratory environment.

● Prepare the rabbit for immunization by shaving the hair at one or two places of thigh.

● For the production of high titre antibodies the following schedule can be followed.

- Day 1 – inject one mL of 1% BSA with Freund's Complete Adjuvant subcutaneously using a 21 gauge needle in the thigh region.

- Day 4 – repeat day 1 injection and allowed the animal to rest for 14 days. During this time primary response may be achieved.

- Day 18 – inject 1 mL of BSA with Freund's incomplete Adjuvant into the thigh of one leg

- Day 25 – repeat 18th day injection in other leg.

- Day 29 – collect blood from the animal.

- Subject collected blood to serum preparation.

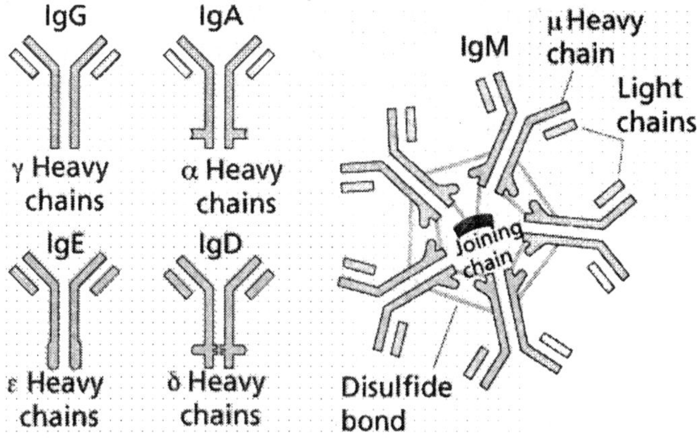

- Serum is subjected to antigen antibody reaction.

- Perform precipitation reaction If the Antigen is soluble; perform agglutination reaction If antigen is insoluble.

Fig. 30.2 – Different types of antibody (imunoglobulins)

Observation and result

After completion of immunization, blood sample is collected and antigen antibody reactions are performed using precipitation method.

Viva Questions

Define the following : antibody , monoclonal antibody , polyclonal antibody , bleeding , immunization, Serum, BSA, Adjutants – Complete and Incomplete.

What is the need of polyclonal antibody production?

What are the materials required for polyclonal antibody production?

What are the differences between monoclonal and polyclonal antibody production.

Spotters: Adjuvant, Polycolonal antibody production, antibody structure (Fig. 30.2).

31. Blood Collection and Serum Preparation

Aim

To collect blood from the patient.
To prepare serum from the blood.
To know the blood collection methodology.

Background Information

Serology, the study of serum, is the science that studied antigen antibody reactions or immunologic reactions of the body, using the serum. Immunology is closely related to serology. It consists of collection of blood and preparation of serum specimens and various immunological tests procedure for specific sero diagnosis. Fresh serum is routinely used for all serological tests.

Box 31.1 - Chyle: A fluid consisting of a mixture of lymphatic fluid (lymph) and chylomicrons that has a milky appearance. Chylomicrons are small fat globules composed of protein and lipid (fat), which are combined in the lining of the intestine. Chylomicrons are found in the blood and in lymphatic fluid where they serve to transport fat from its port of entry in the intestine to the liver and to adipose (fat) tissue.

Serum is to be preferred to plasma for any immune assay due to the tendency of the clotting factors in plasma to form spontaneous clots and so mimics or mask antigen antibody reactions. The fluid that remains after the blood clots is the serum. If the serum has been obtained from an immunized animal and contains the desired antibodies are called **antiserum**.

Blood is collected in the morning, usually by venipuncture. Collection of blood at other time of the day is possible but should not be done for at least 2 hours after meals. If taken sooner, **chyle** (Box- 31.1) is likely to be present, in which case the serum would be unsatisfactory for serological testing. Serum specimen should be tested within 24 hours, if it is not possible, it should be stored frozen. If storage at frozen temperature is not possible add 0.01% w/v merthiolate as preservative. Serum is sterilized by filtration. Combination of two filters (0.45mm and 0.22mm filters) are used to filter higher volume of serum.

Materials Required

Sterile syringe, sterile needle, Tourniquet, Disinfectant, Centrifuge tube or test tube for blood collection

Blood Collection

- Assemble all things required during blood collection.
- Ask patient to sit on a height stool.
- Select the puncture site carefully after inspecting both the arms.
- Place the tourniquet under the patient arm just above the bend in the elbow.
- Using the index finger of your left hand, feel for the vein where you will introduce the needle.
- Disinfect the skin with 70% alcohol. Rub the venipuncture site thoroughly.
- Remove the syringe and needle from the protective wrap and assemble them and fix the needle tightly. Do not touch the tip of the needle.
- Take the syringe in the right hand holding your index finger against the base of the needle. Position the needle and push the needle firmly and steadily, without hesitation, into the center of the vein. Try to enter the skin first then the vein at 30-40⁰ angle. The needle should not pass straight through the vein. Push the needle along the line of the vein to the depth of 1-1.5 cm.
- With your left hand slightly pull back the piston. Blood should appear in the barrel.
- Continue to withdraw the piston and fill the syringe with the requisite amount of blood.
- Release the tourniquet by pulling on the looped end.
- Place a cotton wool over the hidden point of the needle.
- Remove the needle from the syringe and gently expel the blood into the appropriate container.
- Add anticoagulant (if needed) to prevent clotting.

Serum Preparation

- Non-anticoagulated blood yield serum, serum is used in serological and biochemical studies. In order to obtain serum, blood is collected in a tube without anticoagulant.
- Collect blood as per the method described earlier.
- Collect 10mL or 5mL or 2.5mL of blood in a dry glass tube or centrifuge tube without anticoagulant.
- Leave the blood to clot at room temperature for 30 minutes. Do not disturb the clotting blood during this period.
- After 30 minutes but not more than 2 hours, detach clot from the wall and centrifuge the tubes at 2500 rpm for 5 minutes.
- Unstoper the tube, take out the serum by means of a Pasteur pipette, and transfer the serum into another test tube and store in a refrigerator.

- Serum complement interferes with many tests and can be inactivated by heating (56 ° C) the serum sample in a water bath for 30 minutes. Inactivated serum must be used with in 2 hours.

Observation: Blood is collected and subjected for serum preparation. Serum is used to study antigen antibody reactions.

Viva questions

Define Blood, serum , venipuncture and Chyle
What is the role of disinfectant during blood collection?

Spotters: Blood, syringe, serum

32. Isolation and separation of Peripheral Blood Mononuclear cell (PBMC)

Aim

To separate lymphocytes from the human blood

Background information

Blood cell having a round nucleus are called PBMC (Peripheral Blood Mononuclear Cell).Eg., a lymphocyte or a monocyte. These blood cells are a critical component in the immune system to fight infection. The lymphocyte population consists of T cells, B cells and NK cells. These cells are often extracted from whole blood using ficoll, a hydrophilic polysaccharide that separates layers of blood, with monocytes and lymphocytes forming a buffy coat under a layer of plasma. This buffy coat contains the PBMCs. Additionally, PBMC can be extracted from whole blood using a hypotonic lysis which will preferentially lyse red blood cells. This method results in neutrophils and other polymorphonuclear (PMN) cells which are important in innate immune defense to be obtained.

Principle

Ficoll Hypaque method is one of the most reliable method for the separation of PB MC. Ficoll Hypaque is an aqueous solution of density 1.077 + 0.001 g/ml containing Ficoll 400 and sodium diatrizoate with calcium disodium ethylenediamintetraacetic acid. Ficoll 400 is a synthetic high molecular weight (Mw 400 000) polymer of sucrose and epichlorohydrin, which is readily soluble in water. Ficoll 400 has a low intrinsic viscosity (17 ml/g) compared with linear polysaccharides of the same molecular weight solutions. Sodium diatrizoate is a convenient compound to use with Ficoll 400 since it forms solutions of low viscosity with high density. Sodium diatrizoate is the sodium salt of 3,5-diacetamido- 2,4,6-triiodobenzoic acid.

On centrifugation, cells in the blood sample sediment towards the blood/Ficoll-Hypaque interface, where they come in contact with the Ficoll 400 present in Ficoll Hypaque. Red blood cells are efficiently aggregated by this agent at room temperature. Aggregation increases the rate of sedimentation of the red cells, which rapidly collect as a pellet at the bottom of the tube, where they are well separated from lymphocytes. Granulocytes also sediment to the bottom of the Ficoll Hypaque layer. This process is facilitated by an increase in their densities caused by contact with the slightly hypertonic Ficoll Hypaque medium. Thus, on completion of centrifugation, both granulocytes and red blood cells are found at the bottom of the tube, beneath the Ficoll Hypaque. Lymphocytes, monocytes, and platelets are not dense enough to penetrate into the Ficoll Hypaque layer. These cells therefore collect as a concentrated band at the interface between the original blood sample and the Ficoll Hypaque. This banding enables the lymphocytes to be recovered with high yield in a small volume with little mixing with the Ficoll Hypaque medium. Washing and centrifugation the harvested cells subsequently removes platelets, any contaminating Ficoll Hypaque and plasma. The resulting cell suspension then contains highly purified, viable lymphocytes and monocytes and is suitable for further studies.

Materials required

Ficoll – Hypaque solution (Ficoll 400 5.7g; sodium diatrizoate 9g ; calcium disodium ethylenediamintetraacetic acid 0.0231g and Distilled water100mL), Two 10 mL glass test-tubes for each blood sample to be processed (The test-tubes should be siliconized).

Balanced salt solution (At least 20mL for each sample to be processed). The balanced salt solution may be prepared from two stock solutions A and B.

Solution A		Solution B	
Anhydrous D-glucose	- 1.0g	NaCl	- 8.19g
$CaCl_2, 2H_2O$	- 0.0074g	Distilled water	- 1000mL
$MgCl_2.6H_2O$	- 0.1992g		
KCl	- 0.4026g		
TRIS	- 17.565g		
Dissolve in approximately 950mL distilled water and add conc. HCl until pH is 7.6 before adjusting the volume to 1 L.			
To prepare the balanced salt solution, mix 1 volume of solution A with 9 volumes of solution B.			

Pasteur pipettes (3mL) These pipettes should be siliconized, A low speed centrifuge, Glass centrifuge tubes, Syringe with needle.

Anticoagulants - Heparin, EDTA, citrate, acid citrate dextrose (ACD), and citrate phosphate dextrose (CPD).

All glassware that comes in contact with the sample should be siliconized before use. Glassware are siliconized by immersining it in a 1% silicone solution for 10 seconds, washed thoroughly with distilled water and dried in an oven.

Procedure

- Collect fresh blood sample at 18 to 20°C.

- To a 10mL test-tube add 2mL of defibrinated or anticoagulant-treated blood and an equal volume of balanced salt solution (final volume 4mL).

- Mix by drawing the blood and the buffer in and out of a Pasteur pipette.

- Add 3mL Ficoll-Hypaque solution to the centrifuge tube.

- Carefully layer the diluted blood sample (4 mL) onto the Ficoll-Hypaque (Important - When layering the sample do not mix the Ficoll-Hypaque and the diluted blood sample).

- Centrifuge at 4000 rpm for 30–40 min at 18–20 °C.

- Draw off the upper layer using a clean Pasteur pipette, leaving the lymphocyte layer undisturbed at the interface (Care should be taken not to disturb the lymphocyte layer. The upper layer, which contains the plasma, may be saved for later use).

- Using a clean Pasteur pipette transfer the lymphocyte layer to a clean centrifuge tube (It is critical to remove all the material at the interface but in a minimum volume. Removing excess Ficoll-Hypaque causes granulocyte contamination; removing excess supernatant results in platelet contamination).

- Add at least 3 volumes (6mL) of balanced salt solution to the lymphocytes in the test-tube.

- Suspend the cells by gently drawing them in and out of a Pasteur pipette.

- Centrifuge at 6000rpm for 10 min at 18–20°C.

- Discard the supernatant.

- Suspend the lymphocytes in 6–8mL balanced salt solution by gently drawing them in and out of a Pasteur pipette.

- The lymphocytes should now be suspended in the medium appropriate to the application.

Check for cell viability

- Add 50µL of 0.5% tryphan blue in Balanced Salt solution to 50µL of cell suspension.

- Mix and make wet mount.

Observation

Blue and unstained cells may observed

Result

Blue stained cells are dead cells and unstained cells are viable.

Spotters

Ficoll Hypaque, Structure of WBC.

Viva questions

What Type Of Cell is called PBMC?

How PBMC are separated from other blood cells?

What is the role of Ficoll Hypaque in separation of PBMC?

How do you remove RBC from mixture?

33. Antigen antibody reactions

33A. Agglutination Reactions

Agglutination is the visible clumping together of bacterial cells or particles with specific antibody. The resulting clumps are referred as agglutinates. Insoluble antigens are detected with the help of agglutination reactions. Physiological saline used as a suspending medium in most of the agglutination tests. Agglutination tests are performed on slides, in tubes and in micro titration plates. Type of agglutination can be either active or passive.

Active agglutination

These are tests in which there is a direct agglutination of bacterial antigens with its corresponding antibody. Eg. The slide agglutination of *Salmonella* (WIDAL).

Passive agglutination

These are tests in which the specific antibody or known antigen is attached to inert particles or cells. When the known antigen or antibody combines with its corresponding antibody or antigen in the specimen, the particles or cells are agglutinated. The carrier particles or cells used only to show that the antigen or antibody reaction has occurred. Their role in this reaction is therefore passive. The substances and cells used as carriers in passive slide agglutination are Latex particles (Pregnancy test, RPR test), Carbon particles and Stabilized Staphylococcal cells.

Latex particles

These are polystyrene particles that can be coated with either antigen or antibody e.g., ASO Test, Latex agglutination test

Carbon particles

These are coated with cardiolipin antigen used in the *rapid plasma reagin test*.

Stabilized staphylococcal strains

Most strains of Staphylococcus produce protein A on their surface. Killed Staphylococcal cells coated with antibody can be used to identify bacteria and detect soluble extracellular bacterial antigens in specimens and body fluids. The term coagglutination (COAG) is used to describe the agglutination of antibody coated Staphylococcal cells by antigen.

Viva questions

Define Agglutination, active agglutination, passive agglutination.

33 Aa. Pregnancy Test

Aim

To detect HCG in urine for the diagnosis of Pregnancy.

Principle

Human chronic gonadotrophin (HCG) is a hormone produced by placenta very early in pregnancy. It's a glycoprotein and consist of two subunits a and b. The isolated sub units lose their biological activity but are able to generate antibodies. Sub unit a structure of HCG is identical with a chain of TSH, LH, FSH, therefore b HCG forms the most acceptable marker for diagnosis of pregnancy. The secretion of HCG in urine begins approximately 20 days after the last menstrual period and increase rapidly.

The test is based on antigen (b HCG in urine sample) and antibody (anti b HCG antisera reaction. b HCG, is present in urine sample neutralizes anti b HCG antibody and hence does not allow agglutination with HCG agglutinating antigen, however when b HCG is absent in urine sample, the free anti b HCG antibody reacts with HCG agglutination antigen and results in agglutination. Thus a negative sample shows agglutination in less than 2 minutes. Levels of HCG equivalent to 0.5mL/mL and above can be detected in urine specimens. This principle is known as latex agglutination inhibition assay.

Materials Required

b HCG antibody, dropper bottle, HCG agglutination antigen, test sample, Disposable droppers, Reusable glass slides, Disposable applicator sticks.

Specimen collection

For optimal results its best to use the 1st urine voided in the morning as it contain the greatest concentration of HCG. Specimens could be stored at 2 to 8 ^{0}C for 72 hours.

Procedure

- Bring HCG agglutinating antigen and b HCG antibody to room temperature and shaken well for some seconds before use.
- Wash the glass slide and dry with paper towel to remove cell traces of specimens and reagents previously tested. The slide must be clean and dry.
- Place one drop of clear urine sample on the clean slide.
- Add b HCG antibody onto the slide
- Mix the sample and the reagent well.
- Add 1 drop of HCG agglutinating antigen and mix well.
- Gently rock the slide for 2 minutes and observe the results .

Note:

Urine specimen which contain blood and high bacterial contamination shall not be used.

Positive results form very early pregnancy, it is recommended that weak positive result should be re tested with the fresh urine sample 48 hours later.

Improper mixing of the specimens with the reagent can lead to incorrect results.

Result

Absence of agglutination shows positive result in sample A, it is due to the presence of HCG in urine. Hence sample A is positive to pregnancy test.

Viva questions

Expand HCG.

What are the natures of HCG?

What is the principle of pregnancy test?

What is the kind of specimen used to check pregnancy?

How do you interpretate the result?

Spotters: HCG

33 Ab. Anti Streptolysin - O Test

Aim

To determine the ASO in human serum.

Principle

ASO is a rapid agglutination procedure for the direct detection and semi quantitation of ASO from patients blood. The antigen, a latex particle suspension coated with streptolysin O, agglutinates in the presence of specific antibodies with β haemolytic Streptococcus infection. An antistreptolysin-O (ASO) test is a blood test that measures the amount of ASO in the blood. ASO tests are generally used to diagnose and monitor the treatment of a streptococcus infection. A series of tests every 10 to 14 days for six weeks is often required to confirm diagnoses and monitor the progress of an infection. ASO is an antibody generated in response to infection by a specific type of bacteria called *Group A Streptococci*. A serious Streptococcus infection will cause ASO levels to rise significantly. Therefore, a physician may order an ASO test to determine whether the person has a condition (e.g., endocarditis or rheumatic fever) related to a serious streptococcus infection.

Materials Required

ASO KIT, Positive control, Negative control, Physiological saline, Reaction slide, Serum droppers, Applicator stick etc.,

Procedure

Qualitative test

- Allow all reagents as well as the sample to reach room temperature. Mix well before using
- Place one drop of serum onto the slide with the help of disposable serum dropper.
- Add one drop of ASO latex antigen to the above drop and mix with disposable applicator stick.
- Rock the slide gently to and fro for two minutes and examine for agglutination.
- Positive and negative control also maintained.

Semi quantitative test

- Perform semiquantitative test when serum is agglutinate in qualitative test.
- Place 50μL diluted glycine-saline buffer onto each of 5 circles of the slide.
- Using micropipette, add 50ml of the serum sample to the drop of Glycine saline buffer in first circle.
- Using the same micropipette, mix the sample with saline by aspirating back and forth for several times.
- Aspirate 50μL from first circle and transfer to second circle.
- Repeat the same operation upto 5th circle.
- Aspirate 50ml from 5th circle and discard. Add a drop of antigen to all circles.
- Rock the slide gently for 2 minutes and record the results

Table 33.1 - Observation Record

S. No	Circle	Dilution	Observation	Interpretation
1	1st	1:2		
2	2nd	1:4		
3	3rd	1:8		
4	4th	1:16		
5	5th	1:32		

Calculation

Concentration of ASO in serum is calculated

ASO(IU/mL) =200x highest dilution of serum showing agglutination

Sensitivity =200IU/mL

If the qualitative test shows agglutination it indicates ASO level in serum is 200IU/mL

Observation

Agglutination is noted/ not observed

Viva questions

Expand ASO.

How do you perform ASO test?

What kind of bacteria is responsible for Anti streptolysin O production?

Mention the nature of streptolysin O.

Mention method used to perform ASO test.

Spotters : ASO.

33 Ac. WIDAL TEST

Aim

To diagnose a suspected case of enteric fever - serologically

Principle

Widal & Sicard in 1896 described the test called Widal test. It is used for diagnosing typhoid fever. Widal test is essentially an agglutination test where specific antibodies against Salmonella react with the corresponding antigen. It is a most important diagnostic test for the investigation of enteric fever. The etiological agent of enteric fever is *Salmonella typhi, S. paratyphi A* and *S. paratyphi B* which differ physiologically and antigenically. There are two types of antigen, they are 'O' antigen or somatic antigen,"H' antigen or flagella antigen.

When a patient suffers from an infection of enteric fever the antibodies specific to the etiological agents are produced in serum. The concentration increases gradually and the diagnostic titre values appear between seventh or eighth day of infection, therefore the 1st test is done during this period. The second test if required can be done after one week.

Materials required

Test tubes (10x75mm), water bath, saline, patient serum (1mL of positive diseased serum is diluted against 1.9 mL of saline), positive serum, Micropipette

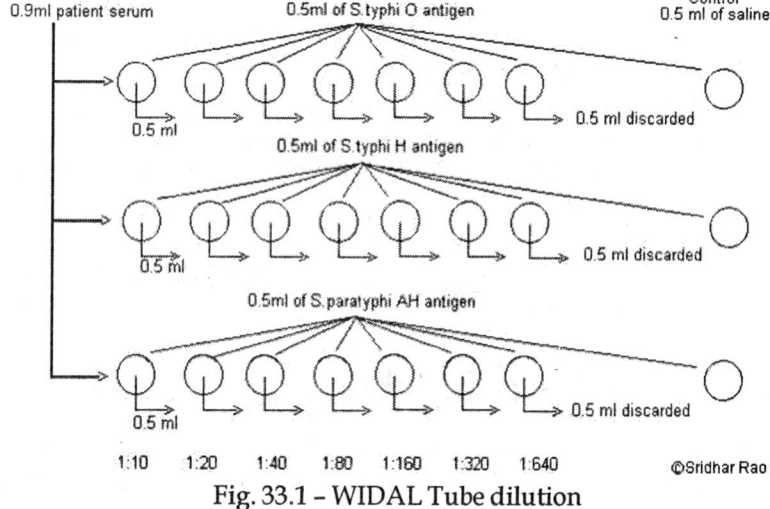

Fig. 33.1 – WIDAL Tube dilution

Procedure

Rapid Slide Test

- Place one drop of undiluted test serum in each of the first four circles and one drop of positive control serum in each of the last two circles (5, 6)

- Place One of the antigen 'O','H' A (H), B (H) in circles 1, 2, 3 and 4 respectively and 'O' antigen in the circle 5 and any one of the H antigen (H, A(H),B(H)) in circle 6.

- Mix the content in each circle with separate applicator stick.

- Rotate the glass slide for one minute and observe for agglutinations.

- When agglutination is visible within one minute, proceeded for quantitative test.

Quantitative tube test (Fig-33.1)

- Take twenty four clean dry test tubes of 10x75 mm size for each serum under test and arranged.

- Dilute Serum sample by adding 0.1ml of saline with 0.9ml of serum (Prepare serum for required quantity).

- Add 0.5ml of saline to all tubes.

- Add 0.5ml of diluted serum to 1st tube and are diluted serially. Discard 0.5ml serum finally.

- Arrange test tubes in 3 rows with 8 tubs each.

- Add 0.5ml each of *S. typhi* O antigen in First row tubes, *S. typhi* H antigens in 2nd row tubes and Salmonella A(H) antigens in 3rd row tubes (Fig 33.1).

- Mix the sample well and incubated at 37⁰C for 16 to 20 hrs and examined for agglutinations.

Observation

Note agglutination in both slide and tubes.

Interpretation

Since positive sera contains antibodies to all the three type of Salmonella.(*S.typhi, S.paratyphiA(H), S.paratyphiB(H)*) agglutination occurred in all the three series up to 1:160 dilution.

Viva questions

Who devised Widal test?
What are the types of antigens are detected through Widal test?
Name the disease, which is diagnosed by Widal test.
What are the principles of Widal test?
Why is widal called agglutination reaction.
Define O antigen & H antigen.
When do you perform slide test & tube test.
Can the result of Widal test result only used for diagnosis of typhoid fever?

Spotters: Widal test, Salmonella typhi and S. parayphi O and H antigens

33 Ad. RPR Test

Aim

To assess the treponemal infection in human beings.

Principle

Rapid plasma reagin is a blood test for syphilis. It is used to look for an antibody against *Treponema pallidum* antigens. The RPR test is a non treponemal preparation specially developed for the rapid detection and semi quantitation by flocculation on a slide of reagins, a group of antibodies detected against tissue components produced by almost every patients infected with *Treponema pallidum*. The test uses the VDRL antigen which employ a standardized cardiolipin antigen coated on to carbon particles, resulting in a reagent that retains the sensitivity and specificity of VDRL and adds stability, reading- ease and convenience. A negative (non reactive) RPR is compatible with a person not having syphilis, but in the early stages of the disease, the RPR often gives false negative results. Conversely, a false positive RPR can be encountered in infectious mononucleosis, lupus, antiphospholipid antibody syndrome, hepatitis A, leprosy, malaria and occasionally pregnancy. A positive test result may mean that patient have syphilis. If the screening test is positive, the next step is to confirm the diagnosis with a more specific test for syphilis, such as

FTA-ABS. The FTA-ABS test will help distinguish between syphilis and other infections. How well the RPR test can detect syphilis depends on the stage of the disease. The test is most sensitive — almost 100% — during the middle stages of syphilis. It is less sensitive during the earlier and later stages of the disease.

Materials Required

RPR kit (Fig-33.2), Positive control, Negative control, Physiological saline.

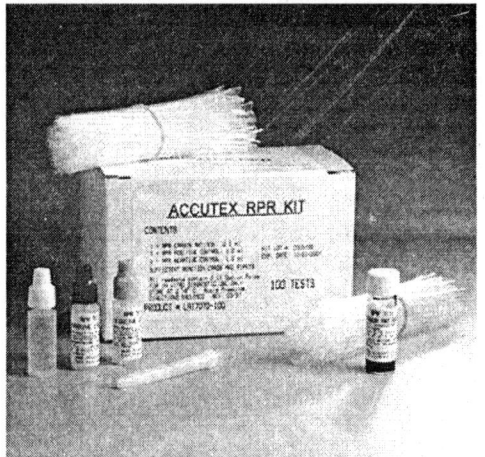

Fig. 33.2 – RPR Kit

Procedure

Qualitative

- Bring the test reagents and samples to room temperature.
- Place one drop of serum (40µL) on slide with the help of disposable serum dropper.
- Add one drop of RPR antigen suspension (18µL) using antigen dropper.
- Spread and Mix entire area of the circle by using disposable applicator stick.
- Rock the slide to and fro for 6 minutes and observed for appearance of carbon particle clumping.

Semi quantitative test

- Perform semiquantitative test when serum is agglutinate in qualitative test
- Place 50µL diluted glycine-saline buffer onto each of 5 circles of the slide
- Using micropipette, add 50µL of the serum sample to the drop of Glycine saline buffer in first circle.
- Using the same micropipette, mix the sample with saline by aspirating back and forth for several times.
- Aspirate 50µL from first circle and transfer to second circle.
- Repeat the same operation upto 5th circle.
- Aspirate 50ml from 5th circle and discard.
- Rock the slide gently for 2 minutes and record the results
- Add a drop of RPR antigen.

Observation

Agglutination was noted/ not observed

Table 33.2 : Observation Record

S. No	Circle	Dilution	Observation	Interpretation
1	1st	1:2		
2	2nd	1:4		
3	3rd	1:8		
4	4th	1:16		
5	5th	1:32		

Result

Agglutination indicates that the patients having Treponema infection. It should be confirmed using specific treponemal tests.

Viva questions

Expand RPR&VDRL.
Define flocculation.
What is cardiolipin antigen?
What type of disease is diagnosed by RPR test?

Spotters

RPR kit, Treponema antigens

33 Ae. CRP Test

Aim

To Determinate of C reactive protein in serum.

Principle

The C reactive protein is a rapid agglutination procedure for the direct detection and semi quantification on slide of C reactive protein. The reagent, a latex particles suspension coated with specific anti human C Reactive protein. Antibodies agglutinates in the presence of C Reactive protein in the patient serum. The CRP test is useful in assessing patients with Inflammatory bowel disease, some forms of arthritis, Autoimmune diseases, Pelvic Inflammatory Disease (PID), Coronary heart disease (CHD), Cardiovascular disease. While the CRP test is not specific enough to diagnose a particular disease, it does serve as a general marker for infection and inflammation, thus alerting medical professionals that further testing and treatment may be necessary. Because CRP increases in severe cases of inflammation, the test is ordered when acute inflammation is a risk (such as from an infection after surgery)

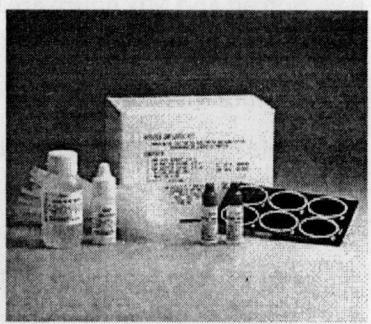

Fig.33.3-CRP kit

or suspected based on patient symptoms. CRP also is used to monitor wound healing and to monitor patients who have surgical cuts (incisions), organ transplants or burns as an early detection system for possible infections. A high or increasing amount of CRP in blood suggests that, patient have an acute infection or inflammation. In a healthy person, CRP is usually less than 10 mG/L. Most infections and inflammations result in CRP levels above 100 mG/L. If the CRP level drops, it means that patient is getting better and inflammation is being reduced. When results fall below 10 mG/L, no longer have clinically active inflammation. CRP levels can be elevated in the later stages of pregnancy as well as with use of birth control pills or hormone replacement therapy (i.e., estrogen). Higher levels of CRP have also been observed in the obese.

Materials Required

CRP kit (Fig – 33.3), Positive control, Negative control, Physiological saline

Procedure

- Allow all reagents as well as the sample to reach room temperature. Mix well before using
- Place one drop of serum onto the slide with the help of disposable serum dropper.
- Add one drop of CRP latex antigen to the above drop and mix with disposable applicator stick.

- Rock the slide gently to and fro for two minutes and examine under good light source for agglutination. Positive and negative control also maintained.

Semi quantitative test

- Perform semiquantitative test when serum is agglutinate in qualitative test
- Place 50µL diluted glycine-saline buffer onto each of 5 circles of the slide
- Using micropipette, add 50µL of the serum sample to the drop of Glycine saline buffer in first circle.
- Using the same micropipette, mix the sample with saline by aspirating back and forth for several times.
- Aspirate 50µL from first circle and transfer to second circle.
- Repeat the same operation upto 5th circle.
- Aspirate 50µL from 5th circle and discard.
- Add one drop of antigen to all circles.
- Rock the slide gently for 2 minutes and record the results

Calculation

Concentration of CRP in serum is calculated

CRP(mG/dL)=0.6X highest dilution of serum showing agglutination

Sensitivity =0.6mG/dL

If the qualitative test shows agglutination it indicates CRP level in serum is 0.6 mG/dL

Observation

Agglutination was noted/ not observed

Table 33.3 Observation record

S. No	Circle	Dilution	Observation	Interpretation
1	1st	1:2		
2	2nd	1:4		
3	3rd	1:8		
4	4th	1:16		
5	5th	1:32		

Results

A C-reactive protein (CRP) test is a blood test that measures the amount of a protein called C-reactive protein in your blood.

Viva Questions

What is the purpose of performing CRP test?

Expand CRP.

Define latex antigen.

Mention diseases diagnosed by CRP test.

Spotters : CRP Kit

33Af. Coombs test

Indirect Coombs test

Aim

To detect presence of Rh-antibodies or other antibodies in patients serum.

To check whether an Rh-negative women has developed Anti Rh-antibodies.

Background information

Anti D may be produced in the blood of any Rh-negative person by exposure to D antigen by-Transfusion of Rh positive blood. In Pregnancy, if infant is Rh positive (if father is Rh-positive) Abortion of Rh-positive fetus may indicated.

Materials required

Test tubes (10x75 mm), Pasteur pipettes, Incubator, Centrifuge

Specimen: Serum (need not be fasting)

Reagents: Antihuman serum, Anti-D serum, Control

Procedure

- Label three test tubes as 'T" (test serum) PC (Positive control) and NC (negative control).

- In the tube labelled as 'T', add two drops of Anti-D serum.

- In the tube 'PC' add one drop of saline.

- Add one drop of 5 % saline suspension of the pooled 'O' Rh (D) positive cells in each tube.

- Incubate all the three tubes for one hour at 37°C.

- Wash the cells three times in normal saline to remove excess serum with no free antibodies, (in the case of inadequate washings of the red cells, negative results may be obtained).

- Add two drops of Coombs serum (anti human serum) to each tube. Keep for 5 minutes and then centrifuge at 1,500 RPM for one minute.

- Resuspend the cells and examine macroscopically as well as microscopically.

Observation and result

Clotting may be observed.

Direct Coombs test (direct antiglobulin test):

Aim

To detect anti-D antibody or other antibodies attached to the red cell surface within the blood stream.

Background information

When there is Rh-positive baby in the womb of a sensitized Rh-negative women; the antibodies produced in the mothers serum cross the placenta and after entering the baby's blood stream, these antibodies will attach to the baby's Rh-positive red blood cells. These coated (or sensitized) cells are clumped and removed from the circulation, causing haemolytic anaemia (Haemolytic Disease of the Newborn: Erythroblastosis Faetalis). When the baby is born, the baby's blood is collected (or cord blood is collected from umbilical cord) and tested by the anti globulin Coombs test (direct) to detect anti D antibodies coated on red blood cells.

Materials required

Test tubes (10x75 mm), Pasteur pipettes, Incubator, Centrifuge

Specimen: Serum (need not be fasting)

Reagents: Antihuman serum, Anti-D serum, Control

Procedure

- Prepare a 5 % suspension in isotonic saline of the red blood cells to be tested.

- With clean Pasture pipette add one drop of the prepared cell suspension to a small tube.

- Wash three times with normal saline to remove all the traces of serum.

- Decant completely after the last washing

- Add two drops of Antihuman serum.

- Mix well and centrifuge for one minute at 1500rpm.

- Resuspend the cells by gentle agitation and examine macroscopically and microscopically for agglutination.

Observation and result

Agglutination may or may not observed.

Viva questions

What is the principle of coombs test?

How do you differentiate direct coombs test from indirect coombs test

What is Erythroblastosis Faetalis

Spotters

Erythroblastosis Faetalis

33 B. Precipitation

Introduction

Precipitation technique is used to detect and identify antigens in specimens, extracts and cultures. In precipitation test, the antigen and antibody are in a soluble form and combined to form a visible precipitate. Electrolytes are usually required for this reaction.

There are three main types of precipitation techniques. These are Tube precipitation test, Gel diffusion and immunoelectrophoresis.

When both antigens and antibodies are diffuse through the gel, this is referred to as double diffusion. When only the antigen or antibody diffuse with corresponding antigen or antibody being contained in the agar, this is called single diffusion. Antigen and antibody diffuse each other and where they meet in optimal proportion a visible line of precipitate forms is called double diffusion. If specific antibody is incorporated into the gel and wells are cut to contain the antigen, which diffuse radially. Ring precipitate forms around the well called single radial diffusion. Counter immunoelectrophoresis (CIE) is referred to as counter current electrophoresis (CCEP) and immunoelectrophoresis (IEOP). Electrophoresis is used to increase the speed with which the antigen and antibody travel in the agar gel. A line of precipitation forms where the antigen and antibody meet in optimal proportion. Factors responsible for precipitation are pH, purity and ionic strength of the gel.

33 Ba. Radial Immunodiffusion Test

Aim

To perform radial immunodiffusion for the given sample.

Principle

When antigen diffuses radially forming a concentration gradient disc in gel containing uniformly distributed antibodies. The antigen antibody complex precipitates in the gel where the diffusion antigen reach on equivalence with the antibody concentration present in the gel, the precipitate formed in the gel appear as an opaque ring. The ring diameter is directly proportional to the antigen concentration.

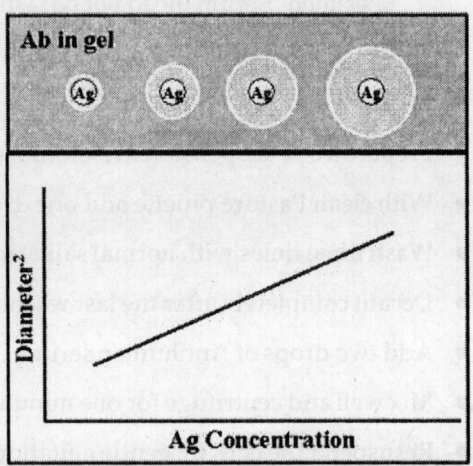

Fig 33.4 – Radial Immuno diffusion

In this method, antibody is incorporated before the gel is made. Thus the antiserum is uniformly distributed through out agar gel. Antigen is then allowed to diffuse from wells into the agar gel. Initially as the antigen diffuse out of the well, it's concentration is relatively high and it forms soluble antigen antibody adducts. However as it diffuses further and further from the well, its concentration decreases. When its concentration becomes equivalent to that of the antibody in the gel, antigen-antibody precipitates and a precipitin ring is formed. Greater the concentration of antigen greater is the diameter of precipitin ring. Thus, by running a range of known antigen concentration on the gel and by measuring the diameter of their precipitin rings, a calibration graph can constructed and quantity of antigen / antibody are calculated.

Materials required

Agarose, Veronelbuffer (Refer Page 149), standard antigen, test antigen, antiserum , gel punch with syringe , glass plates, template, semi log graph sheet, Distilled water, Micropipettes, A box to keep the gel plate, Moist chamber, assay buffer etc.,

Precautions

The glass plate should be wiped grease free with cotton for the even spreading of agarose

The wells should be cut neatly without rugged margins to get a perfect rug of precipitation.

The antiserum should be added to the agar only after it cools to 55°C. High temperature will inactivate the antibody.

After the addition of antiserum to the agar proper mixing is essential for uniform distribution of antibody.

Procedure

- Dissolve one gram of agarose in 100ml of Vernoal buffer by heating.
- Allow the solution to cool and mix 120µL of antiserum with 6ml of the solution.
- Pour the agarose solution containing the antiserum on to a grease free glass plate that had previously been set on a horizontal level.
- Allow the gel to form by cooling.

- Cut the wells of 4 mm diameter into the gel using a gel punch.
- Dilute the antiserum upto 1:16.

Dilution:

- Arrange four 1.5ml micro centrifuge tubes in rack.
- Add 50µL of buffer to all tubes
- Add 50µL antigen to the first tube (1:2).
- Transfer 50µL antigen from 1st tube to 2nd tube (1:4) and continue the same procedure to remaining tube (1:8 and 1:16).
- Add 20µL of diluted antigen to respective wells.
- Keep the gel plate in a box containing wet cotton and incubated overnight at room temperature.
- Measure the diameter of the precipitation disc by marking the edges of the circle.
- Construct a standard graph by plotting the diameter of the precipitation ring against the concentration of the antigen in semi log graph.
- Determine the concentration of unknown by reading the concentration against the ring diameter.

Observation

Precipitation zone indicates the presence of specific antibodies in the serum to the test antigen added. The standard graph is drawn for the ring diameter.

Viva questions

Precipitation , precipitation ring .

What is the principle of radial immuno diffusion.

What are the precautions to be taken during RID.

How do you perform RID .

Mention the nature of agarose .

Spotters : Picture of radial Immuno diffusion.

33 Bb. Double immunodiffusion test (Ouchterlony Double Diffusion test)

Aim

To check antisera for the presence and specificity of antibodies for a particular antigen.

Principle

Double immunodiffusion technique was first described by Ouchterlony. Antigen and antibody placed in adjacent wells in agargel diffuse radially. Initially as the antigen and antibody diffuses out of the respective wells, the concentrations are relatively high nearer to the well, however as they diffuse further from the wells, the concentration decreases at one point where the concentration become equivalent and antigen-antibody complex precipitate to form a precipitant line.

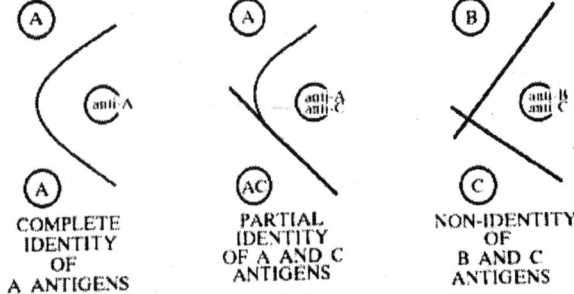

COMPLETE IDENTITY OF A ANTIGENS

PARTIAL IDENTITY OF A AND C ANTIGENS

NON-IDENTITY OF B AND C ANTIGENS

Fig 33.5 – Double immuno diffusion

Materials Required

Agarose, Veronal buffer (Refer Page 149), antigen, test antisera, glass plates, gel-punch with syringe, template, micropipettes, tubes, distilled water, a box to keep the gel plate in moist chamber.

Precaution

The glassplate should be wiped grease free with cotton for the even spreading of the agarose.

Ensure that the chamber has enough wet cotton to keep the atmosphere humid.

Procedure

- Prepare 1% agarose solution in 1x vernoal buffer by heating the dissolved agar completely.
- Cool the solution to about 55 - 60°C and pour required volume on to a grease free glass plate that had previously been set on horizontal level surface.
- Allow the gel to set for 20 - 30 minutes.
- Keep the gel plate on the template provided.
- Punch wells in the gel with the help of a gel punch corresponding to the marking on the template with gentle process.
- Add 20µL of the antigen in the side wells and
- Add 20µL of antiserum to the center well
- Keep the plate in the moist chamber overnight at room temperature.
- Observe the plate for an opaque precipitant line between the antigen and antisera wells.

Interpretation

Precipitant line indicates the presence of antibody in the antiserum to the antigen added.

Viva questions

What is the other name of DID?

What are the difference between RID&DID?

What are the use of buffer in ID?

How do you examine precipitation line?

Spotters : Picture of Double immuno diffusion.

33 Bc. Counter Current Immuno Electrophoresis

Aim:

To check antisera for the presence and specificity of antibodies for a particular antigen by Counter current immunoelectrophoresis.

Introduction

Counter Current Immuno Electrophoresis (CCIE) is a rapid version of Ouchterlony double diffusion technique. This technique is used to check antisera for the presence and specificity of antibodies for a particular antigen. This experiment can be performed within an hour.

Materials Required

Agarose (it is prepared by adding 1.5g agarose in 10µL veronol buffer and 90ml of distilled water. Melt the agarose in boiling water bath), Antigen, Antiserum, Reservoir buffer (Tris-242gm, Glacial acetic acid - 57.1ml, 0.5M EDTA (pH -8)-100ml, Make up the volume to 1 lit using distilled water), , Electrophoresis apparatus, **Veronal buffer** (0.075M) is prepared by mixing 276g dimethyl barbituric acid in 1000mL distilled water & dissolve it by heating. Then add 15.45g sodium dimethyl barbiturate and 1g sodium azide (pH-8.6).

Procedure

- Prepare 10 ml of 1.5 % agarose in 1x buffer by adding dry agarose powder to the buffer and heating slowly to dissolve agarose completely.
- Place the slide in a leveled tabletop and quickly pipette 7-mL agarose on to the slide
- Allow the agarose to solidify
- Place the gel slide in a template and punch 3mm wells.
- Place the slide in the electrophoresis tank and fill the tank with buffer till the buffer just covers the gel surface.
- Add 10 micro liter of antigen in four well's towards negative electrode and 10 micro liter positive control and three test antisera in wells towards positive electrode.
- Apply 50 V and allow the electrophoresis to continue for about 45 minutes
- Observe for precipitin line between antigen and antisera wells.

Observation And Interpretation

Precipitation lines are observed

Viva questions

What are the advantages & disadvantages of CCIE?

List applications of CIE.

What are the stains used in CIE?

Spotters : Picture of C.I.E.

34. Enzyme Linked Immuno Sorbent Assay

Aim

To assess antigen antibody reactions.

To findout microbial infections by antigen antibody reactions

Introduction

The ELISA technique is used for a semiquantitative determination of the concentration of certain antigens/antibodies. It is first introduced in early 1970s by Engvall and Pearlmann. This technique is used to diagnose various infections of human body. This test can detect protein upto 0.0005mG /mL.

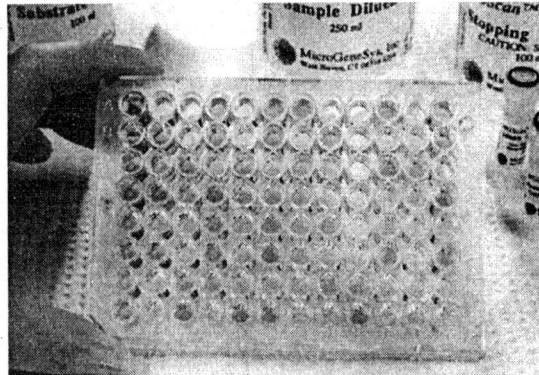

Fig. 34.1 – ELISA Plate

Enzyme can be chemically coupled to either Ag or Ab and retain the biological properties. Once Ag or Ab is bound to the plate they become resistant to vigorous washing in detergent buffer whilst excess unbound reagent is simply removed by this process. In the subsequent steps one or more layers of a solid phase captured immune complex are formed with unbound entities again efficiently washed away. An enzyme conjugate of Ab or Ag when bound in immune complex leaves the enzyme component available for substrate reaction.

Horse radish peroxidase, alkaline phosphatase , acetylcholine esterase, β D galactosidase are some of the enzymes used in ELISA. Substrates used in ELISA are hydrogen peroxide, Acetylcholine, Glucose 6 phosphate, NADP. ELISA is highly sensitive, specific and rapid method to analyze infection but it requires expensive cold store chemicals, instruments and well trained expertise to handle instruments.

Direct ELISA, Indirect ELISA, Sandwitch ELISA and Competitive ELISA are the types of ELISA.

Materials Required

Micro titre plates, Micropipettes, Multichannel pipettes, ELISA reader

Coating buffer

Sodium carbonate	- 7.95g
Sodium bicarbonate	-14.65g
PH	-9.6

Washing buffer (PBS-T)

PBS	-1000mL
Tween 20	-0.05mL

Dilution buffer

PBS-T	-100mL
Bovine serum albumin	-1g
Allow it to dissolve. Do not shake.	

Glycerol saline

Glycerine	-50mL
Normal saline	-50 mL

Substrate buffer

Ortho phenylene diamine	-4mG
Citrate buffer	-100mL

Stopping solution

Add 54 mL of concentrated sulphuric acid to 1000mL distilled water

Normal saline

Sodium chloride	-0.85g
Distilled water	-100mL

PKE saline

Potassium chloride	-14.912g
Potassium dihydrogen phosphate	-6.804g
EDTA	-3.722g
pH	-7.6g

Procedure

Doubles sandwitch

- Coat the plate with 50µL test serum and keeping at 4°C overnight.
- Wash three times in PBS - T.
- Add the purified Antigen to all the wells, incubate at 37°C for 1 hour.
- Wash three times with PBS-T.
- Add 50µL immunoglobulin conjugate and incubate at 37 ° C for 30 minutes.
- Wash three times in PBS-T.
- Add freshly prepared OPD substrate solution (100µL) each to all the wells. Incubate in dark condition for 15 minutes.
- Observe the colour of the wells.
- Read absorbance in ELISA reader.

Indirect ELISA:

- Coat the ELISA plate with purified antigen (50µL). Keep overnight. Discard the contents and wash the plate 3 times with PBS-T. Saturate the wells by addition of 1% BSA in PBS and incubate one hour at 37 ° C.
- Wash the plate 3 times with PBS-T.
- Add Antibody to be tested in two rows starting with a dilution of 1: 10.
- Incubate 1 hour at 37 ° C.
- Wash the plate 3 times with PBS-T.
- Add 50µL of anti-antibody labeled with peroxidase conjugate in a pretitrated dilution.
- Wash the plate 3 times with PBS-T.
- Add 100µL of freshly prepared substrate solution to all the wells and incubate in dark for 15 minutes.
- Read the absorbency in ELISA reader.

Observation And Result

Colour change is noted and read using ELISA reader

Viva questions

What is ELISA?
What are the types of ELISA?
What is enzyme immuno assay?
What are the steps involved in ELISA?
Who introduced ELISA?
What are the principles of ELISA?
What are the advantages & disadvantages of ELISA?

Spotters: H_2O_2, horseradish peroxidase, mirotitre plate/ELISA plate and ELISA reader.

35. Purification of IgG

Aim

To purify immunoglobulin G from the given serum sample.

Introduction

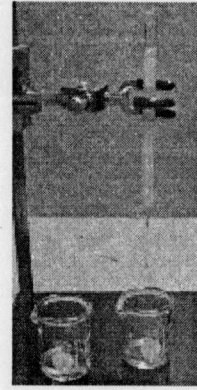

Chromatography consists of two phases that are Stationary phase and mobile phase. In column chromatography the stationary phase is packed in a cylindrical column. Majority of the chromatography is routinely carried out using the column. The apparatus and general techniques used for gel exclusion, ion exchange, adsorption and affinity chromatography have much in common.

Gelfiltration also known as gel permeation and molecular sieving, is a common and simple technique for the separation of compounds of their size. It is first introduced as a laboratory procedure in 1959. Main principle of this experiment is, a solution containing two or more molecular species differing fairly widely in size, is allowed to percolate through a long column placed with the gel matrix. Commonly available gel matrix are used in gel filtration chromatography.

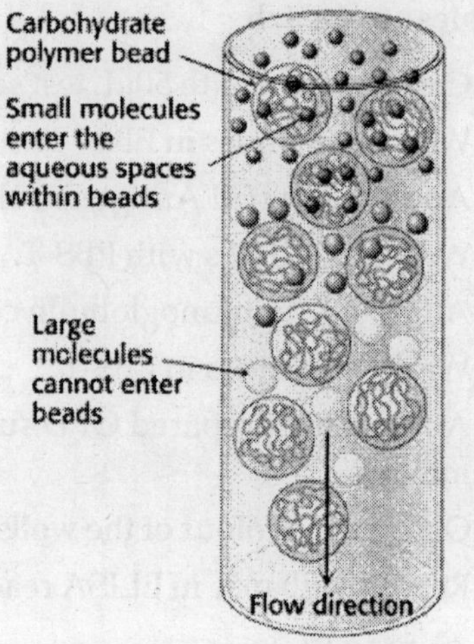

Fig.35.1: Column chromatography

Carbohydrate polymer bead

Small molecules enter the aqueous spaces within beads

Large molecules cannot enter beads

Flow direction

Fig. 35.2: Principles of column chromatography

Chromatography columns are considered to consist of a number of adjacent lenses in each of which there is sufficient space for the solute to achieve complete equilibrium between the mobile and stationary phase.

Materials Required

Glass column, Sephadex G 100, Elution buffer, Fraction collector , Peristaltic pump , Marker proteins.

Procedure

• Weighs about 20g dry sephadex G 100 and suspend in 100mL of distilled water or elution buffer in a beaker. Allow 5 hrs or 8 hrs (depends upon manufactures instructions) for the gel to swell completely.

• Set up a glass or plastic column of dimension 25cm long and 1. 5 inner diameter.

• Pack good quality glass wool at the bottom to a height of about 0.5-1cm. This will prevent leaking of the gel particles during the experiment.

• Make good slurry of the gel in a suitable buffer after proper swelling of the gel.

• Pour small volume of buffer in to the column to avoid trapping of any air bubbles.

• Pour the gel slurry to the full of column.

• Wait until the gel settles down to the desired height by gravitational force (Never allow the column to dry).

• Place the suitable filter disc on top of the gel bed. Equilibriate the column thoroughly by passing through the column buffer.

• Apply the sample in column buffer or to the top of bed. The sample volume should preferably limit to 1-3% of the total bed volume. Sample can be applied carefully by pipette or through automatic buffer injector.

• Continuously add buffer to the column bed to develop the chromatogram.

152

- Protein molecules pass through the gel space while small molecules distribute between the solvent inside and outside the gel and then pass through the column at a slower rate.

- The efficient emerging out of the column can be routed through a suitable spectrophotometer to monitor the absorbency at a particular wavelength 200nm, 250nm and 210nm.

- Standard protein also eluted by the same above-mentioned and the reading is compared and estimate the amount of IgG present in the sample.

Viva questions

Define chromatography

Mention the type of chromatographic method used to purify immunoglobulin

What are the principles of serum chromatography?

Spottors: Column chromatography set up, sephadex

36. Ammonium Sulphate Precipitation of Protein

Aim

Purification of proteins by salt precipitation method

Introduction

The solubility of proteins is markedly affected by the ionic strength of the medium. As the ionic strength is increased, protein solubility at first increases. This is referred to as *"salting in"* however beyond a certain point the solubility begins to decreases and this is known as *"salting out"*.

The charges on a protein in solution can be neutralized by the addition of salts and this also has been used for purification of protein. Ammonium sulfate is used for the precipitation of protein because of its high solubility 840g/l, its dissolution in water and exothermic or the solution get cooled.

Materials Required

Ammonium sulphate, Beaker, Magnetic stirrer, Caprylic acid, Phosphate buffered saline (NaCl – 8g; KCl-0.2g; N_2HPO_4-1.15g;KH_2PO_4-0.2g; Distilled water – 1000mL; pH-7.4).

Procedure

Common to all protein except IgG

- Sample is taken in a beaker

- To this add ammonium sulphate salt in small amount with stirring to give 30% saturation for 15 minutes (Refer Table –36.1).

- Centrifuge the contents at 3000 rpm for 15 minutes.

- To the supernatant add calculated amount of ammonium sulphate to give 50% saturation (Refer Table –36.1).

- Centrifuge the contents at 3000 rpm for 15 minutes.

- To the supernatant add ammonium sulphate to 75 % saturation (Refer Table –36.1).

- Centrifuge the contents at 3000 rpm for 15 minutes.

- Precipitate and supernatant are subjected to protein estimation.

Purification of IgG Fraction From Whole Serum

- Mix 100mL serum with 200 mL of 40% ammonium sulphate (Refer Table –36.1) and 100 mL of phosphate buffered saline.

- Add 8.2 ml of caprylic acid drop wise at room temperature.

- Stir for 30 minutes and remove precipitate by centrifugation at 10,000 rpm for 10 minutes.

- Dialyze the precipitated IgG against 0.9% sodium chloride solution

Table-36.1: The amount of solid ammonium sulphate to be added to a solution to give the desired final saturation at 0°C

Initial con-centration of NH_4SO_4	Final concentrations of ammonium sulphate, % saturation at 0°C																
	20	25	30	35	40	45	50	55	60	65	70	75	80	85	90	95	100
	Gram solid ammonium sulphate added to 100 ml of solution.																
0	10.7	13.6	16.6	19.7	22.9	26.2	29.5	33.1	36.6	40.4	44.2	48.3	52.3	56.7	61.1	65.9	70.7
5	8	10.9	13.9	16.8	20	23.2	26.6	30.0	33.6	37.3	41.1	45.0	49.1	53.3	57.8	62.4	67.1
10	5.4	8.2	11.1	14.1	17.1	20.3	23.6	27.0	30.5	34.2	37.9	41.8	45.8	50.0	54.5	58.9	63.6
15	2.6	5.5	8.3	11.3	14.3	17.4	20.7	24.0	27.5	31.0	34.8	38.6	42.6	46.6	51.0	55.5	60.0
20	0	2.7	5.6	8.4	11.5	14.5	17.7	21.0	24.4	28.0	31.6	35.4	39.2	43.3	47.6	51.9	56.5
25		0	2.7	5.7	8.5	11.7	14.8	18.2	21.4	24.8	28.4	32.1	36.0	40.1	44.2	48.5	52.9
30			0	2.8	5.7	8.7	11.9	15.0	18.4	21.7	25.3	28.9	32.8	36.7	40.8	45.1	49.5
35				0	2.8	5.8	8.8	12.0	15.3	18.7	22.1	25.8	29.5	33.4	37.4	41.6	45.9
40					0	2.9	5.9	9.0	12.2	15.5	19.0	22.5	26.2	30.0	34.0	38.1	42.4
45						0	2.9	6.0	9.1	12.5	15.8	19.3	22.9	26.7	30.6	34.7	38.8
50							0	3.0	6.1	9.3	12.7	16.1	19.7	23.3	27.2	31.2	35.3
55								0	3.0	6.2	9.4	12.9	16.3	20.0	23.8	27.7	31.7
60									0	3.1	6.3	9.6	13.1	16.6	20.4	24.2	28.3
65										0	3.1	6.4	9.8	13.4	17.0	20.8	24.7
70											0	3.2	6.6	10.0	13.6	17.3	21.2
75												0	3.2	6.7	10.2	13.9	17.6
80													0	3.3	6.8	10.4	14.1
85														0	3.4	6.9	10.6
90															0	3.4	7.1
95																0	3.5
100																	0

Viva questions

Define salting out and salting in

What are the principles of protein precipitation by NH_4SO_4?

How does NH_4SO_4 precipitate protein

37. Dialysis

Aim

To remove salt from the sample.

To purify antigens and antibodies from the samples.

Introduction

Dialysis is a process, used to selectively remove small molecules from a sample containing mixture of both small and large molecules. It is commonly used for removing salts from the protein. Dialysis is effectively achieved using a special type of membrane known as semipermeable membrane. The semipermeable membranes allow the small molecules to pass freely through holding the large molecules inside. The membranes are essentially made up of cellulose derivatives. Dialysis membranes are characterized by their Nominal Molecular Weight Cut Off (NMWCO). It depends primarily on the pore size of the membranes. NMWCO is defined as the lowest molecular weight compound retained by the membrane at 90% or more.

Rate of dialysis is mainly based on Solvent, Temperature, concentration gradient, Diffusion constant, Thickness, area, porosity of membranes, Reverse dialysis and Electro dialysis (used to remove salts and nucleic acids).

Materials required

Phosphate buffer, 2% sodium bicarbonate, 10mM EDTA, Sucrose, Dialysis membrane.

Procedure

- Generally dialysis membranes are supplied by the manufactures as dry membranes and contain about 10% glycerol. It is used to prevent brittleness of the membrane and can be removed by soaking.

- Cut dialysis membranes into required size and soak in the clean distilled water to remove 10% glycerol content.

- Remove the heavy metals by boiling the tube in 10mM EDTA.

- Boil the tube in 2% $NaHCO_3$ solution for 10 minutes to remove sulphide.

- Again boil the tube in 10mM EDTA for 20 minutes.

- Wash inside and outside of the tube with the help of distilled water using a squeeze bottle.

- Again boil the tubing's for 10 minutes in 10mM EDTA to remove excess $NaHCO_3$.

- Wash inside and outside of the tube with the help of distilled water using a squeeze bottle.

- Store the tube in 10% ethanol at 4°C.

- Take one piece of dialysis tube.

- Wash inside and outside with distilled water.

- Tied one end securely with a dialysis closure clip.

- Check the tube for leaking.

- If there is no leakage, remove the water and fill 2/3 sample solution that to be dialyzed using a pipette.

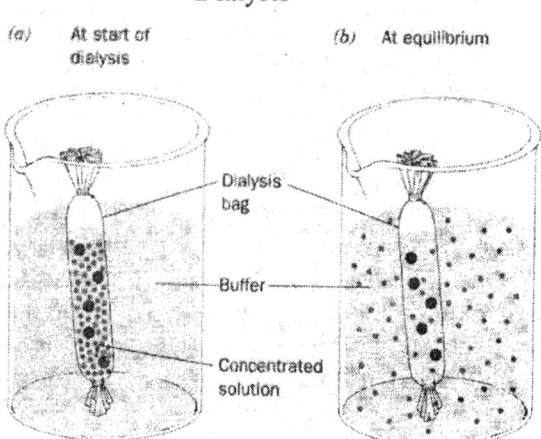

Dialysis

(a) At start of dialysis   (b) At equilibrium

Dialysis bag

Buffer

Concentrated solution

Fig.37.1: Dialysis Process

- Close open end securely by tying with closure clip.
- Place the bag in an appropriate buffer solution and dialyzed for 3-4 hours at required temperature.
- For better results magnetic stirrer also used for dialysis. During this time most of the small molecules will be removed from the bag. Change the buffer, if necessary. During dialysis water being freely permeable, would have entered the bag and diluted the proteins.

Concentration of protein is by the following method

Carefully bury the dialysis bags with solution in a jar containing sucrose and kept it in a refrigerator. Water will move out and get absorbed by sucrose. Now the bag contains desalted protein. This may be subjected to further purification.

Viva questions

Define dialysis

What are the principles of dialysis?

How do you concentrate protein after dialysis?

Spotters: Dialysis membrane

38. Separation of Protein by SDS PAGE

Aim

To separate the proteins from the given sample based on the molecular weight.

Principle

Any charged ion or group will migrate when placed in an electric field. Negatively charged particles in solution move towards positive electrode and vice versa. These particles move at different speeds in solution depending on their net charge and the size of the molecule.

SDS in the presence of reducing agent beta mercapto ethanol dissociates proteins into their sub units and bind large quantities of it to the protein, which completely masks the natural charge of the protein giving a constant charge to mass ratio. The large molecule there fore greater the charge so, the electro protein mobility of the complex depends on the size of the molecular weight of the protein.

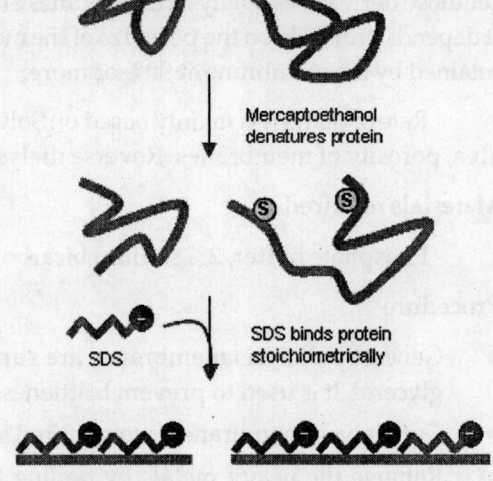

Fig38.1- Applications of SDS and mercaptoethanol

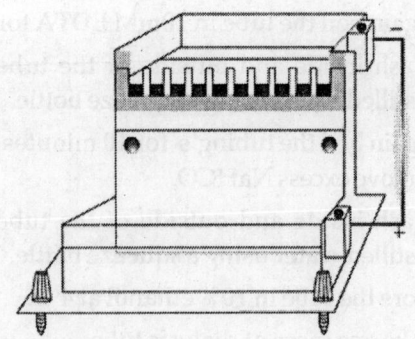

Fig. 38.2: SDS – PAGE Apparatus

Extraction Of Proteins

- Take 5ml of washed bacterial pellet and add 5ml of 10 % cold TCA.
- Incubate in ice for 30 minutes.
- Centrifuged at 12000 rpm for 5minutes.
- Wash the pellet with ethanol : ether (1:1) repeatedly to remove TCA.

- Dissolve TCA precipitate in 0.625 molor TRIS Hcl (pH 6.8)
- The sample is subjected to SDS-PAGE.

Materials Required

Gel electrophoresis apparatus with power pack (Figure 38.2)

Reagents

Acrylamide stock

Acrylamide	-29.2g
NN methylene bis acrylamide	-0.8g
Distilled water	-100mL

Stored at 4 ° C in dark bottle

Separating or Resolving gel buffer (4X)

Tris	-18.15g
SDS	-0.4g

Dissolve the salt in 50 ml of distilled water and adjust the pH with 1N Hcl. Make up to 100 ml with distilled water and stored at 4°C. pH –8.8

Stacking gel buffer (4X)

Tris	-6.05g
SDS	-0.4g

Dissolve the salt in 50 ml of distilled water and adjust the pH with 1N Hcl. Make up to 100 ml with distilled water and stored at 4°C. pH –6.8

Running or Reservoir buffer

Tris	-3g (25mM)
Glycine	-14.4g (192mM)
SDS	-1g (0.1%)

Dissolve and made up to 1000ml with distilled water

Protein stain

Coomassie brillient blue	-0.25 g
Methanol	-50ml
Acetic acid	-7ml

Dissolve and made up to 100ml with distilled water

Destaining solution

Methonol	-5ml
Acetic acid	-7ml

Mix and made upto 100ml with distilled water

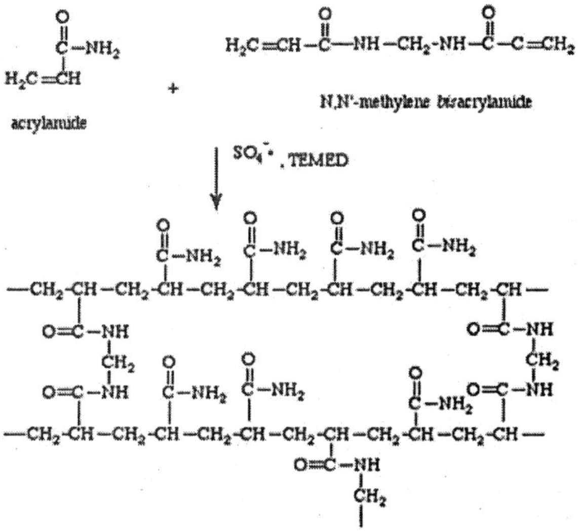

Fig 38.3- Polymerization reaction catalysed by TEMED and NH_4SO_4

Box-38.1 Concentration for X% Separation or stacking gel	
Separating gel concentrations 10%, 12%, 15 %	
Stacking gel concentrations 5%, 7.5%	
Acrylamide stock	-X%/3 ml
Stacking / Separating gel buffer-	2.5 ml
Distilled water	- (7.5-X%/3) ml
Total Volume	-10ml

Storing solution

Methonol	-5ml
Acetic acid	-7ml
Distilled water	-87.5ml

Sample buffer

0.0625mM Tris Hcl	-1.2ml
SDS	-1g
Glycerol	-3ml
Beta mercapto ethanol	-200ml
Bromophenol blue	-2ml
Distilled water	-5ml

10% Ammonium persulphate (APS)

0.5g APS dissolved in 5ml of Distilled water

NNNN Tetra methylene ethylene diamine

Procedure

- Clean the glass plates by soaking them in chromic acid over night.
- Rinsed them with water and then with ethanol.
- Place the plates down on to clean tissue paper with the side which is be contact with the gel upper and swab with an acetone soaked tissue paper held in a gloved hand. After a final rinse with ethanol allow the plates to air dry.
- Fix the gel plate with appropriate spacers on the gel plate.
- To avoid leakage vacuum grease on both sides of the spacers are applied.
- Prepare the resolving gel buffer solution as per the required concentration % and volume required (Table 38.1)

Table 38.1 – Quantity of reagents required to prepare separating gel

10 % Gel	10 ml	20 ml	30 ml	40 ml	50 ml
Acrylamide Stock	3.3	6.6	9.9	13.2	16.5
Distilled water	4.2	8.4	12.6	16.8	21
Separating gel buffer	2.5	5	7.5	10	12.5
10% APS	0.1	0.2	0.3	0.4	0.5
TEMED	0.004	0.008	0.012	0.016	0.02
12 % Gel	10 ml	20 ml	30 ml	40 ml	50 ml
Acrylamide Stock	4	8	12	16	20
Distilled water	3.5	7	10.5	14	17.5
Separating gel buffer	2.5	5	7.5	10	12.5
10% APS	0.1	0.2	0.3	0.4	0.5
TEMED	0.004	0.008	0.012	0.016	0.02
15 % Gel	10 ml	20 ml	30 ml	40 ml	50 ml
Acrylamide Stock	5	10	15	20	25
Distilled water	2.5	5	7.5	10	12.5
Separating gel buffer	2.5	5	7.5	10	12.5
10% APS	0.1	0.2	0.3	0.4	0.5
TEMED	0.004	0.008	0.012	0.016	0.02

- Degas the mixture and add TEMED and ammonium persulphate. Pour this solution in to plate up to the level such that 1 to 2 cm gap is allowed for stacking gel. Remove air bubbles if any.
- Add even layer of iso-butanol on the top of the separating gel solution to get a flat surface on the top of the gel.
- Allow the gel to polymerize for 30 minutes. Remove the iso-butanol layer and washed with water.
- Prepare the stacking gel solution as per as per the required concentration % and volume required (Table 38.2)

Table 38.2 - Quantity of reagents required to prepare Stacking gel

5 % Gel	10 ml	20 ml	30 ml	40 ml	50 ml
Acrylamide Stock	1.6	3.2	4.8	6.4	8
Distilled water	5.9	11.8	17.7	23.6	29.5
Stacking gel buffer	2.5	5	7.5	10	12.5
10% APS	0.1	0.2	0.3	0.4	0.5
TEMED	0.01	0.02	0.03	0.04	0.05
7.5 % Gel	10 ml	20 ml	30 ml	40 ml	50 ml
Acrylamide Stock	2.5	5	7.5	10	12.5
Distilled water	5	10	15	20	25
Separating gel buffer	2.5	5	7.5	10	12.5
10% APS	0.1	0.2	0.3	0.4	0.5
TEMED	0.004	0.008	0.012	0.016	0.02

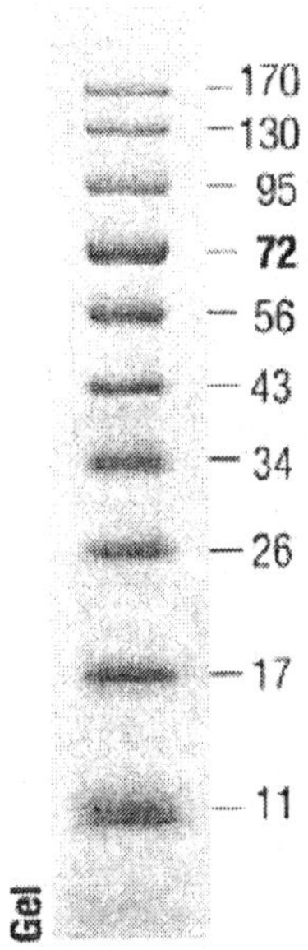

Fig 38.4 – Protein Marker

- Degas the mixture and add TEMED and ammonium per sulphate (Table 38.2).
- Pour the solution carefully on the top of the separating gel.
- After 20 minutes, remove the bottom spacer and fix the gel with slab gel unit. Remove the comb and fill up the wells with reservoir buffer.
- Add equal volume of sample buffer to the sample solution and boiled in a water for 30 minutes.
- Add 100-200µl of the above sample mixture or load into each well.
- Load standard protein mixture to any one of the well to compare the molecular weight of the sample proteins.
- Add reservoir buffer to anode and cathode chambers until the buffer touches the gel.
- Connect the power supply and apply 60v until the marker dye enters the separating gel and then increase the voltage to 100-200v.
- Continue the power supply until the marker dye reaches the bottom of the gel. Disconnect the power supply and remove the slab gel set up.
- Remove the glass plate and place the gel in coomassie brilliant blue stain for 2-4 hrs.
- Destain the gel in destaining solution mixture and obtain clear gel.
- Store the gel is stored in storing solution.

Observation and Result

Samples used: Crude extract from bacteria

Standard : Bovine serum Albumin

Different bands of protein stained with Brilliant Blue were observed.

Spotters: Sodium Dodecyl Sulphate, Acrylamide, Bis acrylamide, PAGE gel apparatus

Viva Questions:

Define electrophoresis

What are the applications of SDS in SDS – PAGE?

Why is this experiment called SDS-PAGE?

What are the uses of beta mercapto ethanol, TEMED, APS in SDS-PAGE?

39. Western Blotting

Aim

To transfer protein from gel to membrane.

To identify protein/ antigen/ antibody through immuno blotting.

Introduction

The transfer of protein bands from an acrylamide gel onto a more stable and immobilizing support is called as protein blotting. A number of supporting materials such as nitrocellulose, diazobenyloxymethyl cellulose sheets, nylon filters etc., are used for this purpose. This technique requires separation of proteins. The separated proteins are buried in polyacrylamide gel and therefore further analysis of proteins or their recovery is manageble. However, the proteins can be effectively transferred from the gel to the supporting medium by blotting. This method is an extension of southern blotting used to transfer DNA from gels to nitrocellulose filter and is called as the western blotting. Western blotting and immunodetection, together is a powerful analytic tool in biological studies.

Principle

The separated proteins are transported out of the gel by the capillary action of buffer in an electric field. The presence of SDS increases the solubility of proteins and thus facilitate the migration of proteins. Once out of the gel, the protein comes in contact with the nitrocellulose membrane, which binds the protein very strongly on to the surface as the thin band thus producing replica of original gel.

Materials Required

Nitrocellulose Membrane

Blotting buffer

0.02M Tris Hcl-2.42g

0.15M Glycine -10.25g

20% methanol-200mL

Water to one litter (can be stored at 4 ° C for 2-3 weeks)

Blocking buffer

Phosphate buffered saline   -100ml

Tween 20   —0.05ml

Bovine serum albumin   -1g

Assay buffer (10x)

Wash buffer

Primary antibody

Antigen

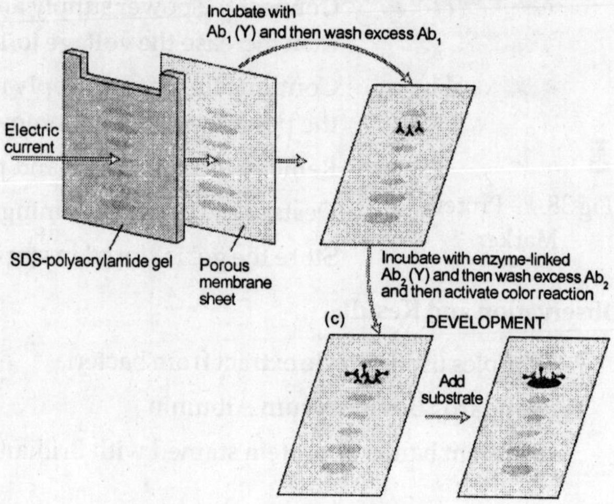

Fig 39.1- Mechanism of protein transfer

Labeled (conjugated) antibody

Preparation of conjugate (Antibody labeling)

- Conjugate means covalent complex of IgG and an enzyme.
- Dissolve 5 mG of horseradish peroxidase in 1 mL of 0.3 molar Na_2CO_3 (pH 8.1). The solution should prepare freshly.
- Add 0.1mL of 1% fluro dinitro benzene in pure alcohol. If the HRP used is not pure, a precipitate may be formed that must be removed by centrifugation (18,000 rpm for 10 minutes).
- Mix thoroughly and incubate for 1 hour at room temperature.
- Add 1mL of 0.16 molar ethylene glycol mix and incubate for another one hour at room temperature. The total volume is now 2.1mL.
- Dialyze the mixture against 0.01 molar sodium carbonate buffer (pH -9.5) for 25 hours. The buffer should be changed at least 3 times.

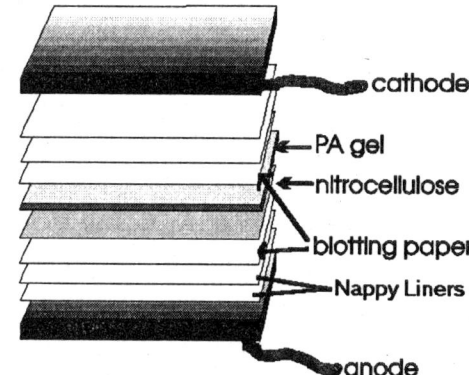

Fig 39.2: Arrangement of Membrane for electroblotting

- Add IgG dissolved in 0.01 molar sodium carbonate buffer (pH -9.5) to the peroxidase aldehyde solution in the following ratio. One volume IgG solution to one volume of activated peroxidase aldehyde or 5mG purified IgG to 3ml-peroxidase aldehyde solution.
- Mix well and incubate 2-3 hours but not longer at room temperature. If any precipitate is formed clarify by centrifugation at 10,000 rpm for 10 minutes.
- Dialyze extensively against 0.01 molar phosphate buffer (pH 7.2) containing 0.9 % sodium chloride at 4 ° C. Store the conjugate in a refrigerator or freezer in small aliquots and use once only

Substrate

- Protein stain : 0.1% amidoblack 10 B in methanol: acetic acid: water (5:1:5)
- Transfer of protein is carried out either by electrophoresis (electroblotting) or by the capillary action of buffer (capillary blotting)

Procedure

Electro blotting

- Assemble the blotting sandwich with in the blotting cassette as shown in Fig. 39.2. Take care to avoid air bubbles between the gel and nitrocellulose membrane.
- Insert the cassette into the apparatus filled with blotting buffer and connect the power supply. The gel should be towards cathode and the membrane towards anode.
- Apply current 35V, overnight or 50 V, 5 hours for blotting.
- During this step transfer of proteins from the gel to the membrane takes place by protein binding property of the nitrocellulose membrane.
- In this method, transfer buffer used have low ionic strength, which allows Electro transfer of proteins without current; this avoids the generation of heat. Methanol used in the buffer to increase binding of protein to nitrocellulose and to reduce the swelling of the gel during transfer.

Immuno detection

- Remove the nitrocellulose membrane from the casette.

- Place the membrane in blocking buffer for 2 hour at room temperature or over night in the cold.

- Suspend 20µL primary antibody in 10ml assay buffer in a suitable apparatus.

- Immerse blot in the primary antibody solution and agitate gently for 30 minutes.

- Wash the blot by immersing in wash buffer for 3-5 minutes. Repeat two more times.

- Prepare a 1:1000 dilution of labeled antibody in assay buffer. Prepare a sufficient (10-ml) volume of diluted antibody to cover the blot.

- Immerse the blot in a labeled second antibody solution and agitate gently for 30 minutes.

- Wash the blot by immersing in wash buffer for 3-5 minutes. Repeat two more times.

- Immerse the washed blot in 10 mL of substrate solution with gentle shaking. Bands should develop sufficient colour with in 5-10 minutes.

- Remove the blot and wash with distilled water and dry.

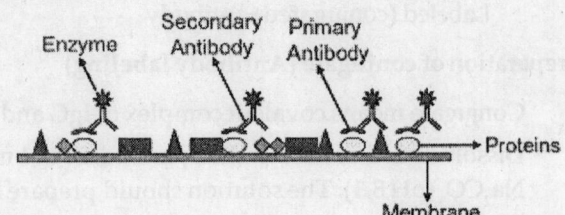

Fig: 39.2 - Reaction occurring on the membrane. Protein binds on the membrane. Primary antibody binds to the specific protein followed by the secondary which has an enzyme linked whose reaction can be visualized

Observation and result

Specific bands of specific proteins are observed and indicated the presence of virus/ antibody.

Spotters: Nitrocellulose membrane, Western blot assembly.

Viva questions

Mention enzymes and chemicals used in western blotting

What are the needs of western blotting?

What are the importance of western blotting in HIV testing?

40. Immunoflurescence test.

Aim

To demonstrate antigen (Bacterial / viral / fungal) by immunofluorescence (IF) test.

Background information

Immunofluorescence (IF) is one of the method adopted to detect antigens from clinical specimen. It is widely used for the rapid diagnosis of antigens as well as antibodies. This test makes use of a fluorescence – labeled antibody /antigen to stain specimens containing specific antigen /antibody, so that the stained cells fluoresces under UV illumination. There are two types of IF, direct IF, and indirect IF. Direct IF detects antigens where as indirect IF detects antibodies. Fluorescein

Box:40.1 – Advantages and disadvantages of IF

Advantages

More rapid and sensitive .

Use full identification of all types of antigens.

More specific.

Disadvantages:

Non quantitative test.

Requires expertise .

Requires expensive equipment .

Fluorescent dye fades faster.

Requires UV radiation for visualization.

isothioacyanate is the most commonly used dye . This dye emits a greenish / yellowish light. Other dye in these tests are Rhodamine (red / orange), dansyl (yellow) and phycoerythrin (red).

Direct IF antibody test used to detect antigens of bacteria, viruses, fungi and parasites in the serum, CSF, urine, faeces, tissues and other clinical samples. Eg. Influenza virus, *Corynebacterium diphtheriae, Niesseria gonorrrhoea etc.*

Principle

Antibody developed against antigens to be tested is labeled with a fluorescent dye and is used to detect unknown antigen. IF antigen is found in the specimen, the antigen will bind the fluorescein labeled antibodies . This specific antigen antibody reaction will emit a fluorescents, which will be observed by a fluorescent microscope using UV radiation .

Materials required

Fluorescent microscope, Acetone, Phosphate buffered saline (pH 7.2), Buffered glycerol (7.2), 10 % Glycerol in PBS, Evans Blue counter stain (1: 10000), BSA, Glass slides, petriplates, Glass rod, filter paper, coplin jar, Commercially available Gp A *Streptococcus pyogenes* culture .

Procedure

- Take clean glass slide.
- Prepare the smear using unknown *Streptococcus pyogenes* culture.
- Fix the smear with acetone or alcohol.
- Add one drop of fluorescent-labeled antibody on to the slide.
- Allow the antibody to spread.
- Keep the Smear with antibody containing slide in petriplate and incubate at 28^0C for 30 minutes.
- Wash the slide with 1 % buffered saline to remove away excess antibody.
- Place the slide in coplin jar containing 1 % buffered saline for 10 minutes at 25 °C.
- Allow the slide to dry.
- Add one drop of buffered glycerol on to the slide and covered with cover slip.
- Examine the slide under fluorescent microscope.

Observation

Slide showed the presence of fluorescence.

Result

Fluorescence on *Streptococcus pyogenes* smeared slide indicated that the sample contains *Streptococcus pyogenes*. The infection is due to the gram positive bacterium *Streptococcus pyogenes* . We may change antigen and antibody to detect / identify specific diseases. 1-10μg / mL of phenylene diamine could be added to the mounting medium to prevent fading of fluorescent dye

Viva questions :

What are the principles of Immunofluorescence test ?
Give examples for fluorescent dye ?
What are the difference between direct IF and indirect IF ?
Mention advantages and disadvantages of IF test ?

Medical Microbiology

A. Clinical Biochemistry and Haematology

41. Total Erythrocyte Count

Aim

To estimate the total erythrocyte count using haemocytometer.

Clinical significance

Dutch biologist Jan Swammerdam is the first person who described RBC from the blood of a frog. Decreased RBC is indicated during trauma, burns, pregnancy, haemolytic anemia, haemorrhagic infections, gastrointestinal (GI) or other vascular bleed, iron deficiency anaemia, vitamin B12 or folate deficiency, bone marrow damage, Metabolic disorders, Chronic inflammation.

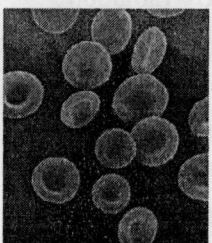

Fig. 41.1:
Structure of RBC

Increased RBC is seen during dehydration, pulmonary disease, congenital heart disease, polycythemia, renal problems, over-transfusion of whole blood, tissue hypoxia.

Principle

A sample of whole blood is mixed with a RBC Diluting fluid (Box 41.2) that acts as Anti-coagulant, Anti-haemolysis, Anti-aggregation, Anti-rouleaux (Box 46.1), Preserve RBC shape and Lyse WBC.

Normal Value

Male-> 4.56million cells/cumm.
Female-> 4 to 4.5 million cells/cumm.

Materials required

Specimen: Capillary blood is recommended.

Miocroscope with low power and high power objective, Neubauer counting chamber with coverslip, shali pipette, test tube, cotton.

RBC diluting fluid (Citrate Formalin Solution or Dacies fluid)

RBC diluting fluid prepared by adding 3g Trisodium citrate and 1mL formalin in 100mL of distilled water.

Box 41.1 – Symptoms and Management

Headache, Chest Pain, Pale skin, Fatigue, Weak, Short of breath, Increased heart rate **indicates that you have low red blood cell count.** Rest between activities, Plan ahead and save your energy for the most important activities, Avoid or stop activities that make you short of breath or make your heart beat faster, Eat a diet with adequate protein and vitamins, Drink plenty of non-caffeinated and non-alcoholic fluids are things to be done **to manage low red blood count**

Box 41.2 RBC Diluting Fluids

Gower's solution is a diluting fluid for red cell counts; an isotonic solution containing sodium sulfate and glacial acetic acid.

Hayem's solution is an isotonic fluid used for diluting blood samples in red blood cell counts. Contains mercuric chloride, sodium sulfate and sodium chloride.

Citrate Formalin Solution is a RBC diluting fluid contains Trisodium citrate and formalin.

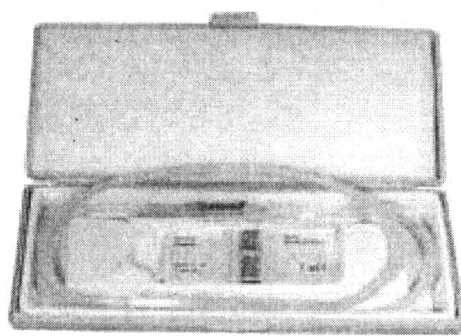

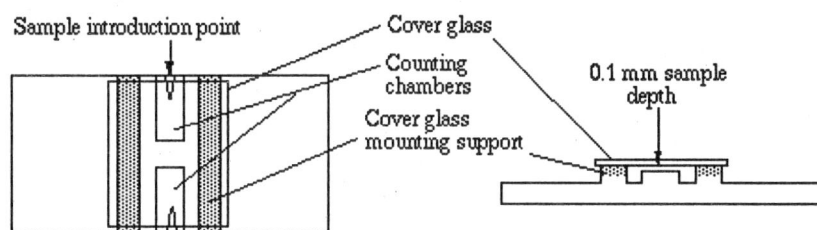

Fig 41.2 : Haemocytometer   Fig 41.3 : Ruling area and method of sample introduction

Procedure

- Fill Red blood cell pipette with capillary blood up to 0.5 mark by holding the pipette horizontally.

- Draw RBC diluting fluid up to the mark 101. While filling the bulb, the pipette should be gently rotated to obtain good mixing.

- Place the cover slip over the Neubauer chamber so as to cover the ruled platform evenly.

- Now load the chamber. This is done in 3 steps.

  ◆ Mix the contents of pipette for 3 minutes.

  ◆ Expell 6 drops from the pipette to remove the fluid in the stem that has not been mixed with the blood.

  ◆ By holding the pipette at an angle of 45⁰ and touching the space between the cover slip and the chamber by the point of the pipette, allow an appropriate drop of the mixture to run under the cover glass by capillary action.

Box 41.3 : Description about Counting chamber

The adjacent **figure 41.4** shows the rulings (improved Neubauer), which are inscribed on the counting chamber. The smallest squares in the large center square (where red cells are counted) have an area of 1/400 mm and are arranged in groups of 16. Each group of 16 squares is set off from the others by triple lines. The middle line is the one, which actually defines the area of the squares adjacent to such a triple line. The inner line, therefore, is included within the area of the square.

Erythrocytes in five of the 25 groups of 16 small squares are counted. These groups are the four corner groups and the one in the center.

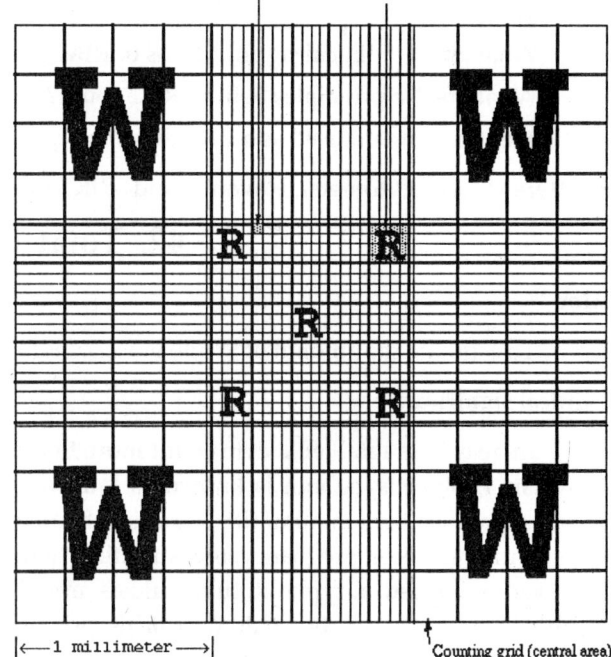

Small square = 1/400 sq. mm.   1/25 sq. mm.

|←—1 millimeter—→| Counting grid (central area)

Fig 41.4 : Neubauer counting chamber

- Allow sample 2 minutes to settle.
- Place counting chamber on the stage of the microscope.
- Switched on the microscope to low power objective adjust the light and locate large square in the center with 25 small square.
- Count the RBC in the four corner squares and in the centre squares.
- Make the total of the all the cells counted in 5 squares and calculate the RBC/cumm by the following equation.

Calculation

$$\text{Number of RBC/mL} = \frac{\text{No. of cells counted X Dilution}}{\text{Area counted X Depth of fluid}}$$

Dilution= 200 ; Area counted = 5 X 0.04 = 0.2; Depth of fluid = 0.1 mm

$$\text{Factor} = \frac{\text{Dilution}}{\text{Volume}} = \frac{200}{0.2 \text{X} 0.1}$$

$$= 10,000$$

So RBC/cumm of the blood = Number of cells counted X 10,000

Result

The given blood sample contains -_____million cells/cumm of red blood cells.

Viva questions

Why there is a need of higher dilution of blood in RBC count?

What are the clinical significations of RBC count?

What are the principles behind RBC count?

Mention reagent used as a RBC diluting agent.

Spotters - Haemocytometer, Hayems fluid/RBC diluting fluid, Neubauer counting chamber, RBC structure.

42. Total Leucocyte Count

Aim

To estimate the amount of White blood cells (leukocyte) in human blood.

Clinical significance

Increased in total leukocyte count more than 10,000 cells/cu.mm is known as **leukocytosis** and decrease of less than 4,000 cells/cu.mm is known as **leucopenia**. Pathological leukocytosis observed in infection such as pneumonia, tonsilitis, meningititis, abscess, rheumatic fever, diphtheria, small pox, chicken pox, erythroblastosis foetalis, uremia, ulcer, pregnancy, menstruation, high temperature, severe pain and muscular exercise. Leukopenia is observed in influenza, typhoid, tuberculosis, measles, brucellosis, agranulocytosis, hepatitis B infection, dengue, sandfly fever, radiation, rheumatoid arthritis, primary bone marrow depressions and megaloblast conditions. Counts that continue to rise or fall to abnormal levels indicate that the condition is getting worse. Counts that return to normal indicate improvement. Pregnancy in the final month and labor may be associated with increased WBC levels.

There are many drugs that cause both increased and decreased WBC counts. Smoking may also cause an increased WBC count.

Principle

The blood is diluted to 1:20 with the WBC diluting fluid. The Glacial acetic acid lyses RBC while the Gentian violet stain the nuclei of leukocytes. A weak acid solution that lyses nonnucleated red blood cells. The cells are counted under low power objective by using counting chamber. The number of white blood cells in undiluted blood are calculated and reported as the number of WBC/ cu.mm of whole blood.

Normal Value

Adult → 4,000 to 10,000 cells/cumm

At birth → 10,000 to 25,000cells/cumm

1 to 3 years → 6,000 to 18,000 cells/cumm

4 to 7 years → 6,000 to 15,000 cells/cumm

8 to 12 years → 4,500 to 14,000 cells/cumm

Box 42.1 – Reason for high and low WBC count

A low number of WBCs is called leukopenia. It may be due to: Bone marrow failure (for example, due to infection, tumor, or abnormal scarring), Collagen-vascular diseases, Disease of the liver or spleen, Radiation

A high number of WBCs is called leukocytosis. It may be due to: Anemia, Infectious diseases, Inflammatory disease, Leukemia, Severe emotional or physical stress, Tissue damage (for example, burns)

Materials required

Capillary blood is recommended for total leukocyte count, Microscope, Neubauer counting chamber with coverslip, shali pipette, WBC diluting fluid (Trucks Fluid) - WBC diluting fluid is prepared by mixing 1% aqueous solution of Gentian violet in 2mL of Glacial acetic acid and 100mL distilled water. Solution is mixed properly with stirrer and the solution is ready for use.

Procedure

- Draws blood in a clean dry pipette upto the mark 0.5.

- Wipe off the outside of the pipette with cotton.

- Now draw the diluting fluid upto the mark 11(dilution 1 in 20).

- Hold pipette horizontally and mix the contents of the pipette for 5 minutes for complete haemolysis of RBCs.

- Expel the first 4 drops of the content.

- Place the haemocytometer on a flat surface with the cover slip on the counting chamber.

- Load the haemocytometer with the mixture, by holding the pipette at 45^0 angle and touching the space between the cover glass and the chamber by the point up the pipette, an appropriate drop of the mixture is allowed to run under the cover glass by capillary action. It must be sufficiently large to cover the whole ruled platform, yet not large enough to fill the moats. Also there must be no air bubbles.

- Leave the counting chamber undisturbed for 3to5 minutes to allow the cells to settle.

- Place the counting chamber on the stage of the microscope. Switch to the low power objective

- Adjust the light and locates the large square on one of the corner with it small squares.

- Scan all large corner squares and count the cells, which are identified by their blue colour with a large nucleus. Make a total of all the cells counted in 4 squares and calculate the WBC/cu.mm by following calculations

Calculation

$$\text{Number of WBC/cumm} = \frac{\text{No of WBC counted X Dilution}}{\text{Area counted X Depth of the fluid}}$$

Dilution = 20,   Area counted = 4, Depth of the fluid = 0.1mm,

I.e. WBC counted in whole blood = No of cells counted x factor

$$\text{Factor} = \frac{20}{4 \text{ X } 0.1} = 50$$

Result

The given blood sample having – – – – – –cells / cumm.

Viva questions

Define leucocytosis, leucopenia.

Mention clinical condition associated with leucopenia.

Reason for leucocytosis.

Mention name of the ingredient present in WBC diluting fluid.

What is Trucks fluid?

Explain the role of gentian violet and glacial acetic acid in WBC diluting fluid.

Spotters – Trucks fluid, Haemocytometer.

43. Total Platelet count

Aim

To count number of platelets present in the given blood sample.

Background information

Platelets or thrombocytes are the cells circulating in the blood of mammals that are involved in haemostasis leading to the formation of blood clots. Like red blood cells, platelets have no nucleus. Primary haemostasis is the immediate response to injury, which involves platelets. Secondary haemostasis is the next response to injury, which involves other components of the clotting system. If the number of platelets is too low, that can cause bleeding. If the numbers of platelets is too high, that can cause blood clots (thrombosis) which block blood vessels and cause strokes and heart attacks. An abnormality or disease of the platelets is called a **thrombocytopathy** which could be either a low number (thrombocytopenia), a decrease in function (**thrombasthenia**) or an increase in number (**thrombocytosis**).

Box 43.1: Drugs suppress platelet function

Oral agents - aspirin, clopidogrel, cilostazol, ticlopidine. Intravenous agents - abciximab, eptifibatide, tirofiban. Others - acetaminophen, quinidine, sulfa drugs, digoxin, vancomycin, valium, and nitroglycerine.

Normal value

In an adult, a normal count is about 150,000 to 450,000 platelets /mL of blood. If platelet levels fall below 20,000 /mL , spontaneous bleeding may occur and is considered a life-threatening risk.

Clinical significance

Disorders leading to a reduced platelet count are Thrombocytopenia, Idiopathic thrombocytopenic purpura - also known as immune thrombocytopenic purpura (ITP), Thrombotic thrombocytopenic purpura, Drug-induced thrombocytopenia, e.g. heparin-induced thrombocytopenia (HIT), Gaucher's disease, Aplastic anemia, Alloimmune disorders, Fetomaternal alloimmune thrombocytopenia. Patients undergoing chemotherapy or radiation therapy may also have a decreased platelet count. Up to 5% of pregnant women may experience thrombocytopenia at term.

Increased platelet counts (thrombocytosis) may be seen in individuals who show no significant medical problems and with significant blood problem called myeloproliferative disorder. Increased platelets may induce sticking, forming clumps that can block blood vessel and cause damage, including death (thromboembolism).

Materials required

Red pipette, Rubber pipe, Plastic syringe, Pipette vibrator, Haemocytometer & cover slip (Counting chamber), Microscope, Rees and Ecker Platelet Diluting Fluid. It is a clear, dark blue liquid. It contains Brilliant Cresyl Blue (0.1g), Formaldehyde (0.2mL), Sodium Citrate Dihydrate (3.8g) and Deionized Water (100mL). Filter the solution each time before use.

Procedure

- Fill blood into red pipette upto 0.5 mark.
- Fill reagent add up into the pipette to 101 mark.
- Rotate the pipette horizontally for complete mixing of blood and diluting fluid.
- Discard the first 3-4 drops.
- Fill in the haemocytometer nicely.
- Allow platelets to set down in moisture chamber for 15 min.
- Count 4 WBC squares under microscope (x400).
- Calculate the Platelet concentration by making use of following formula.

Calculation

Volume of 1 WBC square	$= 1 \times 1 \times 0.1$ cu.mm.
	$= 0.1$ cu.mm.
Volume of 4 WBC square	$= 0.1 \times 4$ cu.mm.
	$= 0.4$ cu.mm.
In 0.4 cu.mm. the Platelet count	$= N$ (counted No.)
In 1 cu.mm. the Platelet count	$= N \times 1 / 0.4$
	$= N \times 2.5$
The dilution for Platelet count	$= 0.5 / 100$
	$= 200$
The final Platelet count	$= N \times 2.5 \times 200$
	$= 500 \, N$ (/cu.mm.)
Calculation Platelet count	$=$ number of Platelets counted (N) x volume factor (=2.5) x dilution factor (=200)
	$= N \times 500$
Normal range	$= 140,000 - 440,000 / $ cu.mm.
	$= 140 - 440 \times 10^3 / $ cu.mm.

Viva questions

Mention the name of platelet diluting fluid.

What are the functions of thrombocytes?

Mention few commercial drugs which supress the function of thrombocytes

Mention about the clinical significance of platelet count.

Define thrombocytopathy, thrombosis, haemostasis, thrombocytopaenia, thromblastenia, thrombocytosis, thromboembolism.

Spotters – Platelet diluting fluid/Rees Ecker fluid

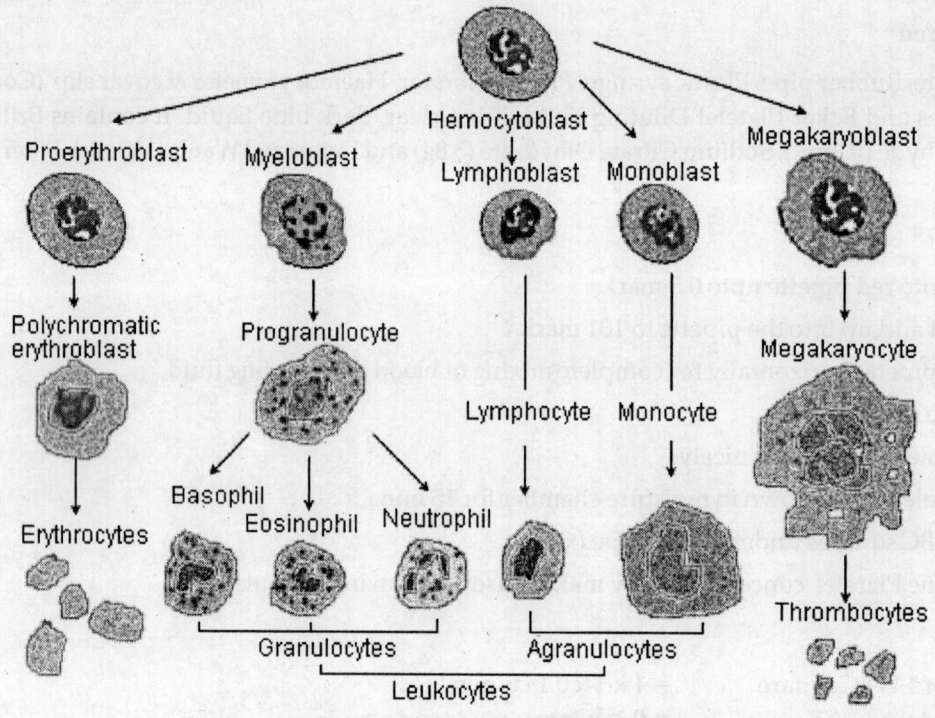

Fig 43.1 : Haematopoiesis

44. Differential Count

Aim

To differentiate leukocytes.

To assesses the ability of the body to respond and fight infection.

To detects the severity of allergic reactions, parasitic and other types of infection and drug reactions.

To identify some types of leukaemia or lymphoma.

Principle

Three major step involved in differential count are preparation of smear, staining of smear, microscopic observation. The smear is made with a drop of blood taken directly from the skin puncture, which gives the true picture of blood morphology. Staining is done with polychromatic stain, that includes methylene blue and eosin

(Leishman's stain). The polychromatic stain induces multiple colours when applying to the cells. The stain is dissolved in Methanol and buffer (pH-7 to 7.2). Methanol act as a fixing agent and also as a solvent. Following staining the basic components of white cell are stained by the acidic eosin dye and they are described as eosinophilic or acidophilic, where the acidic components of blood (nucleus and nucleic acids) take blue to purple shade by the basic dyes and they are called basophilic. The neutral components present in the blood cells are probably stained by both of the dyes.

Clinical significance

Neutrophils can increase in response to bacterial infection, inflammatory disease, steroid medication or more rarely leukaemia. Decreased neutrophil levels may be the result of severe infection or other conditions such chemotherapy. *Eosinophils* can increase in response to allergic disorders, inflammation of the skin and parasitic infections. They can also occur in response to some infections or to various bone marrow malignancies. *Basophils* can increase in cases of leukaemia, long-standing inflammation, the presence of a hypersensitivity reaction to food or radiation therapy. *Lymphocytes* can increase in cases of bacterial or viral infection, leukaemia, lymphoma or radiation therapy. Decreased lymphocyte levels are common in later life but can also indicate steroid medication, stress, lupus and HIV infection. *Monocyte* levels can increase in certain leukaemias, in response to infection of all kinds as well as to inflammatory disorders. Decreased monocyte levels can indicate bone marrow injury or failure and some forms of leukaemia.

Materials Required

Two clean slides, Finger puncture blood, lancet, Spirit, Compound microscope with oil immersion, Buffer (pH – 6.8) etc.

Leishman's stain preparation: it is performed by grinding 2g Leishman stain powder in pestle and mortar by adding small quantity of methanol. After complete grinding and mixing the solution is made up to 100mL using Methanol These two components are mixed thoroughly and warmed up to 50°C. Filter the solution and it is ready to use.

Buffer is prepared as follows- A. Na_2HPO_4 –9.47g /L; B. KH_2PO_4 –9.08g/L. Mix 49.6mL solution A and 50.4mL solution B to get 100 mL Phosphate buffer.

Normal value

Neutrophils – 50-70%
Lymphocytes – 20-40%
Eosinophils-1-3%
Monocytes – 1-5%
Basophils –1%

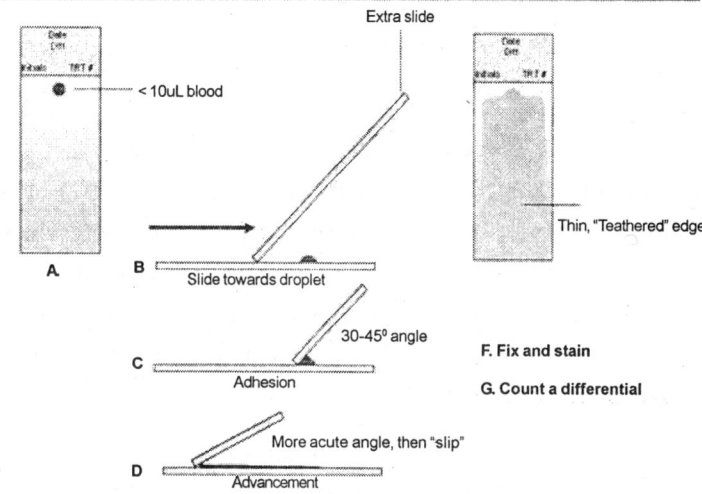

Fig 44.1 : Blood smearing

Procedure

Preparation of smear

• Place a drop of blood onto the center of the slide about ½ inch from the end.

- Holding a second clean slide at a 40° angle, touch the angled end to the midlength area of the specimen slide. Pull the angled slide back into the blood, and allow the blood to almost fill the end area of the angled slide.

- Continue contact with the blood under the lower edge, quickly and steadily moving the angled slide until the blood is used up.

- Dry the blood smear.

Fixing and staining (Methanol present in the stain fixes the smear).

- Keep the slide on the staining rack with the blood smear facing up.

- Apply undiluted Leishmann's stain over the smear and is left undisturbed for 2 minutes.

- Apply buffered water over the stained smear and allow continuing for 5-7 minutes.

- Washed off the slide in the stream of buffered water.

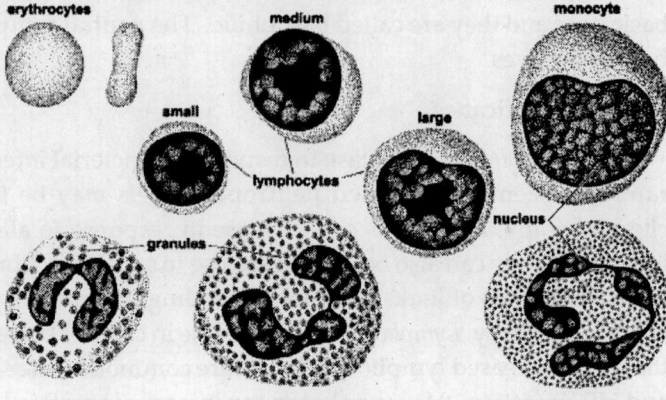

Fig 44.2 : Morphological variations of WBC

Examination of blood smear:

- Examine the stained blood smear under a low power microscope (In an ideal smear 3 zones are identified, the thick area or head following which is the body and the tail with the thin and of smear. The portion of blood smear, which appears slightly before the tail end of the smear is chosen).

- Place a drop of immersion oil on slide (various types of WBC are identified and enumerated based on the staining and morphology of the nucleus Fig 44.2).

Observation

Granulocytes: These are granulated cells, which stained pink and include eosinophils, Basophiles and Neutrophils.

Neutrophils: Pale pink cytoplasm with fine coloured granules includes band and segmented form.

Eosinophils: Cytoplasm stains pink colour and contains red and orange granules.

Basophils: Cytoplasmic granules are large, dark and blue -black coloured.

Lymphocytes: Large size lymphocytes have clear blue cytoplasm on the margin of the nucleus. In smaller size lymphocytes a dark violet colour almost fills the entire cell and has rim of clear cytoplasm.

Result

Different forms of WBC are observed based on nucleus morphology. Number of different WBC present in the sample also counted and compared with normal value. Based on blood WBC picture individual's infectious status are interpretated.

Viva questions

What are the principles of differential count?
Name the major ingredients of leishman's stain.
Mention clinical significance of neutrophils, lymphocytes and monocytes
How do you differentiate different types of WBC?
Differentiate granulocytes from agranulocytes.

Spotters-Blood smear, leishman's stain, neutrophils, lymphocytes, eosinophils.

45. Haemoglobin Estimation

Aim

To determine haemoglobin by shalli haematin method.

Clinical Significance

A decrease in haemoglobin below the normal range is an indication of anaemia. Haemoglobin level is also decreased in pregnancy, blood loss, malnutrition, polycythemia, congenital heart disease due to reduced oxygen supply and in haemo concentration due to loss of body fluids in severe diarrhoea and vomiting.

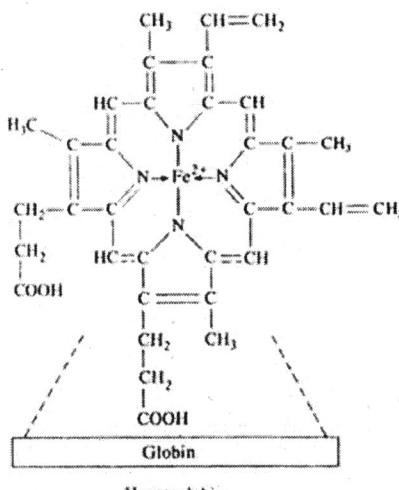

Normal Value

Male   -14-18g/dL

Female   -11.5-16.5g/dL

Children -11-14.5g/dL

Materials Required

Fig 45.1-Structure of Haemoglobin

Specimen-anticoagulated blood, Shali haemoglobino meter, Calibrated tube for haemoglobin measurement, Shali pipette, 0.1N Hcl, Distilled water, Pasture pipette etc.,

Principle

When blood is added to 0.1N Hcl, haemoglobin is converted into brown coloured acid haematin. The resulting colour after dilution is compared with standard reference of haemoglobinometer.

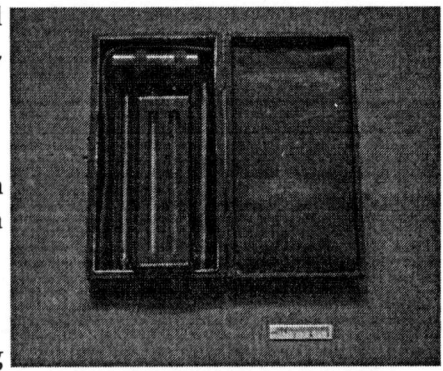

Procedure

- Add 0.1N of Hcl upto the lowest mark of the calibrated tube by using Pasteur pipette

Fig 45.2: Haemometer Kit

- Draw 20µL of the blood in the shali pipette, wiped excess blood with the help of dry cotton.
- Transfer the blood to the acid in the calibration tube
- Mix blood and acid well and allow to stand for at least 10 minutes at room temperature.
- Dilute the solution with few drops of water and mixed well.
- Repeat the dilution until the colour matches with the standard glass in the haemometer
- Match the colour against the natural light.
- Note the level of the fluid at its lowest miniscus and record the reading corresponding level on the scale in the g/dL.

Observation and result

G% of Haemoglobin is observed based on colour of acid haematin in calibrated tube and the results are interpreted as normal or abnormal by referring normal value chart.

Viva questions

Describe the clinical significance of haemoglobin count

Mention the normal haemoglobin content in male/ female / children?

What is the principle of haematin method?

Mention alternate method for haemoglobin estimation

Spotters -Haemometer, structure of haemoglobin.

46. Erythrocyte Sedimentation Rate

Aim

To estimate the Erythrocyte sedimentation rate by Westergren method.

Clinical significance

This test was invented in 1897 by the Polish doctor Edmund Biernacki. ESR is a non-specific test that reflex changes in plasma protein which accompanist most of the acute & chronic infections. These pathological conditions accelerate rouleaux formation of red cells. As a result of rouleaux formation ESR increases which suggest the possible pathological condition. Normalization of ESR indicates possible recovery from the disease. The ESR is increased by any cause or focus of inflammation. The ESR is decreased in sickle cell anaemia, polycythemia and congestive heart failure. The basal ESR is slightly higher in females. ESR is performed to monitor inflammation. ESR rate is high during inflammation.

> **Box 46.1: Rouleaux** are stacks of red blood cells formed (Coin roll formation) because of the unique discoid shape of these cells in vertebrate body. The presence of acute phase proteins particularly fibrinogen interacts with sialic acid on the surface of RBC and allows the formation of rouleaux.

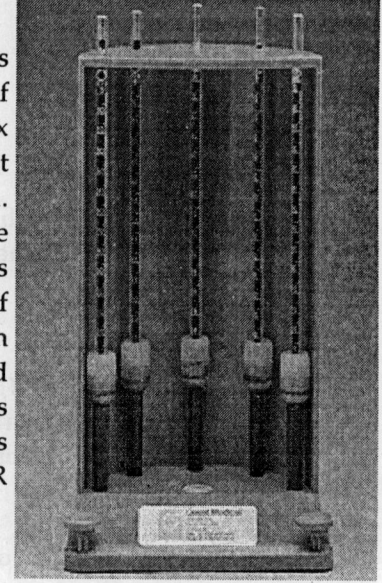

Fig 46.1 : Westergren tube with stand

Principle

The Erythrocyte Sedimentation Rate (ESR) is a nonspecific assay used to screen the presence or absence of active disease. The settling of red corpuscles (red blood cells - RBCs) is due to the differential densities of the RBCs and their medium. Most often, an increased ESR is due to an increased amount of plasma proteins (i.e., acute phase globulins and less commonly to inherent characteristics of RBCs (Wintrobe 30). ESR is measured in mm/hr using the Modified Westergren Method. Normally red cells do not settle far toward the bottom of the tube. Many diseases make extra or abnormal proteins that cause the red cells to move close together, stack up, and form a column (rouleaux). In a group, red cells are heavier and fall faster. The faster they fall, the further they settle and the higher the ESR.

Normal value:

Men - 5-15 mm/hour

Women- 5-20 mm/hour

Materials required

Specimen: Citrate blood (mix 1.6mL blood with 0.4 mL of 3.8% sodium citrate solution), 3.8% sodium citrate solution, Westergren tube calibrated in millimeters, Rack for holding Westerngren tubes (ESR stand), Timer, Vials or test tubes.

Procedure

- Place the Westerngren rack in a leveled plain surface, away from direct sunlight and air-drift.
- Fill the Westerngren tube exactly to the '0' mark.
- Set the timer exactly for 30minutes.
- Note the level to which the red cell column has fallen at the end of 30minutes.
- Repeat the reading upto 60minutes.
- Report the result in mm/30minutes and mm/60 seconds

Observation and result

Settled cells were measured using calibrated westergren tube. Compare normal value before interpretation.

Viva questions

Expand ESR

Clinical significance of ESR

What are the principles behind ESR?

What is the need of citrated blood in ESR estimation?

Mention physiological condition associated with ESR

Spotters - Westergtsen tube, ESR stand.

47. Serum Glutamate Oxaloacetate Transaminase (SGOT)

Aim

To detect the level of SGOT in the given serum sample.

Principle

The method is called as Reitnian and Franked method.

GOT catalyzes the following reactions

α - Ketoglutamate + L - Aspartate $\leftrightarrow$ L. Glutamate + Oxaloacetate

Oxaloacetate is coupled with 2,4,dinitro phenyl hydrazine which gives known colour in alkaline medium and this is measured calorimeterically at 505nm.

Background information

Serum glutamte oxaloacetate transaminase (SGOT) is an enzyme, normally present in liver and heart cells. SGOT is released into blood when the liver or heart is damaged. The blood SGOT levels are thus elevated with liver damage (for example, from viral hepatitis) or with an insult to the heart (for example, from a heart attack). Some medications can also raise SGOT levels. SGOT is also called aspartate aminotransferase (AST). Aspartate aminotransferase (AST), formerly called serum glutamic-oxaloacetate transaminase or SGOT. In liver disease, the AST increase is usually less than the ALT increase. However, in liver disease caused by alcohol use, the AST increase may be two or three times greater than the ALT increase.

AST High levels may indicate liver cell damage, hepatitis, heart attack, heart failure, or gall stones.

Advantages:

Highly popular and simple method.

This method gives reproducible results.

Substrate and standard are specially stabilizes.

It is very economical.

Normal value

AST: 0-35 IU/L

Abnormal SGOT Value indications

20-200 IU/L indicates Coronary infraction, 250-1500 IU/L indicates Hepatic damage and 50-100 IU/L indicates Jaundice.

Materials Required

Test tubes, conical flask, standard measuring flask, pH meter, spectrophotometer.

Phosphate buffer : Dissolve 5.965g of di sodium hydrogen phosphate and 1.09g potassium dihydrogen phosphate in water and dilute to 500 mL (pH-7.4).

Standard solution : Dissolve 0.022g Sodium pyruvate in 100mL of phosphate buffer. Make fresh as needed.

GOT substrate : Transfer 0.146g of α - Ketoglutarate and 13.3 g of DL Aspartic acid to a beaker. Add 1N Sodium hydroxide until the solution is complete. Adjust the pH 7.4 with sodium hydroxide and dilute to 500mL with phosphate buffer.

DNPH colour developer : Dissolve 0.099g of 2,4 dinitrophenyl hydrazine in 500mL of 1N hydrochloric acid. Store in dark bottle in the refrigerator.

NaOH solution 0.4N : Dissolve 8g of NaOH in distilled water and dilute to 500mL with distilled water.

Procedure

- Pipette 0.5mL of GOT substrate into a test tube and place in 37 ^{0}C for 5 minutes in waterbath.
- Add 0.1mL of serum and mix.
- Incubate exactly 60 minutes for SGOT
- Add 0.5mL of DNPH and mix
- Let stand at room temperature for 20 minutes.
- Add 5mL of 0.4N NaOH, mix vigorously and let stand for 5 minutes.
- Read colour calorimetrically at 505nm. Follow Same procedure for standards.

Calibration curve/Standard graph is prepared by using following table 47.1

Table47.1 : Calibration curve

Reagent	Blank	1	2	3	4	5	Incubation
Distilled water	0.2mL	0.2mL	0.2mL	0.2mL	0.2mL	0.2mL	
Substrate	1mL	0.9mL	0.8mL	0.7mL	0.6mL	0.5mL	5minutes / water bath
Standard	— —	0.1mL	0.2mL	0.3mL	0.4mL	0.5mL	60OT / water bath
DNPH	1mL	1mL	1mL	1mL	1mL	1mL	20 minutes / room temp.
NaOH	10mL	10mL	10mL	10mL	10mL	10mL	5 minutes / room temp.

Observation

Table 47.2: Result reporting table

Tube No.	True OD	SGOT/IU
1		22
2		55
3		95
4		150
5		215
TEST		

Results

Colour change is noted and read at 505nm. True OD values are plotted against SGOT/IU. Results are interpreted after comparison with normal value.

Viva questions

Expand DNPH, GOT , SGOT , AST.

What is the clinical significance associated with SGOT.

What are the principles of SGOT detection?

Spotters - DNPH, sodium pyruvate.

48. Serum Glutamate Pyruvate Transaminase (SGPT)

Aim

To detect the level of SGPT in the given serum sample.

Principle

α - Ketoglutarate + L. Alanine ↔ L. Glutamine + Pyruvate

Pyruvate couples with 2,4, dinitro phenyl hydrazine (2, 4 DNPH) to give the corresponding hydrazone, which gives known colour in alkaline medium, which is measured calorimetrically at 505nm.

Background information

Alanine aminotransferase (ALT), formerly called serum glutamate pyruvate transaminase or SGPT, is an enzyme necessary for energy production. It is present in a number of tissues, including the liver, heart and skeletal muscles, but is found in the highest concentration in the liver. Because of this, it is used in conjunction with other liver enzymes to detect liver disease, especially hepatitis or cirrhosis without jaundice. Additionally, in conjunction with the aspartate aminotransferase test (AST), it helps to distinguish between heart damage and liver tissue damage. ALT Values are significantly increased in cases of hepatitis, and moderately increased in cirrhosis, liver tumor, obstructive jaundice, and severe burns. Values are mildly increased in pancreatitis, heart attack, infectious mononucleosis and shock. Most useful when compared with ALP levels.

Normal Reference Values

Male : upto 40 IU/L at 37°C

Female : upto 31 IU/L at 37°C

Abnormal SGPT Value indications

70 -75 IU/L indicates Coronary infraction, 50-1000IU/L indicatesHepatic damage and 100 – 200IU/L indicates Jaundice.

Materials required

Test tubes, conical flask, standard measuring flask, pH meter, spectrophotometer

Phosphate buffer : Dissolve 5.965g of di sodium hydrogen phosphate and 1.09g potassium dihydrogen phosphate in water and dilute to 500 mL(pH-7.4).

Standard solution : Dissolve 0.022g Sodium pyruvate in 100mL of phosphate buffer. Make fresh as needed.

GPT substrate : 0.146g of α - Ketoglutarate and 8.9 g of DL Alanine are taken in a beaker. Add 1N sodium hydroxide until the solution is complete. Adjust the pH 7.4 with sodium hydroxide and dilute to 500mL with phosphate buffer.

DNPH colour developer : Dissolve 0.099g of 2,4 dinitrophenyl hydrazine in 500mL of 1N hydrochloric acid. Store in dark bottle in the refrigerator.

NaOH solution 0.4N : Dissolve 8g of NaOH in distilled water and dilute to 500mL with distilled water.

Procedure

- Pipette 0.5mL of GPT substrate into a test tube and place in 37 °C for 5 minutes in a water bath.

- Add 0.1mL of serum and mix.

- Incubate exactly 30 minutes for SGPT

- Add 0.5mL of DNPH and mix and incubate at room temperature for 20 minutes.

- Add 5mL of 0.4N NaOH, mix vigorously and let stand for 5 minutes.

- Read the colour calorimetrically at 505nm. Follow Same procedure for standards.

Precautions

Serum sample must be free from haemolysis. Since RBC's are rich in this enzyme.

Calibration curve/Standard graph is prepared by using following table 48.1

Table 48.1 : Calibration curve

Reagent	Blank	1	2	3	4	5	Incubation
Distilled water	0.2mL	0.2mL	0.2mL	0.2mL	0.2mL	0.2mL	
Substrate	1mL	0.9mL	0.8mL	0.7mL	0.6mL	0.5mL	5minutes / water bath
Standard	– –	0.1mL	0.2mL	0.3mL	0.4mL	0.5mL	30 PT / water bath
DNPH	1mL	1mL	1mL	1mL	1mL	1mL	20 minutes / room temp
NaOH	10mL	10mL	10mL	10mL	10mL	10mL	5 minutes / room temp

Observation

Table 48.2: Result reporting table

Tube No.	True OD	SGOT/IU
1		25
2		50
3		85
4		135
5		200
TEST		

Results

Colour change was noted and read at 505nm. True OD values are plotted against SGPT/IU. Results are interpretated after comparison with normal value.

Viva questions

Define ALT, AST, and SGPT.

Why increased SGPT relates liver disorders

What are the principles of SGPT?

49. Serum Cholesterol Analysis

Aim

To estimate the amount of cholesterol present in the given sample.

Clinical significance:

Cholesterol occurs in appreciable amounts in the body. Most of the cholesterol is synthesized by the liver from acetyl co A. Cholesterol is concerned with the metabolism of lipids and is an important precursor for steroid hormone synthesis. Serum cholesterol level is increased in diabetes mellitus, Nephrosis, billiary cirrhosis, Hypothyroidism and decreases in severe infection, severe anaemia, hyper thyrodism and malnutrition.

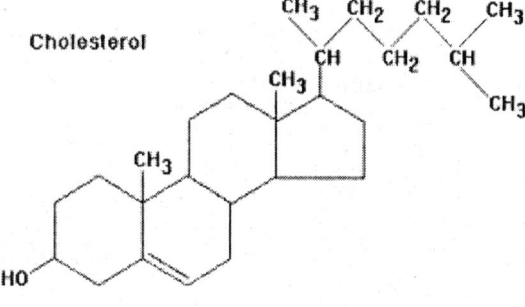

Fig 49.1 : Structure of Cholesterol

Principle

This test is performed by means of oxidation reaction. Two-reaction centers are present in the cholesterol molecules. They are the double bond and the OH group. Cholesterol reacts with strong acid reagents and produce coloured substances chiefly chestadiene sulfonic acid. Acetic acid and acetic anhydride are used as the solvent and dehydrating agent while sulphuric acid as dehydrating and oxidizing agent. In this method cholesterol in the serum is extracted in to the presence of acetic acid. Addition of sulphuric acid gives a blue coloured chromatophore.

Reagents

Stock ferric chloride reagent: 840mG ferric chloride is weighed and dissolved in 100mL glacial acetic acid.

Ferric chloride precipitating reagent : Dilute 10mL stock ferric chloride 100mL glacial acetic acid.

Ferric chloride diluting reagent : Dilute 8.5mL of stock using 100mL of glacial acetic acid.

Standard cholesterol : Dissolve 200mG of cholesterol in 10mL of ferric chloride precipitating reagent and made up to 100mL with glacial acetic acid.

Procedure

- To 0.1mL of serum add 4.9mL of ferric chloride reagent.

- Mix well using glass rod and centrifuge for 15 minutes.

- From this Take 2.5mL of filtrate and add 2.5mL of ferric chloride diluting reagent followed by 4mL of concentrated sulphuric acid with through mixing.

For standard curve, Take various concentration of cholesterol and made upt 5mL using ferric chloride diluting reagent. Then add 4mL concentrated sulphuric acid to all tubes. Mix well and read the colour developments at 560nm. Plot a standard graph and calculate the amount of cholesterol present in the given sample.

Normal Value

150-250mG/100mL of cholesterol.

Calculation

2.5mL of filtrate contain mG of cholesterol

2.5mL came from 5mL of sample = $\dfrac{100 \times 5}{2.5}$

= 200mG

This 5mL made from 0.1mL of the sample

0.1mL sample contain   = 200mG

100mL sample contain   = $\dfrac{200 \times 100}{0.1}$

= 200mG/dL.

Result

The amount of cholesterol present in the given sample is mG/dL.

Viva questions

Clinical significance of cholesterol in blood.

What are the significance of acetyl COA in lipid metabolism.

What are the principles of cholesterol estimation?

What are the difference between cholesterol & lipids?

What are the uses of $FeCl_2$ & H_2SO_4 in cholesterol estimation?

Spotters - Structure of cholesterol, cholesterol powder.

50. Serum Sugar Analysis

Aim

To estimate the amount of sugar present in the given sample by O toludine method.

Principle

The aldehyde group of glucose condenses with O.toludine in glacial acetic acid (colourless). On heating blue green colour is developed which is due to the formation of N- glucosamine.

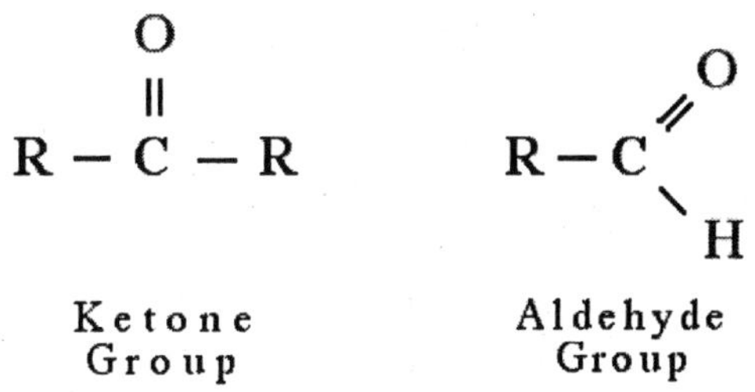

$$O$$
$$\parallel$$
$$R - C - R$$

Ketone Group

$$O$$
$$R - C \overset{\diagup}{\underset{\diagdown}{}} H$$

Aldehyde Group

Fig 50.1: Reaction Points in Sugar

Materials required

Reagents:

O.toludine reagent:

O.toludine, acetic acid and water are mixed in the ratio of 15:75:10. Add 2.5g of boric acid and 2.5g of thiourea and mixed well & keep it in a brown bottle.

10% tri chloro acetic acid.

Stock standard:

Dissolve 100mG of glucose in 100mL of distilled water.

Working standard:

10mL of standard solution are made up to 100mL using distilled water. 100mL of working standard contain 10mG of glucose. Ie., 0.1mL contains 10µG of glucose.

Procedure

- Take Various concentrations of working standard solution ranging from 10µG –100µG (0.1mL to 1mL) into a series of test tubes and make up to 1mL with distilled water.
- Use 1mL of distilled water as blank.
- To 0.1mL of serum, add 2mL of 10% trichloro acetic acid to precipitate proteins. Allow to stand and centrifuge at 5000rpm for 10 minutes.
- Take 1mL of protein free filtrate in a test tube and marked as test.
- Add 3mL of O.toludine reagent to all tube and keep in a boiling water bath for 15minutes.
- Read the greenish colour formed at 620nm.

Result and discussion

Reaction between different chemical reagents leads to colour change, which is read at specific wavelength of light. Results obtained through standard graph is compared with normal value for final interpretation.

Viva questions

What are the principles associated with serum sugar analysis.

Differentiate folin Wu method and O toludine method of serum sugar analysis.

Clinical significance of serum sugar.

What is hypoglycemia, hyperglycemia.

What is the need of TCA in sugar estimation.

Expand TCA.

Spotters - Carbohytrate structure, 'O' toludine

51. Estimation of Urine Albumin

Aim

To estimate the amount of protein present in the urine.

Introduction

Most plasma proteins are too large to pass through the glomeruli of the kidney. The small amount of protein, which does filter through, is normally reabsorbed back into the blood by the kidney tubules. Only trace amounts of protein (less than 0.15g per 24 hours) can there fore be found in normal urine. These amounts are insufficient for detection by routine laboratory tests.

During diseased condition, more than trace amounts of proteins are found in urine, are termed as proteinuria. This condition is often refers to as albuminuria because when there is glomerular damage most of the protein which passes through the glomerular filter is albumin because this protein molecule is smaller than most of the globulin's.

Causes of proteinuria

Tubular urinary disease, Pyogenic/ tuberculus pyelonephritis, Severe lower urinary tract infections, Nephrolic syndrome, Urinary schistosomiosis, Severe febrile illness, Hypertension accompanying haematuria.

Principle

Albumin present in urine gets coagulated when it is heated, by the addition of sulfo salicylic acid. It dilutes the coagulants and forms a cloudy white precipitate at the junction of 2 fluids. Sulfosalicylic acid method is a more sensitive method than TCA method. This produces 4 times more turbidity with albumin.

Materials Required

Sulfo salicylic acid reagent- 5g Sulfo salicylic acid in 25mL of Distilled water, Test tubes, patients Urine sample, Control sample, etc.,

Procedure

● Take two test tubes and labelled one as 'C' for control and other as 'T' for test.

● Add about 2mL of clear urine in to each tube (if the urine is turbid or cloudy, filter or centrifuge it to obtain a clear sample).

● Using the pH paper, test the reaction of the urine. If neutral or alkaline, add a drop of glacial acetic acid to each tube and mixed.

● Add 2-3 drops of Sulfo salicylic acid reagent to tube 'T'

● Holding the tube against a dark background examine for cloudiness in tube 'T'. Report the appearance in tube 'T' as follows.

No cloudiness	- Negative
Slight cloudiness	- +
Moderate cloudiness	- ++

Marked cloudiness	- +++
Cloudiness with precipitate	- ++++

Observation and Result

Presence of albumin in urine is detected based on cloudiness and precipitation. The given urine contains +/ ++/+++/++++ quantities of albumin.

Viva questions

Define Albuminuria.

Why are the causes of proteineuria?

Why there is a difficulty in measuring albumin in normal urine.

Low quantity of protein is present in normal urine –Why?

How do you interpretate the results of urine albumin.

Spotters - Positive result of urine albumin, sulfosalicylic acid.

52. Estimation of Urine Bile Salt

Aim

To determine bile salt in the urine.

Clinical Significance

Bile salt is not present in normal urine. It is detected in urine, when it is unable to leave the blood circulation through haepatic route into the intestine. The yellow to green colouration of the urine recognized bile salt in urine (Hepatitis).

Materials Required

Specimen – Urine, Test tubes, Sulphur powder.

Principle

Bile salt lowers the surface tension of the urine, when sulphur powder is added on the surface of the liver patients urine it sink to the bottom of the tube. In normal urine it float on the surface.

Procedure

● Take about 10mL of urine in a test tube

● Sprinkle a little dry sulphur powder on the surface of the urine.

● Observe the sulfur particle and record the results.

Observation and Result

Sink or floating nature of sulfur powder is noted and the results are reported as normal or abnormal.

Viva questions

Mention the principles of urine bile salt estimation.

What are the clinical significance of urine bile.

Differentiate jaundice and hepatitis.

Why sulphur powder sink in the presence of bile salt.

Spotters - Sulphur powder, bile salt.

53. Estimation of urine sugar

Aim

To determine the urine sugar quantitatively.

Clinical Significance

Presence of glucose in urine (glucosuria) following overnight positive is indicative of diabetes milletus.

Principle

The aldehyde group present in the glucose changes the blue coloured alkaline cupric sulphate to yellow red cuprous oxide. Several other sugar such as lactose, fructose, galactose, pentose and nonsugars such as uric acid, creatinine, ascorbic acid and homogenistic acid having a similar reducing property.

Materials Required

Specimen – urine, Test tubes, Test tube stand, Test tube holder, Dropper, Pipette, Bunsen' burner, Benedict's reagent etc.,

Benedict's reagent preparation

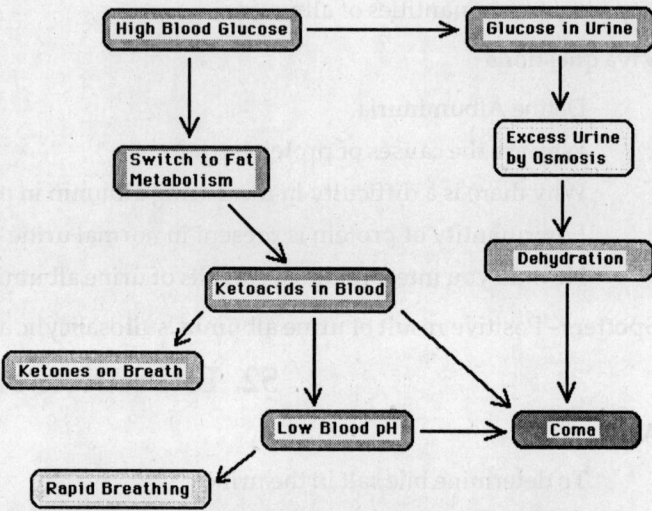

Fig 53.1 : Out come of high sugar in human

Dissolve 100g sodium carbonate in 900mL of distilled water, boil for 2-3 minutes, cool and add 173g cupric sulphate. Dissolve the content and make the final volume to one liter. The reagent is stable at room temperature.

Procedure

- Label the required test tubes and arranged them in a stand.
- Add 5 mL of Benedict's reagent to the test tubes.
- Using Pasteur pipette, add 1 mL of urine to tubes and mix well.
- Heat to boil.
- Cool it in running tap water.
- Positive reaction depends on the presence of fine yellow, orange or brick red precipitation
- Record the results.

Observation and Results

Different colour is noted when different urine sample is tested, which indicates variable concentrations of sugar present in urine samples. Concentration depends on colour.

Viva questions

What is diabetes mellitus?
What are the principles of urine glucose analysis?
Highlight excess glucose metabolism in human.
Mention about the clinical output of high glucose level in blood.
What are the components of benedict reagent?
How do you interpretate urine glucose level by benedicts test.

Spotters : Benedict's reagent.

B. Clinical Bacteriology
54. Isolation of Normal Flora from mouth / oral cavity

Aim

To isolate and understand positive & negative aspects of mouth / oral cavity normal flora.

Background information

Normal microbiota of the oral cavity contains those organisms that are able to resist mechanical removal by adhering to surfaces like gums and teeth. Oral cavity serves as an ideal environment for microbes because it provides moisture and food material. However continuous desquamation of epithelial cell, flow of saliva and mechanical flushing action removes microbes from the oral cavity.

At birth the oral cavity is essentially a sterile, warm and moist cavity containing variety of nutritional substances. The saliva is composed of water, aminoacids, proteins, lipids, carbohydrates and inorganic compounds. The newborne establish its normal flora within few days after birth. The oral cavity is colonized by microorganisms from external environment. Initially, the microbiota consist mostly of the genera Streptococcus, Lactobacillus, Neisseria, Actinomycetes. Some yeast is also present. The number and kinds of microbes present in mouth depends on the diet and to association with other peoples, objects such as towels, and feeding bottles. The only species isolated from the mouth through out the life is *S.salivaris*. It has an affinity to epithelial tissues and appears in large number on upper surface of the tongue.

Until eruption of teeth most microbes present in the mouth are aerobes and facultative anaerobes. As the first teeth erupt the anaerobes become dominant due to the anaerobic nature of the gingival groove. As the first tooth grows *Streptococcus gordonii* and *S.mutans* attach to their enamel surface, *S.salivaris* attaches to the buccal and gingival epithelial surfaces and colonizes the saliva. These Streptococci produce various adherence factors. These factors enhance the attachment of oral bacteria. The aggregation of bacteria on organic matter of the teeth surface is termed dental plaque. These organisms allow the secondary invaders and forms dental caries, gingivitis and periodental diseases. Periodental disease is caused by several groups of bacteria.

Materials required

Sample: 1mL saliva, 2 swabs from tongue, 2 swabs from buccal cavity, 2 swabs from teeth.
Media: Nutrient agar, Streptococcus selection agar, MRS medium, Blood agar, MacConkey agar.
Others: Petriplates, pipettes, inoculation loop, cotton, Cotton swab etc.

Procedure

- Collect 1mL saliva, swab from tongue, swab from buccal cavity and swab / scrap from teeth of normal individual.
- Keep all samples in laminar flow chamber for inoculation.
- Prepare sterile plates of 5 Nutrient agar, 3 MRS medium, 5 Blood agar and 4 MacConkey agar. Also prepare 4 broth tubes of streptococcus selection broth.
- Enrich swabs from tongue, buccal cavity and teeth using streptococcus selection broth and incubate at 37°C for overnight.
- Inoculate a loop full of overnight culture from streptococcus selection broth on two plates of blood agar and incubate one plate aerobicallay and one anaerobically at 37°C for 24-48hours.
- Inoculate 0.1mL of saliva to the plates of Nutrient agar, MRS medium, Blood agar and MacConkey agar and incubate aerobically at 37°C for 24hours.
- Inoculate swabs of tongue, buccal cavity and teeth on Nutrient agar, MRS medium and MacConkey agar as spread and incubate at 37°C for 24hours.
- Observe colony morphology, identify the possible isolates and interpretate the results

Observation and results

Different colonies of bacteria will be observed and subjected for identification.

Viva questions

What are the normal floras of oral cavity?

Listout few nonspecific or innate immunity of oral cavity.

Which bacterium is frequently isolated from oral cavity?

Name the medium used to enrich Streptococcus and to isolate Lactobacillus

What are the similarities and differences of Streptococcus and Lactobacillus

55. Isolation of bacteria from sputum

Aim

To isolate and identify pathogens from sputum.

Introduction

Lower respiratory tract (LRT) infections involves lung and bronchi. Normally Lower respiratory tract is a sterile organ. Any organism that is able to by-pass the host defenses, enter the Lower respiratory tract, and multiply is capable of causing diseases in LRT.

Possible Pathogens

Staphylococcus aureus, Streptococcus pneumoniae, Streptococcus pyogenes, Mycobacterium tuberculosis, Klebsiella pneumoniae, Beta haemolytic group B Streptococci, Haemophilus influenzae, Neisseria species, Pseudomonas aeruginosa, Mycoplasma pneumoniae etc.,

Materials Required

Media : Blood agar, Chocolate agar, Mac Conkey agar, Baired parker agar, Cetrimide agar, LJ medium, Buffered charcoal yeast extract agar, Modified Thayer martin agar, New york city agar medium.

Gram staining reagent, AF staining reagent, Conical flasks, Test tubes, petriplates etc.,

Procedure

Specimen -

Collect Early morning sputum. It contains pooled overnight secretions with concentrated bacteria. A sterile wide mouth jar with a tight screw cap lid can be used to collect sample.

Transporting - For Tubercle bacilli isolation

Sputum is transported or stored by adding cetyl pyridinium chloride - sodium chloride (CPC-NaCl) . It digests sputum and prevents the over growth of other pathogens.

Table 55.1 Bartlett grade of Sputum	
No. of Neutrophils per field	Grade
<10	0
10-25	+1
>25	+2
Presence of mucous	+1
No. of epithelial cells per field	Grade
10-25	-1
>25	-2

Procedure

Gram stain for Lower respiratory tract specimen:

- Gram stain can aid in rapid diagnosis and appropriate treatment. The following cells are observed after staining, they are PMN, squamous epithelial cells, ciliated columnar epithelial cells and bacteria. Bartlett grades the sputum sample using gram staining (Table 55.1). It is performed by the following method.

- Smear the purulent portion of the sputum.

- Fix the smear by heat and methanol fixing procedure.

- Stain the smear by gram stain technique **(Refer experiment No. 14bc).**

- Observe the smear under 40X microscopic objective.

Acid Fast Staining : Refer Experiment No : 14 bf

Culturing

Routine

- Wash the purulent part of the sputum with sterile 5mL of physiological saline.

- Inoculate washed sputum on the plates of blood agar and chocolate agar.

- Add optochin disc to the chocolate agar. This will help to identify *Streptococcus pneumoniae.*

- Incubate the blood agar plate aerobically and chocolate agar plate in a carbon di oxide enriched atmosphere at 35-37 ° C for upto 48 hours.

- Examine the growth and report the result.

For AFB (Acid Fast Bacilli – *Mycobacterium tuberculosis*)

- About 20 minutes before culturing decontaminate the specimen by mixing equal volumes of sputum and NaOH (40g/l solution). Shake at intervals to homogenize the sputum.

- Using a sterile premarked Pasteur pipette, inoculate 200µL of the sputum on a slope of acid Lowenstein Jensen medium. Allow the specimen to run down the slope.

- Slope turn yellow due to alkalinity of the specimen but it will become green again (acid in the medium neutralizes the NaOH).

- Incubate the tubes at 37°C in rack placed at an angle of about 45° to ensure that the specimen is in contact with the full length of the slope.

- After one week, place the slopes in an upright position and continue to incubate the cultures for a further 5-6 weeks, examine twice a week for growth.

For other pathogens

- Streak the sputum on selective and differential medium for the isolation and differentiation, as per clinical diagnosis and recommended by the physician (Table 55.2).

Table 55.2 -Observation - possible growth on Media

Staphylococcus aureus Blood agar – β Haemolytic colony Mannitol salt agar – Yellow colour colony Baired parker agar – Black Colour colony Vogel -Johnson agar -Black Colour colony with yellow background DNase test medium – Pink colour colony **Refer experiment 64**	*Streptococcus pneumoniae* Blood agar – α haemolytic colony Capsulated strains produce α haemolytic mucoid colony. Optochin sensitive Bile solubilizer **Refer experiment 65**
Streptococcus pyogenes, Blood agar – β haemolytic colony Optochin resistant Bile non solubilizer **Refer experiment 65**	*Mycobacterium tuberculosis,* Acid fast Lowenstein Jenson medium – Cabbage coloured colony
Klebsiella pneumoniae Mac Conkey Agar – Mucoid LF colonies Capsulated strain	*Haemophillus influenzae* Levinthols medium- colourless colonies Chocolate agar- grey coloured colonies Satellism
Neisseria meningitides New York City agar medium-Small ash coloured colonies Modified Thayer martin Agar-Small colourless colonies	*Pseudomonas aeruginosa* Cetrimide agar – Greenish blue colonies **Refer experiment 67**
Mycoplasma pneumoniae Mycoplasma isolationmedium – Fried egg appearance	

Viva questions

When did you collect sputum?

What are the specimens used to diagnose respiratory tract infection?

What are the methods available to collect sputum?

Why there is a need for early morning sputum?

What is CPC – NaCl?

What are the uses of CPU- NaCl?

What is Bartlett grading?

Name the medium used for the recovery or tubercle bacilli.

What are the possible bacterial pathogens of LRT?

How do you grade sputum sample?

Name the medium used for the cultivation of haemolytic Streptococcus.

How do you differentiate Staphylococcus & Streptococcus?

Define AFB.

What are all the ingredients of LJ medium?

What are the specialties of chocolate agar?

Spotters - LJ medium, chocolate agar, blood agar, microscopic picture of Staphylococcus, Streptococcus, Mycobacterium.

56. Isolation of bacteria from upper respiratory track (Throat)

Aim

To isolate and identify pathogens from throat

Background infection

Infections affecting the throat (larynx) or the main airway (trachea) or the airways going into the lungs (bronchi) are common. These infections are sometimes called laryngitis, trachitis or bronchitis. Doctors often just use the term URTI (upper respiratory tract infection) to include any or all of these. Cough is usually the main symptom. Other symptoms include fever, headache, aches and pains. Cold symptoms may occur if the infection also affects the nose. Symptoms typically peak after 2-3 days and then gradually clear. However, the cough may persist after the infection has gone. This is because the inflammation in the airways caused by the infection can take a while to clear. It may take up to 4 weeks after other symptoms have gone for the cough to clear completely.

Infections of the upper respiratory tract

Sinusitis, Strepthroat, Otitis media, Diphtheria, Pharyngitis, Supporative parotitis, Laryngitis, Tonsillitis, Pertusis, Scarlet fever, Epiglotitis, Parotitis, Trachitis, Rheumatoid fever

Bacterial Etiological agents

Streptococcus pyogenes, Other beta haemolytic Streptococci, Bordetella pertusis, Streptococcus pneumoniae, Haemophilus influenzae, Corynebacterium diphtheriae, Pseudomonas aeruginosa, Borrelia sp., Bacteroides malaninogenicus, Neisseria meningitidis, Klebsiella sp., Staphylococcus aureus

Materials required

Specimen - Sodium alginate throat swab for Pertusis, Sinus washings, Surgical biopsy, Swab of posterior pharynx, Swab of tonsil, Pernasal swab, **Nasopharyngeal aspirates**- Gently pass a sterile catheter through tonsil as far as the nasopharynx. Attach a sterile syringe to the catheter and aspirate the specimen of mucopus. Dispense the specimen into a sterile container.

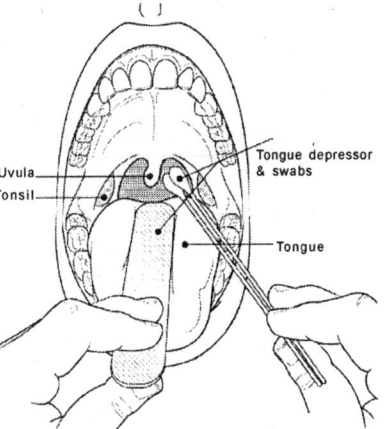

Fig. 56.1 – Throat Swab

Nasopharyngeal swab (Fig. 56.2) - Insert a **STERILE DRY SWAB** into the nasal cavity of the patient and wipe the swab along the sides of the nasal passage. Place the swab with the cotton tip end into the small vial (or leakproof screw top tube with 3-5 ml volume) of virus transport medium.

Throat swab -Bright light from over the shoulder of the patient should be focused in to the oral cavity. The patient is instructed to open the mouth at 'aah' position and breath deeply. The tongue is gently depressed with tongue blade to visualize the tonsillar fossae and posterior pharynx. The swab is extended between tonsillar pillars and behind the vulva. The tonsillar areas and posterior pharynx should be firmly rubbed with the swab. After collection the cotton swabs are placed into sterile Cary Blair transport media to prevent desiccation during transit to the laboratory (Fig. 56.1)

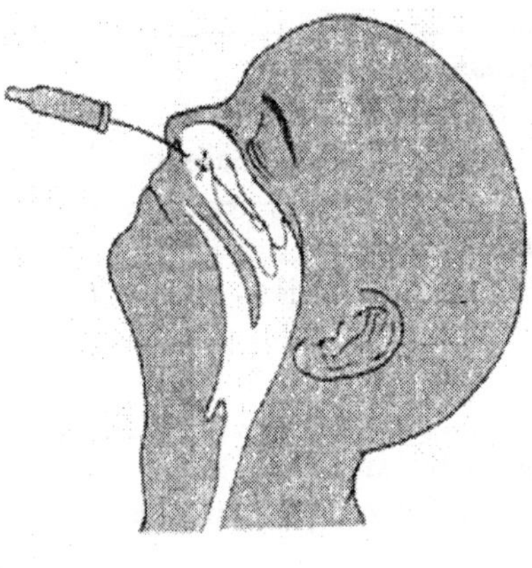

Fig. 56.2 – Nasopharyngeal swab

Media: Blood agar plate, Cystine tellurite blood agar, Loeffler agar slant, Chocolate agar, Charcoal Cephalexin Blood Agar (CCBA), Modified tindsale medium, Saboured dextrose agar, Thayer martin agar, Cetrimide agar, New York City Agar Medium, Baired Parker Agar, Mac Conkey agar.

Alberts staining reagent, bacitracin disc etc.

Procedure

Microscopy

Alberts Staining Technique – Refer Experiment No. 14bg

Culturing

- Inoculate the swab on a plate of blood agar.
- Add a bacitracin disc to the plate. This will help in the identification of *Streptococcus pyogenes*.
- Use tinsdale's medium and Tellurite blood agar for the recovery of *Corynebacterium diphtheriae*
- Use chocolate agar for the isolation of *H.influenzae, N.meningitidis*.
- Use charcoal cephalexin blood agar and Bordet Gengou medium for the recovery of *Bordetella pertusis*.
- Use MacConkey agar to isolate Gram Negative pathogens.
- After inoculation all the plates should be incubated at appropriate temperature for a required time.

Table 56.1 -Observation - possible growth on Media

Staphylococcus aureus	*Streptococcus pneumoniae*
Blood agar – β Haemolytic colony	*Blood agar – α haemolytic colony*
Mannitol salt agar – Yellow colour colony	*Capsulated strains produce α haemolytic mucoid colony.*
Baired parker agar – Black Colour colony	*Optochin sensitive*
Vogel - Johnson agar - Black Colour colonywith yellow background	*Bile solubilizer*
DNase test medium – Pink colour colony	**Refer experiment 65**
Refer experiment 64	
Streptococcus pyogenes,	*Corynebacterium diphtheriae*
Blood agar – α haemolytic colony	Loeffler agar – Luxurious growth
Optochin resistant	Cysteine tellurite blood agar-Black colour colony
Bile non solubilizer	Blood agar- α haemolytic colonies
Refer experiment 65	**Refer experiment 66**
Klebsiella pneumoniae	*Haemophillus influenzae*
Mac Conkey Agar – Mucoid LF colonies	Levinthols medium- colourless colonies
Capsulated strain	Chocolate agar- grey coloured colonies Satellism
Neisseria meningitidis	*Pseudomonas aeruginosa*
New York City agar medium-Small ash coloured colonies	Cetrimide agar – Greenish blue colonies
Modified Thayer martin Agar-Small colourless colonies	**Refer experiment 67**
	Bordetella pertusis
	Bordet –Gengou medium – Glistening mercury like colonies
	Rogen-Lowey medium – Ash coloured colonies

Viva questions

What are the possible pathogens of throat?

Is there any normal flora in throat?

Mention few viral and bacterial infection of throat.

Name the medium used for the cultivation of *C.diphtheriae*.

How do you differentiate *S. aureus* & *C. diphtheriae*

Define colony morphology of pathogen on selective and differential medium.

Spotters - Microscopic picture of *C. diphtheriae*, Staphylococcus, Streptococcus, Neisseria sp. Selective & differential medium.

57. Isolation of bacteria from stool

Aim

To identify the gastrointestinal pathogens

Background information

Normal human intestine harbours more than 500 types of microbes. Among these some of the microbes are considered as pathogens. Pathogens may enter through food and water systems. Most of the intestinal disorders are based on the toxins.

Pathogens of gastrointestinal tract includes, *Escherichia coli, Salmonella enteritis, Shigella sp., Camphylobacter, Vibrio sp., Plesiomonas sp., Aeromonas sp., Yersinia enterocolitica*

Materials Required

Medium : MacConkey agar, GN broth, HE agar, TCBS agar, Alkaline peptone water, Caphylobacter isolation medium, Yersinia selective medium.

Procedure

Specimen: Stool or rectal swab

Transport

The specimen should be transported as early as possible. Don't refrigerate the stool specimen if possible because certain species of *Shigella species* are susceptible to cooling and drying.

Processing

- Observe the nature and colour of the specimen
- Assess Microscopic nature of the specimen by using iodine wet mount technique and gram staining technique.
- Inoculate the Gram negative broth and alkaline peptone water with few loopful of stool specimen and incubate at 37°C for 4-5 hrs. Observe turbidity.
- Streak Haektoen Enteric agar (HE) by using gram negative broth and TCBS agar with alkaline peptone water inoculum. Observe the plates for the pathogens after 24 hours of incubation at 37°C.
- At the same time remaining medium given in the medium section are streaked by direct method.
- After the completion of primary plating techniques, identify the bacterial pathogens using various biochemical tests.

Table 57.1 -Observation - possible growth on Media

Escherichia coli	*Salmonella sp.*
Eosin Methylene Blue Agar – Metallic sheen colonies Xylose Lysine Deoxy cholate Agar – Yellow colour colonies Salmonella Shigella agar – pink colour colonies Rajhans medium – Greenish colonies Hektoein Enteric agar – Salmon colonies Mac Conkey agar- LF colonies Mac Conkey Sorbitol Agar – Colourless indicates EHEC **Refer experiment 61**	Hektoen enteric agar – Dark centered colony with Green margin Xylose Lysine Deoxy cholate agar- Dark centerd colony with Pink margin Salmonella Shigella agar - ark centered colony with Pink margin Bismuth sulphite agar – Black colonies Rajhans medium – Reddish colonies **Refer experiment 62**
Shigella sp.	*Campylobacter sp.,*
Xylose Lysine Deoxy Cholate Agar – Colourless colonies Salmonella Shigella agar– Colourless colonies Hektoein Enteric agar– Colourless colonies Rajhans medium – Colourless colonies **Refer experiment 63**	Campy CVA agar – Colourless colonies Campy Food ID agar – Brown colour colonies
Vibrio cholerae	*Plesiomonas sp.,*
Alkaline peptone water – Luxurious turbid growth TCBS agar – Circular yellow colour colonies	*Chrome agar – Yellow colour colonies*
Aeromonas sp.,	*Yersinia enterocolitica*
Chrome agar – Brown colour colonies Inositol brillient green bile agar – Colourless colonies Blood agar with 20 µL/mL ampicillin – Pale coloured colonies CIN agar – Circular pink colonies	CIN agar – Pink small colonies XLD agar – Yellow colonies Blood agar – Yellowish brown colonies PSTA enrichment broth – Luxurious growth

Viva Questions

How pathogens enters in to human intestinal system?

List bacterial pathogens associated with gastro intestinal system.

When stool is collected for diagnosis?.

List some of the selective medium used for the differentiation EHEC from other *E.coli*.

Name the medium used for the differentiation of EHEC from other E.coli.

How do you confirm pathogenic *E. coli*?

How do you differentiate types of *E. coli*?

Name the medium used for the cultivation of vibrio

Spotters - Picture of *V. cholerae*, Selective & differential medium

58. Isolation of bacteria From Wound (Pus)

Aim

To isolate the pathogenic bacteria from the wound specimens.

Background information

Wound is an abnormal break in the skin or other tissue, which allows blood to escape. Wounds are two types, they are open wound and closed wound. Open wound allows blood to escape from the body. Here the skin is broken. All open wounds are contaminated by germs, which enter from air, fingers and other parts of the body. Any wound, which has not begun to heal properly after 48 hours it, may be infected. Infection may further spread and cause dangerous illness to human beings. *Staphylococcus aureus* mostly isolated from skin wounds, *Pseudomonas aeruginosa* is associated with infected burns and with hospital acquired infections. *Escherichia coli, Proteus species* associated with abdominal abscess. *Clostridium perfringens* is found mainly in deep wounds.

Possible Pathogens

Staphylococcus aureus, Pseudomonas aeruginosa, Clostridium sp., Escherichia coli, , Proteus sp., Bacteroides, Klebsiella spp., Streptococcus pyogenes.

Materials required:

Sterile leak proof container, Sterile cotton swab, Amies transport medium, Blood agar, Neomycin blood agar, Robertson cooked meat medium, MacConkey agar.

Specimen collection

Pus from wound is collected at the time of the abscess is incised and drained or after it ruptured naturally. Collect a sample of the pus on a sterile cotton swab and insert it in a leak proof container of Amies transport medium.

Procedure

Macroscopic and microscopic examination

Colour and nature of the specimen is examined before starting microscopy.

Microscopy – Gram staining – Refer experiment No 14c

Culturing

- Inoculate two blood agar, one neomycin blood agar, one MacConkey agar and one cooked meat medium tube using pus sample.

- Incubate One blood agar and MacConkey agar aerobically at 35-37°C overnight.

- Incubate Neomycin blood agar and 2nd blood agar plate anaerobically at 35-37°C for 48 hours.

- Incubate Cooked meat medium at 35-37°C for 72 hours.

- Observe Colony morphology on different medium and record the results.

- Subject the isolated colonies to biochemical test for species identification.

Table 58.1 -Observation - possible growth on Media

Staphylococcus aureus	Clostridium sp.,
Blood agar – β Haemolytic colony Mannitol salt agar – Yellow colour colony Baired parker agar – Black Colour colony Vogel -Johnson agar -Black Colour colonywith yellow background DNase test medium – Pink colour colony **Refer experiment 64**	Cooked meat medium – saccharolytic or proteolytic growth Blood agar – single or double zone colonies
	Pseudomonas aeruginosa
	Cetrimide agar – Greenish blue colonies **Refer experiment**
Streptococcus pyogenes,	Escherichia coli
Blood agar – β haemolytic colony Optochin resistant Bile non solubilizer **Refer experiment 65**	Eosin Methylene Blue Agar – Metallic sheen colonies Xylose Lysine Deoxy Cholate Agar – Yellow colour colonies Salmonella Shigella agar – pink colour colonies Rajhans medium – Greenish colonies Hektoein Enteric agar – Salmon colonies Mac conkey agar- LF colonies **Refer experiment 61**
Proteus sp.,	
CLED with bromothymol blue – Bluish green colonies XLD agar – Black colonies	
Klebsiella pneumoniae	
Mac Conkey Agar – Mucoid LF colonies	

Viva Questions

Define wound.

What are the types of wound?

Which are the predominant flora of wound.

Name the organism involved in anaerobic wound infection.

Which medium is used for the cultivation of anaerobic wound pathogens?

How do you identify *Pseudomonas aeruginosa* from wound?

Name the medium used for the identification of *Staphylococcus, Streptococcus, Pseudomonas, Klebsiella*.

What are the uses of blood agar?

Is microscopy necessary for wound pathogen isolation?

What are the advantages of microscopy in pathogen identification from clinical samples?

What kind of specimen is used for the recovery of wound pathogen?

How do you identify fungal &protozoan infections in wound?

What are the principles of Mac Conkey agar & blood agar?

Spotters - Microscopic picture Staphylococcus , Streptococcus , Clostridium, Selective & differential medium.

59. Isolation of bacteria from blood

Aim

To isolate the pathogens from the blood.

Background Information

The presence of bacteria in blood is called bacteremia. Transitory bacteremia can occur during the course of many infections. Continuous bacteremia most often suggests an intravascular source of infection. The term septicemia refers to a severe and often fatal infection of the blood in which bacteria multiply and release toxins in the blood stream. The symptoms of septicemia include fever, chills and shock.

Bacteria that can be associated with neonatal septicemia include *Escherichia coli*, Staphylococci, Beta haemolytic group B Streptococci and other coliforms.

Viridans Streptococcus are the commonest cause of sub acute infective endocarditis. In typhoid, *Salmonella typhi* can be detected in the blood of 75-90% patients during the first 10 days of infection.

Possible pathogens

Staphylococcus aureus, Viridans streptococci, Streptococcus pneumoniae, Streptococcus pyogenes, Salmonella typhi, Escherichia coli, Klebsiella pneumoniae, Corynebacterium diptheriae, Yersinia pestis, Leptospira species, Brucella species, Beta haemolytic group B Streptococci, Proteus sp., Haemophillus influenzae, Neisseria species.

Materials Required

Syringe, Sterile needle, 70% ethanol, Thioglycollate broth, Tryptone soya diphasic broth, Blood agar, Chocolate agar, Mac Conkey agar, SS agar, EDTA, Materials for WBC and differential count, Giemsa stain.

Procedure

Sample collection

- Blood should be collected before anti microbial treatment has been started and at the time when the patients temperature begins to rise.
- Blood for culture should be taken by vein puncture.
- 10-20 mL of blood collected from adult
- 1-2.4 mL collected from young infants
- 2.4-5 mL collected from old infants.
- Two-blood culture should be performed from each patient to confirm the causative agent.

Culturing

- Prepare thioglycollate and tryptone soya diphasic medium and sterilize at appropriate temperature.
- Withdraw appropriate volume of blood from patients.
- Divide the blood into three portions. Inoculate two portions into thioglycollate and tryptone soya diphasic medium.
- Inoculate remaining portion into a bottle containing EDTA. This blood is used to perform total, differential count, staining and also streak one loop full of blood into the SS agar.
- Incubate all culture bottles / plates at 37° C.

Examination and sub culturing

For thioglycollate broth

- Examine daily for up to 14 days
- Look for visible signs of bacterial growth such as turbidity above the red cell layer.

Subculturing (A strict aseptic technique must be used to avoid contamination)

- Using a sterile needle and small syringe, insert the needle through rubber liner in the cap, and withdrawn 1mL of broth culture.
- Inoculate the broth on blood agar, chocolate agar and Mac Conkey agar.
- Incubate blood agar and chocolate agar anaerobically for 48 hours and Mac conkey agar plate aerobically for over night.

For tryptone soya biphasic culture

- Examine daily for 7 days and twice a week for upto 4weeks
- Look for colonies on the agar slope and signs of bacterial growth on broth.
- If growth is present subculture on blood agar, chocolate agar and Mac Conkey agar.
- Examine gram stained smear of the colonies.
- If large gram positive rods resembling *Clostridium perfringens* are seen, subculture on Lactose egg yolk milk agar and incubate the plate anaerobically.
- If Brucella is suspected increased attention should be taken and mark as HIGH RISK

Table 59.1-Observation - possible growth on Media

Staphylococcus aureus	*Streptococcus pneumoniae*
Blood agar – α Haemolytic colony	*Blood agar – α haemolytic colony*
Mannitol salt agar – Yellow colour colony	*Capsulated strains produce α haemolytic mucoid colony.*
Baired parker agar – Black Colour colony	*Optochin sensitive*
Vogel -Johnson agar -Black Colour colonywith yellow background	*Bile solubilizer*
DNase test medium – Pink colour colony	**Refer experiment 65**
Refer experiment 64	
Streptococcus pyogenes,	*Mycobacterium tuberculosis,*
Blood agar – α haemolytic colony	*Acid fast*
Optochin resistant	*Lowenstein Jenson medium – Cabbage coloured colony*
Bile non solubilizer	
Refer experiment 65	
Klebsiella pneumoniae	*Haemophillus influenzae*
Mac Conkey Agar – Mucoid LF colonies	Levinthols medium- colourless colonies
Capsulated strain	Chocholate agar- grey coloured colonies
	Satellism
Neisseria meningitidis	*Pseudomonas aeruginosa*
New York City agar medium-Small ash coloured colonies	Cetrimide agar – Greenish blue colonies
Modified Thayer martin Agar-Small colourless colonies	**Refer experiment 67**

Escherichia coli	*Salmonella sp.*
Eosin Methylene Blue Agar – Metallic sheen colonies Xylose Lysine Deoxy Cholate Agar – Yellow colour colonies Salmonella Shigella agar – pink colour colonies Rajhans medium – Greenish colonies Hektoein Enteric agar – Salmon colonies Mac conkey agar- LF colonies **Refer experiment 61**	Hektoein enteric agar – Dark centered colony with Green margin Xylose Lysine Deoxycholate agar- Dark centered colony with Pink margin Salmonella Shigella agar - ark centered colony with Pink margin Bismuth sulphite agar – Black colonies Rajhans medium – Reddish colonies **Refer experiment 62**
Corynebacterium diphtheriae Loeffler agar – Luxurious growth Cysteine tellurite blood agar-Black colour colony Blood agar- α haemolytic colonies **Refer experiment**	*Yersinia pestis,* *Blood agar* – 48-hour *Y. pestis* culture with characteristic "hammered copper" morphology; 72-hour *Y. pestis* culture with characteristic "fried egg" morphology Brain heart infusion broth - suspended flocculent or crumbly clump growth Wayson staining – Biopolar Positive
Proteus sp., CLED with bromothymol blue – Bluish green colonies XLD agar – Black colonies	Clostridium per fringers Lactose egg yolk milk agar - Double zone of haemolygis Cooked meat medium - Proteolysis

Viva questions

Why human blood is not used for the preparation of blood agar?

List out blood borne infection of human.

How do you cultivate typhoid-causing pathogens from blood?

What is biphasic medium?

What are the advantages of thioglycollate medium?

Define Bacteremia, transitory bacteremia, septicemia and toxemia.

Spotters – Tryptone bi phasic medium, Blood agar

60. Isolation of bacteria from Urine

Aim

To analyze the etiology of urinary tract infection.

Background information

The presence of bacteria in urine is called bacteriuria. Significant bacteriuria is usually accompanied by pyuria (pus cells in urine). Infection of the bladder is called cystitis, and infection of kidney is called pyelonephritis. *Escherichia coli* is a commonest cause of urinary tract infection.

Possible Pathogens

Staphylococcus saprophyticus, Pseudomonas aeruginosa, Escherichia coli, Proteus sp., Klebsiella spp., Haemolytic Streptococcus , Enterococcus sp .

Medium used

Blood agar, MacConkey agar, Cetrimide agar, CLED agar, SS agar, KF streptococcus agar, Nutrient agar

Sample Collection

Mid stream urine, Cathedral and Subrapubic aspiration are the common urine collection methods. It is collected in sterile, dry, wide necked, leak proof container. About 20mL of sample should be collected. If immediate delivery to the laboratory is not possible, the urine should be refrigerated at 4^0C. If the delivery of more than 1 hour is anticipated, boric acid should be added to the urine. Specimen containing boric acid need not be refrigerated.

Procedure

Macroscopy

- Note the appearance of the specimen.
- Colour of the specimen.
- Nature of the specimen.
- Normally freshly passed urine is clear and pale yellow-to-yellow depending on the concentration. When left to stand, cloudiness may develop due to precipitation of urates in acid urine or phosphates and carbonates in alkaline urine. Urates may give the urine a pink-orange colour.

Table 60.1-Appearance of urine during infection

S.No	Colour	Infection
1	Cloudy	Bacterial
2	Red and cloudy	Bacterial and urinary Schistosomiasis.
3	Brown and cloudy	Black water fever
4	Yellow brown and green brown	Acute viral hepatitis
5	Yellow orange	Haemolysis and hepatocellular jaundice
6	Milky white	Bancroftian filariasis

Microscopic Examination – Gram staining (Ref experiment 14bc)

Table 60.2 -Findings of microscopic examination

Bacteria	Casts
White cells	Hyaline
Pus cells	Waxy
Red cells	Cellular
Yeast cells	Granular
Epithelial cells	
Casts	
Crystals	
Parasites	

Culturing

- Approximate number of bacteria per mL of urine, can be estimated by using calibrated loop technique (0.002mL capacity or 1/500mL or 20x500=10,000).
- Dilute the Urine up to 10^{-5} and perform Streak plate technique. (normal urine had less than 10^4 bacteria).

- Divide nutrient agar plates into 6 portions and inoculate a loop full of Urine on respective Portion as single line.

- For selective isolation, mix urine properly and inoculate a loopful of urine on blood agar, Mac Conkey agar, CLED agar, cetrimide agar and SS agar.

- Incubate all plates at 37 ° C for 24 hours

- Observe colony and interpretate the result.

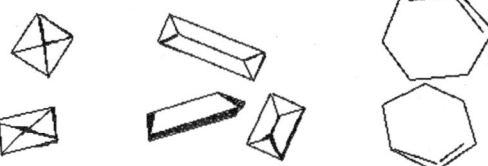

Oxalate   Triple Phosphate   Cystine

Fig 60.1 : Crystals of Urine

Table 60.3 -Observation - possible growth on Media

Staphylococcus aureus	*Escherichia coli*
Blood agar – β Haemolytic colony Mannitol salt agar – Yellow colour colony Baired parker agar – Black Colour colony Vogel -Johnson agar -Black Colour colony with yellow background DNase test medium – Pink colour colony **Refer experiment 64**	Eosin Methylene Blue Agar – Metallic sheen colonies Xylose Lysine Deoxy Cholate Agar – Yellow colour colonies Salmonella Shigella agar – pink colour colonies Rajhans medium – Greenish colonies Hektoen Enteric agar – Salmon colonies Mac conkey agar- LF colonies **Refer experiment 61**
Streptococcus pyogenes, *Blood agar – β haemolytic colony* *Optochin resistant* *Bile non solubilizer* **Refer experiment 65**	*Proteus sp.,* CLED with bromothymol blue – Bluish green colonies XLD agar – Black colonies
Klebsiella pneumoniae *Mac Conkey Agar – Mucoid LF colonies* *Capsulated strain*	*Enterococcus* Azide dextrose broth – Luxurious growth KF sterptococcus agar with TTC – Pinl minute colonies
	Pseudomonas aeruginosa Cetrimide agar – Greenish blue colonies **Refer experiment 67**

Viva Question

Define bacteriuria, pyuria, cystitis, pylonephritis.

What are possible pathogens of UTI?

Why *E.coli* is the commonest cause of UTI?

How do you collect samples to detect UTI?

How colour of specimen gives picture of possible UTI?

What are the microscopic structures are visualized, during suspected UTI?

Why CLED medium is used to recover major UTI pathogens?

Name the commonest medium used for the recovery of G-pathogens.

How do you differentiate *E.coli & Citrobactor?*

In What way *Enterobactor & Klebsiella* are differentiated

Name the medium used for the recovery of Proteus.

Spotters : CLE Dagar.

61. Identification of *Escherichia coli*

Aim

To identify *E .coli* from the given culture.

Background information

E .coli is one of the most important gram negative bacilli of the family Enterobacteriaceae. *E .coli* is considered as a normal flora of healthy human until 1920s. Now it is considered to be a pathogen. On the basis of its pathogenicity five types *E.coli* are described. They are Enteropathogenic *E.coli*, Entero Toxigenic *E.coli*, Entero Invasive *E. coli*, Entero haemarrhagic *E.coli* and Entero aggregative *E.coli*. *E. coli* may cause gastroenteritis and urinary tract infections.

Materials required

Sample : Broth or slant culture.

Chemicals & Media Required

Gram staining reagent, EMB agar, Mac Conkey agar, XLD agar, SS agar, RajHans agar, Hektoein enteric agar, Biochemical test media & reagents, Glass slides, petri plates, test tubes etc.

Procedure

Day I

- Subject the isolated pure culture to simple stain, gram stain and catalase to know the nature of the family of the isolate.

- Streak the isolate on MacConkey agar and incubate at 37ºC for 24 hours.

- Subject the isolate to Motility test, Indole test and TSI test. It is helpful to understand the probable nature of the isolate.

Day II

- Perform MR,VP, Urease, Nitrate, Deaminease, Decarboxylase, Melonate, KCN and carbohydrate fermentation tests along with EMB media inoculation to confirm generic level identification of the isolate.

Day III

- Confirm probably Identified bacterial isolate by streaking on Haektoein enteric agar, XLD agar, SS agar and Rajhans Medium. Incubate all the medium at 37ºC for 24 hours and observed the colony morphology.

- The same procedure is also used to identify Enterobacter and Citrobacter.

- Complete identification is by sero grouping and molecular methods.

Table 61.1 –Observation – Identification characters

S. No	Test	Observation	Result
1	Simple staining	Rod	It may be the member of Enterobacteriaceae.
2	Gram Staining	Gram negative	
3	Growth on MacConkey agar	LF colonies	
4	Catalase	Positive	

5	Motility	Motile	It may be *Escherichia coli*
6	Indole	Positive	It may be *Escherichia coli*
7	Oxidase test	Negative	It may be *Escherichia coli*
8	MR	Positive	It may be *Escherichia coli*
9	VP	Negative	It may be *Escherichia coli*
10	Citrate	Negative	It may be *Escherichia coli*
11	TSI	A/A Gas positive H$_2$S Negative	It may be *Escherichia coli*
12	Growth on EMB agar	Metalic sheen colonies	It confirms *Escherichia coli*
13	Urease	Negative	It confirms *Escherichia coli*
14	Nitrate	Positive	It confirms *Escherichia coli*
15	Growth on XLD agar	Yellow colour colonies	It confirms *Escherichia coli*
16	Growth on HE agar	Salmon coloured colonies	It confirms *Escherichia coli*
17	Growth on SS agar	Pink colour colonies	It confirms *Escherichia coli*
18	Growth on RajHans medium	Bluish green colonies	It confirms *Escherichia coli*

Result

Based on the above observation the given bacteria is identified as *Escheichia coli*

Viva questions

Mention colony morphology of *E.coli* on HE , agar, SS agar, EMB agar, XLD agar, Rajhans medium.
Mention biochemical characters of *E.coli*.
What are the clinical samples are used to isolate *E.coli*.?
Mention about characters of *E.coli*.
List diseases caused by *E.coli* on human.
What are the types of *E.coli*.?
Why *E.coli* is considered as a potential organism.

62. Identification of *Salmonella sp.*

Aim

To identify *Salmonella sp.* from the given culture.

Background information

Enteric fever is a collective term used for invasive infections caused by a small group of bacteria called Salmonella. Salmonella are a group of enteric invasive bacteria. They are responsible for variety of gastrointestinal infections.

Materials required

Sample : Broth or stap or slant culture.

Chemicals & Media Required

Gram staining reagent, Mac Conkey agar, XLD agar, SS agar, RajHans agar, Hektoein enteric agar, Biochemical test media & reagents, Glass slides, petri plates, test tubes etc.

Procedure

Day I

- Subject the isolated pure culture to simple stain, gram stain and catalase to know nature of the family of the isolate.

- Streak the isolate on MacConkey agar and incubate at 37°C for 24 hours

- Subject the isolate to Motility test, Indole test and TSI test. It is helpful to understand the probable nature of the isolate.

Day II

- Perform MR, VP, Urease, Nitrate, Deaminease, Decarboxylase, Melonate, KCN and carbohydrate fermentation tests.

Day III

- Confirm probably Identified bacterial isolate by streaking it on Haektoein enteric agar, XLD agar, SS agar and Rajhans Medium. Incubate all the media at 37°C for 24 hours and observed the colony morphology.

Table 62.1 –Observation – Identification characters

S. No	Test	Observation	Result
1	Simple staining	Rod	It may be the member of Enterobacteriaceae.
2	Gram Staining	Gram negative	
3	Growth on MacConkey agar	NLF colonies	
4	Catalase	Positive	
5	Motility	Motile	It may be Salmonella sp.,
6	Indole	Negative	It may be Salmonella sp.,
7	Oxidase test	Negative	It may be Salmonella sp.,
8	MR	Positive	It may be Salmonella sp.,
9	VP	Negative	It may be Salmonella sp.,
10	Citrate	Positive / Negative	It may be Salmonella sp.,
11	TSI	K/A Gas positive H_2S Positive / negative	It may be Salmonella sp.
12	Growth on SS agar	Black centered pink edged colonies	It confirms *Salmonella sp.,*
13	Urease	Negative	It confirms *Salmonella sp.,*
14	Nitrate	Positive	It confirms *Salmonella sp.,*
15	Growth on XLD agar	Black centered colonies	It confirms *Salmonella sp.,*
16	Growth on HE agar	Black centered colonies	It confirms *Salmonella sp.,*
17	Growth on Bismuth sulphite agar	Jet Black	It confirms *Salmonella sp.,*
18	Growth on RajHans medium	Pink coloured colonies	It confirms *Salmonella sp.,*

Table 62.2 –Differentiation properties of *Salmonella sp.*

Character	*S.typhi*	*S.paratyphi A*	*S.paratyphi B*	*S.paratyphi C*
Glucose	**Acid**	Acid &gas	Acid &gas	Acid &gas
Hydrogen sulphide	+	_	-	-
Lysine	+	-	+	-
Ornithine	-	+	+	-
Rhamnose	-	+	+	-
Xylose	D	-	Acid &gas	Acid &gas
Citrate	-	-	+	-
D-Tartarate	A	-	-	Acid &gas
Mucate	D	-	Acid &gas	-

Result

Based on the above observation the given bacteria is identified as *Salmonells sp.*

Viva questions

Mention few important characters of Salmonella

Which species of Salmonella cause severe typhoid fever?

How do you differentiate Salmonella from *Escherichia coli*

63. Identification of *Shigella sp.*

Aim

To identify *Shigella* from the given culture.

Background information

Gram negative facultative anaerobes of the genus Shigella are the principal agents of bacillary dysentery. Serogoups A, B, and C are very similar physiologically while *S. sonnei* can be differentiated from the other serogroups by positive beta-D-galactosidase and Ornithine Decarboxylase biochemical reactions. The identification of Shigella by species in the clinical laboratory is usually accomplished by slide agglutination using commercially available, absorbed rabbit antisera.

Materials required

Sample :Broth or stap or slant culture.

Chemicals & Media Required

Gram staining reagent, Mac Conkey agar, XLD agar, SS agar, RajHans agar, Hektoein enteric agar, Biochemical test media & reagents, Glass slides, petri plates, test tubes etc.

Procedure

Day I

- Subject the isolated pure culture to simple stain, gram stain and catalase to know nature of the family of the isolate.

- Streak the isolate on MacConkey agar and incubate at 37°C for 24 hours.
- Subject the isolate to Motility test, Indole test and TSI test. It is helpful to understand the probable nature of the isolate.

Day II

- Perform MR,VP, Urease, Nitrate, Deaminease, Decarboxylase, Melonate, KCN and carbohydrate fermentation tests.

Day III

- Confirm probably Identified bacterial isolate by streaking it on Haektoein enteric agar, XLD agar, SS agar and Rajhans Medium. Incubate all the medium at 37°C for 24 hours and observed the colony morphology.

Table 63.1 –Observation – Identification characters

S. No	Test	Observation	Result
1	Simple staining	Rod	It may be the member of Enterobacteriaceae.
2	Gram Staining	Gram negative	
3	Growth on MacConkey agar	NLF colonies	
4	Catalase	Negative	
5	Motility	Non Motile	It may be Shigella sp.
6	Indole	Positive	It may be Shigella sp.
7	Oxidase test	Negative	It may be Shigella sp.
8	MR	Negative	It may be Shigella sp.
9	VP	Negative	It may be Shigella sp.
10	Citrate	Negative	It may be Shigella sp.
11	TSI	K/K No gas noH$_2$S	It may be Shigella sp.
12	Growth on SS agar	Colourless colonies	It confirms Shigella sp.
13	Urease	Negative	It confirms Shigella sp.
14	Nitrate	Positive	It confirms Shigella sp.
15	Growth on XLD agar	Colourless colonies	It confirms Shigella sp.
16	Growth on HE agar	Colourless colonies	It confirms Shigella sp.
17	Growth on RajHans medium	Colourless colonies	It confirms Shigella sp.

Differentiation features of shigella sp.

Characters	S. sonnei	S. dysentriae	S. flexneri	S. boydii
Indole	-	+	+/-	+/-
Ornithine	+	-	-	-
ONPG	+	-	-	-
Nitrate	-	+	+	+
Glucose	A &G	A	A	A
Mannitol	A &G	D	D	D

Result

Based on the above observation the given bacterium is identified as *Shigella sp.*

Viva questions

What are the significance of Shigella?

Name the disease caused by Shigella

Differentiate *Salmonella, Shigella* and *E. coli*

64. Identification of *Staphylococcus aureus*

Aim

To Isolate / identify *Staphylococcus aureus* from clinical samples / from mixed/ pure cultures.

Background information

Members of the genus *Staphylococcus* are facultative anaerobic, nonmotile, gram positive cocci that usually form irregular clusters. *Staphylococci* are responsible for many human diseases. Staphylococci are normally associated with the skin and mucous membranes of warm blooded animals. *Staphylococcus* is located in the order *bacillales*, family Staphylococcaceae of volume 4 of bergeys manual systematic bacteriology second edition but in first edition it is in volume 2, section 12 in the family Micrococcaceae.

Materials required

Culture/ pure culture, gram staining reagents, nutrient agar, blood agar, Mac Conkey agar, Mannitol salt agar, Baired parker agar, DNase test agar, Vogel Johnson Agar, H_2O_2, Serum, Bacitracin, Novobiocin, Frurazolidone, OF basal medium, Glucose, PYR reagent etc.,

Procedure

Day 1

- Check the purity of the culture by streaking the culture on nutrient agar plate, incubate at 37°C for 24 hours and note Colony morphology of the culture (Pure culture showed uniform morphology).
- Perform gram staining (Refer Exp. No. 14⁰C) to look for gram's nature. If the culture is gram positive, perform the following tests.
- Inoculate test organism on blood agar plate and incubate it for 24 hours at 37⁰C aerobically.
- Place Bacitracin, Novobiocin and Furazolidone discs on different corners of blood agar plate and observe for sensitivity pattern.
- Carryout catalase test by inserting a stick containing culture on H_2O_2 solution and observed bubble formation.
- These tests differentiate *Staphylococcus* from Micrococcus

Day 2

- Inoculate test organism on OF basal medium with the carbohydrate glucose.
- Perform motility test, oxidase test and mannitol salt agar for the the differentiate *Staphylococcus* species.

Day 3

- Inoculate test organism on Baired parker agar, Mannitol salt agar, DNase Test medium and vogel Johnson medium to confirm the *Staphylococcus* species and incubate at appropriate temperature for appropriate time duration.
- Perform coagulase test to confirm pathogenic strain of *Staphylococcus aureus*.

Table 64.1 –Observation – Identification characters

S. No	Test	Observation	Result
1	Gram Staining	Gram positive cocci in clusters	It may be *Staphylococcus* or *Micrococcus*
2	Growth on Nutrient agar	Yellowish brown colonies	It may be *Staphylococcus* or *Micrococcus*
3	Catalase	Positive	It may be *Staphylococcus* or *Micrococcus*
4	Growth on OF medium with glucose	Fermentative	It may be *Staphylococcus* sp.
5	Growth on Blood agar	Beta haemolysis	It may be *Staphylococcus* sp.
6	Oxidase test	Negative	It may be *Staphylococcus* sp.
7	Bacitracin	Resistant	It may be *Staphylococcus* sp.
8	Novobiocin	Sensitive	It may be *Staphylococcus* sp.
9	Furazolidone	Resistant	It may be *Staphylococcus* sp.
10	DNase test	Positive	It may be *Staphyloccus aureus*
11	Mannitol salt agar	Yellow colour good growth	It may be *Staphyloccus aureus*
12	Tellurite utilization on Baired parker agar	Black colour colonies	It may be *Staphyloccus aureus*
13	Vogel Johnson agar	Black colour colonies	It may be *Staphyloccus aureus*
14	MacConkey agar	NLF colonies	It may be *Staphyloccus aureus*
15	Cogulase test	Positive	It confirms the pathogenic strain of *Staphylococcus aureus*

Result

Based on the above observation the given bacteria is identified as *Staphylococcus aureus*

Table 64.2 : Differentiation features of Gram positive cocci in clusters

Test	*Micrococcus*	*S. aureus*	*S. saprophyticus*	*S. epidermidis*
Catalase	Positive	Positive	Positive	Positive
Bacitracin	Sensitive	Resistant	Resistant	Resistant
Furazolidone	Resistant	Sensitive	Sensitive	Sensitive
Oxidase	Positive	Negative	Negative	Negative
OF Glucose	Oxidative	Fermentative	Fermentative	Fermentative
Coagulase	Negative	Positive	Negative	Negative
DNase	Negative	Positive	Negative	Negative
Mannitol Fermentation	Negative	Positive	Negative	Negative
Novobiocin	Sensitive	Sensitive	Resistant	Sensitive

65. Identification of *Streptococcus pyogenes*

Aim

To identify *Streptococcus pyogenes* from the given culture.

Background information

S. pyogenes is one of the most common gram positive cocci of the family Streptococcaceae. It is responsible for greater number of infectious diseases. The streptococci are classified by means of two major methods. They are based on their Haemolysis and based on antigens i.e., serotyping. Three types of haemolytic patterns are observed on blood agar, that are alpha haemolysis, Beta haemolysis and gamma haemolysis. Lancefield grouped Streptococci based on antigen as A to O. *S. pyogenes* belongs to the group A. Members of Group A Streptococci is responsible for tonsillitis, scarlet fever, cellulites, rheumatic fever etc.

Materials required

Sample : Broth or slant culture.

Chemicals & Media Required

Gram staining reagent, nutrient agar, Blood agar, Bile esculin agar , Biochemical test media & reagents, H_2O_2, Serum, Bacitracin, Novobiocin, Frurazolidone, Glass slides, petri plates, test tubes etc.

Procedure

Day 1

- Check the purity of the culture by streaking the culture on nutrient agar plate, incubate at 37°C for 24 hours and note Colony morphology of the culture (Pure culture showed uniform morphology). Streptococcus form circular, transleucent to opaque, pinpoint colonies.

- Perform gram staining (Refer Exp. No. 14bC) to look for gram's nature. If the culture is gram positive, perform the following tests.

- Inoculate test organism on blood agar plate and incubate for 24 hours at 37⁰C aerobically.

- Place Bacitracin, Novobiocin and Furazolidone discs on different corners of blood agar plate and observe sensitivity pattern.

- Perform Catalase test by inserting a stick containing culture on H_2O_2 solution and observed bubble formation.

Day 2

- Inoculate test culture on OF basal medium with glucose.

- Perform motility test, oxidase test, SXT test, CAMP test, 6.5% sodium chloride tolerance test, growth tolerance at 10°C and 45°C tests, esculin hydrolysis test to differentiate Streptococcus species.

Day 3

- Perform serogrouping to confirm the *S. pyogenes.*

Table 65.1 –Observation – Identification characters

S. No	Test	Observation	Result
1	Gram Staining	Gram positive cocci in chains	It may be Streptococci
2	Growth on Nutrient agar	Circular Pinpoint translucent colonies	It may be Streptococci
3	Catalase	Positive	It may be Streptococci
4	Growth on OF medium with glucose	Fermentative	It may be Streptococci
5	Growth on Blood agar	Beta haemolysis	It may be Beta haemolytic Streptococci sp.
6	Oxidase test	Negative	It may be Streptococci sp.
7	Bacitracin	Sensitive	It may be Gp. A Streptococci sp.
8	Novobiocin	Negative/ Resistant	It may be Gp. A Streptococci sp.
9	Furazolidone	Resistant	It may be Gp. A Streptococci sp.
10	Bile esculin Hydrolysis	Negative	It may be Gp. A Streptococci
11	Growth at 10°C	No Growth	It may be Gp. A Streptococci
12	Growth at 45°C	No Growth	It may be Gp. A Streptococci
13	Growth in 6.5% NaCl Medium	No Growth	It may be Gp. A Streptococci
14	CAMP test	Negative	It is not a Gp. B Streptococci and confirms Gp. A. Streptococci (S. pyogenes)
15	SXT test	Sensitive	It confirms Streptococcus pyogenes

Result

Based on the above observation the given bacteria is identified as *Streptococcus pyogenes*

To confirm the gram positive chain as Streptococcus pneumoniae it shows the following results

Gram positive cocci in pair
Capsulated
Alpha haemolytic
Characteristic draughtsman colony
Catalase Negative
Optochin sensitive
Bile solubilizer
Inulin fermenter

66. Identification of *Corynebacterium diphtheriae*

Aim

To identify *Corynebacterium diphtheriae* from the given mixed / pure culture.

Background information

Corynebacterium diphtheriae is a pathogenic bacterium that causes diphtheria. It is also known as the **Klebs-Löffler bacillus**, because it was discovered in 1884 by German bacteriologists Edwin Klebs (1834 – 1912) and Friedrich Löffler (1852 – 1915). *C. diphtheriae* is an aerobic, Gram positive organism, characterized by non-encapsulated, non-sporulated, nonmotile, straight or curved rods with a length of 1 to 8 μm and width of 0.3 to 0.8 μm, which form ramified aggregations in culture (looking like "Chinese characters")and sometimes which have clubbed ends. The bacterium may contain polymetaphosphate aggregates called Volutin granules. It is pathogenic only in humans. *C. diphtheriae* produce diphtheria toxin.

Materials required

Sample : Broth or stap or slant culture from throat specimens.

Chemicals & Media Required

Gram staining reagent, Blood agar, tellurite blood agar,Biochemical test media & reagents, H_2O_2, Serum, Glass slides, petri plates, test tubes etc.

Procedure

Day 1

- Check the purity of the culture by streaking the culture on Blood agar plate, incubated at 37°C for 24 hours and note Colony morphology of the culture (Pure culture showed uniform morphology).]

- Perform gram staining (Refer Exp. No. 14bC) to look for gram's nature. If the culture is gram positive, perform the following tests.

- Perform Catalase test by inserting a stick containing culture on H_2O_2 solution and observed bubble formation.

Day 2

- Perform Motility test, Nitrate, Urease, Gelatin hydrolysis, Alberts staining and esculin hydrolysis.

Day 3

- To confirm the Corynebacterium, inoculate test organism on tellurite blood agar and observed for growth.

Table 60.1 –Observation – Identification characters

S. No	Test	Observation	Result
1	Gram Staining	Gram positive rod with irregular arrangements	*It may be Corynebacterium, Listeria, Erysipelothrix, Lactobacilli, Kurthia*
2	Growth on Blood agar	Growth noted	*It may be Corynebacterium, Listeria, Erysipelothrix, Lactobacilli, Kurthia*
3	Catalase	Positive	*It may be Corynebacterium, Listeria, Kurthia*
4	Growth on Blood agar	Beta haemolysis	*It may be Corynebacterium, Listeria*
5	Bile esculin Hydrolysis	Negative	*It may be Corynebacterium*
6	Motility test	Non motile	*It may be Corynebacterium*
7	Nitrate	Positive	*It may be Corynebacterium*
8	Urease	Negative	*It may be Corynebacterium*
9	Gelatin hydrolysis	Negative	*It may be Corynebacterium*
10	Alberts staining	Metachromatic granules present	*It may be Corynebacterium diphtheriae*
11	Tellurite blood agar	Black colour colony	*Corynebacterium diphtheriae*

Result

Based on the above observation the given bacteria is identified as *Corynebacterium diphtheriae*.

67. Identification of *Pseudomonas aeruginosa*

Aim

To identify *Pseudomonas aeruginosa* from the given culture.

Background information

Pseudomonas aeruginosa is an opportunistic pathogen of humans. It is a Gram-negative, aerobic rod belonging to the family **Pseudomonadaceae**. These bacteria are common inhabitants of soil and water. Almost all strains are motile by means of a single polar flagellum. **Infection associated with *Pseudomonas aeruginosa* are Endocarditis,** Pneumonia , **Bacteremia,** **Septicemia,** meningitis and brain abscesses, **otitis,** keratitis, neonatal ophthalmia, osteomyelitis, **Urinary tract infections. Gastrointestinal infections** like pediatric diarrhoea, typical gastroenteritis, and necrotizing enterocolitis, skin infections like burns, trauma or dermatitis; folliculitis, acne vulgaris like symptoms.

Materials required - Sample : Broth or stap or slant culture.

Chemicals & Media Required

Gram staining reagent, Mac Conkey agar, Cetrimide agar, Biochemical test media & reagents, Glass slides, petri plates, test tubes etc.

Procedure

Day I

- Check the purity of the culture by streaking the culture on nutrient agar plate, incubated at 37°C for 24 hours and note Colony morphology of the culture (Pure culture showed uniform morphology).

- Perform gram staining (Refer Exp. No. 14bC) to look for gram's nature and catalase and oxidase.

- Inoculate test organism on Mac Conkey agar plate and incubated it for 24 hours at 37°C aerobically.

- Perform Motility test, Indole test and TSI test. It is helpful to understand the probable nature of the isolate and these will differentate enterobacteriacea from other aerobic family of human pathogens

Day II

- Perform MR, VP, Urease, Nitrate, Deaminease, Decarboxylase, Melonate, KCN and carbohydrate fermentation tests along with EMB media inoculation to confirm generic level identification of the isolate.

Day III

- Probably Identified bacterial isolate is confirmed by streaking it on Cetrimide agar and incubate at 37°C for 24 hours and observed the colony morphology.

Table 67.1 –Observation – Identification characters

S. No	Test	Observation	Result
1	Simple staining	Rod	
2	Gram Staining	Gram negative	
3	Growth on MacConkey agar	NLF colonies	
4	Catalase	Positive	It is not a member of Enterobacteriaceae.
5	Oxidase test	Positive	It is not a member of Enterobacteriaceae.
6	Motility	Motile	It may be *Pseudomonas sp.*
7	Indole	Negative	It may be *Pseudomonas sp*
8	MR	Positive	It may be *Pseudomonas sp*
9	VP	Negative	It may be *Pseudomonas sp*
10	Citrate	Positive	It may be *Pseudomonas sp*
11	TSI	A/K Gas negative H$_2$S Negative	It may be *Pseudomonas sp*
12	Urease	Negative	It confirms *Pseudomonas sp.*
13	Nitrate	Positive	It confirms *Pseudomonas aeruginosa*
14	Growth on Cetrimide agar	Bluish green colonies	It confirms *Pseudomonas aeruginosa*

Result

Based on the above observation the given bacteria is identified as *Pseudomonas aeruginosa*

68. Antibiotic Sensitivity Assay

Aim

To determine the effect of antibiotics on microbial growth.

To assess the sensitivity pattern of the given microbe.

Background information

Antibiotics are synthesized by microbial cells that inhibit or arrest the growth of other microorganisms. This process is often called antagonism. Antibiotics inhibit the growth by various mechanisms. They inhibits protein synthesis, damaging cell wall, interfere PG layer synthesis, inhibit nucleic acid synthesis and prevent the formation of cell membrane. Antibiotics are classified into broad spectrum and narrow spectrum antibiotics on the basis of mode of action. Antimicrobials have increased activity and stability, simpler method of administration, better diffusibility in to the remote area and greater selective toxicity.

> **Box 68.1 – Strokes method**
>
> It is another one disc diffusion method to detect sensitivity pattern of microbes to antibiotics. Both test and control organisms are used in single plate. Only four discs are used in a plate. Radius of zone of inhibition is usually measured.

Antibiotic assay is performed by using disc diffusion technique. Two great scientists **William Kirby and A.W.Bauer** developed it during the year 1966. In this, antibiotics present in disc diffuse in to the remote area. Successfulness of disc diffusion is depends on amount of inoculum, nature of disc, moisture content of media and incubation condition. *This test is done to determine which antibiotic is effective against the particular pathogen. In this method both test and control organisms were used in two separate plates. Maximum of eight disc may be place in a plate. Width of the zone of inhibition is usually measured.*

Materials Required

Culture : 3-4 colonies of pathogen.

Media - Peptone water, Mueller Hinton Agar – this media provide required concentration of Ca++ and Mg ++ ions to growing bacteria. It will avoid false positive and false negative reactions.

Antibiotics - Antibiotic discs for selective pathogens.

General Materials

Petriplates, beakers, test tubes, L – Rod, cotton, Antibiotic Zone Scale / Millimeter scale, pH meter, McFarland Standard etc.,

Procedure

Preparation of inoculum

● Select Three or four colonies of the single species.

● Inoculate test organism in peptone water and incubate for 3 – 4 hours at 35°C.

● Adjust turbidity of the suspension to match 0.5 Mc Farland standard and used for antibacterial sensitivity assay.

Antibiotic assay

● Prepare Mueller Hinton Agar and pour it into petriplates (thickness of medium should be 4 mm).

- Inoculate 0.1mL of turbidity adjusted bacterial culture on the surface of the plate (MHA) and spread by making use of L rod.

- Allow bacterial culture inoculated plates to dry for five minutes.

- Place antibiotic discs on the surface of previously seeded petriplate using appropriate technique (Place 6-8 discs in 100mm dia petriplates).

- Incubate plate at 37°C for 18 - 24 hours.

- Examine the plates for inhibitory zone and measure the zone of inhibition in mm and interpretate the results as per standard. Mention the results as sensitive, moderate and resistant.

- Main causes of error are amount of inoculum, contamination of inoculum, reduction of disc potency, error in measuring the zone of inhibition and poor quality control.

Observation and Result

Organisms growth inhibition is noted as zone of inhibition. It is noted as nil growth around the discs. Rate of zone is compared with standard table given by antibiotic disc manufacturing company and interpretated as sensitive, intermediate or resistant to the antibiotic.

Viva questions

Define MBC, antibiotics, antimicrobial agent, bactericidal, bacteriastatic

How antibiotic discs are prepared.

What are principles of disc diffusion method?

Why antibiotic assay method is called Kirby& bauer methods?

Why Mueller hinton agar is used in antibiotic assay?

What are other methods used in assay of antibiotic?

What is strokes method of disc diffusion?

Compare Kirby bauer method from strokes method.

What factors must be carefully controlled in the Kirby–Bauer method?

What is the difference between an antibiotic and an antimicrobic?

What are some reasons bacteria are becoming more resistant to antibiotics?

Spotters : Mueller hinton agar, Antibiotics, Plates with zone of inhibition

69. Assessment of Minimum Inhibitory Concentrations (MIC)
(DILUTION SUSCEPTIBILITY TEST)

Aim

To assess the minimum bactericidal concentration or minimum inhibitory concentration of antibiotics by agar dilution method.

Background Information

Agar dilution is a quantitative method for determining the MIC of the antibiotics against bacteria to be tested. Minimum inhibitory concentration is the lowest or minimum, concentration of antimicrobials required to prevent bacterial multiplication under specified condition. This technique is performed when a patient does not respond to treatment through to be adequate, relapses while being treated or when there is immune suppression. Dilution technique measures the MIC. They can also be used to measure the MBC, which is the lowest concentration antimicrobial required to kill bacteria. MIC is reported as the lowest concentration of antimicrobial required to prevent visible growth. The MBC is lowest concentration required to produce a sterile culture. Dilution technique requires careful standardization and control of inoculum, broth, anti microbial solutions, incubation time, dilution technique and reading of results. In recent year's **semi automated techniques** have been developed. **E test or Epsilon test** also usually performed to assess MIC. It is a stripe diffusion method but in this different concentrations of antibiotics are impregnated in a single stripe.

Materials Required

Culture	:	Pathogenic bacteria
Media	:	Peptone water
		Mueller Hinton agar
Antibiotic powder:		By the recommendation of the physician.

Water bath, 0.5 McFarland standard, sterile test tubes, 50 mL conical flasks etc. Sterilize all the necessary materials appropriately before starting of the experiment. Strict aseptic condition should maintain while handling the cultures.

Preparation of antibiotics stock

Weigh 200mG of antibiotics powder and dissolve in 5mL of sterile distilled water in sterile screw caped tube (**Stock-200mG/5mL**). Mix 0.5mL of stock solution with 9.5mL sterile distilled water in sterile screw caped tube (Working solution). Concentration of **working solution is 2000µg/mL**.

Procedure

Medium Preparation

- Prepare Mueller Hinton Agar in 500mL conical flasks (180 mL media). Add agar for 200mL concentration.

- Equally dispense entire mediums to ten 50mL conical flask (18mL each) and sterilize at 121°C for 15 minutes in an autoclave.

- Keep ready the media for adding antibiotic solution (Maintain this medium in water bath at 55 – 60°C until use – avoid solidification)

Dilution

- Arrange sterilized test tubes in a test tube rack and label as T1→T10.

- Add 2mL of sterile saline solution to all test tubes under aseptic condition.

- Add one mL of working solution to first tube (T1) using sterile pipette.

- Add one mL of solution from T1 to T2 and continues the dilution upto final. For each dilution separate tip or pipette should be used. Maintain equal volume of saline in all tubes after dilution (2mL).

3. Preparation of bacterial suspension

- Select three or four colonies of the pathogens of the single species.
- Inoculate test organism into peptone water and incubate for 3 – 4 hours at 35°C.
- Adjust the turbidity of the suspension to match 0.5 McFarland standard and used for MIC assay.

4. Preparation of agar plate with different concentration of antibiotics.

- Arrange all the conical flasks (with 18mL MHA), antibiotic dilutions, petriplates and label properly in laminar flow chamber.
- Pour T1 antibiotic solution into one 50mL conical flask containing media.
- Mix Media and antibiotic solution properly and pour into appropriately labeled petriplates. Follow same procedure to remaining solutions T2 to T10. Finally, prepare 10 different antibiotics containing plates and kept ready for inoculation.

5. Inoculation

- Mark a grid depends on the number of culture available for inoculation.
- Inoculate a loopful of culture on the dried surface of the medium.
- Inoculate control plate with the test organisms.
- Allow all the cultures to dry and invert the plates.
- Incubate the Plates at 37^0C for 18 – 24 hrs.
- Observe the plates for visible growth and recorded the results.

Observation

Read the plates for presence or absence of growth. Check the control plate for growth. Control plate must show confluent growth. Read the test plate. The concentration at which growth is completely inhibited is considered as MIC.

Note: In all plates and tubes indicate dilution/ concentration of antibiotic. Express the value as microgram.

Table 69.1: Dilution procedure and concentration of antibiotics

S.No	Tube No.	Volume of Water		Dilution	Intermediate antibiotics in Medium µG/mL	Final concentrationof concentration of antibiotics in µG/mL	Observation
01	T1	2 mL		1:01	1000.00	50.00	
02	T2	2 mL		1:02	0500.00	25.00	
03	T3	2 mL		1:03	0250.00	12.50	
04	T4	2 mL		1:04	0125.00	06.25	
05	T5	2 mL	Serial dilution	1:05	0067.50	03.38	
06	T6	2 mL		1:06	0033.75	01.69	
07	T7	2 mL		1:07	0016.88	00.84	
08	T8	2 mL		1:08	0008.44	00.42	
09	T9	2 mL		1:09	0004.22	00.21	
10	T10	2 mL		1:10	0002.11	00.10	

Result

Presence of growth is noted in any of the concentration of antibiotics. MIC of given antibiotics for test organism is $-----$ µG/mL

Viva questions

What is MIC

What are the alternative methods available to assess MIC

What are the merits and demerits of broth dilution test.

C. Clinical Mycology

70. Isolation of Fungi from Clinical Samples

Aim

To collect proper specimen for the isolation of fungal pathogens.

To perform fungal isolation techniques

Introduction

Fungi are significant, sometimes overlooked, human pathogens. Infection caused by the fungus ranges from mild to life threatening. Diagnosis is based on a combination of clinical and laboratory investigations. Laboratory procedure includes, Demonstration of fungi by microscopy, Identification by culture, Detection of specific humoral response and Detection of fungal antigens and metabolites in body fluids.

Successful of laboratory fungal diagnosis depends on specimen selection, Specimen collection, Specimen transport, Processing, Microscopic examination, Culturing.

Materials Required

Clinical sample, Any one or two media of the following (Dermatophyte fungi - Oatmeal agar; Red yeast-Cornmeal agar; Malassezia - SGA with olive oil; White yeast - Morphology agar; Aspergillus, Penicillium, Paecilomyces - Czapek dox agar; *A.fumigatus* - Sabourau's glucose Agar; Coelomycetes – Brain Heart Infusion medium; Cryptococcus - Niger seed agar), Petriplates, BOD incubator, scalpel etc.

Specimen Selection

Direct specimens are the best choice for fungal infection. Eg. Skin scrapings

Specimen Collection

Specimen collection for the detection of mycoses is very similar to specimen collection for bacteria. But fungal detection requires large quantity of specimen than bacterial identification. Fingernails and toenails suspected of Dermatophytosis should be cleaned extensively with 70% ethanol. Swabs are not optimal specimen collection for fungal identification. Depends on the site of infection, sample collection method and specimen type may vary.

For dermatophytic infection : Skin scrapings, Pus, Nail clippings, Hair plug not cut.

Sucutaneuous infection: Pus, biopsy tissues, Aspirated fluid, Skin scrapings.

Systemic mycosis : Sputum, Bronchial washings, Exudates from cutaneous lesion, CSF, Urine, Tissue biopsy, Vaginal swab, Blood.

Specimen Transport: Fungi are hardy organisms. Their cell wall provides an effective barrier against various toxic agents. Always use aerobic transport media. Transport containers should be sterile, humidified and leak proof. Keep the specimen moist by adding a minimum volume of sterile saline. Desiccation, elevated temperatures, low temperatures and starvation affect viability of some fungi. Bacterial overgrowth is another factor. Transport time should be kept to a minimum (2 hours) because some fungal agents are sensitive to environmental stresses. Specimens from sites with possible contaminating bacteria or leucocytes should be transported rapidly because bacterial overgrowth and leucocytes could cause decreased fungal viability.

Specimens that cannot be transported to the clinical laboratory within 2 hours should be stored at 4°C. Sterile body fluids (30-37°C) and dermatological specimens are not be refrigerated because some dermatophytes are sensitive to cold.

Specimen Processing

Liquid specimens may have low concentration of fungus and will require centrifugation to increase fungal cell concentration. Hard specimens should be minced before inoculation.

Concentration

Large volume of fluid should be concentrated by centrifugation (2000 rpm for 10 min). Use the resulting pellet for culture and KOH examination. Body fluids, Urine, CSF, Sputum are used after digestion with N-acetyl L-cysteine.

Mincing or homogenization

Biopsy samples, tissues and nails must be processed to increase the recovery of fungi. With sterile scalpels, mince specimens into small pieces in a petriplate with a few drops of sterile distilled water. If *Histoplasma* is suspected, specimen is homogenized by using tissue grinder after mincing.

Specimen Examination

Specimen should be evaluated microscopically and macroscopically. Microscopic examination reveals vital information about the relative concentration and type of fungus present in the specimen.

Once a smear is made, several strains can be used to detect fungi. The common staining methods are Calcofluor white, KOH mount, KOH with quink ink, Indian ink, Hanks modified acid-fast stain (Refer 70a, 70b, 70c)

Media selection

Media selection depends on body site, nature of infection and nature of contamination. To prevent bacterial pathogens antibiotics should be used or lower the pH of the medium. Brain heart infusion agar with antibiotics, Potato Dextrose Agar, Mold agar, Sabouraud's Glucose Agar, Niger seed agar, Yeast extract phosphate medium. , Buffered charcoal yeast extract agar, Rose Bengal chloramphenical agar. From the above list of mycotic media, any one or two media selected for cultivation.

Inoculation

Concentrated aspirated body fluids are directly inoculated on to the medium by making use of inoculation loop. Swabs are vortexed in distilled water before inoculation. Vortexed specimens are inoculated on medium after concentration. After inoculation hair and skin scrapings are pressed firmly on the surface of the medium. Nail should be pulverized using scalpels and press fragments firmly onto the medium surface.

Incubation

All fungal media are incubated at 28 to 30°C for 4 weeks, because most fungi will produce colonies by the end of the 3rd Week. Vaginal cultures may be incubated for only 7 days. Observe the media once in two days. *Histoplasma capsulatum* and *Blastomyces dermatidis* may require 4-8 weeks. Aerobic non clinical fungus may produce fruiting bodies within 72 hours.

Examination of Fungal Growth on Primary Media

Read primary plates daily for the first week, every other day for the second week and twice weekly for the remaining two weeks. When growth appears, differentiate yeast from mold by microscopic examination. Once colonies are formed on the media, the organism should be viewed microscopically. Zygomycetes are observed under dissecting microscope. Yeast is observed by Wet preparation, Lacto phenol cotton blue staining and Indian ink preparation. Mold is observed by Wet preparation, Scotch tape, Tease preparation, Slide cultures, Lactophenol cotton blue staining, Ascospore.

Observation

Report the following distinguishing characteristics of fungi during microscopic examinations. Hyphae and yeast cells, Yeast cells only, Yeast cells with capsules, Spherules, Sclerotic cells, Sulfur granules with fungal hyphae.

Result

Fungal species can be identified based on microscopic morphology and culture (Refer Figure 70 a, b, c)

Viva questions

What are the samples used of describe dermatophytes & superficial mycotic infection?

What kinds of transporting methods are adopted to transport fungal sample?

How do you inoculate clinical sample on media?

What are the media used to isolate fungus from clinical samples?

Mention temperature required for fungal cultivation

Mention about incubation condition for fungal isolation.

Spotters – Any one fungal medium, microscopic morphology of mould.

70a. KOH Mount

Aim

To demonstrate fungal elements from the clinical specimens by KOH mount.

Principle

KOH may be used to examine hair, nails, skin scrapings, fluids, exudates or biopsies. The fungal structures such as hyphae, large yeast (*Blastomyces*), spherules, and sporangia may be distinguished. Examine slides with reduced light (narrow the iris diaphragm) and examine negative smears on several consecutive days. The fungal structures may be enhanced by using a phase-contrast microscope. Specimens placed in a drop of 15% KOH will dissolve tissues at a greater rate than fungi because fungi have chitinous cell walls. The clearing effect throughout the clinical specimen can be accelerated by gently heating the KOH preparation.

Materials required.

Microscope, petriplates, slide, coverslip, Bunsen flame, 15% KOH etc.

15% Potassium Hydroxide Solution is prepared by adding 15g potassium hydroxide and 20mL glycerol in 80 mL of distilled water.

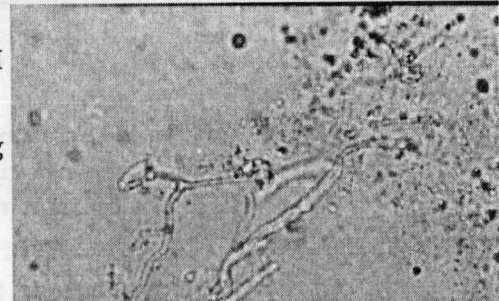

Fig 70.1: KOH mount

Specimen

Pus, aspirates, Skin scrapings, Hair plugging, Nail clipping.

Procedure

- Place the material to be examined onto a clean glass slide.
- Add a drop of 15% KOH to the material and mix.

- Pace a cover glass over the preparation.
- Allow the KOH preparation at room temperature until the material has been cleared. The slide may be warmed to speed the clearing process. Slides that are initially negative for fungi may be re-examined the following day.
- Observe the preparation by brightfield or phase-contrast microscopy.

Observations and Results

Mycelium and spore are observed within the tissue. KOH clears hard tissue and facilitates easy observation. KOH mount provides first hand information about fungal infection in tissues.

Viva questions

What are the uses of KOH?

Mention few application of KOH mount.

How do you interpertate the results of KOH mount?

Spotters - KOH

70b. KOH-DMSO-INK mount / stain

Aim

To demonstrate fungal elements / yeast from clinical samples.

Principle

Specimens placed in a drop of 15% KOH will dissolve tissue at a greater rate than fungi because fungi have chitinous cell walls. The clearing effect throughout the clinical specimen can be accelerated by gently heating the KOH preparation. Addition of Ink to KOH enhances contrast. This method is most useful for detecting *Malassezia furfur* in skin scrapings. DMSO present in staining reagent eliminates the need of heat during staining.

Materials required

KOH-DMSO-INK stain, Slide, Skin scrapings or any other sample, Cover slip, Microscope

Staining reagent

- Potassium hydroxide (15%)
- DMSO (Dimethy Sulphoxide) – 60% - it is prepared by adding 60mL of DMSO to 40mL of distilled water.
- DMSO-KOH reagent–it is generally prepared by adding 20g KOH in 100mL of 60% DMSO solution.
- KOH-DMSO-INK stain- It is prepared by mixing of equal volume of DMSO-KOH reagent and Parkers quink ink.

Procedure

- Take clinical sample in a clean microscopic slide and emulsify with DMSO-KOH-Ink staining reagent.
- Apply cover slip over the preparations and leaves it for 5-10minutes.
- Examine the preparations microscopically.

Observations

Fungal elements and mycelium are observed in clinical samples.

Result

Mycelial elements clearly demonstrated, which indicates the availability of fungal infection in particular tissue. Spore along with conidium describes mould species.

Viva questions

Expand KOH and DMSO

Mention the purpose of using KOH, DMSO and Ink in microscopic examination of fungus.

What are the principles of this technique?

Mention about purpose of this technique.

Spotters – KOH, DMSO, Microscopic picture of ink mount

70c. KOH- Calcoflour fluorescent-stain

Aim

To demonstrate fungal elements from clinical samples

Principle

Calcoflour white stain may be used for direct examination of most specimens using fluorescent microscopy. The cell walls of the fungi bind the stain and fluoresce blue-white or apple-green depending on the filter combination used. The use of calcofluor white (CFW), a fluorescent brightener used in the textile industry, the addition of potassium hydroxide (KOH) will enhance the visualization of fungal elements in specimens for microscopic examination. The CFW nonspecifically binds to the chitin and cellulose in the fungal cell wall and fluoresces a bright green to blue. A substantial amount of non-specific fluorescence from human cellular materials and natural and synthetic fibers should be expected. The CFW highlights suspicious structures but the interpretation of the structures relies on traditional fungal morphologic features.

Materials required

10% Potassium hydroxide, Calcoflour white stain, Slide, Coverslip, Fluoresoent microscope

0.1% Calcofluor White (W/V) Solution - Calcoflour - 1 gm; Distilled water 100 mL

Gently heat if precipitate develops. Filter if precipitate persists. Store at 25° C in the dark.

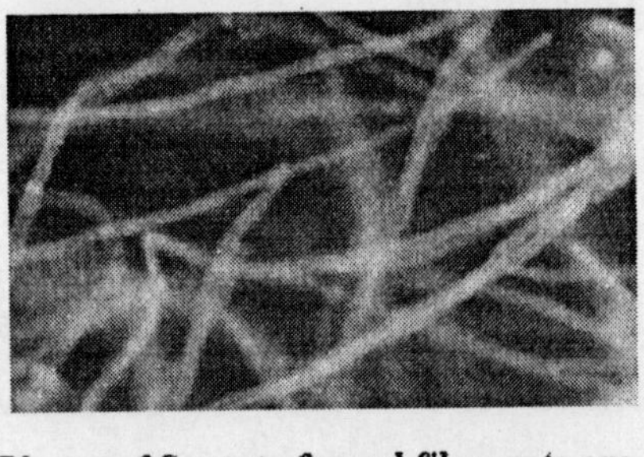

Plenty of Septate fungal filaments are seen

Fig 70.2 : Fungal mycelium

Procedure

- Take small quantity of the specimen on clean slide.
- Add one drop of KOH.
- Also Add one drop of calcoflour stain.
- Place the cover slip on the specimen and incubate for 5-10minutes.
- Examine the slide under fluorescent excitation light of 300-412nm. With a 500nm barrier fungi will appear yellow green. Without an emission filter, fungi will fluoresce bright white.

Expected result

Hyphae, yeast cells and fungal elements will fluoresce.

Viva questions

What are the principles of this technique?

What are the purposes of using calcoflour stain?

Which microscope is used to demonstrate calcoflour white stain?

Spotters - Calcoflour white stain

70d. India ink Preparations

Aim

To identify and differentiate capsulated fungi using India ink.

Principle

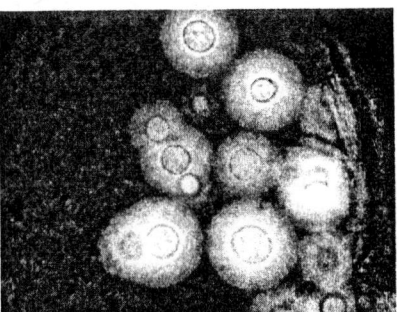

An India ink preparation can be used for the rapid detection of the encapsulated yeasts based on negative staining. The capsule repels the carbon particles of the India ink, giving a clear well-demonstrated halo around each encapsulated stain.

Materials required

India ink and dropper, Blood or CSF sample, Slide, Cover slip, Bright field microscope.

Fig 70.3 – India ink showing *Cryptococcus neoformans*

Procedure

- Place one drop of specimen on clean slide.
- Add one drop of India ink on the specimen
- Place the cover slip on the specimen and allows the ink to diffuse under the cover slip.
- Note the colour of the preparation (Normal Preparation is brownish colour. If preparation is black, add 1-2 drop of sterile distilled water, mix and mount with cover slip).
- Examine the slide under high power objectives

Observation

Presence of budding yeast with clear halos around them indicates capsular materials

Result

Crytococcus neoformans is one of the capsulated yeast.

Viva questions

What are the principles of India ink preparations?

What are the advantages of India ink staining?

What are the organisms identified through India ink?

Spotters – India ink, Microscopic picture of *Cryptococcus neoformans*

70e. Giemsa Stain for *Histoplasma capsulatum*

Aim

To demonstrate *Histoplasma capsulatum* infections in human.

Principle

Giemsa stain is used for examining intracellular structures and is applied to primary specimens of bone marrow tissue and WBC's in which *H.capsulatum* is suspected.

Materials required

Giemsa stain and dropper, Inoculation loop.

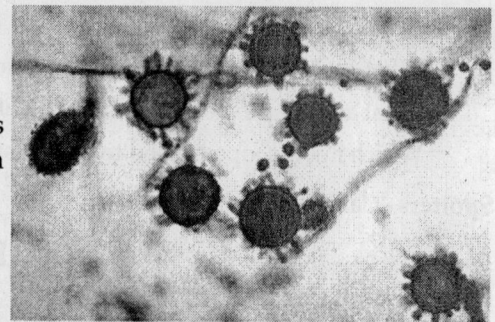

Fig 70.4: *Histoplasma capsulatum*

Procedure

- Prepare thin smear as like differential Leucocyte count procedure.
- Fix the Smear with absolute alcohol for 1 minute.
- Immediately drain off alcohol and allow the smear to dry.
- Flood 1:10 diluted Giemsa stain on the smear and allowed to stain for 5 minutes.
- Wash the slide with water and air dry. Don't blot dry.

Expected result

Necrotic cells in the specimen will have pink cytoplasm.

Normal cell- light blue - violet lavender cytoplasm.

Phagocytised yeast cells will stain light to dark blue, and each will have a clear halo around it.

Look for purple pseudoencapsulated yeast forms of *H.capsulatum* inside PMN cells and monocytes.

Viva questions

Why giemsa stain is used to demonstrate Histoplasma?

How do you differentiate Histoplasma from other fungi?

How do you demonstrate the availability of Histoplasma in tissue?

Spotters – Microscopic picture of Histoplasma, Giemsa stain

71. Identification of Moulds On Primary Culture

Aim

To identify mould on primary isolation media.

Background information

Primary Culture means fungus / mould grown on primary isolati on medium. If an organism is not identifiable on primary culture, subculture should be performed. Yeasts are sub cultured onto yeast morphology agar and inoculated by means of streaking. Molds are sub cultured by several methods. They are Block inoculation, Scarification and Slide culture

Perform all subcultures in a class II biological safety cabinet.

Materials required

Culture of mould on primary isolation medium, Scalpel, Petriplates, Slides, Needle, DTM Media for dermatophyte identification, Czapek dox Agar for aerobic common fungi, Brain Heart Infusion agar for dimorphic fungi, Niger seed agar for Cryptococcus, Sabourauds Dextrose agar, Potato dextrose agar, Rose Bengal chloramphenicol agar

Procedure

Fungal species may subcultured on different commercially available mycological media. On selective and differential medium fungal species grown initially as white/multi coloured mycelium. Fruiting bodies / asexual spores are formed during growth, which is considered as a selective character for identification. Conidium/spores are usually identified by making use of any one of the following methods. Block inoculation, Scarification are the sub culture inoculation methods. Slide culture technique, tease preparation and cellophone tape mount are used to identify conidial structures. All these techniques use Lactophenol Cotton Blue as a clarity stain for clear visualization of fungal elements. Size and shape of the conidia will vary depends up on the genus. The following are different types of conidia present in different fungal species.

Sub culturing

A relatively rich medium (V- 8 Juice agar) and nutritionally poor medium (PDA, Oat meal agar) should be used. BHI is not an optimal spore inducing media but is needed for systemic fungi. A third medium is needed to encourage fruiting body formation. Eg. Cotton seed agar, Hay infusion agar, Water agar. Media lacking antimicrobials should be used for subcultures. For slide culture, clear or moderately translucent media are preferred. Dimorphic fungi convert to yeast more quickly and abundantly on specific media. When conversion is attempted, two plates of the same medium should be inoculated. One is placed at 28°C and the other is at 37°C. All molds should be sub cultured on SGA, PDA and V-8 juice agar.

Mould Identification Based On Spore or Conidium Production

Conidium is one of the asexual parts of mold. Size and shape of the conidia will be vary depends upon the group. Mold conidia may be identified on the basis of slide culture technique. There are seven forms of conidia.

Aleurioconidia

It is usually borne singly, either directly on the hyphae, on short hyphal projections. Eg. *B.dermatitidis, H. capsulatum* and the dermatophytes (*Microsporum, Epidermophyton* and *Trichophyton sp*)

Annelloconidia

It arises from the apex of annelides (flask-shaped or cylindrical) and produced, with the youngest conidium at the base. Eg. *Exophiala werneckii, Exophila spinifera* and *Scopulariopsis sp.*

Arthroconidia

Septation and the disjunction or rounding off of simple or branched conidiogenous hyphae produce them. Eg. *Coccidioides immitis, Trichosporon*

Blastoconidia

They are blown out from another cell, from hyphae. It produced either by simple budding or by germ tube. Eg. *Fonsecae pedrosoi, Cladosporium, Candida sp*

Phialoconidia

They are produced within a conidiagenous cell called phialide. It is a rounded or elongated, vaselike structure. Eg. *Aspergillus, Acremonium, Phialosphora, Penicillum, Phaecilomyces, Exophiala dermatitidis, Mucour and Rhizopus*

Poroconida

They are produced through minute pores in the outer wall of the conidiophore. The conidia may be septate, pigmented and solitary or in chains with the youngest at the tip. Eg. *Alternaria , Curvularia, Bipolaris.*

Sympoduloconidia

It blown out from a conidiophore that enlarges as each new conidium is produced. The primary conidium is produced at the tip of the conidiophore. Successive conidia are produced to the side and above each preceding conidium.Eg. *Fonsecaea pedrosoi, Sporothrix schenckii, Fusarium , Beauvaria , Rhinocladiella*

Observation and results

Hyphae, conidium are looked and referred with standard microscopic picture and confirm for fungal identity (Refer Fig. 70a, b, c).

Viva questions

Name any two fungal subculture medium.

How do you perform fungal subculturing?

Name the methods of fungal culture.

What are the methods adopted to identify fungus?

Give examples for aleurocondia.

Name the conidium produced by Trichosporon.

71a. Block inoculation

Aim

To subculture mould on sporulation or differential media for identification.

Materials required

Culture on primary isolation medium, Differential medium as per fungal type, Scalpel, Petriplate, Incubator etc.,

Procedure

- Cut 0.5cm square block of the fungal colony from primary isolation medium using sterile scalpel.

- Inoculate Fungal block on fresh fungal medium by placing it upside down.

- Incubate plate at 20-28°C for 24-48 hours.

- Examine the fungal growth and observe the morphology using LPCB staining.

Observation and Result

Specified fungal spore and conidium are noted and identified the fungal species.

71b. Scarification

Aim

To subculture mould on differential and identification medium.

Materials required

Blunt needle, Culture on primary isolation medium, Differential medium as per fungal type, Scalpel, Petriplate, Incubator etc.,

Procedure

- Take 24-48 hours grown fungal mould on primary culture medium.

- Scrape the fungus grown on medium surface using blunt sterile needle.

- Inoculate the fungal scrape on specified differential medium by scratching the surface of the medium.

- Incubate the inoculated plate at 20-28°C for 24-48 hours.

- Examine the fungal growth and observe the morphology using LPCB staining.

Observation and Result

Specified fungal spore and conidium are noted and identified the fungal species.

71c. Slide Culture Technique

Aim

To demonstrate fungal morphology for the complete identification.

Background information

Slide culture is a very useful technique to study undisturbed morphological details of fungi, particularly reproductive structures. Conidial structures are clearly demonstrated by this technique.

Materials required.

Petriplates, U shaped glass rod, Cover slip, filter paper, cotton, hot air oven, sabouraud's dextrose agar or potato dextrose agar or Rose Bengal chloramphenicol agar, any one fungal strain etc..

Procedure

- Cut out one cm² agar block from the petriplate.

- Hold the agar block horizontally with the help of sterile scalpel.

- Inoculate one side of the agar block with the spore of the fungus using inoculation needle.

- Place agar block on the center of the slide with inoculated side down and touch on the slide.

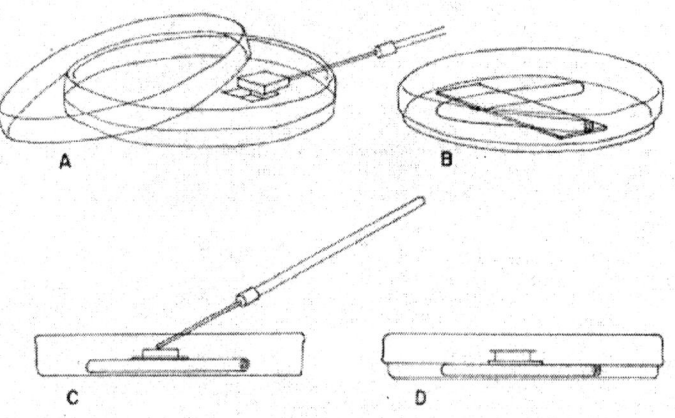

Fig 71.1: Slide culture setup

- Inoculate second side of the agar block with the spore.
- Place the cover slip over the agar block.
- Take sterile petriplate and place a piece of cotton.
- Moisten the cotton with sterile water.
- Place U shaped rod over the cotton to hold the slide culture setup.
- Place the slide culture setup above the rod and closed.
- Incubate the slide culture setup at 25°C for 24 – 48 hours.
- Remove cover slip from the setup and placed in the center of the slide containing lacto phenol cotton blue stain. This is performed after the observation of visual fungal growth.
- Remove agar block from the slide
- Add a drop of lacto phenol cotton blue stain on the slide. Place cover slip over the lacto phenol cotton blue stain.
- Examine both slides microscopically and record the conidial morphology.

Examination

- Fungal spores will develop in the air space between the agar surface and the cover slip.
- Monitor the development of mature spores.
- When sporulation appears, carefully lift the cover slip and stain with LPCB and examine microscopically.
- Determine the spore nature and spore bearing structure nature.

Observations and Results

Mould conidium and mycelium are easily demonstrated and fungal species are identified (Refer Fig. 70 a, b, c)

Viva questions

Mention the requirements for slide culture technique.

What kinds of fungal structures are demonstrated through slide culture?

Why this technique is called slide culture?

What kinds of organisms are identified through this technique?

Spotters – Slide culture set up.

71d. Cellophone tape mount

Aim

To identify moulds using conidium and its spores.

Principle

This method usually maintains the original position of the characteristic fungal structures. Colony should be grown on plated medium.

Materials required

Clear cellophane tape, Lactophenol cotton blue stain, Glass slides, fungal culture etc.,

Procedure

- Take clear cellophane tape.

- Hold the tip of the tape securely with forceps and press the lower, sticky side very firmly to the surface of the fungal colony.

- Gently pulled away the cellophane tape from the fungal colony. Aerial hyphae will adhere to the tape.

- Open up the tape strip and place it on a small drop of LPCB on a glass slide.

- Examine the cellophane tape preparation under the microscope.

Observation and result

Fungal morphology is noted and species of the fungus is identified

71e. Tease preparation

Aim

To observe characteristic fungal morphology for identification.

Principle

A tease preparation is the quickest and most common technique for mounting fungi for microscopic examination

Materials required

Long handled inoculation needle, Two dissecting needles, lactophenol cotton blue stain (LPCB), microscopic slide, cover slip, finger nail polish.

Procedure

- Place one drop of LPCB on E center of the slide.

- Gently remove Small portion of growth midway between the center of the colony and the edge with the help of inoculation needle.

- Place fungal element in the LPCB.

- Gently tease fungal element using the two dissecting needles

- Place the cover slip on the preparations.

- Seal the edges of the cover slip with nail polish to preserve the mount.

Observation

Characteristic fungal conidium and spores are looked through high power objective lens.

Result

Fungal genus and species are identified based on reference microscopic picture (Fig. 70a, b & c).

71f. Lactophenol Cotton Blue Staining (LPCB)

Aim

To identify the filamentous fungi.

To demonstrate fungi and fungal elements.

Background information

Lacto phenol cotton blue is the most commonly used method in a mycology laboratory to identify filamentous fungi. Identification of filamentous fungi is made by their characteristic microscopic morphology such as shape, size, arrangement of spores and hyphae. Different methods are followed to prepare fungal cultures for microscopic examination by LPCB preparation. They are Tease mount preparation, Scotch tape preparation and slide culture preparation.

Materials Required

Compound Microscope, Petri plates , Slide, Cover Glass, inoculation wire and Lacto phenol Cotton blue.

Uses of LPCB – Lactic acid – helps in preserving the morphology of the fungal element

Phenol – acts as disinfectant, Cotton blue- stain fungal element, Glycerol – Hygroscopic agent. It prevents drying.

Procedure

- Place a drop of LPCB on a clean glass slide.
- Remove the small portion of colony with a straight wire and placed it in a drop of LPCB.
- Place the cover glass and apply gentle pressure.
- Allow the preparation for staining for 15 minutes .
- Examine the preparation microscopically and observe mycelium and conidia.
- Compared mycelial and conidial structures with standard for correct identifications (Fig. 70 a, b & c).

Observations and Results

Fungal morphology is noted and identified as _____fungi

Viva questions

How do you prepare LPCB?

What are the uses of LPCB?

How do you perform LPCB staining?

Give importance of LPCB staining.

Spotters – Lactophenol cotton blue stain

71g. Hair Perforation Test

Aim

To distinguish between isolates of dermatophytes, particularly *Trichophyton mentagrophytes* and *Trichophyton rubrum*.

Principle

Dermatophytes and keratinolytic fungi will perpendicularly penetrate hair by hyphae resulting in wedge shaped perforations.

Materials required

Hair cut pieces (1cm)

Sterile distilled water in vial.

Procedure

- Place hair in a vial with water.
- Inoculate with small fragments of the test fungus.
- Incubate at room temperature.
- Individual hairs are removed at intervals up to 4 weeks and examined microscopically in lactophenol cotton blue. Isolates of *T. mentagrophytes* produce marked localized areas of pitting and marked erosion whereas those of *T. rubrum* do not.

Observation

Perforation is observed on hair

Result

The fungal species is identified as *T. mentagrophytes* based on perforation.

72. Identification of yeast

Aim

To identify yeast from unknown culture

Background information

Yeasts are a heterogenous group of fungi that superficially appear to be homogeneous. Yeasts grow as unicellular form that reproduces by fission, budding, or a combination of both. True yeasts reproduce sexually, developing ascospores or basidiospores under favourable conditions. Yeast-like fungi (imperfect yeasts) reproduce only by asexual means. The identification of these fungi is based on a combination of morphological and biochemical criteria. Morphology is primarily used to establish the genera, whereas biochemical assimilations are used to differentiate the various species.

Materials required

Chromogenic yeast agar, Potassium hydroxide, Serum, Test tube, Slide, Cover slip, Microscope, Indian ink, Parkers quink ink, wooden applicators stick.

Procedure

Principal Criteria and Tests for Identifying Yeasts

1. Culture characteristics - Colony colour, shape, texture

2. Asexual structures: a. Shape and size of cells; b. Bipolar, fission, multipolar or unipolar "budding"; c. Absence or presence of arthroconidia, ballistoconidia, blastoconidia, clamp connections, endoconidia, germ tubes, hyphae, pseudohyphae, or sporangia and sporgangiospores.

3. Sexual structures - Arrangement, cell wall ornamentation, number, shape and size of ascospores or basidiospores

4. Physiological studies: a. Assimilation; b. Fermentation c. Nitrogen utilization d. Urea hydrolysis

Cultural characters

Streak Clinical sample on Sabouraud dextrose agar or Rose Bengal chloramphenicol agar plates. Incubate Plates at 25-30⁰C for 48 hours and observed for colony morphology, colour, shape and texture. Record the result and interpretate the results.

CHROM agar test

CHROM agar contains enzymatic substrates that are linked to chromogenic compounds. When specific enzymes cleave the substrates, the chromogenic substrates produce colour. The action of different enzymes produced by yeast species results in colour variations useful for the presumptive identification of yeasts. The test provides only presumptive identification of yeast eg: *C.kruses, C.tropicalis, C.albicans.*

Streak Cultures on the medium and incubate at 35°C in humidified dark chamber for 48-72 hours. After 72 hours observe colour change and interpretate the results.

C.albicans: A medium sized, green, smooth matte colony with a very slight green halo ion the surrounding medium.

C.tropicalois : Smooth medium sized matte colony, which is blue to blue grey with a pale pink edge. The colony may have a dark brown to purple halo, which diffuses into the agar.

C.krusei : A large, spreading, rough pink colony with a pale pink to white edge.

Germ tube test

The germ tube test provides a simple, reliable and economical procedure for the presumptive identification of *Candida albicans.* About 95% of the clinical isolates produce germ tubes when incubated in serum at 35°C for 2.5-3 hours. A germ tube represent the initiation of a hypha directly from the yeast cell.

Indian ink preparations

India ink can be added to specimens such as spinal fluids or exudates to provide a dark background that will highlight hyaline yeast cells and capsular material (halo effect). Hence, it should be used to examine specimens suspected of containing *Cryptococcus neoformans.* White blood cells may be distinguished from *Cryptococcus neoformans* because of the irregular edge of the halo and the pale cell wash

Giemsa Staining

Giemsa stain is used for examining intracellular structures and is applied to primary specimens of bone marrow tissue and WBC's in which *H.capsulatum* is suspected.

Urease test

The rapid urea hydrolysis test is used to screen isolates for *Cryptococcus neoformans.* Under these conditions, *C. neoformans* will rapidly hydrolyze urea, which results in a pink to red colour.

Nitrate test

Yeasts have the ability to use ammonium sulfate, asparagine, peptone, and urea aerobically as sole sources of nitrogen if adequate vitamins are provided. In contrast, aliphatic amines, potassium nitrate, sodium nitrate, and some amino acids are utilized selectively by different yeasts.

Ascospore Induction and Detection

One step in identifying a yeast involves determining whether or not the isolate has the ability to form ascospores. Some yeasts will readily form ascospores on primary isolation medium, whereas others require special media. The ability to form ascospores varies from isolate to isolate and may be lost in old laboratory strains. If only one mating type of a heterothallic yeast is present, no ascospores will be formed. Ascospore media contain small amounts of carbohydrates; this restricts vegetative growth while enhancing ascospore formation.

Modified kinyons Acid fast staining

Modified acid-fast stains are recommended for demonstrating ascospores. Unlike the Ziehl-Neelsen modified acid-fast stain, the modified Kinyoun acid-fast stain does not require heating the reagents used for staining.

Carbohydrate fermentation

It is performed as like bacterial carbohydrate fermentation test (Ref. Experiment   ).

Carbohydrate assimilation

This is performed using the medium phenol red agar base. On the medium spread 0.1mL of yeast culture and place carbohydrate disc. Incubate plates at 37°C for 24 to 48 hours and observed for colour change around disc.

Table 72.1: Identification and differentiation features of Different Yeasts

Organism	Pseudo hyphae	True hyphae	Urease	Blasto conidia	Ascospores	Nitrate	Germ tube
Candida albicans	Present	Present	Negative	Present	Absent	Positive	Positive
Trichosporan	Present	Present	Positive	Present	Absent	Negative	Negative
Saccharomyces	Present	Absent	Negative	Present	Present	Negative	Negative
Crytococcus neoformans	Present	Absent	Positive	Present	Absent	Negative	Negative
Torulopsis	Absent	Absent	Negative	Present	Absent	Negative	Negative
Rhodotorulla	Absent	Absent	Positive	Present	Absent	Negative	Negative
Prototheca	Absent	Absent	Negative	Present	Absent	Negative	Negative
Geotrichum	Absent	Present	Negative	Absent	Present	Negative	Negative
Other Candida	Absent	Absent	Positive	Absent	Present	Negative	Negative
Hanseula	Absent	Absent	Negative	Absent	Present	Negative	Negative

Table 72.2: Differentiation features of Different Yeasts based on carbohydrate assimilation and fermentation

Yeast/ Sugar	Assimilation								
	Glucose	Maltose	Sucrose	Lactose	Galactose	Melibiose	Inositol	Xylose	Trehalose
Candida albicans	Positive	Positive	Positive	Negative	Positive	Negative	Negative	Positive	Positive
Candida lipolytica	Positive	Negative	Negative	Negative	Negative	Negative	Negative	Negative	Negative
Candida krusei	Positive	Negative	Negative	Negative	Negative	Negative	Negative	Negative	Negative
Cryptococcus neoformans	Positive	Negative	Negative	Negative	Negative	Negative	Negative	Negative	Negative

Yeast / Sugar	Fermentation								
	Glucose	Maltose	Sucrose	Lactose	Galactose	Melibiose	Inositol	Xylose	Trehalose
Candida albicans	Fermentative	Fermentative	Negative	Negative	Fermentative	Negative	Negative	Negative	Fermentative
Candida lipolytica	Negative	Negative	Negative	Negative	Negative	Negative	Negative	Negative	Negative
Candida krusei	Fermentative	Negative	Negative	Negative	Negative	Negative	Negative	Negative	Negative
Cryptococcus neoformans	Fermentative	Fermentative	Fermentative	Negative	Fermentative	Negative	Negative	Negative	Negative

Result

Based on the above-mentioned test and microscopic morphology specific type of yeasts are identified.

72a. Germ Tube Test

Aim

To identify *Candida albicans*.

Background informations

Candida are the members of the normal flora of skin. More than 100 species are available in Candida. Among these *Candida albicans* cause most of the human infections. The germ tube test provides a simple, reliable and economical procedure for the presumptive identification of *Candida albicans*. About 95% of the clinical isolates produce germ tubes when incubated in serum at 35°C for 2.5-3 hours. A germ tube represent the initiation of a hypha directly from the yeast cell. They have parallel walls at their point of origin. Germ tube formation is influenced by the medium, inoculum size and temperature of incubation. Fresh normal pooled human sera or a commercially available germ tube solutionare to be used as the medium for the test. The inoculum should result in a very faintly turbid serum suspension. Over-inoculation will inhibit the development of germ tubes. Incubate in at 35°C-37°C for 2.5-3 hours.

Materials required

Wooden applicator stick, Serum, Test tubes, Incubator, microscope, Culture of *Candida albicans* on SDA medium

Procedure

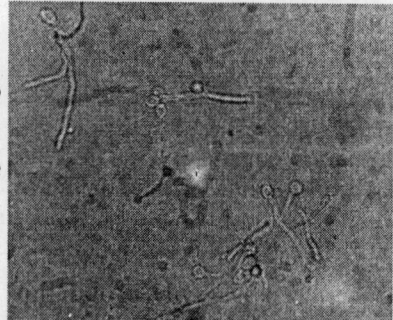

- Label 12 x 75 mm test tubes.
- Using a Pasteur pipette, dispense 3 drops of fresh pooled human serum into the tubes.
- With a sterile wooden applicator stick, lightly touch a yeast colony and place the stick into the serum.
- Suspend the yeast in the serum. Discard the stick in a discard container.
- Incubate the tubes at 35°C for 2.5-3 hours.
- Place a drop of the suspension on a clean microscopic slide.
- Place a clean cover glass over the suspension and then examine it with a microscope using the low power objective. Use high power objective to confirm the presence or absence of germ tubes.

Fig. 72.1 : Germ tube

- Read control and record results.

Observation

Tube like out growth is identified as germ tube (Fig 72.1)

Result

The given culture is found to be *Candida albicans*.

Viva question

How do you perform this test?

What are the requirements of germ tube test?

What are the organisms identified through this technique?

What are the importance of germ tube technique in mycology?

Define germ tube.

Spotter – Structure of Germ tube (Fig 72.1)

Figure 70.a – Microscopic morphology of fungusFigure

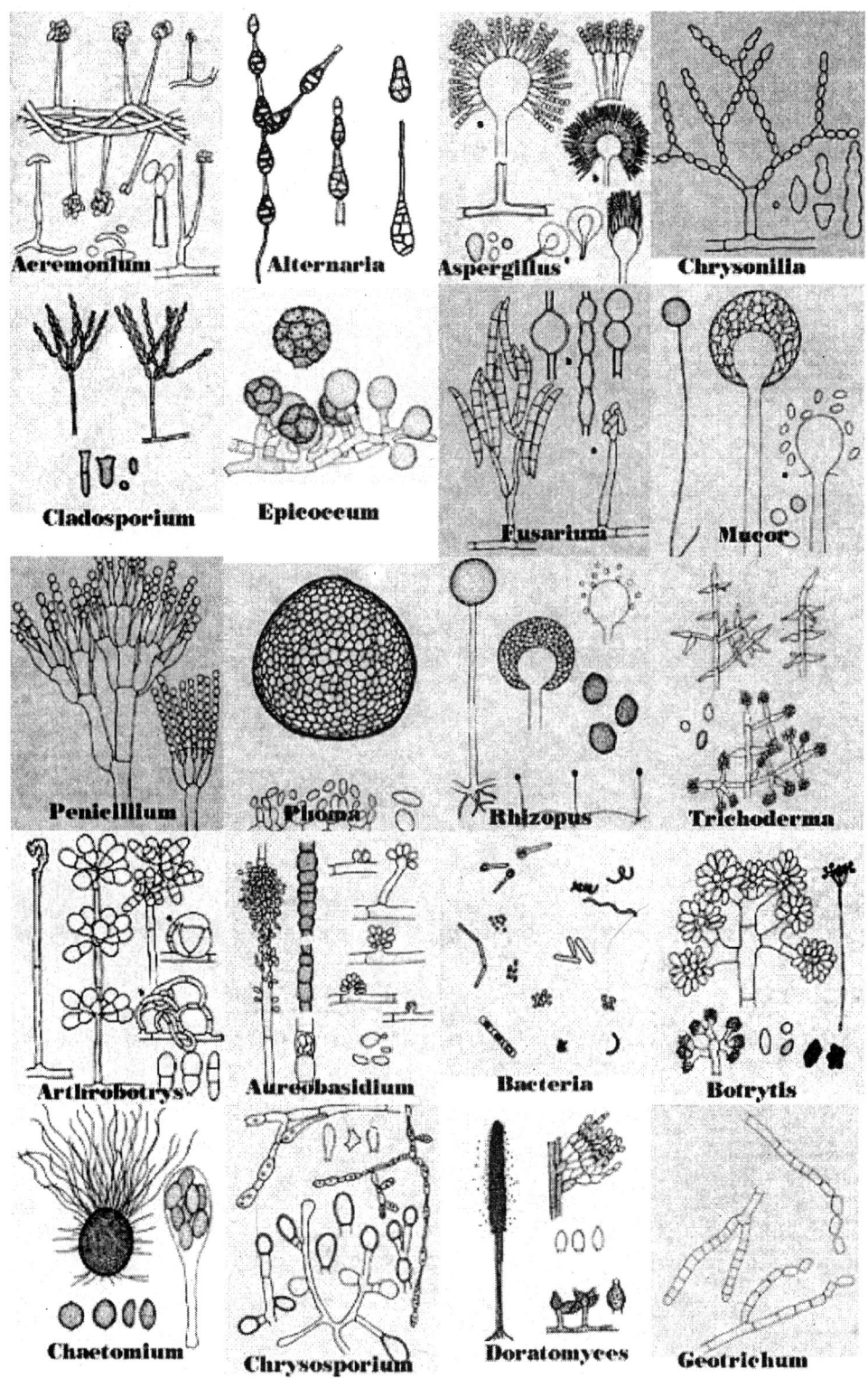

Figure 70.b – Microscopic morphology of fungus

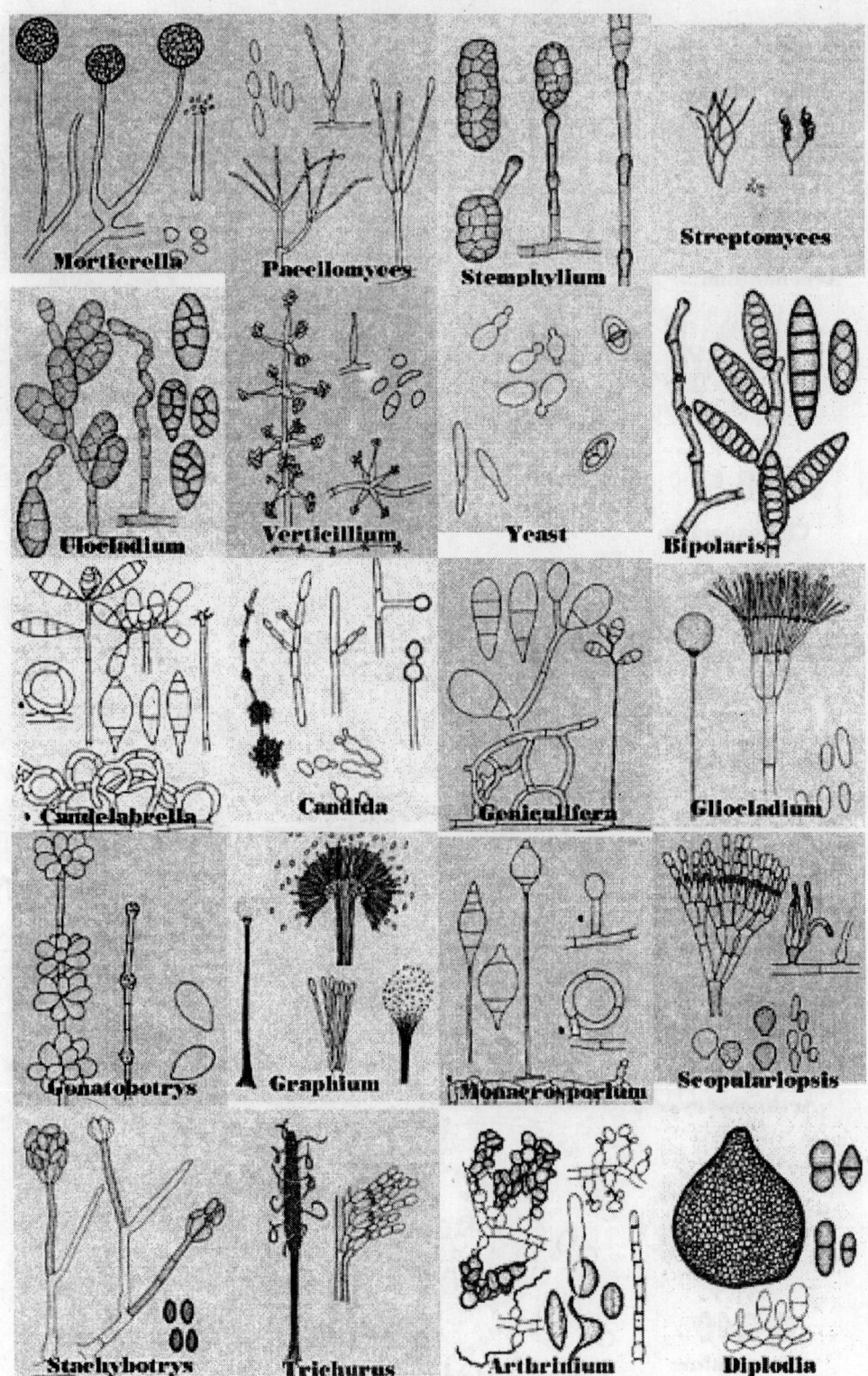

Figure 70.c – Microscopic morphology of fungus

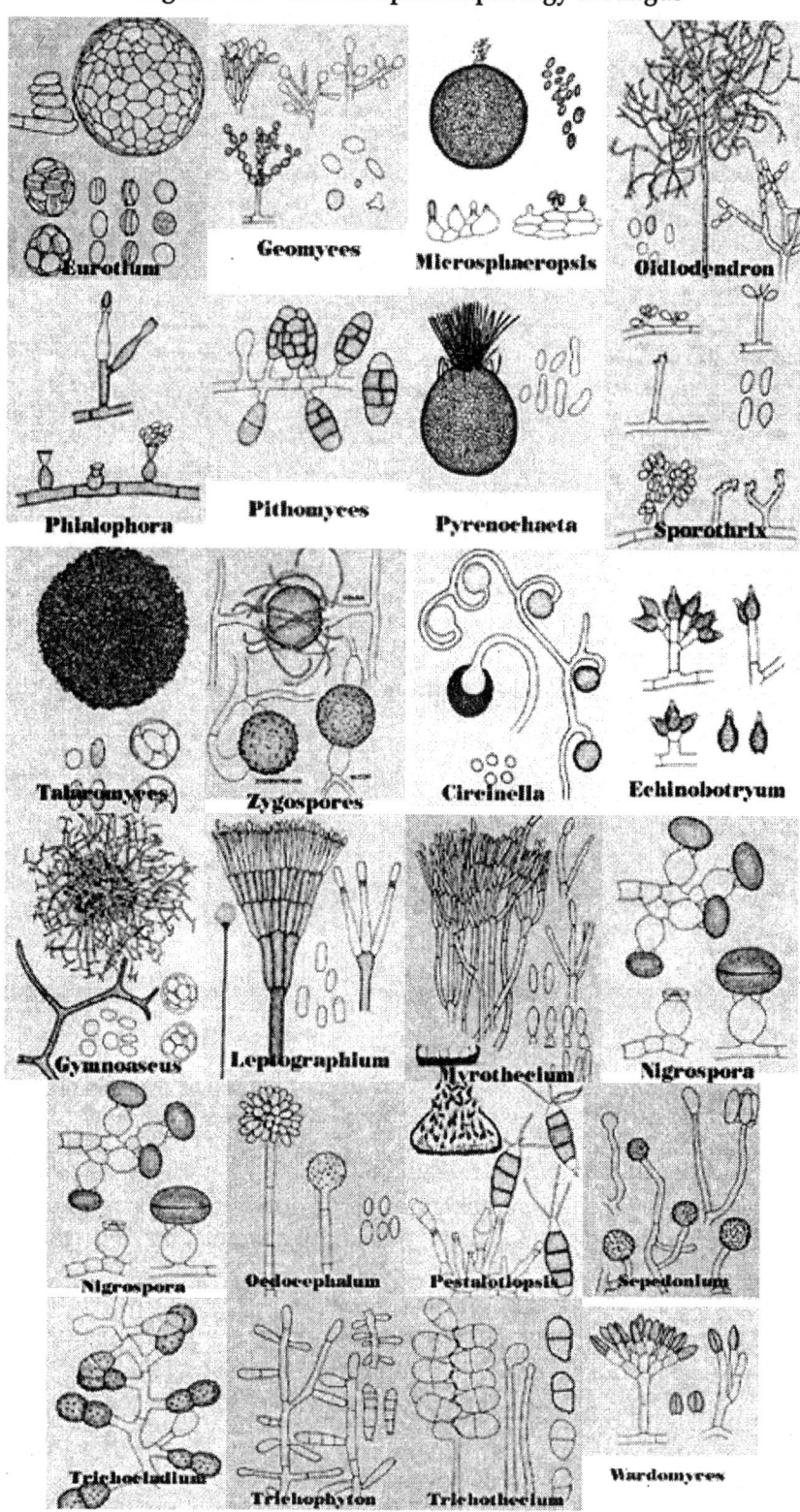

D. Clinical Parasitology

73. Identification of Intestinal Parasites

Introduction

Protozoan and helminthes are two major groups of organisms. They are responsible for varieties of human intestinal infection. Majority of intestinal parasites are detected using stool as specimen. All parasites have distinctive morphology and is studied by microscopic examination of faecal materials. Faecal specimens shows cyst and trophozoites of protozoans, adult worm, segments, larva and eggs of helminthes.

The following parasites may be detected by making use of microscopic techniques. They are *Entamoeba histolytica, Giardia lamblia, Trichomonas hominis, Balantidium coli, Isospora bellei, Taenia solium, Fasciola hepatica, Schistosoma sp, Capilaria, Ascaris lumbricoides, Paragonimus, Enterobius vermicularis, Faciola buski, T. trichura.*

Fresh faecal specimen is important for the detection of parasitic infections. Faecal specimen should be examined within a day (formed stool -1 day, semiformed stool-1 hours, liquid stool-30 min). Faecal specimen should not incubated for parasitic examinations.

Colour, consistency, presence of blood, mucous and segments are to be noted during faecal specimen examinations. Following methods are adopted to diagnose intestinal parasites. They are microscopic methods for morphological identification, concentration methods and culture methods. Microscopic methods include saline and iodine wet mount. Concentration methods are sedimentation method (formal ether, formal detergents) and floatation techniques (Sodium chloride, $ZnSO_4$ and sugar floatation method).

Microscopic methods - Saline wet mount, Iodine wet mount.

Concentration technique – Sedimentation, Floatation.

73a. Microscopic methods

73aa. Saline Wet Mount of Stool

Aim

To examine the faecal specimens for parasitic ova, cyst, trophozoites etc.

To identify intestinal cyst and trophozites of protozoan, eggs and larva of helminthes based on the morphological characters.

Background Information

Stool microscopy is a rapid method employed for the detection of intestinal parasites. Saline wet mount is more advantageous than other wet mount procedure adopted to examine parasites. Saline wet mount maintain viability / motility status of the parasite. It also facilitates demonstration of chromotoidal bodies in the cyst.

Materials Required

Compound microscope, microscopic slide & cover glasses, normal saline (it is prepared by adding 8.5 gms of NaCl in 100mL of distilled water), applicator sticks, Pasteur pipettes, stool Specimen etc..

Procedure

- Take clean microscopic slide.
- Add a drop of Normal saline on the glass slide with the help of Pasteur pipette.

- Take small portion of stool sample in applicator stick and emulsify it in the drop of saline.
- Place the cover glass over the saline preparation.
- Examine the preparation under 10x and 40x objective of the compound microscope.
- Record the findings with the description of morphological characteristics.

Observation and Results

Various morphological features of parasites are observed and recorded and identified(Fig 73a).

73ab. Iodine Wet Mount

Aim

To examine intestinal parasites

To identify cyst, trophozoites, eggs, larva of intestinal parasites on the basis of morphology and internal structures.

Background Information

Iodine wet mount is performed by making use of Dobell's, O'Connor's, lugols and Antoine's Iodine solutions. It is mainly used for the detection of protozoan parasites. This method clearly demonstrates the presence of nuclei as brown dots. It also demonstrates the yellowish cytoplasm and brown glycogen mass present in the cyst. Disadvantages of this technique includes trophozoites are killed by iodine; chromatoidal bars in protozoan cysts are not clearly visible.

Materials required

Compound microscope, microscopic slide, cover glasses, applicator stick, pasteur pipette, iodine Solution (it is prepared by adding 1g potassium iodide and 15g of iodine crystals in 100mL of distilled water), Stool sample.

> **Box 73.1- Nature of helminthic eggs**
> *Ascaris lumbricoides, Trichuris trichura, taenia sp., Echinococcus sp. Schistosoma., Fasciola, Paragonimus are bile stained eggs.*
> *Hook worm, Enterobious vermicularis, Hymenolepsis nana are non bile stained eggs*

Procedure

- Place a drop of Iodine solution on a clean glass slide.
- Emulsify the stool specimen with the help of applicator stick.
- Use the cover glass to cover the emulsified stool sample and blot excess fluid.
- Examine the sample under low power and high power objectives and record the findings.

Result

Cyst, trophozoits, eggs of different Parasites (Fig 73a and b) are observed and identified.

Viva questions

What are the purpose of wet mount?

Why saline wet mount is performed?

What are the advantages and disadvantages of Iodine & saline wet mount?

How do you detect protozoan , helminthic parasite using saline & iodine wet mount?

List different types of iodine used for iodine wet mount.

Spotters – Cyst and Trophozoites of protozoans; eggs of trematodes, cestrodes

73b. Concentration of Stool Parasites

Aim

To demonstrate parasitic burden of an individual.

Background information

Faecal concentration has become a routine procedure as a part of the complete ova and parasite examination and allows the detection of small numbers of organism that may be missed in direct wet smear.

73ba. Sedimentation - *Formalin-Ethyl Acetate*

Principle

Ethylacetate is used as an extractor of debris and fat from the faeces and leaves the parasites at the bottom of the suspension. The formalin-ethyl acetate sedimentation method is recommended, because it is the easiest to perform, allows recovery of the broadest range of organisms and is least subject to technical error.

Materials required :

Stool, 10% formalin, Centri fuge tubes , Centrifuge, 0.85% NaCl, ethylacetate.

Procedure

- Transfer ½ teaspoon of fresh stool into 10mL of 10% formalin in a vial or round bottom tube. Mix the stool and formalin throughly. Let the mixture stand a minimum of 30 minutes for fixation.

- Depending on the amount and viscosity of the specimen, strain sufficient quantity through wet gauze into a conical 15mL centrifuge tube to give the desirable amount of sediment.

- Add 0.85% NaCl almost to the top of the tube and centrifuge for 10minutes at 2000rpm. The amount of sediment obtained should be ½ to 1mL.

- Decant the supernatant fluid and suspend sediment in saline. Add saline almost top of the tube and centrifuge again for 10minutes at 2000rpm.

- Decant the supernatant fluid and suspend the sediment on the bottom of the tube in 10% formalin. Fill the tube half full only. If the amount of sediment left in the bottom of the tube is very small or the original specimen contain lot of mucous, do not add ethyl acetate.

- Add 4-5mL ethyl acetate. Stopper the tube shake vigorously for at least 30 seconds.

- Centrifuge for 10minutes at 2000rpm.

- Four layers should result;

- A small amount of sediment in the bottom of the tube.

- A layer of formalin.

- A plug of Faecal debris on the top of formalin.

- A layer of ehtylacetate at the top.

- Free the debris by rinsing the plug with an applicator stick; decant all of the supernatant fluid. After proper decanting, a drop of or two of fluid remaining on the side of the tube may run down into the sediment. Mix this fluid with sediment.

- If the sediment is still solid, add a drop or two of saline to the sediment mix, add a small amount of material to slides, add a cover slip and examine.

- Systematically scan using the 10x objective. The entire cover slip area should be examined.

Result

Protozoan trophozoite and/or cyst helminthes eggs and larvae maybe seen and identified. Protozoan trophozoites are less likely to be seen (Fig 73a, b and c).

73bb. Floatation Method

Aim

To concentrate parasites presents in the Faecal matter on the basis of specific gravity.

Principle

The floatation procedure permits the separation of protozoan cyst and helmintic eggs from excess debris through the use of liquid with the help of specific gravity. The parasitic elements are recovered in the surface film and the debris remains in the bottom of the tube. This technique yields a preparation than the sedimentation procedure; however, some helminthes eggs do not concentrate well with the floatation method. The specific gravity of the zinc sulphate can be increased, although this usually causes more distortation in the organisms present and is not recommended for routine clinical use. To ensure the detection of all possible organisms, both the surface film and sediment must be examined. For most laboratories, this is not a practical approach.

Specific gravity of hookworm egg-1.055

Specific gravity of zinc sulphate is over 1.2

The zinc sulfate flotation technique is a clinical method to determine the presence or absence of parasitic organisms and also the approximate parasite burden. The zinc sulfate floatation technique breaks up faeces and using differential specific gravities, isolates the protozoan cysts and helminth ova and larvae. MgSo4 and sheathers sucrose floatation are few other floatation methods used to concentrate stool specimens.

Materials required

Formalin (5 or 10%), 0.85% NaCl, Zinc Sulphate (33%). Slide, Coverslip, Test tube

Procedure

- Mix one to a few grams of faeces with 10 times its volume of distilled water.

- Strain 10 mL through gauze into a centrifuge tube.

- Centrifuge at 2500 RPM for one minute.

- Discard the supernatant and add 2-3 mL of water to the sediment, breaking up the sediment.

- Repeat this procedure until the supernatent is nearly clear (Usually 2-4 washings).

- Pour off the supernatant and mix the sediment with 2 mL of zinc sulfate (38.6 g/100 mL of distilled water). Fill the centrifuge tube to within 5 mm of the top.

- Centrifuge again for 5 minutes.

- Let the sample stand for 5 minutes.

- Using a bacteriological loop, remove several loopfuls and examine microscopically.

- Add a drop of Lugol's iodine to stain.

● Examine for protozoan cysts and helminth egg capsules and larvae.

Observation

Protozoan trophozoites and cyst and helminthic eggs and larvae may be seen and identified (Figure 73a, b and c).

Result

Based on the morphology and size parasitic burden is identified as – – –

Viva questions

What are the needs of stool concentration?

Mention few floatation methods.

What are the principles of floatation methods?

Fig 73a – intestinal Protozoans

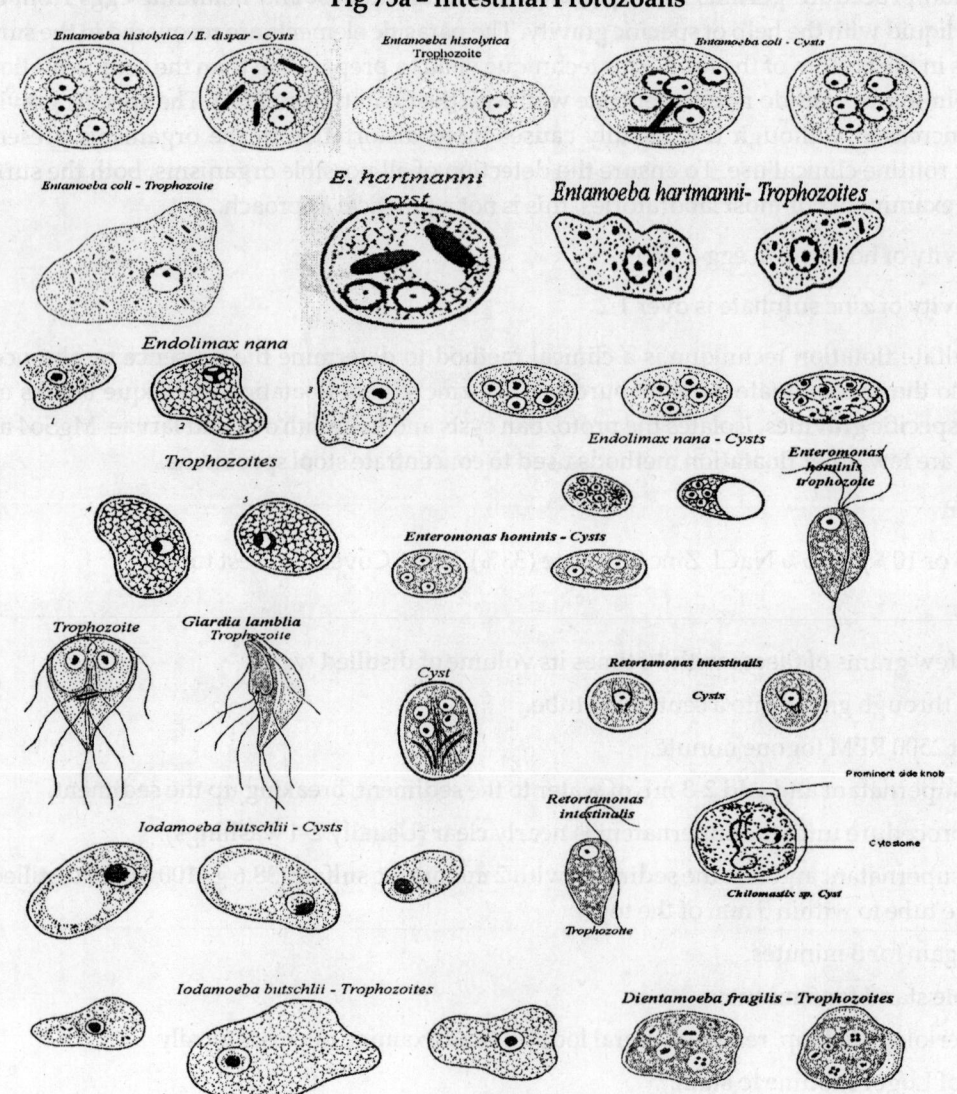

Fig 73b – Intestinal, Tissue protozoans and helminthes

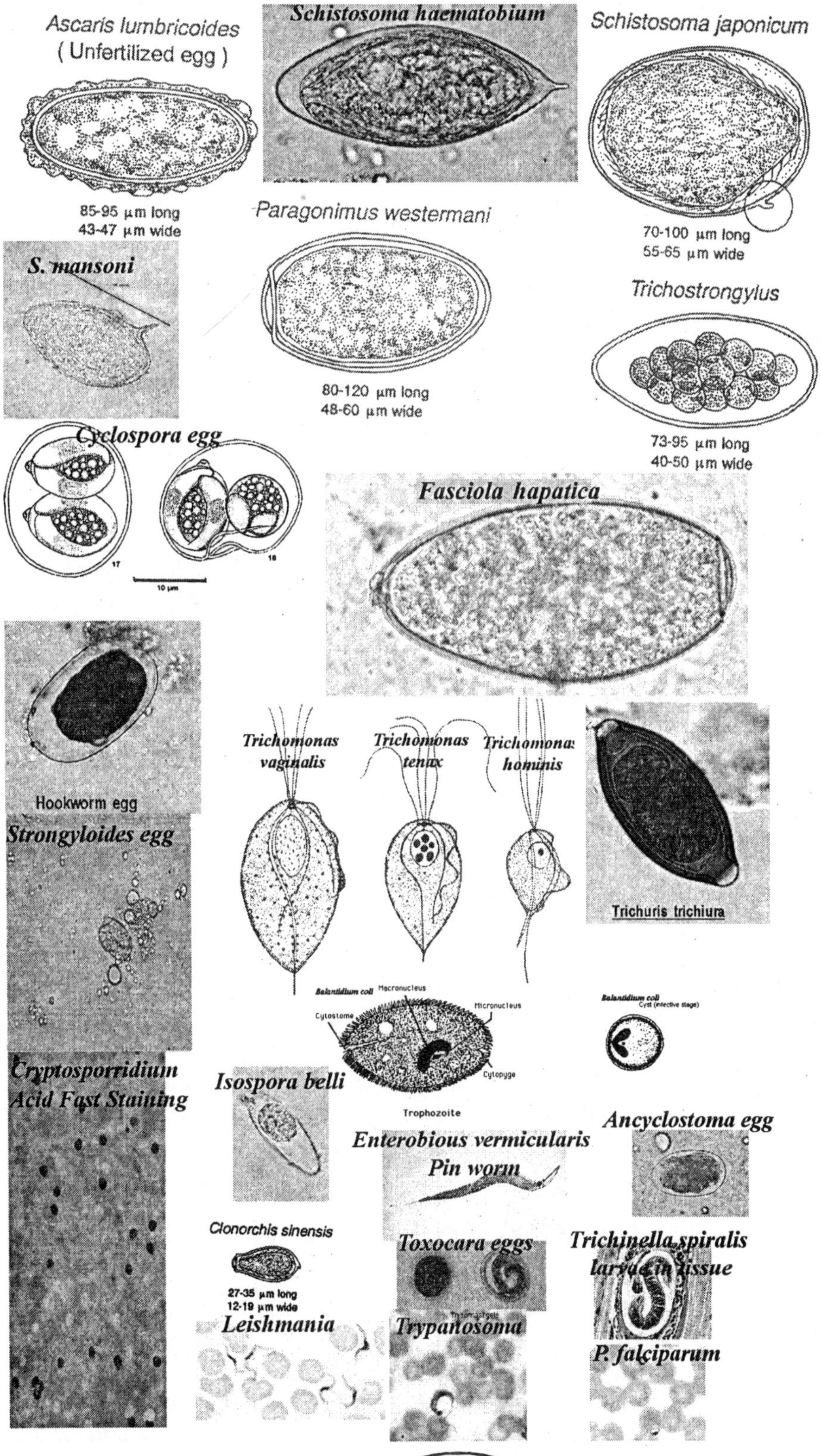

Ascaris lumbricoides
(Unfertilized egg)

85-95 µm long
43-47 µm wide

Schistosoma haematobium

Schistosoma japonicum

70-100 µm long
55-65 µm wide

S. mansoni

Paragonimus westermani

80-120 µm long
48-60 µm wide

Trichostrongylus

73-95 µm long
40-50 µm wide

Cyclospora egg

10 µm

Fasciola hapatica

Hookworm egg

Strongyloides egg

Trichomonas vaginalis

Trichomonas tenax

Trichomonas hominis

Trichuris trichiura

Balantidium coli Macronucleus
Cytostome
Micronucleus
Cytopyge

Balantidium coli Cyst (infective stage)

Cryptosporridium Acid Fast Staining

Isospora belli

Trophozoite

Enterobious vermicularis Pin worm

Ancyclostoma egg

Clonorchis sinensis

27-35 µm long
12-19 µm wide

Toxocara eggs

Trichinella spiralis larvae in tissue

Leishmania

Trypanosoma

P. falciparum

241

Fig73c. Intestinal helminthes eggs

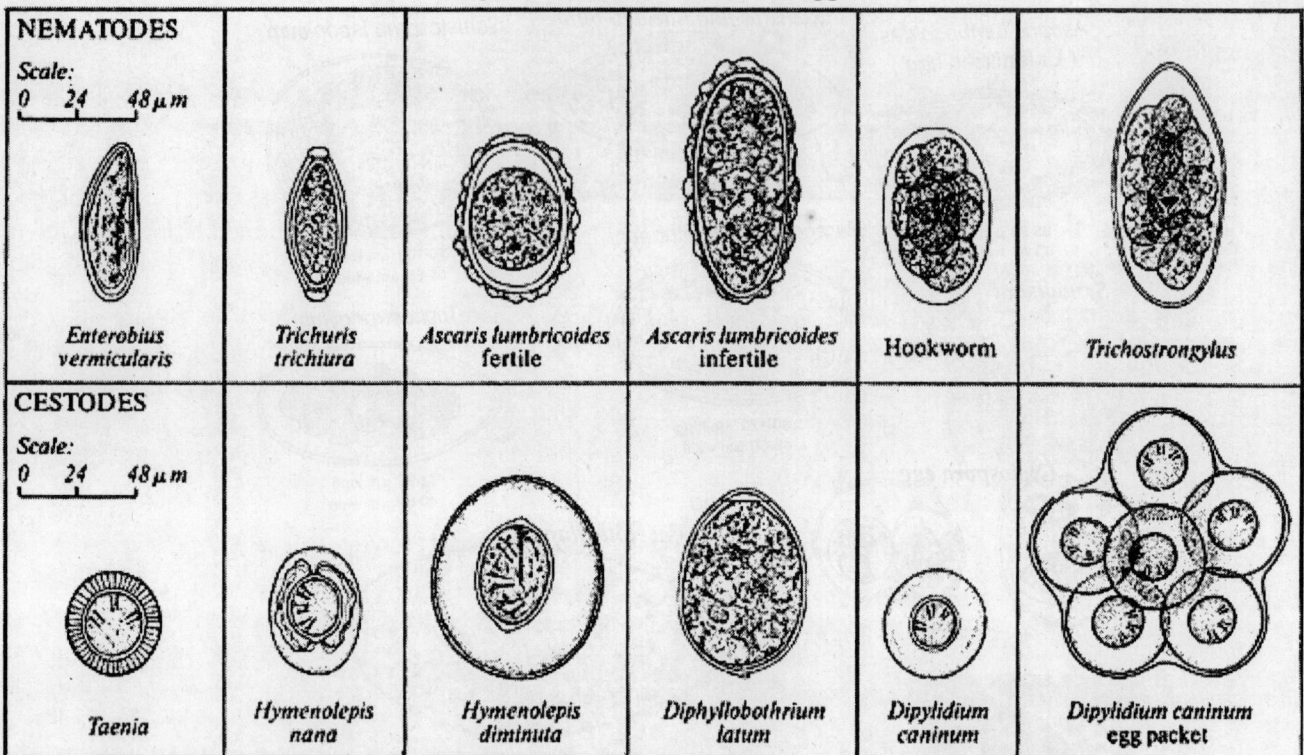

Fig73d. Segments of helminthes present in human stool

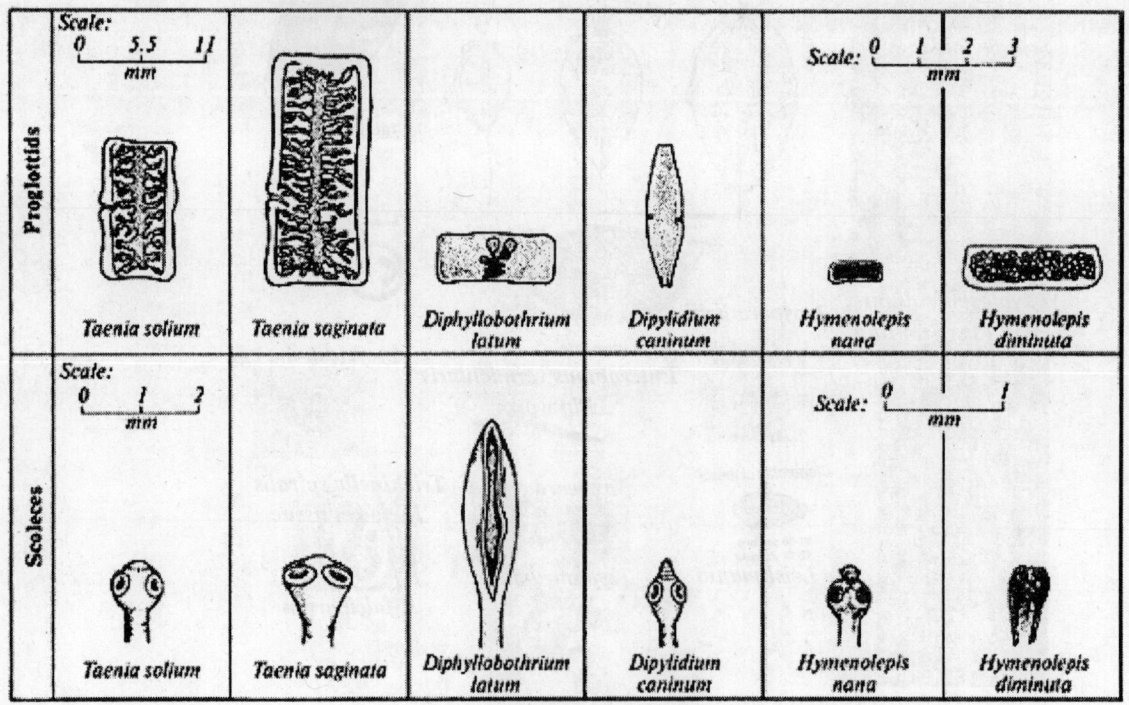

74. Identification of blood and tissue parasites

Introduction

Different types of protozoans and lesser number of helminthes played a vital role in blood and tissue infections. *Plasmodium sp, Tryphanosoma sp,Leishmania sp, T. vaginalis, W. bancrofti, Loa loa, Schistosoma, Paragonimus, Enterobius vermicularis, Taenia sp*, are some of the parasites usually detected using blood, urine, sputum, CSF, bone marrow, spleen, skin tissue, deodinal aspirate, corneal scrapes samples. Thick and thin blood smears from peripheral blood is used to screen blood parasites. Microscopic methods are the best methods to screen. Stained blood films are the most reliable and efficient means for definitive diagnosis.

Blood parasite can be detected by means of giemsa and wrights staining. It is used to differentiate nuclear or cytoplasmic morphology of platelets, RBCs, WBCs and parasites. Blood film should be prepared to observe clear morphology of blood parasites. There are two types of blood films , they are thin blood film and thick blood film. Stained blood films are the most reliable and efficient means for definitive diagnosis of nearly all blood parasites. For some parasites it is recommended to prepare a thin film in one slide, a thick film on other slide and combination on third slide.

74a. Thin blood film preparation

Aim

To prepare thin blood film for parasite examinations.

Background information

This is identical to a differential blood cell count film. It provides a good area for examining the morphology of parasites and RBCs and is used to confirm identity of parasites. This is less sensitive than thick film.

Materials Required

Blood from finger puncture or EDTA blood, Slide 2 nos, Lancet or syringe, Methanol

Procedure

- Place a drop of blood onto the center of the slide about ½ inch from the end.

- Holding a second clean slide at a 40° angle, touch the angled end to the midlength area of the specimen slide. Pull the angled slide back into the blood, and allow the blood to almost fill the end area of the angled slide.

- Continue contact with the blood under the lower edge, quickly and steadily moving the angled slide until the blood is used up.

- Label the slide appropriately and allow it to air dry.

- If the film is stained with giemsa stain after the film is completely dried, fix it with methanol and allow to air dry

Observation

Thin blood smear is stained with giemsa/wrights/ leishmans staining procedure.

74b. Thick blood film preparation

Aim

To prepare thick blood smear for the examination of parasitic infection.

Principle

The thick film essentially condenses into an area suitable for examination above 20 times more blood than thin film. The RBCs are lysed during the staining process so that only parasites, platelets and WBCs remain visible. It is used to differentiate a low parasitemia.

Procedure

For finger puncture blood

- Touch a clean glass slide to a large drop of blood standing on the finger until the circle of blood is nearly 1.8 - 2cm.

For vein puncture blood

- Place a drop of blood in the centre of the slide. Using either the corner of the another slide or an applicator stick, spread the blood into a circle about 1.8-2cm.

- Allow the film to air dry. Do not fix the thick film.

- If it is stained with methanol based stain dip smear in buffered water for 10 min.

Observation

Thin blood smear is stained with giemsa/wrights/ leishmans staining procedure.

74c. Giemsa stain

Aim

To stain and differentiate blood parasites.

Principle

In 1891, Giemsa stain was discovered by Ramanowsky, the Russian protozoologist. Giemsa stain is also called Ramonowsky stain. Until 1960s, Giemsa stain is used to describe chromosomes of cells. Giemsa stain is used to differentiate nuclear & cytoplasmic morphology of platelets (pink), RBC(pink), nuclei and granules of PMN (purple), parasite (blue), flagella of parasites (red). Giemsa stain is most useful to stain thick blood film. Giemsa stain must be diluted with buffered water pH 6.5 or 7 or 7.2 before using.

Materials required

Specimen - Finger puncture blood or vein puncture blood containing EDTA (0.020 g/10 mL of blood).

Reagents - Giemsa stain and Giemsa buffer (Phosphate Buffer)

Glass slides, alcohol, Glass marker, Applicator stick.

Equipment -Microscope, binocular with mechanical stage; calibrated ocular micrometer.

Procedure

Wear gloves when performing this procedure.

Thin blood films (only)

- Fix air-dried film in absolute methanol by dipping the film briefly (two dips) in a Coplin jar containing absolute methanol.

- Remove and air dry.

- Stain with diluted Giemsa stain (1:20, vol/vol) for 20 min (For a 1:20 dilution, add 2 mL of stock Giemsa to 40 mL of buffered water in a Coplin jar).

- Wash by briefly dipping the slide in and out of a Coplin jar of buffered water (one or two dips). *Note: Excessive washing will decolourize the film.*

- Let air dry in a vertical position.

Thick blood films (only)

- Allow film to air dry thoroughly for several hours or overnight. Do not dry films in an incubator or by heat, because this will fix the blood and interfere with the lysing of the RBCs. *Note: If a rapid diagnosis of malaria is needed, thick films can be made slightly thinner than usual, allowed to dry for 1 h, and then stained.*

- Do not fix.

- Stain with diluted Giemsa stain (1:50, vol/vol) for 50 min (For a 1:50 dilution, add 1mL of stock Giemsa to 50 mL of buffered water in a Coplin jar).

- Wash by placing film in buffered water for 3 to 5 min.

- Let air dry in a vertical position.

Observation

If *Plasmodium* is present, the cytoplasm stains blue and the nuclear material stains red to purple.

Schüffner's stippling and other inclusions in the RBCs infected by *Plasmodium* spp. stain red.

Nuclear and Cytoplasmic colours that are seen in the malarial parasites will also be seen in the trypanosomes and any intracellular leishmaniae that are present.

The sheath of microfilariae may or may not stain with Giemsa, while the body will usually appear blue to purple.

Results

Report any parasite, including the stage(s) seen. Examples: *Plasmodium falciparum* rings and gametocytes, rings only. *Plasmodium vivax* rings, trophozoites, schizonts, and gametocytes. *Wuchereria bancrofti* microfilariae. *Trypanosoma brucei gambiense/rhodesiense* trypomastigotes. *Trypanosoma cruzi* trypomastigotes. *Leishmania donovani* amastigotes

74d. Wrights stain

Aim

To stain thin blood film for the differentiation of blood parasites.

Principle

Wright stain is the combination of acid dye (Eosin) and a basic dye (Methylene blue) for use of staining the blood smear. It highlights the differences among different types blood leukocytes for easier recognition of eosinophils and basophils. Wrights stain can be used to stain thin blood films. Wrights stain also called ramanovsky dye.

Materials required

Wright stain – grind 0.9g of wright stain powder with a portion of methanol in clean mortor, as the dye is dissolved in the methanol and pour this to tightly stoppered glass bottle. Shake vigorously several times daily for atleast 5 days. Filter through whatman no.1 paper into a brown bottle, shelf life is 36 months.

Stock Buffer

Alkaline buffer - Na_2HPO_4-9.5g; Distilled water –1000mL

Acid buffer - NaH_2PO_4-9.2; Distilled water –1000mL

Buffered water - Acid Buffer-50mL; Alkaline buffer- 50mL; Distilled water –900mL; pH-6.8±0.1

Coplin jar, Mortar and Pestel, filter paper, volumetric flask, Microscope, Brown bottle, pH meter, staining rack etc.,

Procedure

- Prepare thin and thick blood film.
- Add stain drop by drop. Count the number of drops needed to cover the surface.
- Let stand 1 – 3 minutes.
- Add the same drop of buffered water and mix the stain.
- After 4 – 8 minutes, flood the stain from the slide with buffered water.
- Wipe the stain.
- Air dry.
- Observed under microscope.

Observation

If *Plasmodium* is present, the cytoplasm stains blue and the nuclear material stains red to purple.

Schüffner's stippling and other inclusions in the RBCs infected by *Plasmodium* sp. Stains red.

Nuclear and Cytoplasmic colours that are seen in the malarial parasites will also be seen in the Trypanosomes and any intracellular leishmaniae that are present.

The sheath of microfilariae may or may not stain with Giemsa, while the body will usually appear blue to purple.

Results

Report any parasite, including the stage(s) seen (do not use abbreviations). Examples: *Plasmodium falciparum* rings and gametocytes, rings only. *Plasmodium vivax* rings, trophozoites, schizonts, and gametocytes. *Wuchereria bancrofti* microfilariae. *Trypanosoma brucei gambiense/rhodesiense* trypomastigotes. *Trypanosoma cruzi* trypomastigotes. *Leishmania donovani* amastigotes

74e. Leishman's Stain

Aim

To differentiate blood parasites.

Principle

It is also called Romanowskys stain. Leishman stain is a combination of eosin and methylene blue. It also contain oxidation product of methylene blue called azures. These azures provide further contrast in smears of peripheral blood.

Materials required

Leishman's stain – it is prepared by grinding 150µg of leishman stain powder in Mortar and Pestle by adding 100mL methanol. This stain matures in 2 or 3 days.

pH 6.8 phosphate buffer

Working stain: Leishman's stain diluted 1:4 with buffer

Xylene

Procedure

For thin smear

- Cover the smear with 5-10 drops of leishman working stain and stained for 2 minutes.
- Add Buffered water to dilute the stain and allowed for 10 – 15 minutes.
- Wash the stain with buffered distilled water.
- Dry the slide and examine under high power objectives.

For thick smear

- Perform staining as like thin smear
- Finally, immerse the smear in water until red colour disappeares.

Results

Report any parasite, including the stage(s) seen. Examples: *Plasmodium falciparum* rings and gametocytes, rings only. *Plasmodium vivax* rings, trophozoites, schizonts, and gametocytes. *Wuchereria bancrofti* microfilariae. *Trypanosoma brucei gambiense/rhodesiense* trypomastigotes. *Trypanosoma cruzi* trypomastigotes. *Leishmania donovani* amastigotes

Note :

Leishmen and Wright stain has both fixatives & stain. Giemsa stain, field stain has only staining reagent. Dehaemoglobination should be done on thick blood film. This is done by immersing slide in distilled water for few minutes. JSB (Jaswant singh bhattacharjee) stain also used for staining of blood film. Thick blood film should not be fixed because fixation with methanol prevents lysis of RBC & dehaemoglobilization.

Viva questions

Name different Romanowsky stains.

Name the parasites present in blood and tissues.

How do you identify malarial parasites

What are the differences between thick and thin blood film

List any four blood parasites

Why leishman stain is called as Romanowsky stain

What are the principles of giemsa staining.

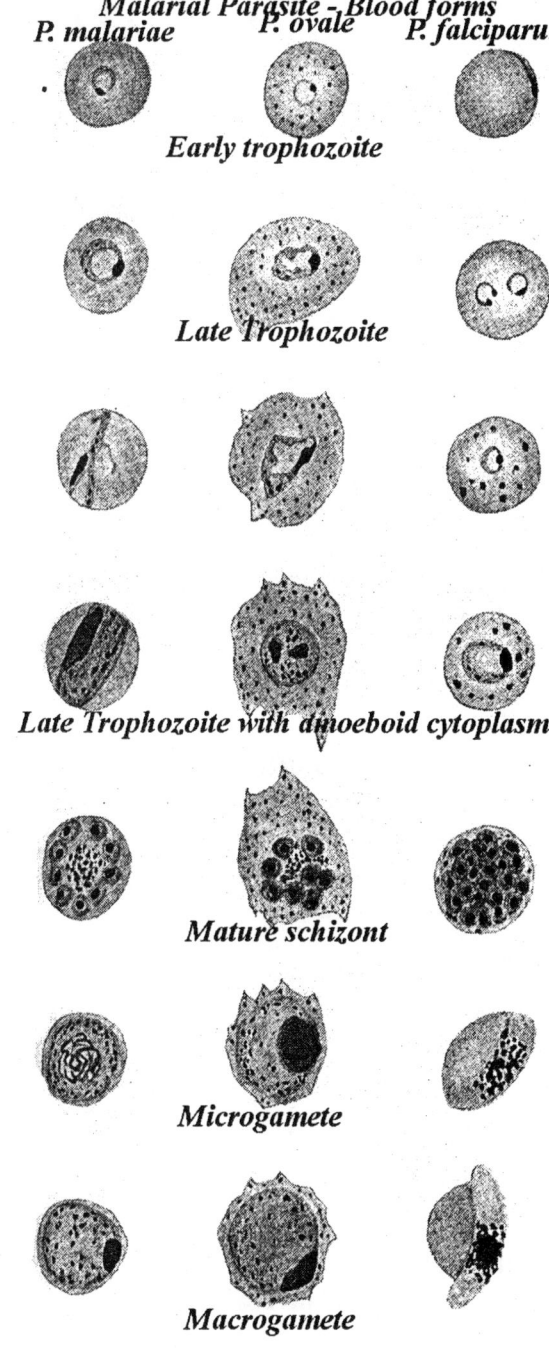

Malarial Parasite - Blood forms

P. malariae   *P. ovale*   *P. falciparum*

Early trophozoite

Late Trophozoite

Late Trophozoite with amoeboid cytoplasm

Mature schizont

Microgamete

Macrogamete

Figure 74.1- Malarial parasite

Soil Microbiology

CHAPTER 5

75. Isolation of Bacteria from Soil

Aim

To isolate and enumerate soil bacteria.

Background Information

Soil is the outer covering of the earth, which consists of loosely arranged layers of materials composed of inorganic and organic constituents in different stages of organization. Different types of macro and micronutrients of soil provide a natural environment for the survival of living things. The fertility of soil depends not only on its chemical composition, but also on the qualitative and quantitative nature of microbes. Winogradskey may rightly be considered as the pioneer of soil bacteriology. In 1925, Winogradskey classified soil bacteria into two broad categories-the *autochthonous* and the *zymogenous* organisms. Indigenous populations always uniform and constant in soil. When specific nutrients are added to soil zymogenous population will increases and gradually decreased when the substrate is exhausted.

> **Box 75.1 Colony morphology of Azotobacter and Rhizobium**
>
> Azotobacter grown on Jensen medium as white glistening colonies. Rhizobium grown in YEMA medium as mucoid, gummy, colourless colony.

Most common soil bacteria are *Pseudomonas, Arthrobacter, Clostridium, Achromobacter, Bacillus, Micrococcus, Flavobacterium, Corynebacterium, Sarcina, Azospirillum, Azatobacter, Rhizobium* and *Mycobacterium. Escherichia coli* is encountered rarely in soil. *Aerobacter* and *Agrobacterium* are frequently encountered. *Myxococcus, Chondrococcus, Archangium, Polyangium, Cytophaga* and *Sporocytophaga* are also encountered in soil. *Nitrosomonas, Nitrobacter, Klebsiella* are available in soil rarely.

Materials Required

Soil sample, Media (Nutrient Agar, Yeast extract mannitol agar for Rhizobium, Jensens medium and Ashby medium for *Azatobacter, Azospirillum* medium for *Azospirillum*)., 100mL sterile water blank, 9mL sterile water blanks, Sterile pipettes, Sterile petriplates, Marker, Match box, Bunsen burner, Alcohol etc.

Procedure

Soil sample collection

Soil sample is collected normally at the depth of 15 cm and transferred to clean containers. Three to five samples are taken from different area of one field and mixed evenly. From the mixed sample at least 10- 25-g of soil is taken as a representative sample of the particular field.

Soil dilution and plate count

Common isolation

- Prepare one 100mL sterile water blank and five 9ml water blanks and arranged properly in a rack.
- Add 10g of soil sample to the 100 mL of sterile water and considered it as stock solution (1:10)
- Take 1mL stock solution using sterile pipette and serially diluted up to 1:10000000 (10^7).

- Plate sample from 10^{-5}, 10^{-6} and 10^{-7} diluents on nutrient agar medium by pour plate method.
- Allow plates to solidify
- Incubate plates at 37 °C for 24 hours.

Azatobacter isolation

- Inoculate 0.1mL of 1:10 diluted sample on Jensen's medium or Ashby's medium by spread plate technique
- Incubate plates at 37 °C for 24 hours.

Azospirillum isolation

- Inoculate 10mL of 1:10 diluted sample to the Azospirillium isolation medium.
- Incubate medium aerobically for 96 hours at room temperature.

Rhizobium isolation

- Inoculate 0.1mL of 1:10 diluted sample on YEMA medium by spread plate technique
- Incubate plates at 30°C for 10 days

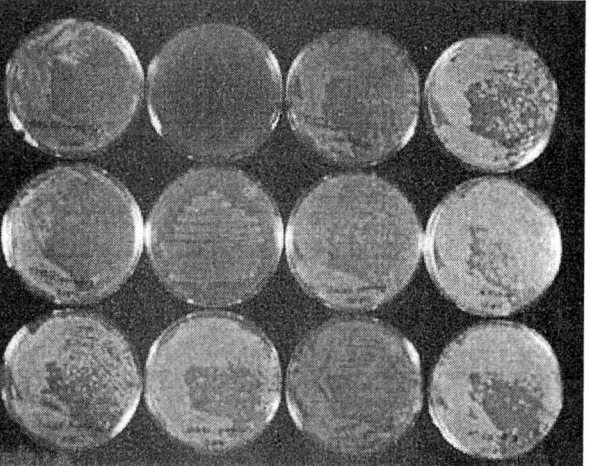

Fig 75.1 : Different types of Soil bacteria on different media

Observation

Observe the number and distribution of bacterial colonies.

Select plates from the appropriate dilution with countable colories (30-300)

Average total number of Colonies

Note colour and nature of colonies selective isolation medium

Table 75.1- Observable record on bacterial isolation

S.No	Medium	Dilution	Number of CFU/mL		Average
			Original	Replicate	
1	Nutrient agar	10^{-5}			
		10^{-6}			
		10^{-7}			
2	Azospirillum medium	10^{-1}			
3	Jenson medium / Asbhys medium	10^{-1}			
4	YEMA medium	10^{-1}			

Calculation

Calculate the number of organisms per gram of soil by applying the formula.

$$\text{Viable cells / g of soil} = \frac{\text{Mean plate count X dilution factor}}{\text{Dry weight of soil}}$$

Result

The given soil sample contains – – – – – – – – – – – – –CFU/g

Viva questions

Define Autochthonous, allochthonous and Zymogenous microorganisms.

Name the medium used for the isolation of Azatobacter.

Mention colony morphology of Azatobacter and Rhizobium on the specified medium.

Why we selected 10^{-5}, 10^{-6} and 10^{-7} dilution to isolate bacteria?

Mention few contributions of Winogradsky.

Why there is a larger population of microbes in soil?

Spotters: Nutrient agar, Jensens medium, YEMA medium, Azospirullum medium etc.

76. Isolation of Fungi from the Soil

Aim

To isolate and identify soil fungus.

Background Information

Fungi are classified into Phycomycetes, Ascomycetes, Basidiomycetes and fungi imperfecti. Many fungi, which are isolated from soil, come under the class fungi imperfecti by virtue of the fact that they produce abundant asexual spores and lack sexual stage. Fungi imperfecti are distinguished from others by their septate mycelium and a structure called **conidiophore** from which conidia or spores are continuously produced. Other three classes have both sexual and asexual characters. The quality and quantity of organic matter present in soil have a direct bearing on fungal numbers in soil since most fungi are heterotrophic in nutrition. Fungi are dominant in acid soil. Most common fungi found in Indian soil are, *Aspergillus, Botrytis, Cephalosporium, Gliocladium, Monilia, Penicillium, Scopulariopsis, Spicaria, Trichoderma, Trichothecium, Verticillium, Alternaria, Cladosporium, Pullularia, Cylindrocarpon, Fusarium, Mucor, Rhizopus, Zygorinchus, Phythium, Chaetomium, Rhizoctonia, Helminthosporium, Humicola, Metarhizhium* etc..

Materials Required

Media (Potato Dextrose Agar / Rose Bengal Chloromphenicol Agar/ Sabouraud Dextrose Agar/ Czapec Dox Agar), Water blanks (100mL and 9mL), Pipettes, Petriplates

Procedure

Soil sample collection

Soil sample is collected normally at the depth of 15 cm and transferred to clean containers. Three to five samples are taken from different area of one field and mixed evenly. From the mixed sample at least 10- 25g of soil is taken as a representative sample of the particular field.

Soil dilution and plate count

- Prepare one 100mL sterile water blank and four 9mL water blanks and arranged properly in a rack.
- Add 10g of soil sample to the 100 mL of sterile water and considered it as stock solution (1:10)
- Take 1mL stock solution using sterile pipette and serially diluted up to 1:100000 (10^{-5}).
- Plate 0.1mL of sample from 10^{-3}, 10^{-4} and 10^{-5} diluents on any one of the fungal isolation medium (Potato Dextrose Agar / Rose Bengal Chloromphenicol Agar/ Sabouraud Dextrose Agar/ Czapec Dox Agar), by spread plate method.

- Allow plates to solidify
- Incubate plates at 25-30 °C for 48 hours.

Observation

Fungal colonies are observed and identified by slide culture technique (Refer Experiment 65 and figure 64a,b c for identification of fungi).

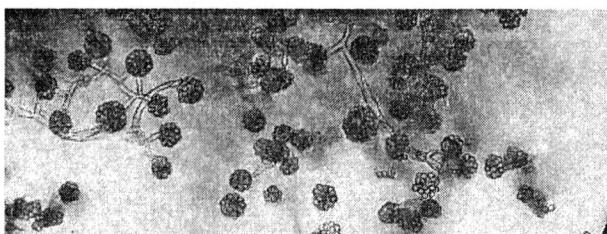

Fig. 76.1 – Microscopic View of *Trichoderma sp.*

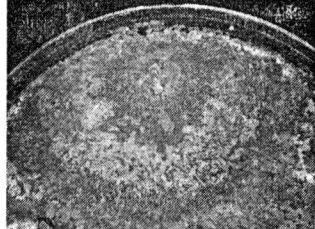

Fig. 76.2 : Green colour Spore bearing *Trichoderma sp.* used as Biofertilizer

Table 76.1- Observable record on fungal isolation

S.No	Medium	Dilution	Number of CFU/mL		Average
			Original	Replicate	
1	Any one fungal medium	10^{-3}			
		10^{-4}			
		10^{-5}			

Calculation

Calculate the number of organisms per gram of soil by applying the formula.

$$\text{Viable cells / g of soil} = \frac{\text{Mean plate count X dilution factor}}{\text{Dry weight of soil}}$$

Result

The given soil sample contains — — — — — — — — — — — — CFU/g of fungi

Viva questions

What are the major groups of fungi?

How fungi differ from bacteria?

List few agriculturally important fungi.

Name any one fungal selective media.

How PDA does not allow the growth of bacteria?

How do you detect mould growth on media?

Mention method by which fungi are identified.

Spotters: PDA, SDA, RBCA, CDA, *Aspergillus, Fusarium, Trichoderma.*

77. Isolation of Actinomycetes from Soil

Aim

To enumerate the number of actinomycetes present in the given soil sample.

Background Information

Actinomycetes are soil microorganisms, which have common characteristics to bacteria and fungi. On agar plates they can easily distinguished from other bacteria. Unlike slimy distinct colonies of true bacteria, which grow quickly, actinomycetes colonies grow slowly show powdery consistency and stick firmly on the agar surface. A closure look at a colony under bright field microscopy reveals slender unicellular-branched mycelium forming asexual spores for propagation. Actinomycetes differ from fungi in the composition of their cell wall. They don't have chitin and cellulose. The number of actinomycetes increases in the presence of decomposing organic matter. Waterlogging of soil is unfavorable for the growth of actinomycetes. The percentage of actinomycetes in the total microbial population increases with the depth of soil. The commonest genera of actinomycetes found in soil are *Streptomyces, Nocordia* and *Micromonospora*.

Materials Required

Soil sample, Media (Actinomycetes isolation medium, Kenknight and Mundiers Medium, Starch casein nitrate agar (Kurstars agar), Asparagine mannitol agar, Soil extract agar), Saline or water blank, Petriplates, Pipettes, laminar air flow, bunsen burner, inoculation loop etc.,

Procedure

Soil sample collection

Soil sample is collected normally at the depth of 15 cm and transferred to clean containers. Three to five samples are taken from different area of one field and mixed evenly. From the mixed sample at least 10- 25g of soil is taken as a representative sample of the particular field.

Soil dilution and plate count

- Prepare one 100mL sterile water blank and four 9mL water blanks and arranged properly in a rack.
- Add 10g of soil sample to the 100 mL of sterile water and considered it as stock solution (1:10)
- Take 1mL stock solution using sterile pipette and serially diluted up to 1:10000000 (10^4).
- Plate 0.1mL sample from 10^{-1}, 10^{-2} and 10^{-3} diluents on Actinomycetes isolation medium by spread plate method (Use triplicates for each dilutions).
- Incubate plates at 25-30°C for 48 hours

Table 77.1- Observable record on Actinomycetes isolation

S.No	Medium	Dilution	Number of CFU/mL		Average
			Original	Replicate	
1	Actinomyces isolation medium	10^{-1}			
		10^{-2}			
		10^{-3}			

Modified procedure for actinomycetes isolation

- Weigh 1g of soil sample and add to 9mL of saline in a test tube.
- Shake vigorously.
- Allow the suspension to settle for 1minute
- Kept ready the medium at 55 ° C

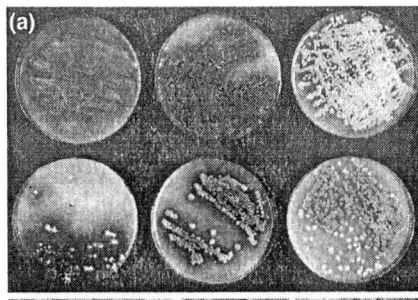
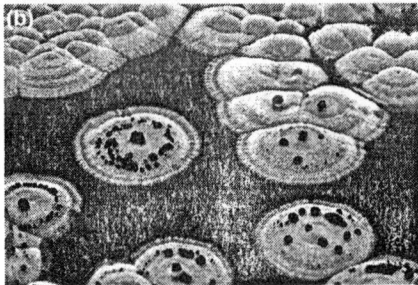

- Transfer 5mL of suspension to 100mL of starch casein nitrate agar
- Mix the contents gently, do not shake
- After 5 minutes, Pour the suspended soil dilution into the Petri plates.
- Incubate all plates at 25 °C for 4-5days

Note:

To suppress the growth of competing bacteria and fungi incorporate cycloheximide in the isolation medium (50μg/mL). Exposing soil organism at 55 °C for 5 minutes will kill many sensitive gram negative bacteria and make it easier to isolate pure culture.

Observation

Observe the plates for number and distribution of actinomycetes colonies

Make an average of each triplicate

Observe colonies for its nature

Fig 77.1- a – Growth of Actinomycetes on actinomycetes isolation medium (Rough dry colonies). B. Close view of Streptomyces sp.,

Result

The given soil sample contains – – – – – – – – – – – – –CFU/g of actinomycetes

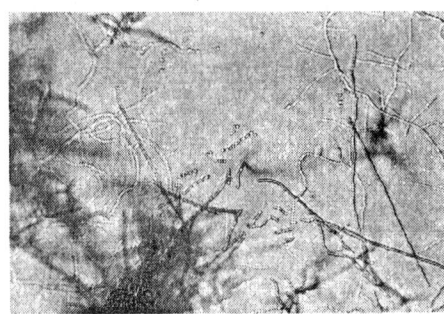

Fig 77.2 – Microscopic view of Streptomyces sp.

Viva questions

Define Actinomycetes.

List differentiation properties of bacteria and actinomycetes.

How actinomycetes differ from fungi?

How do you detect actinomycetes on agar medium?

How do you reduce bacterial growth on Actinomycetes medium?

Mention few important generas of Actinomycetes.

Mention importance of streptomyces in agriculture and other fields.

What is geosmin.

Spotters: Actinomycetes isolation medium

78. Isolation of Cyanobacteria from soil

Aim

To isolate Cyanobacteria from soil

Background information

Cyanobacteria, also known as **blue-green algae, blue-green bacteria. It belongs to phylum Cyanophyta** of bacteria that obtain their energy through photosynthesis. The name "cyanobacteria" comes from the colour of the bacteria. They are a significant component of the marine nitrogen cycle and an important primary producer in many areas of the ocean, but are also found on land. Many cyanobacteria can fix nitrogen and photosynthesize. Cyanobacteria are found in almost every conceivable environment, from oceans to fresh water to bare rock to soil. Most are found in fresh water, while others are marine, occur in damp soil, or even temporarily moistened rocks in deserts. A few are endosymbionts in lichens, plants, various protists or sponges and provide energy for the host. Cyanobacteria include unicellular and colonial species. Colonies may form filaments, sheets or even hollow balls. Some filamentous colonies show the ability to differentiate into several different cell types: vegetative cells, the normal, photosynthetic cells that are formed under favorable growing conditions; akinetes, the climate-resistant spores that may form when environmental conditions become harsh; and thick-walled heterocysts, which contain the enzyme nitrogenase, vital for nitrogen fixation. Heterocysts may also form under the appropriate environmental conditions (anoxic) wherever nitrogen is necessary. Common cyanobacteria found in soil are *Nostoc.*, *Anabaena*, *Scytonema*, *Calothrix etc*

Materials required

Soil sample from rice field., Chus medium / Prinsheims broth, Pipette, Conical flask, Illuminated growth chamber, Polythene bags, Inoculation loop, Burner etc.,

Procedure

- Collect soil or water from rice field and transport to the laboratory.
- Prepare any one of the cyanobacterial isolation medium in 100mL conical flasks (25mL medium) and sterilize at 121°C for 30minutes.
- Inoculate 1g of sample in to cyanobacterial isolation medium (maintain duplicate)
- Incubate all flasks at 30±2°C for 2-3 weeks in an alternate light and dark regime of 12 hours.
- Algal growth appear in broth after 2-3 weeks.
- Perform wet mount and note the nature of Cyanobacteria.
- In the mean time prepare Chus agar and pour into pertriplates.
- Inoculate Cyanobacteria from broth to plate by streak plate technique.
- Incubate plates at 30±2°C for one week in an alternate light and dark regime of 12 hours.
- Select individual colonies and maintain in agar slants.

Observation

Several types of Cyanobacteria grown on broth as green or bluish green coloured mucilagenous sheat. It may be unicellular or multicellular. Isolated colonies are maintained.

Result

Isolated Cyanobacteria are identified as _____. (It is based on Fig 78.1).

Fig 78.1 Microscopic Picture of some important Cyanobacteria

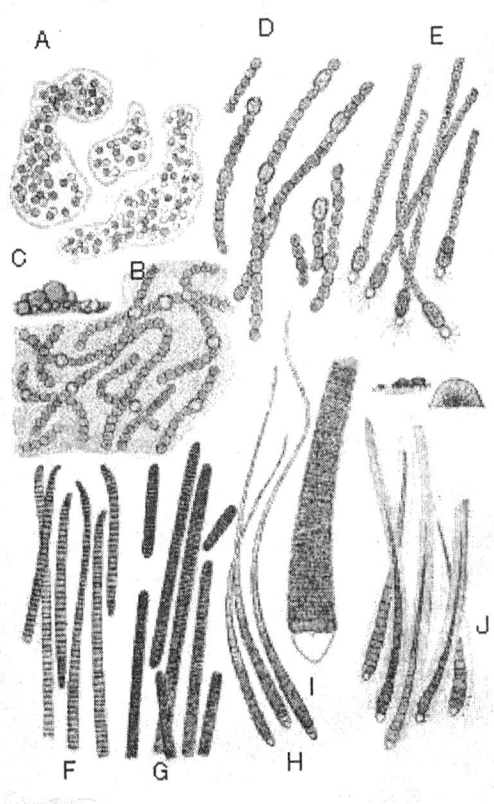

A : Microcystis B : Nostoc

C : The whole of Nostoc

D : Anabaena

E : Cylidrospermum

F : Oscillatoria

G : Oscillatoria

H : Calothrix

I : The magnifying figure of the adhered part of Calothrix

J : Rivularia

Viva questions

Define photosynthetic bacteria.

Give examples for photosynthetic bacteria.

Mention media used for the cultivation of Cyanobacteria.

How do you isolate Cyanobacteria from soil.

How do you identify Cyanobacteria.

Name structure found in cyanobacteria responsible for N_2 fixation.

Give examples for nitrogen fixing Cyanobacteria.

Name Cyanobacteria used as a biofertilizer.

Spotters – Microscopic picture of Nostoc, Anabaena and Oscillatoria

79. Isolation Phosphate solubilizers from soil

Aim

To isolate phosphate solubilizing microorganisms from soil.

Background information

A considerable number of bacterial species are able to exert a beneficial effect on plant growth. Mostly they are associated with the plant rhizosphere, so they are called as rhizobacteria. This group of bacteria has been termed plant growth promoting rhizobacteria, Eg., *Alcaligenes, Acinetobacter, Arthrobacter, Azospirillum, Bacillus, Burkholderia, Enterobacter, Erwinia, Flavobacterium, Paenibacillus, Pseudomonas, Rhizobium, and Serratia.* They are used as biofertilizers or control agents for agriculture. Phosphorus is second only to nitrogen in mineral nutrients

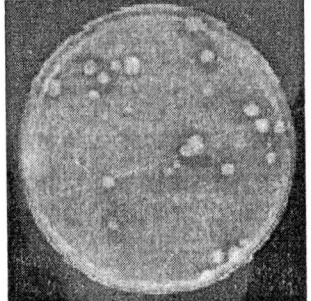 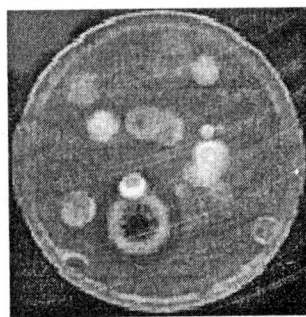

Fig 79.1 Picture showing Phosphate solublizing microorganisms Left- Bacteria on Pikovskaya medium Right – Fungus on Rose Bengal agar – Clearance around colonies showing phosphate solubilization

most commonly limiting the growth of crops. Phosphorus is an essential element for plant development and growth making up about 0.2 % of plant dry weight. Plants acquire P from soil solution as phosphate anions. However, phosphate anions are extremely reactive and may be immobilized through precipitation with cations such as Ca^{2+}, Mg^{2+}, Fe^{3+} and Al^{3+}, depending on the particular properties of a soil. In these forms, P is highly insoluble and unavailable to plants. As the results, the amount available to plants is usually a small proportion of this total. Several scientists have reported the ability of different bacterial species to solubilize insoluble inorganic phosphate compounds, such as tricalcium phosphate, dicalcium phosphate, hydroxyapatite, and rock phosphate.

Mechanisms of phosphate solubilization

The principal mechanism for mineral phosphate solubilization is the production of organic acids and acid phosphatases play a major role in the mineralization of organic phosphorus in soil. It is generally accepted that the major mechanism of mineral phosphate solubilization is the action of organic acids synthesized by soil microorganisms. Production of organic acids results in acidification of the microbial cell and its surroundings. The production of organic acids by phosphate solubilizing bacteria has been well documented. Gluconic acid seems to be the most frequent agent of mineral phosphate solubilization. Also, 2-ketogluconic acid is another organic acid identified in strains with phosphate solubilizing ability. Strains of *Bacillus* were found to produce mixtures of lactic, isovaleric, isobutyric and acetic acids. Other organic acids, such as glycolic, oxalic, malonic, and succinic acid, have also been identified among phosphate solubilizers. Strains from the genera *Pseudomonas*, *Bacillus* and *Rhizobium* are among the most powerful phosphate solubilizers. Chelating substances and inorganic acids such as sulphuric, nitric, and carbonic acid are considered as other mechanisms for phosphate solubilization.

Materials required

Pikovskaya agar, Rose Bengal agar, Soil sample, Saline, L Rod, Test tubes, Pipettes, Laminar air flow etc.

Procedure

- Collect soil sample from agricultural field.

- Weigh 1g of soil in clean paper or aluminium foil.

- Transfer soil to 100mL sterile saline and considered as 1:100 dilution.

- Inoculate 0.1mL of sample on Pikovskaya agar plate to detect bacterial phosphate solubilizers and Rose Bengal Chloramphenicol agar with calcium phosphate to detect fungal phosphate soulbilizers

- Incubate Pikovskoya medium at 37^0C for 24 hours and fungal medium at 25^0C for 48 hours

- Phosphate solubilizers produce clearing zones around the colonies in media.

Observation

Clearing zones around the colonies are observed .

Result

Presence of clearing around colonies indicates the bacterium or fungi are the phosphate solublizer.

Viva questions

Define phosphate solubilizers.

Mention few examples for phosphste solubilizers.

Explain how microbes solubilize phosphste

Mention the importance of phosphate in soil fertility.

Spotters: Pikovskaya medium

80. Assessesment of VAM Colonization and its Staining

Aim

To demonstrate the existence of mycorrhizal association in the given root.

To stain the given plant roots for its VAM colonization.

Background information

Mycorrhizae are a phenomenon of fungal association with plant roots. German botanist Frank first described it. There are three types of association namely ectomycorrhizae, endomycorrhizae and ectendomycorrhizae. The differences between these three are self-explanatory. Mycorrhizal association is universal and found in almost all climatic conditions involving all except few plants. It increases nutrient supply, mineral and water supply to the plants. VAM belonging to the family Endogonaceae (Zygomycetes) are among the more common and widely distributed of the soil borne fungi. *Endogone, Glomus, Gigaspora, Acaulospora, Glaciella, Sclerocystis* and *Enterophospora* are the common genera of VAM fungi. The Vascular Arbuscular Mycorrhizae (VAM) is an important type of association, as it satisfies the nutrient requirement of the host by forming vesicles and arbuscles. These special structures help in the transfer of nutrients from the soil to root system. Many plant especially belonginging to the family Graminaceae and legumes are highly susceptible to VAM fungi colonization. As VAM fungi are obligate endosymbionts, the isolation of organisms in pure culture is nearly not possible, but it can be demonstrated by special techniques.

Materials Required

Scissors, Forceps, Distilled water, FAA solution (it contains 5mL formaline; 5mL 38-40% acetic acid and 90 mL 70% ethyl alcohol), 10% potassium hydroxide, 2% hydrochloric acid, **Lactic glycerol blue stain**, **Destaining solutions for VAM** (Lactic glycerol solution), Any one-plant root.

Lactic glycerol blue stain (Tryphan blue-0.5g; Lactic acid -400mL; Glycerol -500mL; Distilled water -100mL); **Destaining solutions** (Lactic acid-10mL; Glycerol-20mL).

Procedure

● Choose the roots, clean by washing in tap water and cut into small pieces of about one cm in size.

● Store the cleaned pieces of roots in the FAA solution to facilitate fixation.

● Transfer the root pieces in a conical flask containing 10% KOH solution.

● Heat the root at 90°C for 1-3 hour and cooled.

● Wash repeatedly with water.

● Transfer the washed root to a beaker containing 2% HCL and retained for 2-5 minutes

● Stain acid washed roots with lactic glycerol blue stain by applying heat at 90 °C for 5-10 minutes.

● After satisfactory staining, destain the root pieces with lactic acid solution

● Examine the stained root pieces under microscopically for the presence of stained VAM fungal hyphae.

Observation

Blue coloured Vesicles and Arbuscles are noted with in the root (Fig. 80.1).

Results and Discussions

Processed root is examined for the availability of arbuscles and vesicles and indicate the availability of VAM and discuss the importance of VAM in agriculture.

Viva Questions

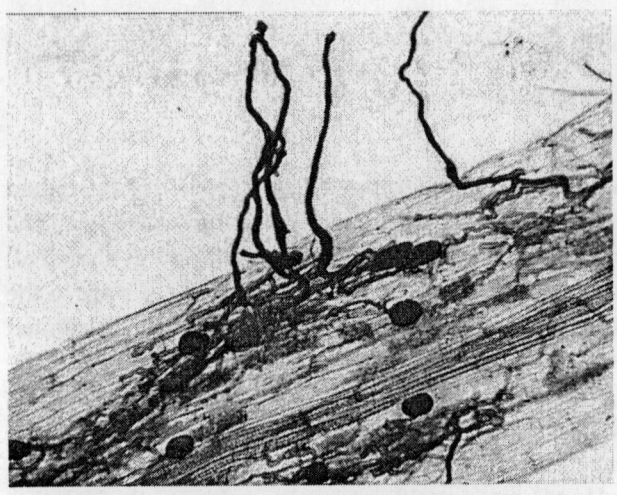

Fig. 80.1- Arbuscular mycorrhiza, showing arbuscules and vesicles within the root cortex and hyphae radiating from the root surface.

Define VAM.

Define ectomycorrhizae, endomycorrhizae and ectendomycorrhizae.

Differentiate VAM from endomycorrhizae.

What are Arbuscles and vescicles?

Name the stain used to assess VAM colonization.

What are the uses of VAM?

What are FAA?

What is Hartig net?

Is VAM a example for mutualistic relationship?

What are the uses of KOH in VAM Assessment?

Name the fixative used to assess VAM colonization.

Spotters – Picture of VAM, lactic glycerol blue stain

81. Isolation and cultivation of Rhizobium from legumes

Aim

To cultivate Nitrogen fixing Rhizobium from root nodules of legumes.

Background Information

Rhizobium is a type of nitrogen fixing bacteria that lives in soil and forms a symbiotic association with the root cells of leguminous plants. Legumes are herbaceous woody plants that produce seed in pods. The relationship between *Rhizobium* and legume root is called mutualism. Rhizobium was first isolated by Beijerinick, a Dutch scientist, from root nodules of legumes in 1888 and named it as *Bacillus radicicola*, now placed under the genus Rhizobium.

Characters of Rhizobium are, Gram negative, Rod shaped cells, 0.5-0.9mm x 1.2-mm in size, Nonspore forming, Contain enzyme nitrogenase. PHB granules are available, Strictly aerobic, Motile by single polar flagellum, Chemoorganotrophic, white, Colonies are circular, convex, semi translucent, raised and mucilaginous and also host specific.Isolation of Rhizobia is relatively easy if it is isolated from the host plant nodule but difficult if isolated from the soil. It doesn't grow well on the peptone medium. Yeast extract mannitol agar is commonly used for the isolation, cultivation and identification of Rhizobia. Mannitol is often used as the carbon source. Bromo thymol blue act as a pH indicator when added to the standard YEMA medium. Fast growing Rhizobia produce an acid reaction while slow growers produce alkaline reaction. congo red also used to differentiate Rhizobia from Agrobacterium. Three main species of Rhizobia are *Rhizobium leguminosarum, Rhizobium meliloti, Rhizobium loti*. Isolation was performed by serial dilution prepared from the root nodules or the fluid from crushed nodules is spread on the surface of YEMA medium with the help of smooth glass rods. Cultures are maintained on YEMA medium and sub cultured regularly and identified by specific tests.

Materials Required

Root nodules, YEMA medium with and without congo red, 0.1% mercuric chloride, 70% ethyl alcohol, 10mL sterile water blanks, 90mL sterile water blanks, Petriplates , YEMA medium with bromothymol blue, Peptone water, Kovacs indole reagent , Nitrate medium, Sulphanilic acid, Alpha naphthalamine, YEMA with lactose, YEMA with pH 11, Cover glass,Cavity slide, Ordinary slide, Gram staining reagents,Giemsa stain

Procedure

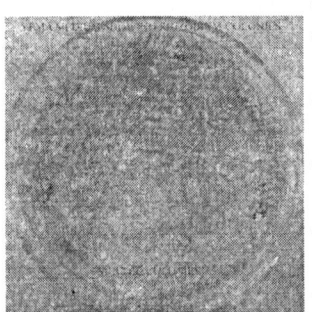

Fig 81.2 – Rhizobium on YEMA

- Prepare and Sterilize YEMA medium.
- Uproot the roots of leguminous plants and brought to the laboratory.
- Wash root systems in running tap water to remove adhering soil particle.
- Select and wash healthy pink unbroken and firm root nodule.
- Immerse nodules in 0.1% mercuric chloride for 5minutes for surface sterilization.
- Place nodules in 70% ethyl alcohol for 3 minutes.
- Wash nodules repeatedly by using sterile water.
- Crush nodules using glass rod in 1mL of water.
- Make uniform suspension of nodule with help of sterile water.
- Spread 0.1mL of the each suspension from various dilutions on YEMA plates or Streak loopfull of Suspension.
- Incubate all plates at 26 °C for 10 days.

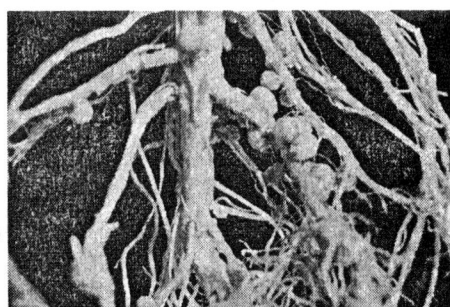

Fig 81.1: Nodules formed where Rhizobium bacteria infected soybean roots.

Cultivation and Identification

Isolated bacteria was streaked on YEMA medium with Congo red and YEMA with bromothymol blue medium and differentiated. Then it was identified by microscopic and biochemical methods. After completion of these processes, Rhizobium is cultivated on YEMA medium and sub culture regularly.

Observation

On YEMA medium Rhizobium grown as colourless Mucoid colony.

Table 81.1 Characteristic features and differentation features of Rhizobiun & Agrobacterium.

S.No	TEST	RESULT	
		Rhizobium	Agrobacterium
1	Gram staining	-	-
2	Giemsa staining	+	-
3	Motility	+	+
4	Indole	+	+
5	Nitrate	+	+
6	Lactose agar	-	+
7	Hoeffers alkaline	-	+
8	On YEMA	+	+
9	On YEMA with Congo red	-	+
10	On YEMA with bromothymol blue	+	-

Results

The isolated organism belongs to the genus Rhizobium

Viva questions

Name symbiotic N2 fixing bacteria.

Name the medium used for the cultivation of Rhizobium.

What are the enzymes of plant and bacteria responsible for N_2 fixation?

Is there any possibilities of natural atmospheric N_2 fixation?

Rhizobium is a aerobic bacterium but it survive within a root nodule. How?

Mention few important characteristic features of Rhizobium.

Define mutualism.

Mention about contributions of Beijerinick.

What are the major difference between Rhizobium and Agrobacterium?

Why mercuric chloride, alcohol treatment is given to nodule?

Mention colony morphology of Rhizobium on YEMA medium.

Mention importance of Rhizobium in agriculture.

Spotters: YEMA medium, Legume plant with root nodule, YEMA medium with rhizobium

82. Testing antagonistic activity of soil microbes

Aim

To check the antimicrobial activity of antagonistic soil microorganisms.

Background Information

In nature microbes grow with various interactions. It ranges from commensalism to antagonism. These interactions may exist within or between different groups of microbes. Some of the microbes produce toxin or antimicrobials that act on other microbial natures and are called antagonism.

Materials Required

Kursters agar (Starch casein agar – Kusters & Williams ; 1964), Test organisms, Antimicrobial substance producing microbe.

Procedure

- (Antimicrobial substance producers and test organisms are kept ready before the starting of an experiment).

- Prepare and sterilize Kusters agar medium & allow to solidify.

- Inoculate antimicrobial substance producing bacteria (Bacillus strain) / fungi at center of the plate (Fig. 82.1).

- Incubate the plate at 30 ° C for 24 hours.

- After 24 hours of incubation, various test organisms are streaked as shown in Reg. 63.1 (Streak should starts from the adjacent region of the antimicrobial substance producing microorganism).

- Incubate the plates again at 30°C for 24 hours.

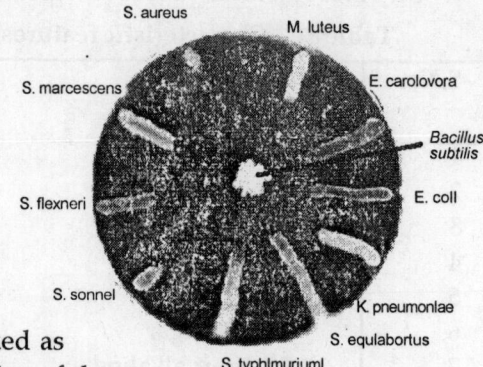

Fig 82.1 Antagonistic Activity of *B.subtilis* Strain

●   Observe for Zone of inhibitance.

Observations and Result

    Zone of inhibitance is noted / not observed between two groups of microorganisms. If zone of inhibitance is noted that organisms are the good source of antimicrobial substances.

Viva questions

    Define antagonism.

    Name the medium used to assess antagonistic activity.

    How do you assess antagonistic activity of soil microorganisms?

    What are the economic importance of screening antagonistic activity?

    Name few organisms having antagonistic activity.

    What is the other name for Kusters agar?

Spotters : Antagonistic activity showing plate.

83. Isolation of bacteria from rhizosphere, rhizoplane and non rhizosphere region

Aim

    To isolate microorganisms from rhizosphere, rhizoplane and non rhizosphere region

    To estimate the rhizosphere effect of soil microbes.

Background Information

    The German scientist Hiltner denoted that region of the soil, which is subject to the influence of plant roots, introduced the term rhizosphere in 1904. It is characterised by greater microbiological activity than the soil away from plant roots. The term rhizosphere effect indicates the overall influence of plant root on soil microorganisms. Soil type, moisture, pH, temperature, age of the plant and conditions of the plant are influence the rhizosphere effect. Root secretes exudate, which has sugars, amino acids vitamins and other growth factors. These factors serve as a nutrient for microbes in the rhizosphere region. The rhizosphere effect is helpful to plants in two ways. They Provide nutrients and helps plants in compeating root diseases. Greater rhizosphere effect is seen in bacteria (R:S value ranging from 10-20 or some times more) than with actinomycetes and fungi. The rhizosphere effect increases with the age of the plant and normally reached its maximum at the stage of greater vegetative growth. Some fungi inhabit the root surface in a mycelial state. They belongs to the genera *Mortierella, Cephalosporium, Trichoderma, Penicillium, Gliocladium, Gliomastix, Fusarium, Cylindrocarpon, Botrytis, Coniothyrium, Mucor, Phoma, Phythium* and *Aspergillus*. The following methods are available to find out the number of microbial population present in soil. Soil dilution and plate count, Soil plate technique, Fluorescent antibody technique, Slide box technique and Contact slide technique. Soil dilution and plate count is widely used for the better enumeration of microbial population in soil. R/S ratio is a rhizosphere effect.

Materials Required

    Freshly collected roots, Soil along with root, Non rhizosphere soil, Nutrient agar, Czapec dox agar, Starch casein nitrate agar, Sterile 100 mL distilled water, Screw cap bottle, 10 mL pipettes, 1mL pipettes, 90mL water blanks, Sterile petriplates etc.

Procedure

Isolation of microbes from rhizosphere soil

●   Collect rhizosphere soils from the roots of 3-4 plants with the help of brush in a Petri plate.

●   Add 10g of rhizosphere soil to 100-mL sterile water and shake for 15 minutes in a magnetic shaker.

- Serially dilute the sample up to 10^{-7}.
- In the mean time, prepare all necessary media and perform pour plate technique for bacteria, spread plate technique for actinomycetes and fungus.
- Plate sample from 10^{-3} 10^{-4} 10^{-5} and 10^{-6} diluents on nutrient agar medium by pour plate method.
- Plate 0.1mL of sample from 10^{-3} 10^{-4} 10^{-5} 10^{-6} and 10^{-4} diluents on Rose Bengal Chloramphenicol agar by spread plate method for isolation of fungi.
- Plate 0.1mL of sample from 10^{-2} and 10^{-5}, diluents on the actinomycetes isolation agar by spread plate method.
- Incubate all plates at appropriate environment.
- Observe plates and record the results.

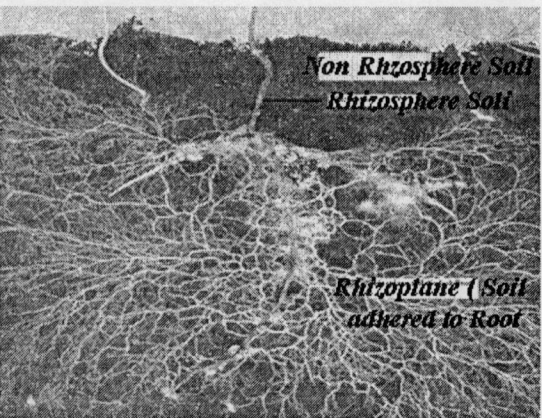

Fig 83.1 – Root regions

Isolation of microorganisms from non-rhizosphere soil

- Collect 10g of non rhizosphere soil and add it to the 100mL sterile distilled water.
- Then follow *isolation of rhizosphere soil microorganisms* procedure.

Isolation of microbes from rhizoplane

- Collect fresh roots and cut into small pieces
- Add root pieces into sterile 100mL of distilled water and it was considered as 10^{-1} dilution

Then follow isolation of rhizosphere soil microorganisms procedure

Also Inoculate root pieces on Nutrient agar, Czapec dox agar and Starch casein nitrate agar for the isolation of rhizoplane microbes.

Calculation of R/S ratio

$$R:S = \frac{\text{Number of microbes in rhizosphere soil}}{\text{Number of microbes in non rhizosphere soil}}$$

Table 83.1 Observation record

S. No	Soil type	Medium	No. of colonies		Average	R/S ratio
			Original	Replicates		
1	Rhizosphere	Nutrient agar Czapec dox agar Starch casein nitrate agar				
2	Non-rhizosphere	Nutrient agar Czapec dox agar Starch casein nitrate agar				
3	Rhizosplane	Nutrient agar Czapec dox agar Starch casein nitrate agar				

Observation

Different types of microorganisms are isolated from rhizosphere, non rhizosphere and rhizoplane region and R/S ratio is calculated.

Result

Increased rhizosphere effect shows good rhizosphere microbial load when compared to non rhizosphere region.

Viva questions

Define rhizosphere and rhizosplane

What is R: S ratio

What is rhizosphere effect

Why the microbial activity is high in rhizosphere region

What is root exudate

84. Analysis of Sodium and Potassium by Flame Photometer

Aim

To analyse Sodium and Potassium contents of the soil.

Background information

The amount of sodium and potassium can be determined by Flame Emission spectroscopy (FES) at a wavelength of 589 nm for sodium and 766.5 nm for potassium. The sample is sprayed into a gas flame and excitation is carried out under carefully controlled and reproducible condition. The desired spectral line is isolated by the use of interference filter or by a suitable silt arrangement in light, dispersing devices such as prisms or gratings. The intensity of light is measured by a phototube potentiometer or other appropriate circuit. The intensity of light at particular wavelength is approximately proportional to the concentration of the element.

Materials required

Instrument

Flame Photometer

Reagents

Sodium standard solution (1000ppm)

Dissolve 2.5422 g of AR grade of sodium chloride (previously dried at 140°C for 1 hour) in little double distilled water and make up to 1000mL in a volumetric flask (1mL = 1.0mG Na).

Potassium standard solution (1000ppm)

Dissolve 1.90g of AR grade of potassium chloride (previously dried at 140°C for 1 hour) in little double distilled water and make up to 1000mL in a volumetric flask (1mL = 1.0mG K).

Procedure

- Prepare calibration curve for sodium and potassium by using standard solutions in the range of 0 to 100 PPM separately at a wavelength of 589 nm for sodium and 766.5 nm for potassium. Use double distilled water as blank in every experiment.

- Spray the samples into a gas flame of flame photometer and determine the sodium and potassium separately.

- Obtain the results directly as concentrations of sodium and potassium present in the sample with the help of calibration curves.

Results

The results are expressed in mG/L as Na for Sodium and mG/L as K for potassium.

Spotters

Flame photometer

85. Trace Element Analysis by Atomic Absorption method

Aim

To estimate Cadmium, Chromium, Cobalt, Copper, Iron, Lead, Manganese, Nickel and Strontium trace elements using AAS.

Background information

The atomic absorption spectrometry is most common method for examination of a large number of inorganic and organic substances. In this technique, the sample is aspirated into a hot flame to convert the element to its atomic vapour. However in this case the absorption of specific radiation by the atom is measured rather than the emission spectra. After atomization of the element in the flame, most of the atoms remain in their ground state. Majority of them can be raised to the excited state, if they are given some specific radiation. The specific radiation which they would otherwise emit while coming to ground state from their excited state. Such radiation is possible to obtain from a hollow cathode lamp made up of the same element. The absorption of this radiation follows Beer's law as applicable to the absorption spectrometry. The concentration of the element can be determined by using a calibration curve.

Materials required

Instrument

Atomic Absorption Spectrophotometer

Soil sample, concentrated Nitric acid, 0.5N Hydrochloric acid.

Procedure

Pretreatment of sample

- Filter the sample and acidified with Conc. HNO_3 to a pH less than 2 immediately after collection of sample.

- Take 1.5litre of filtered sample in a beaker and add 5mL of Conc. HNO_3.

- Evaporate the sample to dryness on a hot plate preventing boiling.

- Add another 5mL of the Conc. HNO_3 after cooling. Heat, by adding some additional HNO_3 until light coloured residue forms.

- Dissolve the residue by adding 0.5 N HCl. Wash the wall of the beaker with 0.5 N HCl and filter the contents.

- Makeup the filtered content up to 50mL with 0.5 N HCl.

After pretreatment of the sample, the sample is aspirated into the flame for estimation of elements as per the Instrument instruction manual.

86. Estimation of soil mineral contents

Note : Use deionized water for mineral content estimation

Soil sample Preparation

Collect soil from a garden / any other area and weigh about 10g of soil. Dissolve 10g of soil in 1000mL of deionied water. Shake vigorously and filter through whatman No. 1 filter. Filtrate is subjected to chemical analysis.

86a. Estimation of pH of Soil

Aim

To assess pH of the given soil sample

Principle

pH is the measure of the relative acidity or alkalinity of the solution and is represented as the negative logarithm of the concentration of free hydrogen ions in a solution. The 'p' of pH denotes the power of the hydrogen ion activity in mole per litre.

$$_p^H = log10 \ [H^+]$$

When two electrodes are dipped in two solutions of different pH levels and connected, a potential difference is set up between the two electrodes, which is measured by the potentiometer. This is directly related to the pH of the solution.

Materials required

p^H meter, beaker, soil sample, pipette

Reagents -Prepare all the solutions in previously boiled and cooled distilled water.

Standard buffer solutions / buffer tablets for $_p^H$ 4.4, 7 and 9.2.

Procedure

- Warm up the instrument for 15 min.

- Calibrate the instrument with the known buffer solutions. (Calibration is done by a buffer solution whose pH is close to that of the sample).

- Immerse the electrode in the unknown sample and stir for minutes and note the pH.

    Note : Instead of preparing buffer solutions commercially available buffer tablets can be used for calibrating the pH meter.

Observation and results

p^H of the given sample is _____

86b. Nitrate

Aim

To estimate the quantity of nitrate available in the given soil sample.

Principle

Nitrate reacts with burcine in strong sulphuric acid solution to form a yellow colour which is measured spectrophotometrically at 410 nm. 1,2,4-phenol sulphuric acid produces 6 nitro 1,2,4 phenol disulphuric acid is the reaction point

Materials required

Soil sample, Beaker, Dark chamber, pipette, pH meter, conical flask, spectrophotometer etc.

Reagents

Nitrate standard solution

Dissolve 0.722 g of potassium nitrate (KNO_3) in 1 litre of distilled water   (1 mL = 0.1 mG NO_3-N). From the above stock solution, prepare standard solutions in the range of 0.1 to 1 mG/L of NO_3-N.

Brucine-sulphanilic acid solution

Dissolve 1g brucine sulphate and 100 mG sulphanilic acid in 70 mL hot distilled water. Add 3mL. Conc. HCl, cool and dilute to 100 mL with distilled water

Sulfuric acid solution

Add carefully 500 mL Conc. H_2SO_4 to 75mL distilled water and cool to room temperature.

Procedure

- Prepare a standard graph in the range of 0.1 to 1.0 mG /l of NO_3-N at the interval of 0.2 mG/l. Distilled water used as blank.

- Take 5 mL of sample in a 50mL beaker and add 1 mL brucine-sulphanilic acid solution to the sample.

- Add 10 mL sulfuric acid solution through the side wall of beaker and mix well.

- Keep the beakers in dark for 10+1 minutes.

- While the colour is developing, add 10 mL distilled water to this solution (but not before 10 minutes).

- Allow to cool in the dark for another 20-30 minutes.

- Read the optical density of the solution at a wavelength of 410 nm and findout the concentration of nitrate nitrogen from the calibration curve.

- If the concentration of sample is higher than upper range of calibration curve, sample is diluted with distilled water. Calculate nitrate / g of soil by the following calculation.

Calculation

5mL of sample contains _____-quantity of Nitrate.

i.e., 1liter contain _____-X200

10g sample is dissolved in one liter of water

10g of sample contains – – – – – – – mG of nitrate

1g of sample contains – – – – – – – mG of nitrate

Result

The result is expressed in mG/g as NO_3-N.

86c. Nitrite

Aim

To estimate the quantity of nitrite available in the given soil sample.

Principle:

Sulphanilic acid is diazotised by nitrite and the diazo compound is coupled with α - naphthylamine hydrochloride to form a reddish purple azo dye at a pH of 2.0 – 2.5.

Materials required

Soil sample, Beaker, Neslers tube, Dark chamber, pipette, pH meter, conical flask, spectrophotometer etc.

Reagents

EDTA solution.

Dissolve 500 mG disodium ethylene diamine tetra acetate dihydrate in distilled water and dilute to 100 mL.

Sulphanilic acid solution

Dissolve completely 600 mG of sulphanilic acid in 70 ml hot distilled water, cool and add 20 mL Conc. HCl dilute to 100 mL with distilled water.

α - Napthylamine hydrochloride solution

To 50 mL distilled water in a beaker, add 1 mL of Conc. HCl. Add 600 mG of α naphthylamine hydrochloride & dissolve and dilute to 100 mL with distilled water.

Sodium acetate buffer solution, 2M

Dissolve 16.4 g sodium acetate or 27.2 g sodium acetate trihydrate in distilled water and dilute to 100 mL.

Nitrite standard solution

Dissolve exactly 493 mG sodium nitrite in distilled water and make up to 1000 mL in a volumetric flask (1 mL = 100 mg of NO_2-N). From the above stock solution, prepare standard solutions in the range of 5 to 50 mg/l of NO_2-N.

Procedure

- Prepare a standard curve in the range of 1.0 to 50.0 mG/l of NO_2-N at the interval of 5 mG/l, by using the following method. Distilled water used as blank.

- Transfer 50 mL of the sample into a Nessler's tube. Add 1 mL of EDTA solution to this solution and stir well.

- Then add 1.0 mL sulphanilic acid to the above solution and mixed thoroughly. After 10 minutes, add 1.0 ml of α napthylamine hydrochloride solution and 1mL sodium acetate buffer solution and mixed thoroughly.

- Read the optical density of the solution at 520 nm after 10 minutes.

- Find out the concentration of nitrite nitrogen from the calibration curve.

- If the concentration of sample is higher than upper range of calibration curve, the sample is diluted with distilled water. Calculate nitrite/ g of soil by the following calculation.

Calculation

50mL of sample contains _____-quantity of Nitrite.

i.e., 1liter contain _____-X20

10g sample is dissolved in one liter of water

10g of sample contains – – – – – – –mG of nitrite

1g of sample contains – – – – – – –mG of nitrite

Result

The result is expressed in mG/g as NO_2-N.

86d. Sulphate

Aim

To estimate the quantity of sulphate available in the given soil sample.

Principle

Sulphate ion is precipitated by barium chloride and form Barium sulphate in hydrochloric acid medium. The concentration of sulphate can be determined from the absorbance of the light by Barium sulphate and then comparing it with a standard curve.

Materials required

Barium chloride, Soil sample, Beaker, pipette, pH meter, conical flask, spectrophotometer etc.

Regents

Conditioning reagent

Mix 75 g of NaCl, 30 mL Conc. HCl (Sp. Gr. 1.18), 100 mL 95 % ethyl alcohol in 300 mL of distilled water. Add 50 mL glycerol to this solution and mix thoroughly.

Hydrochloric acid solution (1 + 1)

Standard Sulphate solution

Dissolve 1.479 g of anhydrous Na_2SO_4 in distilled water to make 1 liter of solution. (1 mL = 1 mG SO_4). From the above stock solution, prepare standard solutions in the range of 5 to 40 mG/l of SO_4.

Procedure

- Prepare a standard graph in the range of 1.0 to 40.0 mG /l of SO_4 at the interval of 5 mG/l, by using the following method. Distilled water used as blank.

- Take 20 mL of sample in a conical flask and add 1 mL of conditioning reagent.

- Stir the solution on a magnetic stirrer and during stirring add a spoonful of $BaCl_2$ crystals. Stir only 1 minute after addition of $BaCl_2$.

- Read the optical density of the solution at 420 nm after 4 minutes and find out the concentration of sulphate from the standard graph.

- If the concentration of sample is higher than upper range of standard graph, sample is diluted with distilled water. Calculate sulphate/ g of soil by the following calculation.

Calculation

20mL of sample contains _____ quantity of sulphate.

i.e., 1liter contain _____ X 50

10g sample is dissolved in one liter of water

10g of sample contains — — — — — — —mG of sulphate.

1g of sample contains — — — — — — —mG of sulphate.

Result

The result is expressed in mG/g as SO_4.

86e. Phosphate

Aim

To estimate the quantity of phosphorus available in the given soil sample.

Principle

Ammonium molybdate reacts with phosphate present in water to form molybdophosphoric acid at low pH which is reduced to a blue coloured complex, "molybdenum blue" by the addition of stannous chloride.

Materials required

Soil sample, Beaker, Dark chamber, pipette, pH meter, conical flask, spectrophotometer etc.

Reagents

Ammonium molybdate solution

(a) Dissolve 25.0g of ammonium molybdate in 175mL of distilled water

(b) Add 280 mL of Conc. H_2SO_4 to 400mL of distilled water and cool

Mix two solutions (a) and (b) and make up the volume to 1 litre with distilled water.

Stannous chloride solution

Dissolve 2.5g of stannous chloride in 100mL glycerol by heating on a water bath.

Standard phosphate solution

Dissolve 0.22 g of pre-dried anhydrousdi potassium hydrogen phosphate (K_2HPO_4) in distilled water and make up the volume to 1 litre, (1 mL = 50 mg PO_4-P). From the above stock solution, prepare standard solutions in the range of 20 to 200 mg/L of PO_4-P.

Procedure

- Prepare a standard graph in the range of 10 to 200mg/L of PO_4-P at the interval of 20.

- Take 50 mL of filtered water sample in a conical flask. (If the sample in having colour and colloidal impurities, remove them by adding a spoonful of activated charcoal and filter it. If colour is not removed, add 2 ml of perchloric acid after evaporation of 50 mL of sample to dryness and made up to 50 ml with distilled water.)

- Add 2 mL of ammonium molybdate solution and 5 drops of stannous chloride reagent to this sample.

- A blue colour will appear in the presence of phosphate.

- After 5 minutes but before 12 min., read the optical density of the solution at 690 nm on a spectrophotometer. (If the concentration of sample is higher than upper range of standard graph sample is diluted with distilled water). Calculate phosphorus / g of soil by the following calculation.

Calculation

50mL of sample contains _____-quantity of phosphorus

i.e., 1liter contain _____ X20

10g sample is dissolved in one liter of water

10g of sample contains – – – – – – –mG of phosphorus

1g of sample contains – – – – – – –mG of phosphorus

Result

The result is expressed in mG/G as PO_4-P.

86f. Calcium

Aim

To estimate the quantity of calcium available in the given soil sample.

Principle

In a solution containing both calcium and magnesium can be determined directly with EDTA. When the pH is made sufficiently high (12 to 13) so that the magnesium is largely precipitated as the hydroxide and an indicator is used which combines only with calcium.

Materials required

Soil sample, Beaker, Dark chamber, pipette, pH meter, conical flask, spectrophotometer etc.

Reagents

Murexide (ammonium purpurate) indicator

Grind 0.2g Murexide with 100g of NaCl.

NaOH solution (1 N)

40 g of NaOH is dissolved in 1 litre distilled water.

Standard EDTA solution (0.01M)

Procedure

- Take 25mL of the sample in a conical flask and add 2.0 mL of NaOH solution.

- Add approximately 100mG of Murexide in the solution and titrate this solution with standard EDTA solution until the pink colour changes to dark purple.

- Calculate calcium/ g of soil by the following calculation.

$$\text{Calcium(mg/l)} \atop \text{[as Ca]} = \frac{T \times E \times 1000}{V}$$

where,

T - Titrate value in mL.

E - Mass in mG of calcium ions equivalent to 1ml of EDTA solution

(1ml EDTA = 0.4008mG Ca)

V - Volume of sample taken

1000ml of sample contains _____-quantity of Calcium.

10g sample is dissolved in one liter of water

10g of sample contains — — — — — — — mg of calcium

1g of sample contains — — — — — — — mg of calcium

Result

The result is expressed in mG/G as Ca.

86g. Magnesium

Aim

To estimate the quantity of magnesium available in the given soil sample.

Principle

When water sample containing both calcium and magnesium is titrated with EDTA at pH 10, using Eriochrome Black - T indicator which estimates calcium and magnesium. In a separate titration against EDTA at pH 12 to 13 range using Murexide indicator, calcium is selectively estimated. From these two values, magnesium concentration may be calculated.

Calculate Magnecium / G of soil by the following calculation.

$$\text{Magnesium (mg/1)}_{\text{(as Mg)}} = \frac{(TH-Ca) \times E \times 1000}{V}$$

where,

TH - Titrate value for total hardness

Ca - Titrate value for Calcium

E - Mass of magnesium equivalent to 1mL of EDTA (1ml = 0.243mG magnesium)

V - Volume of sample in mL.

Calculation

1000mL of sample contains _____quantity of Magnecium.

10g sample is dissolved in one liter of water

10g of sample contains — — — — — — — mg of Magnecium

1g of sample contains — — — — — — — mg of Magnecium

Result

The result is expressed in mG/G as Mg.

86h. Chloride

Aim

To estimate the quantity of chloride available in the given soil sample.

Principle:

Silver Nitrate reacts with chloride in neutral or alkaline solution to form silver chloride. Potassium chromate used as indicator in the silver nitrate titration of chloride estimation. Potassium chromate also reacts with silver nitrate to form red silver chromate. However, this potassium chromate reaction is less favourable than the chloride reaction. So potassium chromate only reacts with silver nitrate in the absence of free chloride ions in the water sample.

When no free chloride is left in the solution at the end point, addition of a drop of silver nitrate titrant results in the formation of silver chromate producing a pink end point.

Materials required

Soil sample, Beaker, Dark chamber, pipette, pH meter, conical flask, burette etc.

Reagents

Silver nitrate (0.02N)

3.40g of Silver nitrate is dissolved in double distilled water and make upto 1 litre.

Potassium chromate indicator

5% Aqueous solution of pure K_2CrO_4

Procedure

- Take 5 mL of sample in a conical flask and diluted to 25 ml with distilled water
- Add 5 to 6 drops K_2CrO_4
- Titrate this solution with standard $AgNO_3$ solution till the first brick red tinge appears
- Calculate Chloride / g of soil by the following calculation.

Calculations

$$Chloride\ (mg/l)\ (as\ Cl) : \frac{T \times N \times E \times 1000}{V}$$

where,

T - titrate value

N - normality of silver nitrate (0.02)

E - equivalent weight of chloride (35.45)

V - volume of sample taken in mL.

Calculation

1000mL of sample contains _____ quantity of Chloride.

10g sample is dissolved in one liter of water

10g of sample contains — — — — — — —mG of Chloride

1g of sample contains — — — — — — —mG of Chloride

Result

The result is expressed in mG/G as Cl.

Viva questions

What is the meaning of P in pH?

Define pH.

What is the need of pH measurement in soil?

What are the significance of pH in agriculture?

What are the methods available to assess pH?

Name the indicator used in pH paper?

Mention electrode available in pH meter?

What are the principle of Nitrate test?

Provide the use of Brucine sulphate in nitrate estimation.

How can you estimate sulphate content of soil?

What is the principle of sulphate estimation?

How do you detect Nitrate, Phosphate, Chloride, Calcium and magnesium?

What are the uses of silver nitrate in chloride estimation?

What are difference between murexide and ammonium purpurate?

What are the uses of Ammonium purpurate and erichrome or solochrome Black T?

Name the indicator used to assess chloride content of soil.

What are the principle of phosphate estimation?

What are the significance of minerals in soil?

What is the need of deionized water in mineral estimation?

Spotters: pH meter, soil, Brucine sulphate, sulphanilic acid, Barium chloride, EDTA, muroxide/ Ammonium purpurate, Solochrome black T/ Erychrome black T, Stannous chloride, silver nitrate, Potassium dichromate.

86i. Fluoride

Aim

To estimate fluoride content of the soil.

Background informations

The SPADNS spectrophotometric method is based on the reaction between fluoride and a zirconium-dye lake (SPADNS dye). Fluoride reacts with the dye lake in the presence zirconyl acid, dissociating a portion of it into a colourless complex anion and the dye. As the amount of fluoride increases, the colour produced by the dye progressively lighter.

Materials required

Reagents

SPADNS solution

Dissolve 958mG of SPADNS [Sodium 2- (Parasulphophenyl Azo) -1, 8-Dihydroxy - 3, 6-Naphthalene di Sulphonate trisodium salt] in distilled water and dilute to 500mL.

Zirconyl - acid reagent

Dissolve 133mG zirconyl chloride octahydrate in 25mL distilled water. Add 350mL of Conc. HCl and dilute to 500mL with distilled water.

Acid zirconyl - SPADNS reagent

Mix equal volumes of SPADNS solution and zirconyl acid reagent.

Standard fluoride solutions

Dissolve 221mG anhydrous sodium fluoride in distilled water and dilute to 1 litre (1mL = 100mG of F^-). From the above stock solution, prepare standard solutions in the range of 0.2 to 1.4mG/Lof F.

Procedure

- Prepare a calibration curve in the range of 0.0 to 1.4mG/L of F at the interval of 0.2, by using the following same method. Distilled water used as blank.

- Take 50mL of the sample in a conical flask.

- Add 10mL of acid zirconyl-SPDANS reagent to the sample and mix well.

- After 1hour, read the optical density of the solution on spectrophotometer at 520nm (If the concentration of sample is higher than upper range of calibration curve, sample is diluted with distilled water).

Result

The result is expressed in mG/L as F.

86j. Silica

Aim

To estimate silica content of the soil.

Principle

Ammonium molybdate at pH 1.2 reacts with silica and any phosphate present in the water sample to produce heteropolyacids. Oxalic acid is added to destroy the molybdophosphoric acid but not the molybdosilicic acid.

Materials required

Reagents

Hydrochloric acid (1+ 1)

Ammonium molybdate solution (10%)

Dissolve 20g of ammonium molybdate in distilled water and make up the volume to 200mL. Adjust the pH between 7 and 8 by adding Ammonium hydroxide. Keep the solution in a polyethylene bottle.

Oxalic acid solution (10%)

Dissolve 20g of oxalic acid in distilled water and make up to 200mL

Standard silica solution

Dissolve 4.73g of sodium meta silicate monohydrate in distilled water and dilute to 1 litre with distilled water (1mL = 1mG SiO_2). From the above stock solution, prepare standard solutions in the range of 2 to 10mG/L of SiO_2

Procedure

- Prepare a calibration curve in the range of 0.00 to 50.0mG/L of SiO_2 at the interval of 5mG/L, by using the following method. Distilled water used as blank.

- Take 50mL of the water sample in a conical flask and add 1mL of Hydrochloric acid and 2mL of Ammonium molybdate solution to the sample.

- After 10 minutes, add 1.5mL of oxalic acid solution to this above solution.

- Mix thoroughly and read the optical density of the solution on Spectrophotometer at 410mn and find out the concentration of silicate from the calibration curve (If the concentration of sample is higher than upper range of calibration curve, the sample is diluted with distilled water).

Result

The result is expressed in mG/L as SiO_2.

86k. Ammonia

Aim

To estimate ammonia content of the soil.

Principle

The sample is buffered at pH 9.5 with a borate buffer to decrease hydrolysis of cyanates of organic nitrogen compounds. It is distilled and absorbed into a solution of boric acid and ammonia is determined with standard mineral acid.

Materials required

Kjeldahl flask, conical flask, burette, piepette, etc.,

Reagents

Hydrochloric acid (0.01N)

Boric acid cum indicator solution

Dissolve 4g of boric acid in 100mL of warm distilled water. Prepare 0.5% bromocresol green solution and 0.1% methyl red solution in ethyl alcohol. Mix bromocreol green and methyl red solution in the ratio of 2:1 to make a mixed indicator. Add 5mL of this mixed indicator to 100mL of boric acid solution. If the colour of solution becomes blue add 0.01N Hydrochloric acid until it turns faint pink to brown.

Borate buffer solution

Add 88mL of 0.1 N of sodium hydroxide to 500mL of 0.025 M sodium tetra borate solution and dilute to 1 litre with distilled water.

Sodium hydroxide solution (6 N)

Procedure

- Take 250mL of sample in a Kjeldahl flask. Add 15mL borate buffer and 6 N sodium hydroxide (Add NaOH until pH 9.5 is reached).

- Place 25mL of boric acid solution containing 2-3 drops of mixed indicator in a conical flask below the condenser so that the tip of outlet of the condenser is dipped in contents of conical flask.

- Heat the kjeldhal flask containing solution and continued the distillation until about 200mL of distillate in collected in the conical flask.

- Remove the conical flask containing distillate after distillation, which turns blue for dissolution of ammonia.

- Titrate the distillate against 0.01N Hydrochloric acid until blue colour changes to pink.

- Run a blank with distilled water in a similar way.

Calculation

$$\text{Total Organic Nitrogen (mg/L)} = \frac{(T-B) \times N \times E \times 1000}{\text{Volume of sample}}$$
$$\text{(as NH}_4\text{-N)}$$

Where,

T - volume of titrant (HCl) used against sample (ml).

B - volume of titrant (HCl) used against blank (ml).

N - normality of HCl (0.01).

E - equivalent weight of nitrogen (14).

The result is expressed in mG/L as NH_4-N.

Result :

The amoung of NH_4 present in sample is expressed as mg/g

Environmental Microbiology

CHAPTER 6

87. Isolation and identification of air borne bioparticles

Aim

To isolate and identify the air borne microorganisms by specific techniques.

Background Information

Air is the simplest one. The relative quantities of various gases in air, by volume percentage are nitrogen 78%, oxygen 21%, argon 0.9%, carbon dioxide 0.03%, hydrogen 0.01% and other gases in trace amounts. Air is mainly a transport or dispersal medium for microorganisms. They occur in relatively small numbers in air when compared to soil and water. The air in the atmosphere, which is found outside the buildings, is referred to as outside air. The dominant flora of outside air is fungus. The commonest fungi are Deuteromycetes, *Cladosporium* and the Basidiomycete Yeast, Sporobolomyces. Widely occuring Bacterial forms are spores of *Bacillus,Clostridium*, resistant nonspore formers such as *Sarcina lutea* and *Micrococcus luteus*, nonpathogenic species of *Corynebacterium* and few gram negative rods such as coliforms and Achromobacteriaceae. About 2-500 cells per m^3 were detected upto the height of 4 kms from the earth surface. Number of microorganisms may vary from place to place. For eg. About several hundreds of bacteria found per cubic meter in country where as several thousands of bacteria are seen per cubic meter in cities. The air found inside the building is referred an indoor air. The commonest flora are *Penicillium, Mucor* and *Aspergillus*. The frequent bacterial species are Staphylococcus, Bacillus and *Clostridium perfringens* . Sources of air microbes are man made activities like digging and plugging of soil, aerosols (droplet nuclei) and air currents brings microbes from plant or animal sources . The optimum rate of Relative Humidity for the survival of most microbes is between 40-80%. Viruses survive at RH 17-25%.

Methods of air sampling

Hesse's method, Settle plate method, Wells centrifuge method, Reuter centrifugal air sampler, Tube sampler, Raised impfinger, Bead bubbler device, Lemon sampler, Hollaender and Dalla Valle sampler, Slit sampler, Size grading slit sampler, Sieve sampler, Litten air sampler.

Airborne pathogens

An adult inhales about 15 cubic meter of air per day. Less than 1% air microbes are pathogens.

Staphylococcus aureus, Streptococcus pneumoniae, Pseudomonas aeruginosa, Enterobacter sp, Klebsiella pneumoniae, Escherichia coli, Chlamydia sp, Haemophillus influenzae, Serratia marcesens, Citrobacter freundii, Acinetobacter, Xanthomonas, Legionella, Mycobacterium tuberculosis

Air borne diseases

Brucellosis, meningititis, anthrax, pharyngitis, scarlet fever, rheumatic fever, erysipelas, puerperal fever, pneumonia, psittacosis, diphtheria, tuberculosis, legionellosis, cryptococcosis, blastomycosis, coccidioidomycosis, histoplasmosis, aspergillosis, common cold, measeles, influenza, mumps, adenovirus infections. For the isolation of airborne pathogens or airborne bioparticles peoples follows settle plate method and air-sampling methods.

Settle plate method

The principle behind this method is that the bacteria carrying particles are allowed to settle onto the medium for a given period of time and incubated at the required temperature.

Materials Required

Nutrient agar, Blood agar is used If Streptococcus assessment is indicated, Rose Bengal chloramphenical agar, Petri plates etc.

Procedure

- Prepare and sterilize media as per a type of microorganisms to be enumerated.
- Pour the molten agar into the petri plates and allow to solidify.
- Dry the agar surface before the starting up of an experiment.
- Label the plates appropriately (Mention place and time of the sampling, duration of exposure etc).
- Open the plates in the selected area for a required period of time (during sampling it is better to keep the plates one meter above the ground).
- Close the plates immediately after exposure for the given period of time.
- Incubate the plates for 24 hours at 37^0C for aerobic bacteria and 3 days for saprophytic bacteria.
- For molds incubation temperature varies from $10\text{-}50^0C$ for 1 to 2 weeks.
- After incubation, count the number of colonies and record the results.

Table 87.1 – Observation record table

S.No	Medium	Time of exposure (in minutes)	No of colonies		Average
			Original	Replicate	
1	Nutrient agar	5 10 15 20			
2	Rose bengol chloramphenicolAgar	5 10 15 20			

Disadvantage

In this method, only the rate of large particles from the air, not the total number of bacteria carrying particle per volume is measured.

Air Sampling Method

Modern air sampler was called *Reuter centrifugal air sampler*. It is portable and battery powered instrument. It resembles large cylindrical torch with open-ended drum at one end. The drum encloses impeller blades, which can be rotated by battery power. Advantage of this method is very convenient for transportation and use.

Procedure

- Assemble air sampler as per the manufacturer instruction

- Insert a plastic strip coated with culture medium along the inner side of the drum.
- Switch on the drum. Air is drawn into the drum and subjected to centrifugal acceleration. That causes the suspended particle to impact on the culture medium.
- Remove the strip after sampling from the instrument and incubated at appropriate environment for up to 72 hours
- Count Colonies grown on media strip and tabulated.

Observation

Different groups of microbial cells / colonies are observed.

Result

Indoor air is more contaminated than out door.

Viva questions

Explain the nature of air

Name the media used for the cultivation of air borne microorganisms

List any 5 air borne microorganisms and diseases.

Name the methods used to assess microbial population in air.

List different methods of air sampling

What are the uses of Rose begal chloramphenicol agar in air flora assessment?

Spotters : Air sampler

88. Effect of high salt concentration on microbial growth

Aim

To analyze the effect of sodium chloride concentration on growth

To assess the effect of osmotic pressure of the environment.

Background information

Growth of bacteria can be profoundly affected by the amount of water entering or leaving the cell. Solution is composed of two parts, that which is dissolved (the solute) and the fluid in which the solute is dissolved (the solvent). The solute concentration is related to a phenomenon known as osmotic pressure. On the basis of solute concentration the medium is divided into three types. They are hypotonic (low solute content), isotonic and hypertonic (high solute content). In hypotonic solution, the solute concentration of the protoplasm is higher than outer side, therefore the osmotic pressure inside of the cell is higher than outside. This internal pressure pushes the cells plasma membrane against the cell wall. As a result, water enters inside of the cell. In hypertonic solution, protoplasm concentration is lower than outer environment concentration, so fluid is effluxed from the cell. In isotonic solution, both cell and outer environment solute concentration are same. Physiological saline is an example for isotonic solution. Blood also act as a isotonic solution. Generally the bacterial cellwall has sufficient strength to withstand the difference in solute concentration. During the differentiation of osmotic pressure cell will burst or shrinked. This phenomenon is known as *Plasmolysis*. It doesnot occur in all bacteria. Those bacteria that withstands higher sodium chloride concentration are called halophills or halotolerent.

Material Required

Bacterial cultures, 0.5%,1%,2%,5%,10% and15% sodium chloride containing nutrient agar medium, Petriplates, Pipettes etc.,

Procedure

- Prepare nutrient broth and inoculate with test organism and incubate for 24 hours at 37°C

- Streak test organism on various concentration of sodium chloride containing nutrient agar plates as single line streak (Fig 88.1).

- Streak atleast four organism in a single plate

- Incubate all plates at 37 °C for 24 hours.

- Observe and record the results.

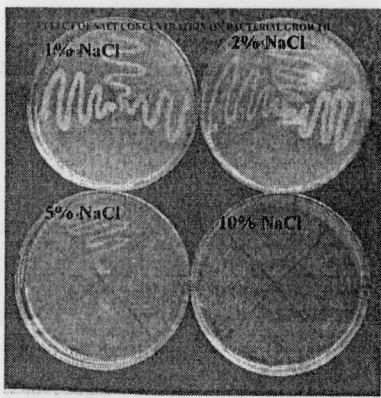

Fig 88.1: Effect of Nacl Concentration on Bacteria

Table 88.1: Observation record table

S.No	Test organism	Salt concentration %					
		0.5	1	2	5	10	15
1	S. aureus						
2	E. coli						
3	Rhizobium						
4	Salmonella sp						

Result

Staphylococcus withstand higher concentration of soil

Viva questions

Define osmotic pressure, hypertonic; hypotonic and isotonic environment

What is plasmolysis

Explain halophils and halotolerant

Name few halophilic bacteria

Mention adoptations of halophilic bacteria.

Spotters: sodium chloride

89. Oligodynamic action of heavy metals on microbes

Aim

To determine the activity of heavy metals on microbial growth.

Background Information

Oligos means little, dynamics means power. The ability of heavy metal compound to exert antimicrobial activity is called as Oligodynamic activity. Various forms of metallic elements like mercury, silver, gold, copper, arsenic and zinc have been applied in microbial control over several centuries. These are often referred to as heavy metals because of their relatively high atomic weight. Silver is used as an antiseptic in a 1% silver nitrate solution. The solution is bactericidal for most organisms. Example: for newborns 1% silver nitrate is added to the eye to prevent gonococcal infection called gonorrhoeal *opthalmia neonatorum*. Inorganic mercuric compounds, such as mercuric chloride probably have the longest history of use as disinfectants. Copper in the form of copper sulfate is used chiefly to destroy green algae (algicide) that grow in reservoirs, swimming pools, and fish tanks. Another metal used, as an antimicrobial is zinc. Zinc chloride is a common ingredient in mouthwashes, and zinc oxide is probably the most widely used antifungal in paints. "When the metal ions combine with the -SH groups on cellular proteins, denaturation results". During experimental demonstration small amount of heavy metal diffuse in the medium. **Disadvantages** are Metals are very toxic to humans if ingested, inhaled or absorbed through the skin. They commonly cause allergic reactions. Commonly used Heavy Metal preparations are *Merthiolate*, Metaphen, Silver sulfadiazine ointment, 1% silver nitrate solution

Materials Required

Nutrient broth, Nutrient agar, 1%Silver nitrate, Zinc chloride, Mercury chloride, Test tubes, Petri plates, Cotton swabs.

Procedure

- Prepare midlog cultures of *Escherichia coli* and *Staphylococcus aureus* in 100mL conical flask containing 50mL medium.

- Pour sterile nutrient agar to the Petri plates and allow to solidify.

- Inoculate 0.1mL test organism on the surface of nutrient agar plates and spread using L – Rod..

- Cut 4mm well using sterile well borer at different places on the plate.

- Add enough quantity of heavy metal solution to the respective wells.

- Incubate all plates at 37°C for 48 hours.

- Observe zone of inhibition.

- Record the result.

Observation and Result

Zone of inhibition is noted and indicates the oligodynamic action of heavy metals.

Viva Questions

Define *oligodynamic* action.

What are the principles of oligodynamic action?

Name few heavy metals.

Name heavy metal used in children.

Mention few diseases cured by heavy metals.

Define antiseptic.

What are the disadvantages of heavy metals in human?

Give few examples of heavy metal preparations available in market.

How do you perform oligodynamic action?

Spotters: Silver nitrate, Zinc chloride, Mercury chloride, Copper.

90. Isolation of coliforms from sewage

Aim

To isolate indicator microorganisms (Coliforms) from the sewage.

Background Information

Sewage or wastewater is defined as used water of a community and it consists of domestic waste, atmospheric water and surface wastewater. Wastewater from city is collected by sanitary sewers; Strom sewers and combined sewers. Waste water exhibits a great diversity in physical, chemical and microbiological character. Wastewater consists of approximately 99.9% of water. Untreated wastewater contains millions of bacteria per mL, which include coliforms, Streptococci, Proteus and anaerobic spore forming bacilli. Detection of indicator microorganisms are the major part of sanitary microbiology. If we consume the polluted water or sewage may leads to intestinal disorder like gastroenteritis, diarrhoea and dysentery. To avoid microbial diseases, microbial monitory is necessary than chemical monitory. Various techniques are available to detect microbial flora of sewage. Among this standard plate count using selective and non-selective media play an major role. In this experiment coliform bacteria are detected by making use of EMB agar.

Materials Required:

Sample : Sewage water; **Media :** Eosin methylene blue agar; **Other material:** Test tubes, Pipette, Petri plates, conical flasks etc.

Procedure

- Collect sewage sample and transport to the laboratory within an hour.
- Serially dilute the sample up to 10^{-6}
- Inoculate 0.1 ml sample from 10^{-4}, 10^{-5} and 10^{-6} dilution on EMB agar by spread plate method.
- Incubate all plates at 37 °C for 24 hours
- Observe the plates and record the results.

Table 90.1: Observation record

S. No	Medium used	Dilution factor Colonies	Metallic sheen Colonies	Non metallic sheen
1	EMB agar	10^{-3}		
		10^{-4}		
		10^{-5}		

Observation

Metallic sheen, dark centered (nucleated) and colourless colonies are observed.

Result

Metallic sheen and dark centered colonies are belongs to coliform group.

Viva questions

Define sewage and waste water.

What are the chemical constituents of sewage?

Why microbial analysis in sewage so important?

Mention about characters of sewage.

What happened if you consume sewage contaminated water?

What is coliforms?

How EMB agar selects only coliforms?

Expand EMB agar.

Is *E.coli* is considered as coliforms? Why?

How do you differentiate coliforms and non coliforms on EMB agar?

What is the purpose of this experiment?

Spotters: EMB agar

91. Estimation of total solids in the effluent sample

Aim

To determine the amount of total solids in the effluent sample

Background information

Residues are settled when potable water is evaporated to dryness. All of the materials forming this residue are grouped together under the term "total solids". The total content of suspended and dissolved solids in water is called total solids. Total solids (some times called total residue) is related to turbidity, except that it includes not just suspended solids, but also dissolved solids such as the mineral ions, calcium, phosphorus, iron, sulfur and bicarnonate. A certain level of these ions is essential for life. Cells also depend on the density of total solids to determine the amount of water that flows in and out of the cell. However, too much dissolved solids in water can affect humans by inducing a laxative effect and giving the water a mineral taste. Increased total solids has a similar effect to turbidity in that water clarity is reduced, water temperature can rise, oxygen levels can fall as a result of less photosynthesis, and solids can bind to toxic compounds and heavy metals.

Materials required

Beaker, conical flask, balance, desicator, Silica crucible, water / effluent sample, Hot air oven etc.

Procedure

● Accurately weigh a clean dry silica crucible and record this weight as W_I

● Transfer unfiltered 100mL sample in the silica crucible

● Evaporate the sample by placing it in a hot air oven at 105^0C for 1 hour.

● Cool it in a desicator

● Take a crucible out of the desicator and record its weight (W_F) (Repeat cycle of drying, cooling, desiccating, and weighing until a constant weight is obtained)

● Calculate the total solids of the given sample as follows

$$\text{Total solids (mG/L)} = \frac{(W_I) - (W_F)}{\text{Sample volume, mL}} \times 1000$$

Where,

W_I – Initial weight of the crucible.

W_F – Final weight of the crucible.

Result

The given sample contains — — — — mG/L of solids

92. Analysis of TDS of effluent

Aim

To determine total dissolved solids in the effluent sample.

Background information

Total Dissolved Solids (often abbreviated TDS) is a measure of the combined content of all inorganic and organic substances contained in a liquid in molecular, ionized or micro-granular suspended form. A total dissolved solid (TDS) is the term used to describe the inorganic salts and small amounts of organic matter present in solution in water. The principal constituents are usually calcium, magnesium, sodium, and potassium cations and carbonate, hydrogencarbonate, chloride, sulfate, and nitrate anions. The presence of dissolved solids varies between the waste water. Potable water consists mostly inorganic salts, dissolved gases and organic matter in low or trace quantities. Majority of these contents are available in dissolved form. Maximum permissible limit of TDS in potable water is 20 – 1000mG/L.

Materials required

Silica crucible, balance, Hot air oven, Effluent sample etc.

Procedure

- Weigh clean dry silica crucible and transfer 100mL of the filtered sample in the silica crucible (W_I)

- Evaporate the crucible in a hot air oven for one hour at 180⁰C. Cool it in a desicator and record its weight. Let it be W_F (Repeat cycle of drying, cooling, desiccating, and weighing until a constant weight is obtained)

- Now calculate the TDS of given sample using the formula

    Calculation

    $$\text{Total dissolved solids (mG/L)} = \frac{(W_I) - (W_F)}{\text{Sample volume, mL}} \times 10,00$$

Where,

W_I – Initial weight of the crucible.

W_F – Final weight of the crucible.

Result

The given sample contains — — — — mG/L of dissolved solids.

284

93. Estimation of total suspended solids of the effluent

Aim

To determine the amount of total suspended solids in the effluent sample

Background information

Suspended solids can clog fish gills, either killing them or reducing their growth rate. They also reduce light penetration. This reduces the ability of algae to produce food and oxygen. When the water slows down, as when it enters a reservoir, the suspended sediment settles out and drops to the bottom, a process called siltation. This causes the water to clear, but as the silt or sediment settles it may change the bottom. The silt may smother bottom-dwelling organisms, cover breeding areas, and smother eggs. Indirectly, the suspended solids affect other parameters such as temperature and dissolved oxygen. Because of the greater heat absorbency of the particulate matter, the surface water becomes warmer and this tends to stabilize the stratification (layering) in stream pools and reservoirs. This, in turn, interferes with mixing, decreasing the dispersion of oxygen and nutrients to deeper layers. **Total suspended solids** in a water quality measurement usually abbreviated **TSS.**

Procedure / Calculations

- Total suspended solids can be obtained by subtracting the total dissolved solids from total solids.

- Total suspended solids = total solids – total dissolved solids

Result

The given sample contains – – – –mG/L of suspended solids.

94. Determination of BOD

Aim

To determine BOD of given effluent sample.

Background Information

The BOD is the way of expressing the amount of organic compound in sewage as measured by the volume of the oxygen required by bacteria to metabolize it under aerobic condition. It is the good index of pollution. If the amount of organic matter in sewage is more, more O_2 will be utilized by bacteria to degrade it. BOD is generally measured by incubating the sample at 20° C for 5 days in the dark under aerobic conditions. Nitrification also consume some quantity of O_2 and it must be checked by adding 1ml of 0.5% allyl thiourea. Sewage should be aerated properly before the commencement of experiments.

Principle - Dissolved Oxygen Method

This method depends on the oxidation of manganese dioxide by oxygen dissolved in water resulting in the formation of tetravalent compound. It is acidified with sulphuric acid, which release free iodine from the oxidation of potassium iodide. The free iodine is chemically equalant to the amount of dissolving oxygen present in the sample and it is determine by titration with a standard solution of sodium thiosulphate.

$$MnSO_4 + 2KOH ——> Mn\,[OH]_2 + K_2SO_4$$

This reaction results in the formation of precipitation.

If the precipitate is white there is no dissolved oxygen in the sample. A brown precipitate indicates the oxygen is present and reacts with manganese hydroxide forming manganese oxide.

$$2MnOH + O_2 ——> Mn\,O(OH)_2$$

Addition of sulphuric acid dissolves precipitate and forms manganese sulphate.

$$Mn[OH]_2 + 2H_2SO_4 --> Mn(SO_4)_2 + 2H_2$$

There is an immediate reaction between this complex and potassium iodide and resulting in the typical iodine colouration of the water (slight brown).

$$Mn(SO_4)_2 + 2KI --> MnSO_4 + K_2SO_4 + I_2$$

The number of molecules iodine liberated by the reaction is equal to number of molecule oxygen present in the sample. The quantity of iodine can be determined by titrating a portion of solution with a standard Sodium thio sulphate solution.

$$2Na_2S_2O_3 + I_2 --> Na_2S_4O_6 + 2NaI$$

Materials Required

BOD bottle, Conical flask, Pipettes, pH meter, BOD incubator.

Reagents

Manganous sulphate solution:

Dissolve 40g $MnSO_4$ in 100mL distilled water.

Alkaline Iodide Acyl solution

Dissolve separately 25g NaOH and 6.75g NaI in distilled water. Mix then make the volume up to 500mL Add 0.5g of sodium azide as a preservative.

Sodium thiosulphate (0.25N)

Dissolve 3.72 g of Sodium thiosulphate in freshly boiled and cooled dissolved water and dilute to 500mL.

Starch Indicator:

Dissolve 1g of starch in 100mL of hot water and add few drops of toluene as a preservative

Procedure

- Collect sewage & add 50mL sewage sample to one litre of 8mg/L O_2 containing water sample.
- Rinse BOD bottle clearly with water.
- Neutralise the pH of the water using acid or alkali.
- Fill Two BOD bottle with water / sewage / effluent sample. Avoid air bubble. Use one BOD bottle for DO estimation.
- Add 2mL of manganese sulphate and 2mL of alkaline iodine azide solution to the bottle.
- Close the Bottle and observe for brown coloured precipitate and allowed to settle at half way.
- Add 2 to 3 drops of sulphuric acid.
- Titrate 50 mL of acidified sample against sodium thio sulphate solution. After the formation of pale yellow colour, add one or two drops of starch indicator to the sample.
- Titrate the sample again up to the disappearance of blue colour (Initial oxygen)
- Incubate remaining bottle at 20-27°C for 3-5 days.
- Estimate oxygen concentration after 5 days of incubation (Final oxygen).
- Dissolved oxygen of the given sample is calculated by the following formula :

$$O2mg/L \quad \frac{\text{Titrant value} \times 0.025 \times 8 \times 100}{\text{Volume of the Sample}}$$

0.025 - normality of the titrant

8 = Molecular weight of Oxygen

BOD of the effluent was calculated by the formula : **BOD = D1-D2**

Observation and result

Colour change is noted and calculated BOD of given sample

Viva questions

Expand BOD.

Define BOD.

How do you perform BOD?

How BOD indicates pollution?

What happened on BOD if microbial load is high in sewage?

How do you reduce nitrification in sewage?

What are the principles of dissolved oxygen measurement?

What is iodimetry?

Why BOD bottles are incubated at 20°C?

What is the purpose of adding starch indicator?

Spotters: BOD bottle, Starch indicator, Sodium thio sulphate

95. Determination of COD

Aim

To determine the chemical oxygen demand of the given polluted water sample by Reflux titration method.

Principle

In recent times, with the increase of pollution by discharging large amount of various chemically oxidisable organic substance of different nature entering the aquatic systems. BOD alone does not give clear picture of the organic matter content of the water sample. In addition the presence of various toxicants in the sample may affect the validity of the BOD test hence COD is the better estimate of the oranic matter, which needs no sophistication and time saving. However COD is the oxygen consumed does not differentiate the stable organic matter from the unstable form. There fore , the COD values are not directly comparable to that of BOD.

The amount of organic matter in water is estimated by their oxidation by chemical oxidants such as $KMnO_4$ or potassium di chromate. The carbon and hydrogen are oxidized and not nitrogen, in the permanganate method. Organic matter is first oxidized with a known volume of $KMnO_4$ and excess of oxygen is allowed to react with potassium iodide to liberate iodine, which is estimated titrimetrically with sodium thio sulphate solution using starch as an indicator

Background information

The chemical oxygen demand (COD) is used as a measure of the oxygen equivalent of the organic matter content of a sample that is susceptible to oxidation by a strong chemical oxidant. Most types of organic matter are oxidized by a boiling mixture of chromic and sulfuric acids. A sample is refluxed in strong acid solution with a known excess of potassium dichromate. After digestion, the remaining unreduced potassium dichromate is titrated with ferrous ammonium sulfate to determine the amount of potassium dichromate consumed and the oxidizable organic matter is calculated in terms of oxygen equivalent.

Materials required

Burette, pipette, conical flask

Reagents

Potassium dichromate solution (0.25N)

Dissolve 12.259 g of potassium dichromate, in distilled water and dilute to one litre

Dry powder of silver sulphate

Dry powder mercuric sulphate

Conc.H_2SO_4 (Sp. Gr. 1.84)

Ferroin indicator solution

Standard ferrous ammonium sulphate solution (0.25N)

Dissolve 98 g of ferrous ammonium sulphate in distilled water, add 20mL of sulphuric acid, cool and dilute to 1L by further adding distilled water. To standardize this solution, dilute 25mL of potassium dichromate solution to about 240 mL with distilled water, add 20mL of sulphuric acid, and cool it. Add 5-6 drops of ferroin indicator solution and titrate against ferrous ammonium sulphate solution. The colour changes from blue green to reddish blue at end point. The exact normality of FAS is calculated as,

$$\text{Normality of FAS} = \frac{\text{Volume of } k_2Cr_2O_7 \text{ (mL)} \times 0.25}{\text{Volume of FAS (mL)}}$$

Procedure

- Take 20 mL of sample in the flask of reflux unit and add 10mL of potassium dichromate solution, a pinch of each silver sulphate and mercuric sulphate and 30mL of sulphuric acid.

- Reflux the contents for 2 hrs.

- Cool the flask, detach from unit and dilute to about 150mL by adding distilled water.

- Add 2-3 drops of ferroin indicator solution and titrate against ferrous ammonium sulphate solution.

- At the end point blue green colour of contents changes to reddish blue.

- Run simultaneously distilled water blank in similar manner.

Calculation

$$\text{Chemical Oxygen Demand (mG/l)} = \frac{(B-T) \times N \times E \times 1000}{\text{Volume of sample (mL)}}$$
$$\text{(as } O_2\text{)}$$

where,

T= volume of titrant (FAS) used against sample (mL).
B= volume of titrant used against blank (mL)
N= normality of Ferrous Ammoniam Sulphate
E = equivalent weight of oxygen (8)

Result

The result is expressed in mG/l as O_2.

Viva questions

Define and expand COD

What are the importance of COD

What are the principles of COD

How do you perform COD

What are the relationship between COD and dissolved oxygen.

Spotters :Potassium dichromate

96. Microbial degradation of cellulose.

Aim

To test cellulose degrading ability of the test organisms.

Background information:

A prominent carbonaceous constituents of higher plant is cellulose. It is a polysaccharide composed of glucose unit in a long linear chain together by β-1,4 glycoside bond. Degradation of cellulose is brought about by fungi, bacteria and actinomycetes by the secretion of extra cellular enzyme composed of at least three components. They are endogluconase, exogluconase and β-glucosidase. The cooperative action of these enzyme is required for complete hydrolysis of cellulose to glucose. *Trichoderma, Cellulomonas, Clostridium, Cytophaga, Bacillus* and some strains of *Pseudomonas* and *Vibrio* have the capability to produce cellulase enzyme. Cellulase degradation is detected in different ways. In solid medium, it is detected by adding aqueous solution of hexa decyl trimethyl ammonium bromide. This reagent precipitates carboxy methylcellulose and produced a clear zone around the colony.

Materials required

Media : Czapek minimal salt agar medium.

Reagent : 1, 5 Hexa Decyl Trimethyl Ammonium Bromide

Culture : *Bacillus, Cellulomonas, Trichoderma viridae*

Others: Petriplates, inoculation loop, test tubes, conical flask, Pasteur pipettes

Procedure

• Prepare and sterilize Czapek mineral salt agar medium.

• Pour the medium into Petri plates.

- Labell the plates with respective microorganisms & Inoculate.
- Incubate inoculated plates at 35°C for 2-5 days
- Flood 1% of aqueous solution of hexa decyl trimethyl ammonium bromide on the plates.
- Observe the plates for zone of clearance.

Observation and Result

A clean zone around colony indicates cellulose degradation

Viva Questions

What is cellulose?

Mention about cellulose degrading enzymes?

Name the microorganisms involved in cellulose degradation.

What are the applications of cellulose degradation?

Name the media used for detecting cellulose degradation.

Mention raw material used for cellulose degradation.

What are the chemical reagent used to detect cellulose degradation?

Spotters: Carboxy methyl cellulose, Hexa decyl trimethyl ammonium bromide.

Food and Dairy Microbiology

CHAPTER 7

97. Bread preparation

Aim

To prepare bread using yeast.
To understand leavening activities of bread.

Background information

Food made from dough of flour or meal are usually raised with yeast or baking powder and then baked called bread. Breads are more amenable to variation in the formulation to meet a wide spectrum of consumer demands with respect to taste and nutritional requirements. Bread is often made from a wheat-flour dough that is cultured with yeast, allowed to rise, and finally baked in an oven. Leavening is the process of adding gas to a dough before or during baking to produce a lighter, more easily chewed bread. Many breads are leavened by yeast. The yeast used for leavening of bread is *Saccharomyces cerevisiae*. This yeast ferments carbohydrates in the flour, including any sugar, producing carbon dioxide.

Types of Bread

White bread is made from flour containing only the central core of the grain (endosperm).

Brown bread is made with endosperm and 10% bran.

Wholemeal bread contains the whole of the wheat grain (endosperm and bran).

Wheat germ bread has added wheat germ for flavouring.

Roti is a whole wheat based bread eaten in South Asia. Chapatti is a larger variant of Roti. Naan is a leavened equivalent of roti and chappati.

Granary bread is bread made from granary flour.

Rye bread is made with flour from rye grain of variable levels.

Importance of materials used in bread preparations

Flour: Wheat is the type of flour used in bread baking. Wheat flours are especially rich with complex **gluten forming proteins**. When mixed with moisture, usually water, form gluten strands, necessary for bread making.

Yeast: Yeast is the heart of the bread making process called **fermentation**. It's the essential ingredient that makes the dough rise and gives home-baked bread its wonderful taste and aroma.

Salt: It is an important ingredient in bread baking (NaCl).

Liquids: Water, Milk: Liquids are an important ingredient in bread baking, with tap water being the most commonly used, but can also include milk. It is important to have the liquid at the correct temperature. In bread recipes, water stimulates the growth of both the yeast and the development of gluten. It dissolves and activates the yeast; it activates the protein in the wheat flour and blends with it to create a sticky and elastic dough. Milk gives bread a more tender crust than water.

Sugar: Sugar adds flavour and rich brown colour to bread's crust. Table sugar is commonly used, but brown sugar, honey, molasses, jams and dried fresh fruits may also be used. Fruit juices also add significant amounts of sugar.

Eggs: Eggs add food value, colour and flavour to breads. They also help make the crumb fine and the crust tender. Eggs add richness and protein.

Fats: Butter, olive oil and margarine are some of the fat used to make a bread tender and moist; they help to prevent the formation of excess **gluten** and increase the keeping qualities of a bread loaf, preventing it from drying out too quickly.

Flavour: Orange, lemon or grape fruit peel as well as alcohol.

Raisins, Dried Fruit and Nuts: Many yeast bread recipes have added raisins, dried fruit and nuts

Bread improvers are frequently used in the production of commercial breads to reduce the time that the bread takes to rise, and to improve the texture and volume of bread. Chemical substances commonly used as bread improvers include ascorbic acid, hydrochloride, sodium metabisulfate, ammonium chloride, various phosphates, amylase, and protease

Materials required

Commercially available wheat flour (Maida), Sugar, Yeast, Dalda, Oven, Bread board, egg, salt, sodium benzoate, edible oil

Procedure

- Gather required items for bread making.

- Select 5L capacity pan or bowl and 45cmX60cm bread board for flour mixing.

- Grease bowl and board using edible oil.

- Pour 150 g flour on bread board and add 8g sugar, 4g salt, 8g dalda, 2 eggs and mix properly by pouring enough quantity of water (125- 130mL).

- Dissolve 4g dry yeast in approximately 25mL of water, poured and mixed with wheat flour.

- On lightly floured bread board, knead dough until smooth and elastic. About 8 to 10 minutes.

- Cover dough with moistened cloth and let rest for 10 minutes (The prepared dough is set a side for 2 hrs while fermentation proceeded. The dough was covered with moistened cloth to prevent moisture loss).

- After 2 hrs "Knocked back" the dough. i.e. manipulated to push out the gas that had been involved in order to even out the temperature and give more thorough mixing. (After "Knock back" the dough were again rested for about 1 hr).

- Then the dough divided into loaf size portion (i.e.100-200g) and these are roughly shaped.

- Rest the dough pieces at about 27°C for 10-15 minutes (1st proof) and molded into final.

- Again rest the dough in the baking pan for the final proofs of 60 minutes at 18°C and then baked in the oven at a temperature of 110°C for 40 min.

- The loaves were allowed to cool for a minimum of 2 hrs at 24°C before cutting.

Observation

Edible bread may come out of oven.

Spotters

Bread, *Saccharomyces cerevisiae,* sodium benzoate, bakers yeast.

Viva questions

How do you prepare yeast?

What is leavening?

Define bread, glutan forming protein, fermentation.

98. Enumeration of microorganisms from bread

Aim

To analyze the quality of the given bread or bakery product.

To know the nature of microbes in bread.

Background Information

Foods are highly susceptible to microbial contamination and decomposition because they are rich in nutrients that support the growth of microbes. Contaminated foods are often inedible and may also be the source of human diseases if the contaminating organisms are pathogen or toxin producer. Some of the important food poisoning caused by bacteria are Botulism; Staphylococcal food poisoning and enteric poisoning which are serious and sometimes fatal. The sanitary control of food quality is concerned with examination of foods for the presence of pathogens. The examination of food is performed for the presence of total number of bacteria in the food is by standard plate count because presence of large number of bacteria in it increases the changes of food quality. Presence of coliforms indicates faecal contamination and may suggest the presence of pathogens. Direct lactophenol cotton blue mounting expresses the fungal contamination.

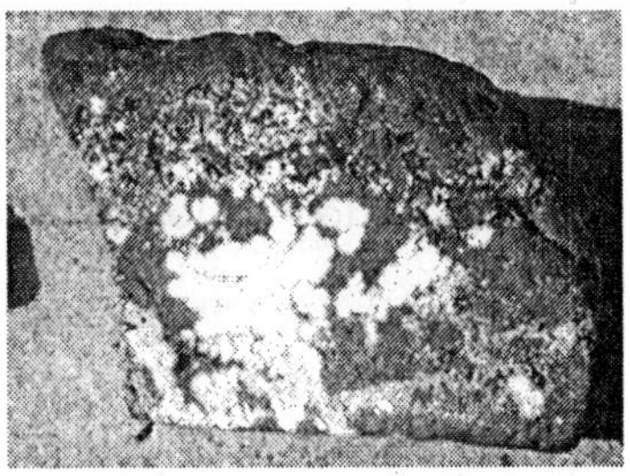

Normal value

Bacteria – Upto 10^3 CFU/g

Fungi -   Upto 10^2 CFU/g

Coliforms- Nil

Materials Required

Fig 98.1 : Spoiled Bread

Sample : Bread or any bakery products.

Petriplates, Pipettes, Test tubes containing sterile water blanks, Conical flasks, Bunsen burner, Pestle and Morter, Slide, Quebec colony counter etc.

Media: Nutrient agar medium, EMB agar, Rose bengol chloromphenicol Agar.

Reagent: Lactophenol cotton blue stain

Procedure

Lactophenol cotton blue staining

- Place one drop of lactophenol cotton blue stain in a clean microscopic slide.
- With the help of sterile forceps take small piece of sample and place on a drop of lactophenol cotton blue stain.
- Place the cover slip on the surface of sample and press gently.
- Examine the slide under 40 x microscopic field.

Standard plate count

- Prepare 10g of bread as semisolid paste using a pestle and morter.
- Add semisolid bread to 90mL of water and make up the volume up to 100mL (Stock)
- Serially dilute 1ml of the stock upto 1:10000 (10^{-4}).
- Pour 1mL of 1:100, 1:1000 and 1:10000 dilution sample into sterile nutrient agar plates as pour plate method.
- Inoculate 0.1 mL sample from 1:10 and 1:100dilution into sterile Rose Bengal Chloramphenicol Agar by spread plate method.
- Inoculate 0.1mL of stock sample into EMB agar plate by spread plate method.
- Incubate, Nutrient agar & EMB agar plates at 37^0c & Rose bengal Chloramphenicol agar plates at 25, 30^0C for 24-48 hours.
- Observe plates for the qualitative measurement of bread quality.

Observation

Bacterial growth is noted on nutrient agar plates. Less fungal growth is noted in fungal plate but there is no growth in EMB agar.

Results

Bacterial, fungal and coliforms growth is within the limits of standard. Hence the bread is fit for human consumption.

Viva questions

What are the possible pathogens in bread?

What type of fungus are predominant in normal bread?

Why fungus is more common in bread than bacteria?

How do you detect fungal element in bread using microscopic method?

Spotters: Lactophenol cotton blue, Nutrient agar, Rose Bengal chloramphenicol agar

99. Microbial examination of curd

Aim

To understand microbial flora of curd.

To isolate *Lactobacillus sp.* from curd.

Background information

Lactobacillus is one of the most important organisms responsible for curd production. Curd is a dairy product obtained by *curdling* (coagulating) milk with rennet or an edible acidic substance such as lemon juice or vinegar and microorganisms. The increased acidity causes the milk proteins (casein) to tangle into solid masses or curds. Spoiled curd may contain different types of faecal bacteria.

Materials required

De Man, Rogosa, and Sharpe medium (MRS) for Lactobacilli, Baired parker agar for micrococcus and Staphylococci, Rosebengal Chloramphenicol agar for Yeast and fungal isolation, Nutrient agar for common hetrotrophic mesophilic bacteria isolation, XLD agar to detect enteric pathogens, Curd sample, Petriplates, pipettes, inoculation loop, L- Rod etc.,

Procedure

- Collect curd samples and transported to the laboratory.

- Prepare & sterilize MRS medium, Baired parker agar, Rosebengal Chloramphenicol agar, Nutrient agar & XLD agar and poured into sterile petriplates.

- Inoculate approximately 0.1g of curd and spread using sterile L-Rod under aseptic condition.

- Incubate Nutrient agar, Baired parker agar and XLD agar plates at 37°C for 24 hours and MRS medium, Rosebengal Chloramphenicol agar at 25°C for 48 hours.

Observation

Observe colony morphology and count number of colonies on each plate. Isolated colonies are subjected to identification.

Result

Lactobacilli are isolated from normal curd.

Spotters

Microscopic view of Lactobacilli, curd, MRS medium.

Viva questions

What is curdling?

Define coagulation?

What are the roles of Lactobacilli in curd formation?

100. Yogurt Production

Aim

To prepare yogurt from milk using Lactobacillus and Streptococcus

Background informations

Yogurt is produced by the fermentation of warm milk by *Lactobacillus bulgaricus* and *Streptococcus thermophilus*. These two bacteria are able to grow at 40-45°C, during which they produce lactic acid and various other byproducts that give its unique flavour.

Materials required

Cow milk, concentrated skim milk, nonfat dry milk, whey, lactose.

Sweeteners: glucose or sucrose, high-intensity sweeteners (e.g. aspartame)

Stabilizers: gelatin, carboxymethyl cellulose, locust bean Guar, alginates, carrageenans, whey protein concentrate. **Starter Culture** :*Streptococcus salivarius* subsp. *thermophilus* (ST) and *Lactobacillus delbrueckii* subsp. *bulgaricus* (LB).

Procedure

- Take 500mL sterile beaker.
- Add 100mL of whole milk and heat to boily.

- While stirring constantly, add 4gms of powdered milk and Mix properly using sterile glass rod.
- Add required quantity of sweetners, stabilizer and flvouring agents.
- Cool to 45°C and inoculate with 1 teaspoon of the commercial yogurt or 10mL culture.
- Cover with plastic wrap.
- Incubate at 45°C for 24 hours.

Examination and observation

Examine the product and record the colour, aroma, texture, and if desired the taste. Make slide preparations of the yogurt. Fix and stain with methylene blue. Examine under oil immersion and record results.

Spotters

Yogurt.

Viva questions

Name the organisms responsible for yogurt production

How do you differentiate yogurt from curd.

101. Production of Sauerkraut

Aim

To make Sauerkraut.

To understand the effects of fermentation on food.

Background information

Sauerkraut is very healthy food. It is also considered as a good source of medicine, diet and it prevents cancer. **Sauerkraut** controls the human digestion. It contains vitamins , minerals (iron, calcium), trace elements, roughage, lactic acid. The first micro-organisms to start acting are the gas-producing cocci (*Leuconostoc mesenteroides*). These microbes produce acids. When the acidity reaches 0.25 to 0.3% (calculated as lactic acid), these bacteria slow down and begin to die off, although their enzymes continue to function. The activity initiated by the *L. mesenteroides* is continued by the *Lactobacilli* (*L. plantarum and L. cucumeris*) until an acidity level of 1.5 to 2% is attained. The high salt concentration and low temperature inhibit these bacteria to some extent. Finally, *L. pentoaceticus* continues the fermentation, bringing the acidity to 2 to 2.5% thus completing the fermentation. The end products of a normal kraut fermentation are lactic acid along with smaller amounts of acetic and propionic acids, a mixture of gases of which carbon dioxide is the principal gas, small amounts of alcohol and a mixture of aromatic esters. The acids, in combination with alcohol form esters, which contribute to the characteristic flavour of sauerkraut. The acidity helps to control the growth of spoilage and putrefactive organisms and contributes to the extended shelf life of the product.

Materials required

Cabbage, cabbage cutter, salt, required taste spices, silo, *Leuconostoc mesenteroides, Lactobacillus plantarum, L. cucumeris, Air tight container, pasteurization vessel etc.,*

Procedure (Procedure described in this experiment is an industrial process. Same procedure also applied for small scale and laboratory scale production)

- Select Good quality cabbage.

- Cut cabbage into small slices.
- Add required quantity of salt (1.5Kg salt / 50Kg Cabbage) and spices to the cabbage.
- Fill cabbages in Silo (A **silo** is a structure for storing bulk materials).
- Inoculate 10% fermentation organism like *Leuconostoc mesenteroides, Lactobacillus plantarum* and *L. cucumeris, Lactobacillus pentoaceticus.*
- Apply mechanical pressure to the cabbage to expel the juice, which contains fermentable sugars and other nutrients suitable for microbial activity.
- Incubate the entire preparations at 20 – 25°C and allowed for fermentation (The optimum temperature for sauerkraut fermentation is around 21°C).
- At the end of the fermentation, lift out the sauerkraut from the silo by means of a mechanical action.
- Pack sauerkraut into pouches of 500g or 750g. Check each pouch individually with regard to its weight.
- Pasteurise sauerkraut by means of continuous pasteurisation.
- After the pasteurisation, check the pouches individually for tightness of pack.

Observation

Prepared Sauerkraut is subjected to microbial examinations.

Spotters

Sauerkraut, Leuconostoc, Lactobacilli.

Viva questions

What is Sauerkraut?

What are the principles behind Sauerkraut production?

Is microbes are responsible for flavour of Sauerkraut

102. Isolation and identification of microbes from fruits and vegetables

Aim

To check the quality of fruits and vegetables.

To identify the isolated microbes.

To know kinds of microorganisms present in fruits and vegetables.

Background Information

Microorganisms present on the surface of freshly harvested fruits and vegetables include not only those of the normal surface flora but also those from soil, water and perhaps plant pathogens. Vegetables and fruits may be dried, frozen, fermented, pasteurized and canned. Generally fruits and vegetables have low number of microbes. During transportation and processing mechanical damage may increase contamination. Precooling of the product and refrigeration during transport may reduce the growth of contaminated microorganisms. Possible sources of contamination are trays, tanks, tables, aprons and filters.

Possible Isolates

Vegetables- **Bacteria:** *Pseudomonas sp., Alkaligens sp., Erwinia sp., Xanthomonas Sp., Micrococci., Coryneforms., Bacillus sp.,* and Other enterobacteriaceae members.

Fruits-

Fungi: *Fusarium; Alternaria; Aureobasidium; Penicillium; Rhizopus*

Bacteria : *Pseudomonas sp., Alkaligens sp., Erwinia sp., Xanthomonas sp., Micrococci sp., Bacillus sp.,*

Fungi : *Fusarium; Alternaria; Aureobacidium; Penicillium., Rhizobus ., Cladosporium; Trichoderma; etc.,*

Normal range of mould in fruits and vegetables

1000-10000 cells /g

Table – 103.1 Range of bacteria in fruits and vegetables

S.No	Classification	A	B	C	D
1	Total viable count	<500000	<5000000	<10000000	>10000000
2	Coliform count	<2500	<5000	<100000	>100000
3	*E.coli*	Absent	Absent	Absent	Absent
4	*S. aureus*	<100	<150	<1000	>1000
5	Salmonella	Absent	Absent	Absent	Absent
6	Yeast	<5000	<10000	<100000	>100000
7	Mould	<5000	<10000	<100000	>100000
8	Vibrio	Absent	Absent	Absent	Absent

A.Excellent   <less than

B. Good   >greater than

C.Satisfactory

D.Poor

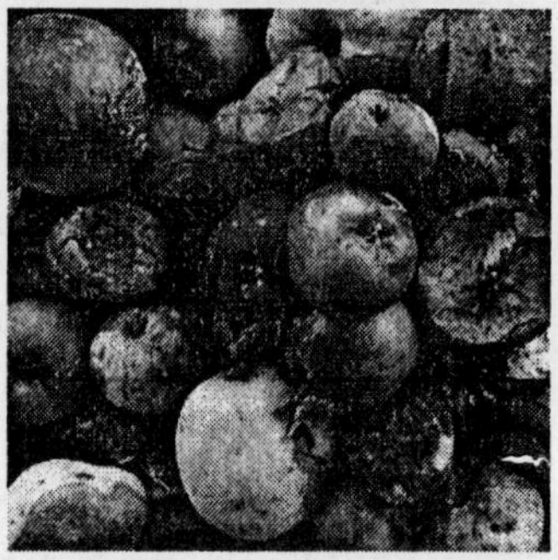

Materials Required

Sample : Vegetable, fruits or its by products.

Media : Nutrient agar, Gram Negative Broth, SS agar, Baired parker agar, EMB agar, EC broth, Azide dextrose broth, Violet Red Bile Agar, KF streptococcus agar, TCBS agar, Alkaline peptone water.

Others : Water / Saline blank, Test tubes, Petriplates, Conical flasks, etc.,

Fig 102.1 : Spoiled fruits and Vegetables

Procedure

1. Preparation of sample

- weigh 10g of sample and blend with 90mL of sterile saline in a sterilized jar.

2. Total viable count of bacteria

- Dilute the sample up to 1:100000 (10^{-5})
- Add 1mL of diluent from 1:1000, 1:10000 and 1:100000 dilutions to sterile petriplates.
- Pour 20 mL of sterile nutrient agar or plate count agar.
- Gently rotate the plates in clockwise and anti clockwise direction and allow solidify.

- Incubate all plates at 35 ° C for 18 -24 hours.
- Examine the plates for its number and nature of colonies.

3.Coliform isolation

- Add 1mL of sample from 1:100 and 1:1000 dilutions to Violet Red Bile Agar plates & perform pour plate method.
- Observe the plates after 24 hours of incubation at 37 ° C for its red coloured colonies.

4. Faecal coliform isolation

- Inoculate 1 mL of sample from 1:10 dilution to EC and Azide Dextrose Broth tubes and incubates at 44 ° C for 24 hours.
- Inoculate a loop full of culture from EC broth and Azide Dextrose Broth into EMB and KF streptococcus agar respectively and incubated at 37 ° C for 24 hours
- Observe plates for its specific colony morphology.

5. Isolation of *Staphylococcus aureus*

- Spread 0.1 mL of sample on the surface of Baired Parker agar and incubate at 37 °C for 24 hours. Observe plates for black coloured colonies.

6. Isolation of Salmonella

- Transfer 1 mL of blended sample to 10mL of gram negative broth and incubate at 37 ° C for 4-6 hours
- Streak a loop full of culture from gram negative broth on SS agar and incubated at 37 ° C for 24 hours

7. Isolation of Vibrio

- Inoculate 1 mL of blended sample in to 10mL of alkaline peptone water and incubate at 37 ° C for 18 hours
- Streak a loop full of culture from Alkaline peptone water on TCBS agar and incubate at 37 ° C for 24 hours

8. Isolation of yeast and moulds

- Inoculate 1 mL of sample from 1:100 dilution into the Rose Bengal chloramphenicol agar as pour plate method and incubated at 28-30 ° C for 48 hours. Examine plates for the growth of eucaryotic microorganisms.

Table 102.1 – Observabel Results

S. No	Sample	Test	Result	Interpretation
1	Fruits	Total viable count		
2		Coliform count		
3		*E.coli*		
4		Stap. aureus		
5		Salmonella		
6		Yeast		
7		Mould		
8		Vibrio		

1	Vegetables	Total viable count		
2		Coliform count		
3		E.coli		
4		Stap. aureus		
5		Salmonella		
6		Yeast		
7		Mould		
8		Vibrio		

Results

Given vegetable / fruit is found to be poor/ good

Viva questions

What are the possible pathogens of fruits and vegetables?

Why enterobacteriaceae members are common in fruits and vegetables?

How do you reduce microbial burden in fruits and vegetables?

What are the source of microbes in fruits and vegetables?

How do you isolate Staphylococcus from fruits?

Spotters : Spoiled fruits, spoiled vegetables, microscopic mould morphology.

103. Isolation of Salmonella from Poultry products

Aim

To isolate *Salmonella sp.* from chicken meat and egg.

Background information

Chicken meat and egg are the important poultry products. Eggs are routinely used by most of the world population. Sometimes egg may be contaminated with *Salmonella typhimurium*, which is a normal flora of hen's intestine. As the eggs are laid along with faecal matter, egg shell is enriched with Salmonella. *Pseudomonas, Alkaligens, Proteus, Serratia* are some of the organisms responsible for egg and meat spoilage. Salmonella is a gram negative bacteria responsible for human enteric fever (Typhoid).

Materials required

10g chicken meat, one egg, homogenizer / Mixie, Gram negative broth, XLD agar, Bismuth sulphite agar, Raj Hans medium, Saline, Autoclave, Hot air Oven, Laminar air flow etc.

Procedure

● Collect 10 g chicken meat and egg from the market and transported to the laboratory.

● Place chicken meat in a homogenizer / mixie and add 10mL of sterile saline to a homogenizer and minse properly.

● Collect egg contents in a sterile beaker and mix properly.

● Inoculate one mL of meat and 1mL of egg contents individually to Gram negative (GN) broth (. to enrich Salmonella) and incubate at 37°C for 3-4 hours.

- Inoculate contents from GN broth to XLD agar and incubate at 37°C for 24 hours.
- Observe any dark centered and pink edge colonies on XLD agar.
- Inoculate dark centered and pink edged colonies from XLD agar to Raj hans Medium and Bismuth sulphite agar.
- Observe for Pink and black colonies respectively on Raj hans Medium and Bismuth sulphite agar.
- Confirm the isolates for Salmonella by performing biochemical and carbohydrate fermentation test.

Results

Salmonella sp. Identified / not identified.

Spotters

Egg, growth of Salmonella on any one of the selective medium.

Viva questions

List out the importance of poultry products
Why egg is easily contaminated wit salmonella?

104. Isolation of microorganisms from grains

Aim

To enumerate the microorganisms from the given food grain.

Background Information

Grains include maize, millet, sorghum, barley, wheat, rice etc. Finished cereal product include flour, cornflakes, bread etc. The microflora of raw cereal grains are found in air, soil and on animals. The number and type of microbes found on any given food grain depend on several factors such as the climate, soil, biological environment, methods and equipment's of harvesting, transport and storage. The survival of microorganisms in food grain depends on moisture and temperature. The higher moisture favours the growth of moulds. The normal bacterial content of flour may range from 20,000 to 50,000 per gram. *Flavobacterium, Aerobacter, Staphylococci* etc. are usually found in food grains.

Materials Required

25 g sample, buffered peptone water, Plate count agar, Rose bengal chloramphenicol agar, Petriplates, Pipettes, Test tubes etc. and other selective medium if needed

Procedure

- Weigh 25 g of sample aseptically into a sterile blender and add 225 mL of buffered peptone water.
- Serially dilute the sample up to 1:1000000 (10^{-6}).
- Plate 1:10000, 1:100000 and 1:1000000 dilution on plate count agar by pour plate method
- Plate 1:10, 1:100 and 1:1000 dilution on Rose bengal chloramphenicol agar by spread plate method.
- Incubate plate count agar plates at 37 ° C for 24 hours
- Incubate Rose bengal chloramphenicol agar plates at 30°C for 42 hours.
- After incubation observe plates and interpretate the results.

Observation and Result

Growth is noted and the results are reported as normal / good/ poor

Viva questions

Mention few important examples of grain products.

Name factors that influence microbial survival in grains.

Name the media used for the isolation of bacteria from grain.

What are the sources of microbial contamination in grains?

Spotters: Plate count agar, Rose bengal Chloramphenicol agar

105. Determination of Thermal Death Point (TDP) and Thermal Death Time (TDT)

Aim

To find out the TDP and TDT of the given bacteria.

Background information

Temperature is one of the important physical factor affecting the microorganisms. Because of the absence of homeostatic mechanism, the bacterial enzyme systems are directly affected by environmental factors. Enzymatic reactions proceeded at maximum speed and efficiently at optimum temperature, which vary with microbial species. Beyond the maximum and minimum temperatures, the enzymes become inactive. High heat generally denatures proteins. Heat resistance varies among different microbes; these differences can be expressed through the concept of Thermal Death Point (TDP). TDP is the lowest temperature required to kill all of the microorganisms in a liquid suspension within 10 minutes.

Another factor to be considered in sterilization is the length of time required for the material to be rendered sterile. This is expressed as Thermal Death Time (TDT), the minimal length of time in which all bacteria in a liquid culture will be killed at a given temperature.

Materials Required

Nutrient broth, Nutrient agar, Petriplates, Pipettes, Water bath, *Escherichia coli, Salmonella, Shigella etc.*

Procedure

Thermal death point

- Prepare 18 tubes of nutrient broth and sterilize at 121°C for 15 minutes.
- Inoculate *E.coli, Salmonella* and *Shigella sp* in 6 tubes each.
- Incubate all tubes at 37 °C for 24 hours.
- Setup a water bath at 40 °C initially, then 50°C, 60°C, 70°C, 80°C and 90°C constantly for 10 minutes.
- Place a 1st set of bacterial suspension in a water bath at 40° C for 10 minutes.
- After 10 minutes remove the culture from the water bath and inoculate on a nutrient agar plates as a single line streak.
- Discard the 40° C broth tube.
- Place a 2nd set of bacterial suspension in a water bath for 10 minutes at 50° C.
- After 10 minutes remove the culture from the water bath and inoculate on a nutrient agar plates as a single line streak inoculation. Discard the tubes.
- Continue to raise the temperature of water bath.

- Expose the culture for 10 minutes
- Inoculate treated culture on nutrient agar plates
- Similarly treat cultures at 60°C, 70°C, 80°C and 90°C and incubate plates at 37°C for 24 hours.
- Observe the plates for bacterial growth and interpretate the results.

Observation

Table 105.1

S.No.	Culture	Temperature (°C)					
		40	50	60	70	80	90
1	Escherichia coli						
2	Salmonella sp.						
3	Shigella sp.						

Thermal death time

Procedure

- Perform the test as mentioned in TDP section

For TDT calculation

- Consider two constant temperature i.e., 40° & 50°C
- Maintain water bath at 40°C
- Place one tube culture in to the water bath at different time intervals. (2,4,6,8,10,12,14,16,18 and 20 minutes).
- Take a loop full of culture from these culture tubes at different time intervals and inoculate in to specific nutrient agar plates as single line streke.
- In the same way, perform test with 50° C.
- Incubate the plates at 37 °C for 24 hours.
- Observe plates and interpretate the results.

Note

For TDP- Use 6 tubes for each temperature and culture

For TDT- Use 1 tube for each temperature and culture

For TDP- Require 1 plate for each temperature and culture.

For TDT- Use more than one plates for each temperature and culture.

Table 105.2 Observation

S.No	Culture	Temperature in ° C	Time interval in minutes									
			2	4	6	8	10	12	14	16	18	20
1	E. coli	40										
		50										
2	Salmonella sp.	40										
		50										
3	Shigella sp.	40										
		50										

Results

Thermal death Point : Growth of bacteria is checked on different temperature treated cultures. Some bacteria tolerates higher temperature and are called thermophiles.

Thermal death time : Continueous exposure of bacteria beyond optimum temperature also reduce the growth activities. This experimental result may useful to setup temperature control point for food borne bacteria.

Viva questions

Define TDT and TDP.

What are the responsibilities of temperature on microbial growth?

What are the needs of performing TDT and TDP?

How do you perform TDP and TDT?

106. Analysis of aflatoxin by Thin Layer Chromatography

Aim

To analyze the availability of aflatoxin in grains

Background Information

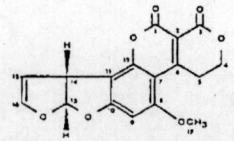

(a) Aflatoxin B₁ (b) Aflatoxin B₂

A wide spectrum of fungi infects most of the agricultural products including food grains and feed stuffs under warm humid condition, especially when the moisture content of the foodstuff is high. Some of the fungi available in the environment get contaminated with food material and make them unfit for human/ animal consumption. During growth fungi produce certain secondary metabolites called mycotoxin. The syndrome resulting from the ingestion of toxin in a mold-contaminated food is referred to as mycotoxicosis.

(c) Aflatoxin G₁ (d) Aflatoxin G₂

Mycotoxin produced by *Aspergillus flavus* is called aflatoxin. Four major aflatoxins have been designated B1, G1 and B2, G2 because they fluoresce blue (B1) and green (G1), when exposed to UV light. It was discovered in the early 1960s. These toxins retain its toxic and carcinogenic ability in many animals. M1 aflatoxin has also been detected in the urine of Philippine women who had consumed peanut butter containing aflatoxin.

Materials required

Glass plate 20x20 cm or 20x10cm, Glass tank with lid, Spreader, Developing solvents, Silica gel G, UV chamber, Mechanical shaker, Toluene, Ethyl acetate, Formic acid, Chloroform. Separation funnel.

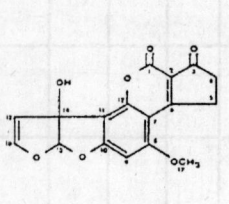

(e) Aflatoxin M₁

Fig. 106.1 Chemical structures of the Aflatoxin group of mycotoxins

Procedure

Extraction of toxin:

- Weigh exactly 50g of ground sample material and transfer it into a 250mL conical flask

- Moist the material uniformly by adding 10-15mL of distilled water and add about 200mL chloroform, stopper mouth with a cotton plug aluminium foil.

- Shake the flask for one hour mechanically.

- Filter the slurry through a Separation funnel under mild suction.

- Transfer the filtrate and shake with water one half volume of chloroform. After the phases separate, drain the bottom phase into a flask containing about 10g sodium sulphate to absorb any water.

- Concentrate the clear, chloroform extract under vacuum over a warm water bath.

Preparation of plate:

- Add 30g silica gel G in stoppered flask containing 60mL distilled water (1:2).

- Make slurry by stirring for 1-2 minutes and pour into the applicator positioned on the head glass plate.

- Coat the slurry over the glass plates at a thickness of 0.25mL for chemical analysis by moving the applicator at a uniform speed from one end to the other. Leave the plates to dry at room temperature for 15-30minutes.

- Heat the plates in an oven at 100-120 ° C for 1-2 hours to remove the moisture and to activate the adsorbent on the plate.

- Leave 2.5cm from one end of the glass plate and atleast an equal distance from the edges.

- Spot different known volumes (5,10μL etc) of the sample extract in various lanes carefully with a micropipette. Similarly spot standard aflatoxin mixture in the concentration range 0.0025 to 0.0125μG in parallel lines.

- Develop the plate in a solvent system of toluene: Ethylacetate: formic acid (6:3:1) in a chromotographic tank for about 50 minutes.

- Dry the plate at room temperature to remove the solvent.

- Visualize the fluorescing spots of toxin under UV light in a cabinet.

- Identify each spot by comparing with the standard toxin spot.

- Determine Rf value of each spot.

$$Rf: \frac{\text{Distance moved by the solute from the origin}}{\text{Distance moved by the solvent from the origin}}$$

Observation

Fluorescent spot is noted on TLC plate, when it is exposed to UV.

Result

Aflatoxin is detected from the rice sample.

Viva questions

Define mycotoxin and mycotoxicosis.

What is Aflatoxin?

What are the sources of Aflatoxin?

What are the principles of aflatoxin detection?

What are the types of aflatoxin?

Name the fungi which secretes aflatoxin.

What are the nature of aflatoxin?

Mention about mobile and stationary phase used to detect aflatoxin.

How do you detect aflatoxin in TLC plate.

Spotters: Aflatoxin structure

107. Qualitative analysis of milk

Aim

To determine the number of bacteria present in the given milk sample by using direct microscopic method and standard plate count method.

Background Information

Milk because of its high nutritive value is one of the most important food products. Not only milk gives nutrient to human beings but also forms an excellent medium for microbes. Unless the animal is diseased the udder milk is virtually sterile. Hence the contamination is usually exogenous. Milk from animals with mastitis characerically has large number of WBC and bacteria

Possible Pathogens from Milk

Alkaligens viscolyticus, Mycobacterium tuberculosis, Mycobacterium bovis, Brucella sp., Toxoplasma sp., Rickettsia., Leptospira., Staphylococcus aureus.

Normal Value of Milk bacteria

Aseptically drawn milk	-500-1000 CFU/mL
Bulk milk tank	-5000-20000CFU/mL
Milk pail or milking machine	-1000-10000CFU/mL

107a. Direct Microscopic examination of milk

Aim

To count microbial population of milk.

Principle

In this experiment a measured volume of milk is spreaded over an area of a slide, fixed, stained and examined microscopically. Since the area of a single microscopic field and volume of milk examined are known, the number of microscopic field can be determined and total number of bacteria / mL is computed.

Materials Required

Milk sample, microscope, methylene blue stain, clean microscopic slide.

Procedure

- Mark 1 cm^2 area on a clean glass slide.
- Spread 0.01mL of milk uniformly over this area.
- Air dry the smear.
- Immerse smear in xylene solution to remove fat materials for 1 minute.
- Wash with ethyl alcohol to remove xylene.
- Stain with methylene blue for 1-2 minutes.
- Examine the slide under oil immersion microscope.
- Count the number of microorganisms / field.

Calculations

Diameter of one oil immersion field	=0.6mm
Area of microscopic field	=πr^2
π	=3.14
r^2	=0.3mm^2
	=3.14 x 0.09 = 2.83
1cm^2	=10mm^2

That is 100/2.83 = 35 fields / 1 cm^2

$\qquad\qquad\qquad\qquad\qquad\qquad$ =35 fields/cm^2

1/100mL was spreader over 1cm^2

Each microscopic field has1/100 x area 1 = 1/3,500

Total number of cells in one mL of milk

$\qquad\qquad$ =Number of cells in one field x 3500

$\qquad\qquad$ =Answer

Result

Methylene blue stained bacterial cells are counted and enumerated. Compare the cells present in one mL of milk with normal microbial flora of milk and interpretate as good quality / poor quality.

107b. Standard Plate Count

Aim

To enumerate microbial population of milk.

Materials Required

Milk sample, plate count agar, petriplates , pipettes etc.

Procedure

- Dilute one mL of milk sample up to 1:100000 using sterile saline under aseptic condition

- Plate one mL diluted sample from 1:100,1:1000 and 1:10000 on plate count agar by using pour plate method.
- Duplicate should be maintained during the performance of this technique.
- Incubate all plates at specific environment for 24 hours
- Observe the plates and interpretate the results.

Observation and Result

Table 107.1

S . No	Technique & medium	Dilution	No of colonies		
			Original	Duplicate	Average
1	Plate count agar	1 : 100			
2	Pour plate	1 : 1000			
3		1 : 10000			

Result

Result of milk quality is interpreted after comparing normal value. Result will be given as good or poor quality.

Viva questions

Mention few important pathogens frequently found in milk.

Give the importance of milk.

Why milk is considered as natural food for microorganisms?

What is the normal microbial flora of milk?

What are the principles behind microbial analysis of milk?

How the bacteria present in milk is enumerated?

What type of media are used for the isolation of bacteria from milk?

Spotters: Plate count agar, methylene blue

108. Quantitative examination of milk

108a. Methylene Blue Reductase Test (MBRT)

Aim

To determine the quality of the given milk sample by Methylene blue reductase test.

Principle

Large number of bacteria present in milk indicates poor methods of production or handling. From the time the milk leaves the udder, until it is dispensed into containers, everything which comes in contact with potential source of contamination. The bacterial content can be reduced by strict sanitary practice. Bacteria present in the milk utilize the oxygen present in the sample thus lowering oxidation-reduction potential due to the exhaustion of dissolved oxygen when methylene blue is mixed with contaminated milk; it loses its colour. The colour disappearance of methylene blue is directly proportional to the number of bacteria present in the milk sample.

Materials Required

Methylene blue(1:2500), Milk sample, Screw cap tubes, Pipettes, etc.,

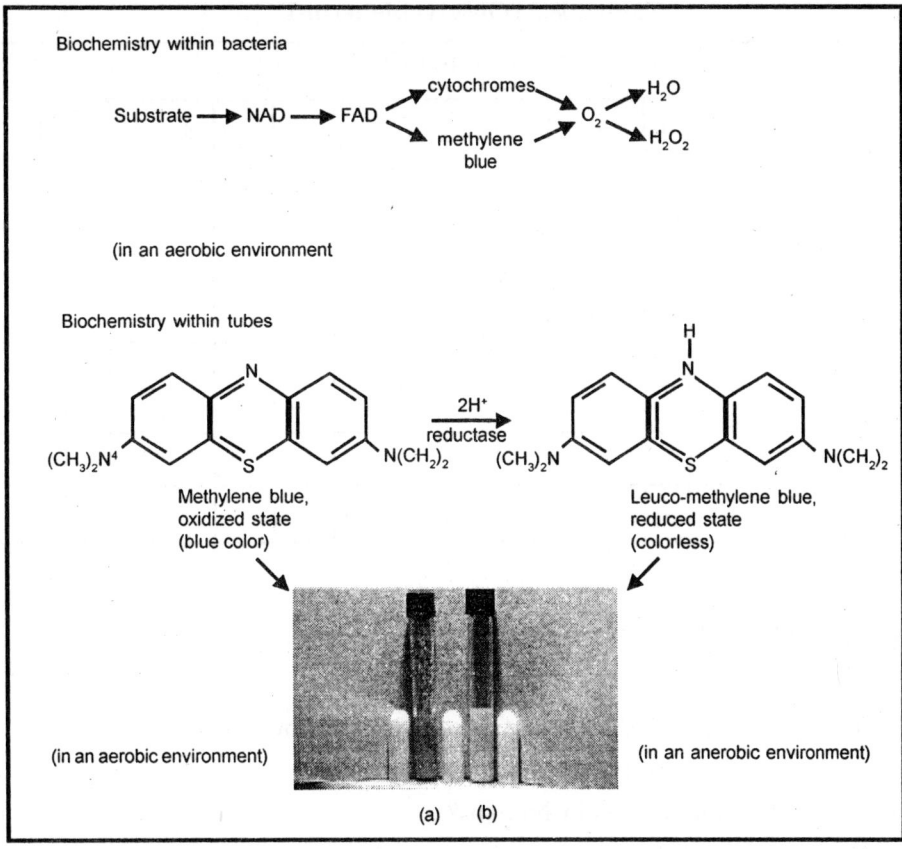

Fig 108.1 – Chemistry and reactions of methylene blue in milk

Procedure

- Collect raw milk sample in a sterile conical flask.
- Transfer 10mL milk sample to sterile screw cap tube.
- Add 1mL of methylene blue solution to all screw capped tubes.
- Close the tubes with rubber stoppers and gently inverted thrice to mix all contents.
- Control tubes with and without dye also maintained.
- Incubate all tubes in water bath at 35 ° C for up to eight hours.
- Observe colour change every half an hour. Quality of milk sample is assessed on the basis of standard given in table 109.1.

Table 108.1: Quality standard of milk by methylene blue reductase test

Class	Interpretation
I	Excellent-not discolourised upto 8hours
II	Good -discolourise after 6 hours but with in 8 hours.
III	Fair- discolourise after 2 hours but with in 6 hours
IV	Poor - discolourise with in 2 hours

Table 108.2 : Observable record

S. No	Sample	Time of discolouration in minutes																Milk quality
		30	60	90	120	150	180	210	240	270	300	330	360	390	420	450	480	
1	A																	
2	B																	
3	C																	
4	D																	
6	Control-1																	
7	Control -2																	

Result

The given milk is found to be excellent/ good / fair/ poor

Viva questions

What is the function of the methylene blue in the reductase test for milk quality?

Why does milk sour when it is not refrigerated?

How can a milk sample be contaminated by humans?

Why is milk pasteurized and not sterilized?

What are the differences in methylene blue reduction time between the different classes of milk? What do these differences signify?

What are some bacteria normally found in milk?

Spotters : Methylene blue

108b. Resazurin Test

Aim

To assess the quality of the given milk sample.

Background Information

Milk contains relatively few bacteria when it leaves the udder of the healthy cow. Milk is an excellent culture medium for many kinds of microorganisms, being high in moisture, nearly neutral in pH and rich in microbial food. This test is to measure the ability of the microorganisms to reduce the resazurin in to other component.

Resazurin purple — — — —>lavender — — —>hydro resazurin

If the bacterial load is high the reduction time is low.

Materials Required

Milk sample, Resazurin dye(1:20,000), Screw capped tubes, Pipettes, Water bath etc

Procedure

- Collect raw milk sample in a sterile conical flask.
- Transfer 10mL milk sample to sterile screw cap tube.
- Add 1mL of Resazurin solution to all screw capped tubes.
- Close the tubes with rubber stoppers and gently inverted thrice to mix all contents.
- Control tubes with and without dye also maintained
- Incubate all tubes in water bath at 35 ° C for up to 60 minutes.
- Observe colour change after one hour of incubation and record the results. Quality of milk sample was assessed on the basis of standard given in table 108.3.

Table 108.3 - Standard milk quality based on resazurin test

S . No	Grade	Colour	Quality
1	I	Purple	Excellent
2	II	Lavender	Good
3	III	Pink	Fair
4	IV	White	Poor

Observation and result

Colour change is observed within an hour and compare the standard, interpretate the results.

Viva questions

What are the principles of rezasurin test

How do you perform this test

Differentiate rezasurin test and MBRT test

What are the significance of this test

Spotters : Rezasurin

109. Potability test of water

109a. Most Probable Number Test (MPN)

Aim

To check the quality of water using MPN technique.

To assess microbial burden of the given water sample.

Background Information

Coliforms or total coliforms refers to the gram negative oxidase negative non spore forming rods capable of growing aerobically on medium containing bile salt and able to ferment lactose within 48 hours at 37 ° C. Aquatic organisms have a great variability in their physiological requirements. No single medium, pH or temperature is ideal for all types of organisms. Water is a very good essential part of life. From time to time it was well recognized that if improperly handled water could be deadly source of epidemic. Usually domestic sewage, animal excreta and industrial

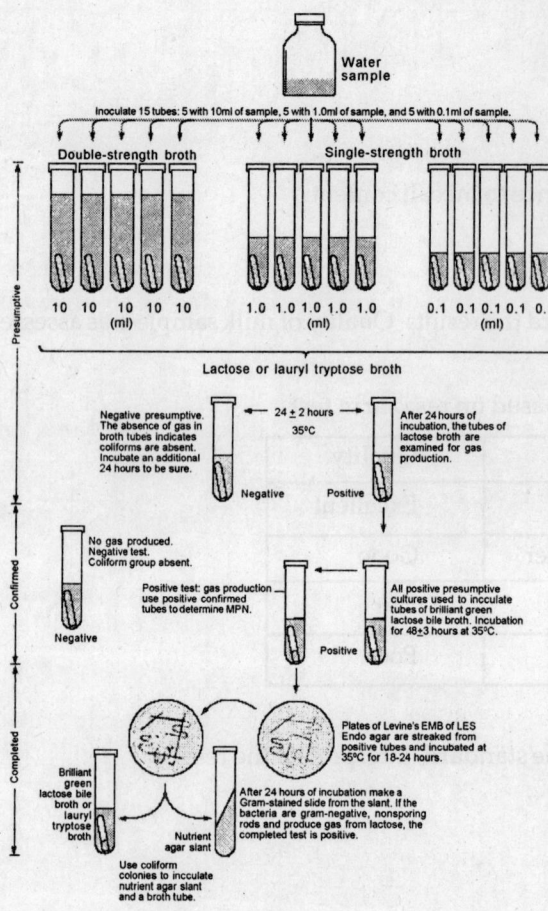

Fig 110.1 : MPN

wastes contaminate water. Main source of biological contamination is the infected symptomatic, convalescent and asymptomatic carries. These pathogens may be shed in water, use up the suspended organic matter and proliferate till it finds entry into another system. Coliforms are the main source of contamination, the presence of coliforms indicates the fall of water quality and need for treatment procedure. MPN technique is used to detect the presence of total coliforms in water. Good quality of water is odorless, colourless, tasteless and free from faecal pollution. Standard plate count (serial dilution/TVC), presence absence test and membrane filter technique also used to check water quality.

Principle

The number of total coliforms (*Enterobacter, Klebsiella, Citrobacter, Escherichia*) in a water sample can be determined by **most probable number (MPN) test**. This test involves a multiple series of Durham fermentation tubes. This test is categorized into three parts; they are the **presumptive, confirmed** and **completed tests**. In the presumptive test, dilutions from the water sample are added to lactose or lauryl tryptose broth fermentation tubes. After 24 to 48 hours of incubation at 35°C, and look for lactose fermentation with gas production. (The lauryl tryptose broth is selective for gram-negative bacteria due to the presence of lauryl sulfate). Confirmed test, showed growth and gas production into brilliant green lactose bile broth, which is selective and differential for coliforms. Gas formation in the Durham tube is a confirmed test for total coliforms. Completed test, confirms Coliform groups.

Collection of sample

Samples of water for bacteriological testing must be collected in sterile bottles. Glass bottles used for water sampling should have a capacity of at least 200mL. They should be fitted with ground glass stoppers or aluminum foil. Using sterile technique collect water. Immediately after collection sample should be placed in a cool box for transport and examine as soon as possible, (It must be within 6 hours).

Materials required

Sample : Drinking water

Media : Lauryl tryptose broth (single & double strength), Brilliant green 2% bile broth, Eosin methylene blue agar, Peptone water, MR-VP broth, Simmons citrate agar, TSI agar, Nutrient agar., Nutrient broth

Reagents : Kovacs indole reagent, Methyl red, 40% KOH, Alpha naphtol, 3% hydrogen peroxide, Gram stain kit

General materials : Test tubes, Petriplates, Conical flasks, Cavity slide, Slide, Pasteur pipette, Vaseline, Cotton, Aluminium foil, durham's tube, Bunsen burner, pipette etc.,

Procedure

Isolation of Total coliforms

Three tube and five tube MPN test may be performed based on the type of water. For known polluted water 5 tube technique is followed. For normal water we may follow 3 tube technique

Presumptive test

- Prepare single and double strength lauryl tryptose broth and pour it into test tubes (10 tubes single strength and 5 tubes of double strength for 5 tube technique and 6 tubes single strength and 3 tubes of double strength for 3 tube technique).

- Sterilize Lauryl Tryptose Broth tubes with Durham's tube.

- Arrange presumptive tubes in 3 rows (five tubes each for 5 tube technique 3 tubes each for three tube technique).

- Aseptically inoculate 0.1mL, 1mL and 10 mL sample into each set of the Lauryl Tryptose Broth tubes and incubated at 35°C for 24 hours (10mL of the sample to the double strength broth).

- Examine the tubes for gas production and record the results. (The negative tubes are further incubated for another 24 hours. Tubes, which exhibit positive result after 48 hours, are also taken for subsequent analysis).

Confirmatory test

- Inoculate one loop full of the inoculum from positive tubes of lauryl tryptose broth into the sterile brilliant green 2% bile broth tubes individually and incubated at 37 ° C for 24 hours

- Examine all tubes for gas production. (Negative tubes are further incubated for 24 hours. The tubes exhibiting positive results are also taken for further analysis). Note the numbers of positive tube results and compute in the MPN table to obtain the value of MPN/ 100mL.

Completed test

The test is aimed for the identification of coliforms through various biochemical means. Streak One loop full of the positive confirmed culture on the sterile EMB agar plate and incubated at 37 ° C for 24 hours. Nucleated colonies with or without metallic sheen are marked as typical colonies and transfer to sterile Lauryl Tryptose Broth and nutrient agar slants. Observe gas production on LT broth. Gas production on LT broth indicates completed test.

Differentiation of coliforms:

Nutrient agar slant colonies are subjected to biochemical test and microscopic examination.

Table 109.1 Observation report

S. No.	Test	Most probable number															MPN index	
		0.1mL					1mL					10mL					lowest	highest
		1	2	3	4	5	1	2	3	4	5	1	2	3	4	5		
1	24hrs Presumptive 48 hrs																	
	24 hrs Confirmatory 48 hrs																	

Isolation of faecal coliforms

Presumptive test	*-lauryl tryptose broth*
Confirmed test	*-EC broth*
Completed test	*-EMB agar*

Incubation temperature - 44 ° C

Isolation of faecal streptococci

Presumptive test	*-Azide Dextrose Broth*
Confirmed test	*-Ethyl Violet Azide Broth*
Completed test	*-KF Streptococcus Agar*

Incubation temperature - 37 ° C

Table 109.2. MPN index and 95 % confidential limits for various combinations of positive tubes in a 3 tube dilution series using inoculum quantities of 10, 1 and 0.1 mL

Combination of Positive tubes	MPN index per 100 mL	95 % confidential limit	
		Lower	Upper
0-0-0	< 3.00	– – –	9.50
0-0-1	3.00	0.15	9.60
0-1-0	3.00	0.15	11.00
0-1-1	6.10	1.20	18.00
0-2-0	6.20	1.20	18.00
0-3-0	9.40	3.60	38.00
1-0-0	3.60	0.17	18.00
1-0-1	7.20	1.30	18.00
1-0-2	11.00	3.60	38.00
1-1-0	7.40	1.30	20.00
1-1-1	11.00	3.60	38.00
1-2-0	11.00	3.60	42.00
1-2-1	15.00	4.50	42.00
1-3-0	16.00	4.50	42.00
2-0-0	9.20	1.40	38.00
2-0-1	14.00	3.60	42.00
2-0-2	2.00	4.50	42.00
2-1-0	15.00	3.70	42.00
2-1-1	20.00	4.50	42.00
2-1-2	27.00	8.70	94.00
2-2-0	21.00	4.50	42.00
2-2-1	28.00	8.70	94.00
2-2-2	35.00	8.70	94.00

2-3-0	29.00	8.70	94.00
2-3-1	36.00	8.70	94.00
3-0-0	23.00	4.60	94.00
3-0-1	38.00	8.70	110.00
3-0-2	64.00	17.00	180.00
3-1-0	43.00	9.00	180.00
3-1-1	75.00	17.00	200.00
3-1-2	120.00	37.00	420.00
3-1-3	160.00	40.00	420.00
3-2-0	93.00	18.00	420.00
3-2-1	150.00	37.00	420.00
3-2-2	210.00	40.00	430.00
3-2-3	290.00	90.00	1000.00
3-3-0	240.00	42.00	1000.00
3-3-1	460.00	90.00	2000.00
3-3-2	1100.00	180.00	4100.00
3-3-3	> 1100.00	420.00	— —-

Viva questions

Why are coliforms selected as the indicator of water potability?

Does a positive presumptive test indicate that water is potable?

Why is the MPN test qualitative rather than quantitative?

What is the function of the following in the MPN test?

a. lactose broth, b. Levine's EMB or LES Endo agar, c. nutrient agar slant, d. Gram stain

What does a metallic green sheen indicate on an EMB plate? Pink to dark red colonies with a metallic surface sheen on LES Endo agar?

What bacterial diseases can be transmitted by polluted water?

Spotters : MPN set up; MPN diagram; MPN chart; lauryl tryptose broth; Brillient green 2% bile broth; EMB agar; Durhams tube.

109b. The presence-absence (P-A) coliform test.

Aim

To check the quality of water using PA test

Background information

The P-A test is a modification of the MPN procedure in which a large water sample (100 mL) is incubated in a single culture bottle with triple-strength broth containing lactose, sodium lauryl sulfate and bromcresol purple indicator. The P-A test is based on the assumption that no coliforms should be present in 100 mL of drinking water. Sodium lauryl sulfate inhibits many bacteria, but not coliforms. A positive test results in the production of acid from lactose fermentation (bromcresol purple changes from purple to yellow) and constitutes a positive presumptive test.

As with the MPN test, it requires confirmation. If there is no colour change, the results are negative for coliforms in the 100-mL water sample.

Materials required

Sample : Drinking water

Media : Triple strength Lauryl tryptose broth, Brillient green 2% bile broth,

General materials : Test tubes, Petriplates, 500mL Conical flasks, Cavity slide, Slide, Pasteur pipette, Vaseline, Cotton, Aluminium foil, durhams tube, Bunsen burner, pipette etc.,

Procedure

Presumptive test

● Inoculate 100 mL of the water sample into a 250- mL P-A culture bottle containing 50 mL of triplestrength P-A broth. Mix thoroughly by inverting the bottle five times to achieve even distribution of the triple-strength medium throughout the sample.

● Incubate at 35°C. (Inspect the P-A culture bottle after 24 and 48 hours for acid production. A distinct yellow colour forms in the medium when acid conditions exist following lactose fermentation. If gas also is being produced, gently shaking the bottle will result in a foaming reaction.)

Confirmatory test

Transfer a loop full of culture (a positive presumptive test) to a tube of brilliant green lactose bile (BGLB) broth containing a Durham tube. Incubate at 35°C and observe for growth and fas production.

Result :

1. Turbidity in the BGLB broth and gas in the Durham tube within 48 hours confirm the presence of coliform bacteria (e.g., *Escherichia coli*).

2. Record results as presence-absence test positive or negative for coliforms in 100 mL of water sample.

Viva questions

What bacterial diseases can be transmitted by polluted water?
What does a positive presence-absence test indicate? A negative presence-absence test?
What are the significance of PA test
Why there is a need of triple strength medium

Spotters: Lauryl tryptose broth, brillient green 2% bile broth.

109c. Membrane filter technique for the quality analysis of water

Aim

To assess the quality of water by membrane filter technique.

Background information

Membrane filter technique is a reliable method for the detection of coliforms in water. The filter discs are 150 micron thick and have pores of 0.45 micrometer with 80% perforation. It facilitates rapid filtration. To detect the coliforms in water, the water is passed through filters. The bacteria larger than 0.45 μm are retained in the filter. Then the filter is placed on an absorbent pad saturated with liquid media and incubated for 24 hours. The organism on filter disc form colonies that can be counted using magnifying instrument.

Advandages of this technique includes good reproducibility, single step results often possible filter can be transferred between different media large volume can be processed to increase assay sensitivity. Save time considerably ability to complete filtration on site and lower total cost when compared to MPN technique.

Disadvantages of this technique are

> High turbidity waters limit volumes sampled,
> High population of bacteria cause overgrowth and
> Metals and phenols can adsorb to filters and inhibit growth.

Materials Required

Water sample, 20 mL of m FC agar for faecal coliforms, 20 mL of m Endo agar for coliforms, 20 mL of KF agar for faecal Streptococci, Sterile 0.45 micrometer filter, Sterile petriplate, 1 liter suction flask, Absorbent pad, Sterile water, Millipore membrane apparatus, Forceps, Suction pump , Dissection microscope etc…

Procedure

- Aseptically assemble the filter apparatus and insert membrane filter as follows
  Place the filter holder aseptically in the Buchner flask. Attach the flask to the vacuum pump line through a rubber hose. Using a flamed forceps place a sterile membrane filter disc, grid side up, on the porous glass support of the filter holder. Set the funnel on the filter holder and fasten in place.
- Shake the water sample and pour 100mL of water sample in to the funnel.
- Filter under vacuum
- When the entire sample has been filtered, wash the inner surface of the funnel with 100mL of sterile water.
- Carefully remove the filter from the filter holder using sterile forceps.
- Place sterile absorbent pad to the sterile petriplates.
- Aseptically add, 2 mL of the medium to the pad to saturate it.
- Aseptically transfer the membrane filter on to the medium saturated pad in the petri dish.
- Incubate all plates at appropriate temperature for 24 hours
- Remove the filter disc from the petriplate and allow to dry on absorbent paper for 1 hour.
- Examine filter paper disc under a dissecting microscope for the presence or absence of coliforms and count number of colonies.

Calculation

Number of coliform per
100mL of water = $\dfrac{\text{colony count}}{\text{Volume of sample used}} \times 100$

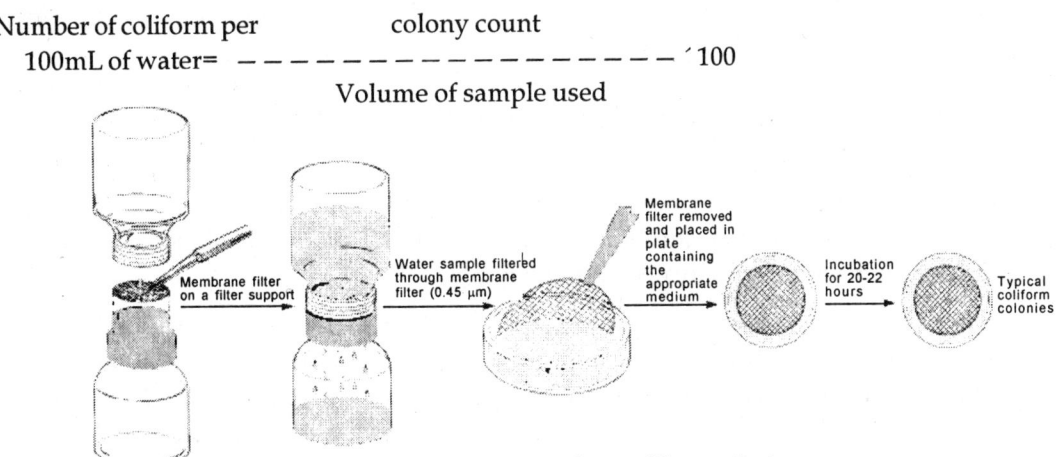

Fig. 109.2 Membrane filter technique

Result : Quality of drinking water is assessed and reported.

Viva questions

Define membrane filter technique.
What are the advantages and disadvantages of this technique?
Why is 0.45mm pore size filter used in this technique.
Mention colony morphology of *Streptococcus faecalis* on KF streptococcus agar.

Spotters: Membrane filter; membrane filteration unit; endo agar; KF agar.

110. Mushroom cultivation

Aim

To know cultivation technology of edible mushrooms.
Cultivation of oyster mushroom.
Spawn production.

Background Information

Mushrooms are fleshy fungi, which constitute a major group of lower plant kingdom. The mushroom is a common fungal fruit body that produces basidiospores at the tip called bacidia. The mushroom first appear as white tiny balls consisting of short stem (stalk) and a cap (pileus) which begins to open up like umbrella. India is the second most popular country of the world with a population of over 100 crores. Mushrooms provide a rich addition to the diet in the form of proteins, carbohydrates, minerals and vitamins.

Nutrient value of mushroom include 91.1% Moisture, 29.9% Protein, 4.4% Carbohydrate, 0.3% Fat and 16K Calories.

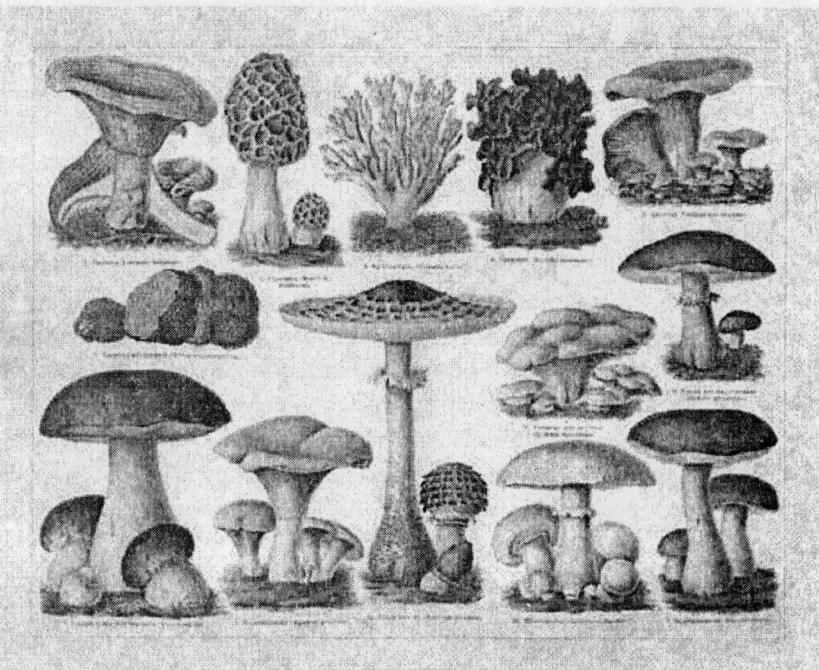

Fig 110.1 – Different varieties of Mushromm grown in India

Presently about a dozen fungi are cultivated in over 100 countries with a production of 2.2 million tons. *Agaricus bisporus*(56%)-white button; *Lentinus edodes*(14%)-shiltake; *Volvariella volvacea*(8%)-paddy straw; *Pleurotus sp*(7%)-oyster; Flammulina(5.5%)-winter mushroom; Tremmula sp(4.6%)-silver ear; Phillota (1.8%)-nameka and Others(1.1%) are the mushroom varieties cultivated for human usage.

Species of the genus Pleurotus called oyster mushroom or Dhingri or Wood Fungus is ranked as the fourth important mushroom of the world amoung the five most important cultivated mushrooms with a production of 15,000 tonnes per annum. The genus contains over 50 species. Of these *P.ostreatus, P.flabellatus, P.sajor caju, P. sapidus, P. fossulatus, P. squarrosules, P. cornucopieae, P. sapathulatus* and *P.florida* have been cultivated in India.

Oyster Mushroom cultivation

Spawn production

Successful cultivation of any mushroom on a small scale, one of the most important requirements is the seed. Spawn is a pure culture of the mycelium grown on a special medium. It is mushroom seed, comparable to the vegetative seed in crop plants. Spawn production mainly consists of three steps. They are Substrate preparation, Substrate inoculation and Incubation of the inoculated substrate.

Materials Required

Pure culture of Pleurotus, Cereal grain, Calcium sulfate, Calcium carbonate, Glucose bottles, Cotton, Cooker , Laminar flow cabinet, Incubator, Wire gauge, Balance, Bunsen burner, Water etc.,

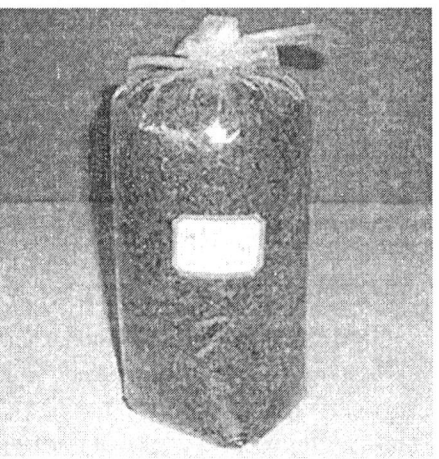

Fig 110.2 : Spawn

Procedure

- Take 600gm of grain in 400-600mL of water in a container.

- Boil the grain for 15-20minutes to bring the moisture content of grain to 40-50%.

- Remove the excess water of grain by spreading the grain in the sieve.

- Allow the grain to surface dry by spreading over the dry surface, in shade, for a few hours.

- Mix the grain thoroughly with chemicals (2% calcium sulfate and 0.5% calcium carbonate on dry weight basis), to adjust the pH of the grain.

- Fill the grain -chemical mixture in 500mL glucose bottles / plastic bag (Fig 110.2).

- Plug the bottles with non-absorbent cotton.

- Sterilize the substrate by autoclaving at 121 ° C for 30 minutes.

- Repeat the process of the sterilization after 24 hours of first autoclaving.

- Allow the substrate container to reach room temperature. Now the substrate is ready for inoculation.

- Inoculate the substrate with the mycelium of the mushroom grown on a specific medium by transferring mycelium in agar on the grain under aseptic conditions.

- Shake the containers, after plugging, to distribute fragments of the mycelium.

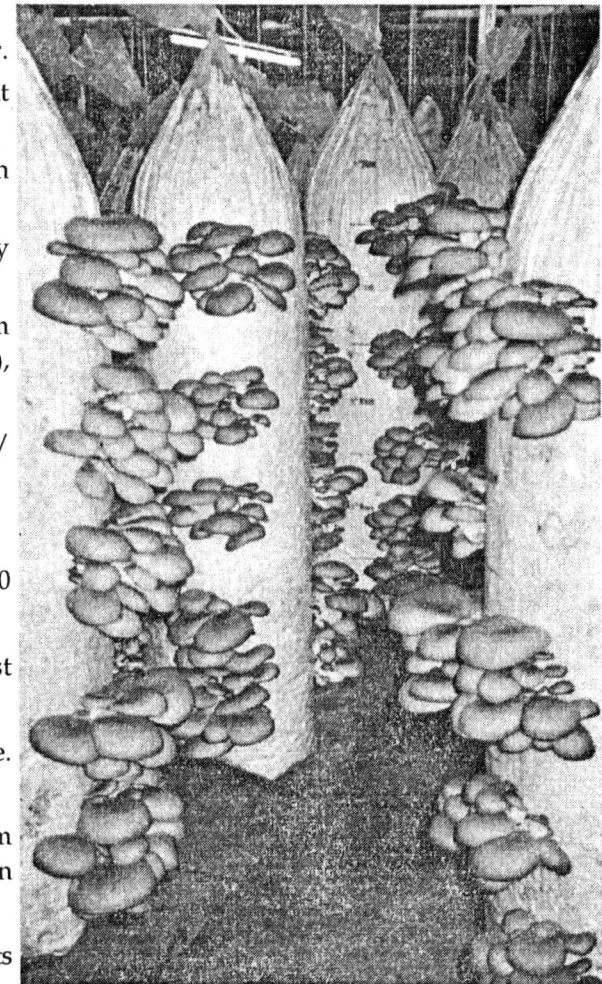

Fig 110.3: Cultivation of Pleurotus

- Store the inoculated containers at 20-25°C in darkness for 3 weeks.
- Shake the containers for an even distribution of mycelium, after a few days of incubation or as soon as mycelium is visible on grain.

Observation and results:

White coloured mycelial growth is noted. This indicated seed of mushroom is completely grown and utilized for oyster mushroom production.

Oyster Mushroom Cultivation

The oyster mushrooms are rich in proteins, mineral contents, devoid of starch and low in calories and carbohydrates. These are ideal food for diabetic and heart patients and those who do not want to put on weight. The various substrates utilized for the cultivation of *Pleurotus* are banana pseudostems, wheat straw, paddy straw, ragi straw, compost prepared from straw, saw dust, beech saw dust, sunflower stalks, rice husk and karad hay. However, the highest yields are obtained on rice straw. These can be grown in any container, e.g. earthen pot, cane gasket, polyethylene bags, iron baskets or in wooden trays.

Materials required

Thatched hut/polyethylene chamber, mud/pucca house, Dry paddy straw (chopped) or other agro-wastes - 100kg , Horse gram powder - 4kg , Spawn bottles of *Pleurotus* sp. , Polyethylene bags - 1kg , Water sprayer.

Procedure:

- Take dried paddy straw.
- Chop the straw into 1 to 2 cm bits.
- Soak the chopped straw into water overnight.
- Drain off the excess water.
- Add horse gram powder at the rate of 8g/kg.
- Add spawn at the rate of 30g/kg.
- Mix all the constituents.
- Fill the mixture into polyethylene bags with holes.
- Incubate the field bags in a room at 21 to 35°C with sufficient light and ventilation for 15-16 days for spawn running (Fig 110.3).
- Spray water over the bags twice a day.

Observation:

Observe for the mushroom crop after 3 to 4 days of opening the polyethylene bags (Fig 110.2).

Harvesting:

First harvesting is to be done 20-22 days after spawning, 2nd harvesting 27-29 days after spawing and 3rd harvesting 34-36 days after spawing.

Precautions:

For better yields, temperature of the room should be in the range of 20-26°C and relative humidity of 70-90%.

Provide light for 15-20 minutes during cropping period.

Polyethylene bags with holes should be used.

Result

Oyster mushroom is cultivated and harvested.

Viva questions

Name biological name of oyster mushroom

Mention the other name of seed of mushroom

Name the grain used to produce spawn

Why polythene bags are used to generate oyster mushroom?

What are the purposes of using paddy straw in mushroom cultivation?

Spotters : mushroom picture, spawn

111. Alcoholic fermentation of fruit juice (Wine preparation)

Aim

To prepare consumable alcohol from grape juice by using yeast.

Background Information

Wine is defined as a product formed by normal alcoholic fermentation of grapes by yeasts and subsequent aging process. The biochemical conversion of juice of grapes to wine occurs when yeast cells enzymatically degrade the fructose and glucose into aldehyde and alcohol as illustrated below,

$$\text{Sucrose} \xrightarrow{\text{Invertase}} \text{glucose/fructose} \xrightarrow{\text{EMP path way}} \text{pyruvic acid} \xrightarrow{\text{Co2 release}} \text{acetaldehyde}$$
$$\downarrow$$
$$\text{Alcohol}$$

Grapes containing 20-30% sugar concentration and yield approximately 10-15% alcohol and acids , minerals also available whose concentration is increased in finished products.

Materials Required

Grapes (white or red) *Sacharomyces cerevisiae*, 1N Hcl, Phenolphthalein, Dinitrosalicylic acid, Rose bengal agar, Conical flask, Cotton etc.,

Procedure

- Wash one kg of white grapes and crushed well with ample amount of water in the sterilized mixer.

- Filter the resulting mixture and whey through a piece of clean cotton cloth.

- Make up the filtrate to 750 mL with distilled water.

- Sterilize 50 mL of filterate and inoculate *Saccharomyces cerevisiae*. Incubate for 24hours at 30°C (Seed culture).

- Sterilize remaining portion and inoculate 50mL of seed culture in the next day and allow for fermentation.

- Add 20g sugar on the second and fourth day after inoculation.

- Periodically perform sugar content estimation, acidity and yeast content count for three weeks and also check the nature of wine.

Yeast count

- Perform Yeast count using Rose Bengal Chloramphenicol Agar.

Acidity test

- Take 20mL of sample in a beaker and add 5 drops of phenopthalein.

- Titrate the contents against 0.1 N NaOH

- Note the colour change (permanent pink).

- Calculate total acidity and volatile acidity using the following calculation

$$\text{Total acidity (Percentage of tartaric acid)} = \frac{\text{ML. of alkali added} \times 7.5 \times N}{\text{volume of juice added}}$$

$$\text{Total acidity (Percentage of acetic acid)} = \frac{\text{ML. of alkali added} \times 6 \times N}{\text{volume of juice added}}$$

Sugar content estimation

- Estimate Sugar content of the juice through Di Nitro Salycylic Acid (DNS) method (Refer experiment 148).

- Compare the results of DNS method with standard graph and estimated the percentage of reducing sugar present in the given sample.

Estimation of alcohol

- Ethanol content of the fermentation medium was estimated through chromic acid method.

- This method was developed by Caputi *et.al.,* in 1968 (Refer experiment 160).

Result

Taste and nature of wine is good and used for human consumption.

Viva questions

Define wine

Mention about biochemical process of wine production

How do you estimate acidity of wine?

Name the medium used to cultivate yeast

Mention about morphology of yeast on fungal isolation medium.

What is the principle of reducing sugar estimation?

Mention method to estimate reducing sugar

Spotters: Yeast., Alcohol

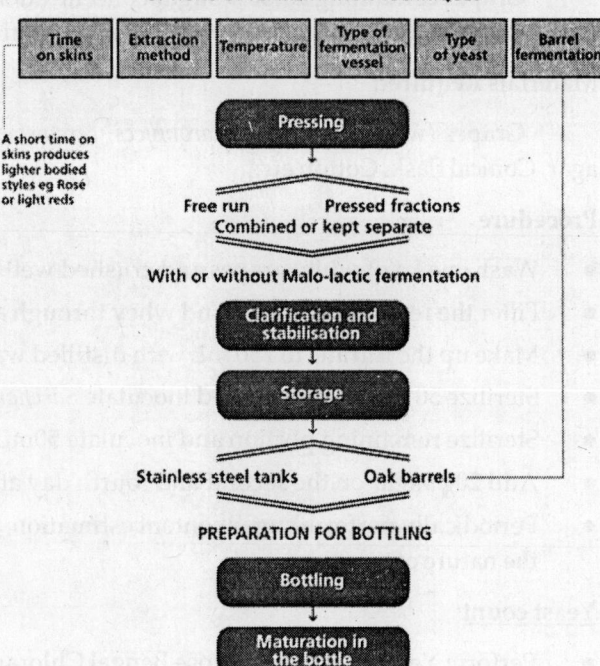

Fig 111.1: Commercial wine making process

112. Preparation of Beer

Aim

To make beer.

To understand the effects of fermentation on food.

Background information

Beer is probably one of the most ancient fermented foods used by man. Beer is produced when the sugars are anaerobically fermented, usually by yeast. In the absence of oxygen the sugars are metabolized by yeast and produced ethanol and carbon dioxide. Some acid is also produced resulting in a low final pH. Beer can be made from any plant material that contains free sugar, but generally beer/whiskey are made from grains.

Materials required

Malt powder, boiler, brewers yeast, hydrometer, corn sugar, materials for alcohol estimation (refer experiment No. 160).

Procedure

- Dissolve the contents of one package (50g) of prehopped malt powder in 1.5 liters of water.
- Boil the mixture. It will foam because of the protein content.
- Cover the pot and cool the mixture rapidly to 49°C
- Bring the volume to 3L with sterile cool water.
- Inoculate 10% yeast directly to the wart (Check the wart with a hydrometer and label fermentation vessel - The initial reading should be about 1350).
- Fill the labeled sterile fermentation vessel with the wart.
- Add a trap to the vessel. The trap consists of a rubber stopper with an attached length of latex tubing. Insert the end of the tube in a flask of water so the gas formed during the fermentation bubbles off in the water.
- Ferment the wart down to a reading of about 1011. This should take 5-7 days. Look for the same low hydrometer reading 2 days in a row.
- Add one level ½ teaspoon of corn sugar to each sterile 100mL bottle. Fill with beer and cap properly.
- Shake each bottle to dissolve the sugar.
- Maintain (condition) the beer at the same temperature as the fermentation for 7-10 days (At the end of the conditioning period either chill and drink or store in the refrigerator until tasting time).
- Check percentage of alcohol and taste. Record findings and report.

Observation and result

Within 15 days beer will be produced and the results are recorded.

Spotters

Beer, *Saccharomyces cerevisiae*.

Viva questions

Define beer

What are the difference between beer and wine?

What is beer conditioning?

Define wart in beer?

Industrial Microbiology

113. Bioethanol Production

Aim

To prepare ethanol from sugar by using brewers yeast.

To estimate alcohol content of the fermentation medium.

Background Information

Ethanol is one of the common solvent and raw material used in the laboratory and in the chemical industry. Alcohol fermentation is an biological degradation of carbohydrates (glucose, sucrose, fructose) to carbon di oxide and ethanol. The amount of ethanol production depends on the following factors, that are the amount of fermentable sugar, organisms capability and fermentation temperature. Yeast is one of the facultative anaerobe occurs as single or in pairs or in short chains or in clusters. Pseudohyphae may be formed. Yeast synthesizes alcohol through EMP pathway.

$$\text{EMP path way} \qquad CO_2 \text{ release}$$
$$\text{Sucrose} \rightarrow \rightarrow \rightarrow \rightarrow \text{glucose/fructose} \rightarrow \rightarrow \rightarrow \rightarrow \text{pyruvic acid} \rightarrow \rightarrow \rightarrow \rightarrow \text{acetaldehyde}$$
$$\downarrow$$
$$\downarrow$$
$$\downarrow$$
$$\text{Alcohol}$$

Materials Required

Brewers yeast, *Growth media, Fermentation medium, Chromic acid, Alcohol distillation apparatus,* Spectrophotometer

Procedure

Seed culture preparation

- Prepare growth media.
- Add 2% glucose.
- Inoculate a loopful of yeast from slant culture.
- Incubate at 37°C for 18 hours.

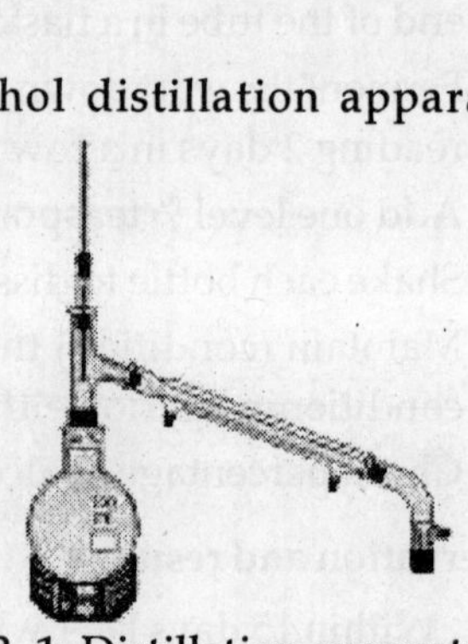

Fig.113 .1: Distillation apparatus

Fermentation process

- Carryout batch fermentation in 500mL of conical flask containing 250 mL sterile fermentation medium.
- Inoculate fermentation medium using 10 % of seed culture.
- Perform Fermentation at room temperature under static process.
- Allow fermentation for 18-24 hour. At the end, collect 10mL fermented broth & estimate alcohol content and reducing sugar of fermentation medium.

Estimation of alcohol

- Ethanol content of the fermentation medium through chromic acid method

- This method was developed by Caputi *et.al.,* in 1968 (Refer experiment 160 - Page 408).

Analysis of reducing sugar from sample

Estimate Reducing sugar content of the fermentation medium through Di Nitro Salycylic Acid (DNS) method (Refer experiment 148 - Page 391 & 392).

Compare the results of DNS method with standard graph and estimate the percentage of reducing sugar present in the given sample.

Result

Alcohol content is detected using chromic acid. Quantity of alcohol production is analysed using alcohol standard graph. In general, yeast produce 1% alcohol from 1g of glucose.

Viva questions

Define alcohol

Give importance of alcohol

How do you estimate alcohol?

List factors affecting alcohol production

Name the medium used for the fermentation of alcohol

Which chemical is converted to alcohol during fermentation?

Is fermentation is a aerobic process or anaerobic process.

Define Pasteur effect

Spotters: chromic acid; glucose; yeast; distillation apparatus

114. Immobilization of yeast cell by using sodium alginate

Aim

To entrap the live cells in a solid matrix and analyze its activity.

Background information

Whole cell immobilization has been defined as "the physical confinement or localization of intact cells to a certain defined region of space with preservation of some desired catalytic activity" (Karel et al., 1985). Many microorganisms own the capability to adhere to different kinds of surfaces in nature on which way are in close proximity to nutrients and easy realize a food supply. Therefore, we can say that these biological systems in their natural state are immobilized. However, many biotechnological process needs to be carried out using immobilization of biocatalysts. Thereby several different techniques and support materials have been proposed for the

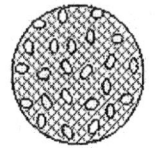

ENTRAPMENT WITHIN A MATRIX

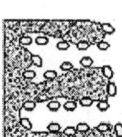

ATTACHEMENT OR ADSORPTION TO A PREFORMRD CARRIER

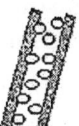

SELF AGGREGATION OF CELLS

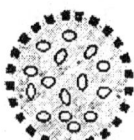

CELLS CONTAINED BEHIND A BARRIER

Fig 114.1 Principal methods of cell immobilization

cell immobilization in vitro. Fig 115. 1 illustrates basic methods for immobilization. These techniques can be divided into four major groups based on the physical mechanism causing immobilization: physical entrapment within a porous matrix, attachment or adsorption to a pre-formed carrier, self aggregation by floculation (natural) or crosslinking agents (artificially induced) and cell contained behind barrier.

All of these methods have the same purpose: to retain high cell concentrations within "a certain defined region of space" such as a bioreactor giving increased volumetric productivity of a system.

During the last thirty years a numerous different kinds of cell-supporting materials for immobilization have been developed, such as polymeric matrices (alginate, agar, gelatin, k-karrageenan, chitosan, pectin, polyacrylamide, epoxy resin, silica gel) and porous and non-porous preformed support materials (wood chips, stainless steel, volcanic rock, cotton cloth, porous glass particles, DEAE cellulose, porous silica, porous ceramics, diatomaceous earth). The choice of cell-supporting material for any specific application is related to the following points: bioreactor configuration, high carrier activity, availability of the carrier in commercial qualities, low cost of immobilization, immobilization, easy and controllable, ease of operating scale-up, excellent mechanical strength during long-time operation, physiological and environmental safety of the materials used and low affinity to contaminations.

Principle

This technique involves a reaction between sodium alginate and calcium chloride forming calcium alginate. With the optimum concentrations of the reactants, the product particles coagulates resulting in the formation of beads. This property could be used as a suitable technique to immobilize microbial cells in the form of beads. Entrapment in insoluble Ca alginate gel is recognized as a rapid, nontoxic, inexpensive, versalite and the most often used method for immobilization of cells (more than 80% of cell immobilization processes are still carried out using alginate). Immobilization offers many potential advantages over free cell systems, such as Higher cell densities and cell loads, Increased volumetric productivity, Shorter overall reaction times, Smaller fermenter sizes which may lower capital costs, The reuse of the same biocatalysts for prolonged period of time due to constant cell regeneration, A continuous process which may be performed beyond the nominal washout rate, Improved substrate utilization, Reduced risk for microbial contamination, Process design simplified, Constant product quality and Improved tolerance or protection of cells from substrate and end-product inhibition.

Materials required

Sodium alginate- 5.5gm; Cacl$_2$- 4%

Culture: any one type of yeast / Seed culture for fermentation.

Medium: Potato dextrose broth, *Growth medium*, fermentation medium

Procedure

Preparation of seed culture

- Prepare Growth medium and sterilize at 110 ° C for 10 minutes
- Inoculate a loop full of yeast culture from slant or 1 mL of culture from broth.
- Incubate at 37°C for 18 hours.

Preparation of immobilized cells

- Prepare sodium alginate slurry by adding 5.5g sodium alginate to150mL of 0.1 % sodium chloride solution with continuous stirring.
- Allow the slurry to stand for 6-8 hours and add 15mL of seed culture.

- Prepare the beads by controlled drop wise addition of slurry to the 4% calcium chloride solution.
- Keep the beads in calcium chloride solution about 30 minutes for *gelation*.

Activation of immobilized beads

- Perform activation of immobilized beads with the help of Growth medium.
- Inoculate required volume of beads into the rich medium and kept it for 30 minutes
- Note the movements of beads.

Fermentation of alcohol using immobilized beads

- Add 25 mL of beads to 250 mL of fermentation medium and carryout the fermentation under static condition at room temperature.
- Estimate alcohol content through chromic acid method (Refer experiment 160 - Page 408).
  (Measure volume of beads using water displacement method).

Observation

Spherical shaped immobilized beads are prepared and activated in Growth medium.

Result

Immobilized *Saccharomyces cerevisiae* cells produces alcohol, which is estimated through chromic acid method.

Viva questions

What is immobilization?
What are the purposes of immobilization?
What are the types of immobilization?
What are the principles of cell immobilization?
What is gelation?
Name the chemicals used in immobilization of cells?
How do you activate immobilized cells

Spotters: Calcium chloride, sodium alginate., immobilized beads.

115. Amylase Production

Aim

To produce amylase from microorganisms.

Background Informations

Amylase is an enzyme that break down starch or glycogen. Amylase is produced by a variety of living organisms, ranging from bacteria to plants and humans. Bacteria and fungi secrete amylase to the outside of their cells to carry out extra-cellular digestion. When they have broken down the insoluble starch, the soluble end products such as (glucose or maltose) are absorbed into their cells. Amylases are classified based on how they break down starch molecules

i. α-amylase (alpha-amylase) - Reduces the viscosity of starch by breaking down the bonds at random, therefore producing varied side chains of glucose.

ii. β-amylase (Beta-amylase) - Breaks the glucose-glucose bonds down by removing two glucose units at a time, thereby producing maltose.

iii. Amyloglucosidase (AMG) - Breaks successive bonds from the non-reducing end of the straight chain, producing glucose.

Many microbial amylases usually contain a mixture of these amylases.

Humans exploit microbial amylases for the following purposes, they are High Fructose Corn syrup preparation, Additives to detergents for removing stains, Saccharification of starch for alcohol production and Brewing. Most commonly used for their industrial production are *Bacillus subtilis, Bacillus licheniformis, Bacillus amyloliquifaciens* and *Aspergillus niger*.

Materials Required

Autoclave, Microwave oven , Nutrient Agar, Potato Dextrose Agar, Soluble starch, Balance, Shaker , Spectrophotometer, Water bath, disposable spoons, micro pipettes, sterile water, Petri dishes , inoculation, Dissecting needle or Cork borer, Bunsen burner, matches, Glass spreader , 95% ethanol.

Amylase production medium (g/1)

Bacteriological Peptone 6g; $MgSO_4$- 0.5g; KCL 0.5g; Starch 1g. Sterilize by autoclaving at 121°C for 15 minutes

Procedure

Isolation of Amylase producers

- Collect 100g of the top soil and transfer into a "Ziploc" bag.
- Suspend about 10 grams of soil in 100 mL sterile distilled water, mix properly (10^{-1})
- Pipette 10 mL of the above and transfer to another 90 mL of water (10^{-2})
- Dilute further in two more 90 mL sterile water blanks (10^{-3} and 10^{-4}).
- Spread 0.1 mL of the diluted samples (10^{-1} and 10^{-2}) on Nutrient Agar plates (4 plates) containing 1 % w/v soluble starch and incubate at 30°C for 24 hours
- Starch-hydrolysing colonies will have an area of clearing around them.
  (It is confirmed by flooding plates with Gram's iodine.)
- Transfer distinguishable amylase-producing bacteria by streak on a fresh plate of Nutrient Agar containing 1% starch.
- Transfer isolated amylase-producing bacteria to Nutrient Agar and allow to grow for 24 hours, then store in the refrigerator until needed.

Amylase production

Seed culture

- Prepare amylase production medium, sterilize properly.
- Inoculate loopful of amylase producing *Bacillus sp.*,
- Incubate for 24 hours at 37°C

Fermentation

- Prepare 250mL of amylase production medium in 500mL conical flask.
- Sterilize at 121°C for 15 minutes.
- Inoculate 25mL of seed culture.

- Incubate at 37°C for 24 hours under shaking condition.
- Withdraw culture and subject to extraction of enzyme.

Extraction of Enzyme from bacteria

- Pour the bacterial culture into centrifuge tubes, and spin for 20 minutes at 5000 rpm.
- Decant the supernatant in to a sterile beaker, which is the crude enzyme extract.

Enzyme Activity

i. Pipette 1 mL of culture extract "enzyme" into a test tube.

ii. Add 1 mL of 1% soluble starch in citrate-phosphate buffer (pH6.5).

iii. Incubate in a water bath at 40°C for 30minutes

iv. Set up a blank consisting of 2mL of the enzyme extract that has been boiled for 20 minutes (boiling inactivates the enzyme), added to the starch solution and treated with the same reagent as the experimental tubes.

v. Stop the reaction by adding 2 mL of DNS reagent and estimate reducing sugar (Refer experiment No 148).

Enzyme activity may be defined as the amount of glucose produced per mL in the reaction mixture per unit time.

Result

Isolated soil bacteria have the capability to produce amylase. Quantity of amylase may vary on the basis of environmental condition. Unit of amylase production is studied indirectly by analyzing reducing sugar by DNS method.

Viva questions

What is amylase?

What are the uses of amylase enzyme?

Mention types of amylase enzyme

Mention about the sources of amylase

Name any two organisms responsible for amylase production

How do you check amylase production in laboratory?

Mention media used for amylase production

Spotters : Starch, Iodine

116. Protease Production

Aim

To Produce Protease from microorganisms

Background Informations

Proteases and metalloprotease constitute one of the most important groups of industrial enzymes, accounting for about 60% of the total enzyme market . Among the various proteases, bacterial proteases are the most significant, compared with animal and fungal proteases and among bacteria, *Bacillus* sp are specific producers of extra-cellular proteases . These enzymes have wide industrial application, including pharmaceutical industry, leather industry, manufacture of protein hydrolizates, food industry and waste processing industry. Thermostable proteases are advantageous in some applications because higher processing temperatures can be employed, resulting in faster reaction rates, increase in the solubility of nongaseous reactants and products, and reduced incidence of microbial contamination by mesophilic organisms. Proteases secreted from thermophilic bacteria are thus of particular interest and have become increasingly useful in a range of commercial applications.

Materials required

Autoclave Microwave oven , Nutrient Agar, Casein, Gelatin, Balance, Shaker, Spectrophotometer, Water bath, disposable spoons, micro pipettes, sterile water, Petri dishes, Inoculation loop, Dissecting needle, Bunsen burner matches , Glass spreader , 95% ethanol.

Protease production Media (g/L of distilled water):

$MgSO_4$-0.5, K_2HPO_4-2.0, KCl-0.3,NH_4NO_3-10.0, Peptone-1.0. Trisodium citrate-10.0.

Adjusted PH to 6.9-7.0 with 1.0 M NaOH and this basal medium is sterilized by autoclaving at 121°C for 15 min. Peptone is sterilized separately and aseptically added to the flasks containing the liquid medium, after cooling.

Procedure

Isolation of Protease producers

- Suspend about 10 grams of soil in 100 mL sterile distilled water, mix properly (10^{-1})
- Pipette 10 mL of the above and transfer to another 90 mL of water (10^{-2})
- Dilute further in two more 90 mL sterile water blanks (10^{-3} and 10^{-4})
- Spread 0.1 mL of the diluted samples (10^{-1} and 10^{-})on Gelatin hydrolysis medium (4 plates) and incubate at 30°C for 24 hours
- Gelatin utilizing colonies will have an area of clearing around them.
- It is confirmed by flooding plates with Mercuric chloride solution.
- Transfer distinguishable, protease-producing bacteria, streak on a fresh plate of Nutrient Agar containing 1 % gelatin.

Protease production

Seed culture

- Prepare protease production medium, sterilize properly.
- Inoculate loopful of protease producing Bacillus sp.,
- Incubate for 24 hours at 37°C

Fermentation

- Prepare 250mL of protease production medium in 500mL conical flask.
- Sterilize at 121°C for 15 minutes.
- Inoculate the above medium with 1ml of an overnight culture and incubated 37°C for 24 hours in a rotary shaker operated at 150 rpm. At time intervals, the turbidity of the cultures is determined by measuring the increase in optical density at 470 nm with a spectrophotometer
- Withdrew culture and subject to extraction of enzyme

Extraction of Enzyme from bacteria

- Pour the bacterial culture into centrifuge tubes, and spin for 20 minutes at 5000 rpm.
- Decant the supernatant in to a sterile beaker, which is the crude enzyme extract.

Enzyme Activity

i. Pipette 1 mL of culture extract "enzyme" into a test tube

ii. Add 1 mL of 1% soluble casein in citrate-phosphate buffer (pH6.5)

iii. Incubate in a water bath at 40°C for 30minutes

iv. Set up a blank consisting of 2mL of the enzyme extract that has been boiled for 20 minutes (boiling inactivates the enzyme), added to the casein solution and treated with the same reagent as the experimental tubes.

v. Estimate protein content by using Folin method (Refer experiment No 152 - Page 396, 397)

Enzyme activity may be defined as the amount of casein produced per mL in the reaction mixture per unit time.

Result

Isolated soil bacteria produced protease enzyme by utilizing protein and quantity of protease is estimated, compared with standard graph and interpreted as unit of enzyme at the particular time

Viva question

How do you screen protease procucers from the environment.
Mention about chemical source which induce protease production.

Spotters

Gelatin, Casein, Mercuric Chloride

Microbial Genetics Molecular Biology and Microbial Biotechnology

117. Isolation of Chromosomal DNA from Bacteria

Aim

To isolate DNA from the given bacterial sample.

Principle

Nucleic acid is vital macromolecule in all living cells. The cell contains basic genetic information. Single strand of DNA is considered as the genetic materials in some viruses. But in higher organisms the DNA is present as nucleoprotein in the chromosome. The DNA occurs almost exclusively in the nucleus with trace amount of mitochondria and chloroplast. The efficiency and recovery of extraction depends on the amount of starting material to be used, the mode of homogenizing or breaking up the cell and the presence of degradative enzymes likes RNase, DNase. *E. coli* chromosomal DNA is a large circular molecule containing approximately 3,000,000 base pairs attached to the bacterial cell wall at several points. Large DNA is very sensitive to mechanical shear, which causes random breaks in the phosphodiester backbone of the molecule. However, if the extraction procedure is performed carefully, large fragments of chromosomal DNA can be obtained with an average fragment length of 100,000 to 200,000 base pairs. Since the average length of a gene is about 2,000 base pairs, there is a high probability that genes of interest will remain intact in one of the fragments of DNA. The procedure explained below is essentially that of Murmur's method.

Materials Required

Midlog bacterial culture, Extraction medium (10 mM Tris. pH 8.2; 10mM EDTA; 200mM NaCl, 0.5% SDS; 200 μG/mL Proteinase), Lysozyme solution (10mG/mL), 25% sodium dodecyl sulphate solution, 5M sodium per chloride, Chloroform: isoamyl alcohol, 24:1, 95% ethanol, Saline citrate 1X, (0.15M sodium chloride, 0.015M tri sodium citrate), 3M sodium acetate, Isopropanol

Sodium chloride is used for causing osmotic shock and had been used for release of hydrolytic enzymes and binding proteins from periplasmic space of gram negative bacteria.

Ethylene diamine tetra acetic acid (EDTA) : Strongly chelates divalent metallic ions (Zn^{2+}, Ca^{2+}, and Mg^{2+}). EDTA causes non- specifies increase in the permeability of gram negative bacteria.

Lysozyme : It is an enzyme which hydrolyses the N- acetyl $1 \rightarrow 4$ β linkages in peptidoglycon. Gram positive bacteria cell wall rigidity depends on peptidoglycon and gram positive bacteria are highly susceptible to lysozyme.

Sodium dodecyl sulphate (CH3 (CH2),O SO3+ Na-) - Anionic detergent causes the denaturation of many proteins

Sodium per chloride ($NaclO_4$) - Causes denaturation and precipitation of proteins

    Isoamyl alcohol: chloroform - Causes precipitation of proteins
    Ethanol (CH_3CH_2OH) - DNA gets precipitated when treated with ethanol.
    Saline citrate - Preserve DNA
    Isopropyl alcohol - Denatures ethyl alcohol
    Sodium acetate - $C_2H_3NaO_2$ - The DNA gets stabilized in this for several months.

Procedure

- Grow bacterial culture at 37⁰C for 24hours in LB broth and take 10mL of culture and centrifuged at 5000 rpm for 10minutes. Add 1mL extraction medium.

- Add 1mL of lysozyme solution to the above suspension; incubate at 37° C for 30minutes shaking occasionally.

- After the incubation, complete the lysis by adding 2mL of 25% SDS solution.

- Heat this preparation for 10 minutes at 60°C in a water bath, finally cool to room temperature.

- Add sufficient 5 M perchloride to the lysed preparation to the final concentration of 1M.

- Add an equal volume of chloroform:iso amyl alcohol to the lysed preparation suspended in 1M perchloride and slowly shake(30-60 oscillations/min) in a highly stoppered flask for 30 minutes at room temperature.

- Separate the resulting emulsion by centrifuging for 5min at 10000rpm at room temperature.

- After centrifugation carefully pipette out the top clear aqueous phase from the coagulated protein emulsion, at the inner phase.

- Place the aqueous phase containing the nucleic acid in the beaker.

- Gently stir the nucleic acid solution with the sterilized glass rod, while slowly adding 2 volume of 95% ethanol down the side of the beaker. So that the ethanol is layered over the viscous aqueous phase. Continue the stirring upto the preparation to mix throughout the phase and spool all of the gelatinous thread like DNA rich precipitate on the glass rod.

- Drain off excess fluid from the spooled crude DNA by pressing the rod against the wall of the beaker until no further fluid can be squeezed from the spooled preparation if the squeezing is not done sufficiently, the alcohol adhering the DNA will make it difficult to dissolve the DNA.

- Dissolve the crude DNA in 9mL of diluted saline citrate.

- To the even suspension add 1mL of 3 M acetate, 1M EDTA and transfer the preparation to 100mL beaker containing 5.4 mL of isopropanol.

- For the storage of DNA, dissolve the crude DNA in 9mL of saline citrate and Store at 2°C with few drops of chloroform.

Result

Isolated DNA is estimated by making use of diphenylamine method and are separated using agarose gel electrophoresis.

Alternative method of DNA isolation
117a. Isolation and Purification of chromosomal DNA from *Escherichia coli*

Aim

To understand how to isolate genomic DNA from the bacterium, *Escherichia coli*

To explain why different protocols are needed for DNA isolation from various taxa.

Principle

Isolation and purification of DNA are essential procedures in molecular biology. Extraction and purification of genomic DNA from procaryotic organisms such as *E. coli* have facilitated the study of complex genomes. This has also led to the construction of genomic DNA libraries for many species.

Materials required

LB medium, 10–12 hour (log phase) broth culture of *Escherichia coli*, 0.5- to 10 μL micropipettes, sterile tips, 10- to 100 μL micropipettes, 100 to 1,000 μL micropipettes, Eppendoff tubes, Centrifuge, 1 mL pipettes, Pasteur pipettes, disinfectant (70% ethanol or 3% hydrogen peroxide), 80°C modular dry bath incubator, 37°C incubator, heating block modules, 65°C water bath

20-mG/mL RNase A solution (DNase free; dissolve 1 mG/mL in 1 X TE [10 mM Tris, pH 7.4 + 1 mM EDTA, pH 8.0], boil 10–30 min, Cool to room temperature, store at -20°C)

Cell lysate solution (Tris-EDTA-SDS) : Tris HCl- 25mM; EDTA- 50mM; SDS - 1%; Lysozyme - 4mG/mL

Protein precipitation solution (Ammonium acetate or potassium acetate or Sodium acetate 1M to 3M)

100% isopropanol, 70% ethanol, 100% absolute ethanol, vortex mixer

Hydration solution (1 X Tris-EDTA hydration solution-TE buffer): TRIS *Hcl*- 10mM; EDTA- 1mM

Procedure

- Prepare 10- to 12-hour broth culture of *E. coli*.

- Label an eppendoff tube. Using a pipette, transfer 1 mL of the *E. coli* culture into the eppendoff tube.

- Spin the tube at 10000rpm for 5 minutes

- Carefully decant the supernatant.

- Add 600 μL of cell lysate solution and gently pipette up and down to resuspend the bacterial pellet (The SDS in the lysis solution is a detergent that disrupts the plasma membrane of the *E. coli* cells).

- Incubate at 80°C for 5 minutes.

- Slowly cool the sample in the eppendoff tube at room temperature (The sample must reach room temperature before adding RNase since heat will denature the enzyme).

- Add 3 μL of RNase solution to the bacterial cell lysate.

- Mix by inverting the microcentrifuge tube 25 times and incubate at 37°C for 30 minutes.

- Cool the sample to room temperature. Add 200 μL of protein precipitation solution and vortex **very gently** for 20 seconds. (The ammonium acetate in the solution precipitates the protein leaving the genomic DNA in solution).

- Centrifuge the sample for 3 minutes at 14,000 rpm to pellet the protein.

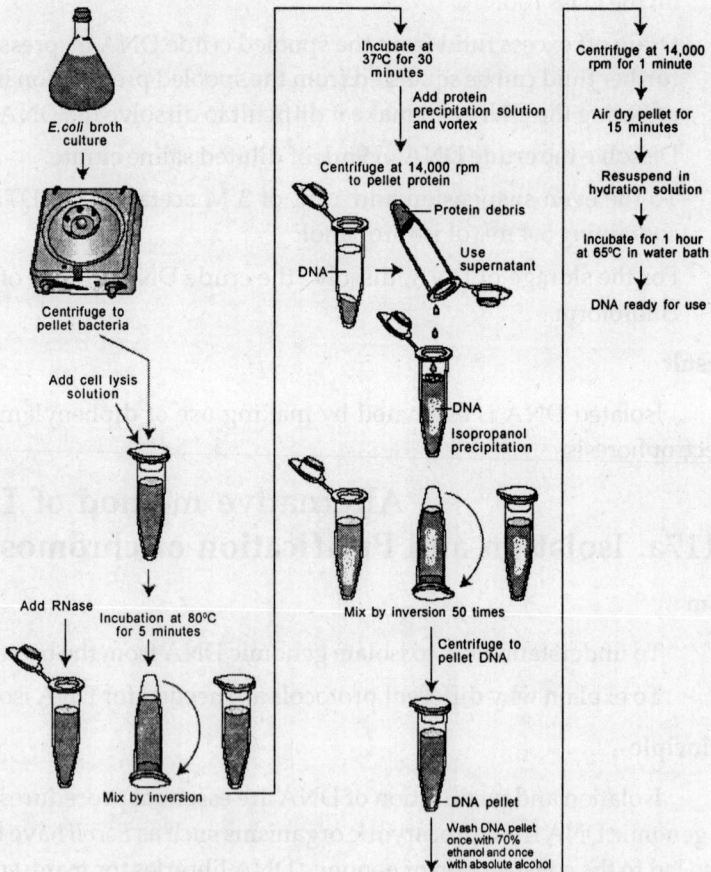

Fig. 117.1 - Steps in Chromosomal DNA isolation.

- Pour the supernatant into a clean 1.5 mL tube leaving the protein pellet behind.
- Add 600 μL of 100% isopropanol, cap the tube, and mix **very gently** by inverting the tube at least 50 times. Vigorous mixing will break the DNA into small fragments.
- Centrifuge in the microcentrifuge at 10,000 rpm for 5 minute to pellet the DNA.
- Pour off the supernatant and drain the liquid onto an absorbent paper. The pellet will appear offwhite to yellow.
- Add 600 μL of 70% ethanol and invert the tube several times to wash the pelleted DNA. Decant the 70% ethanol and add 600 μl of absolute alcohol. Invert the tube several times to wash the pelleted DNA. The *alcohol washes remove any salts* from the DNA.
- Centrifuge at 10,000 rpm for 5 minute.
- Pour off the supernatant very **slowly and carefully** watching the pellet so that it does not come out of the microcentrifuge tube.
- Air dry the DNA pellet for at least 15 minutes. Air drying removes any residual alcohol, which will interfere with any subsequent analyses.
- Add 100 μL of hydration solution to the pellet and place the microcentrifuge tube in a water bath at 65°C for 1 hour or incubate overnight at room temperature.
- The DNA from *E. coli* is now ready to use.

    Isolated DNA may subject to any one of the following technique for characterization.
    - Amplification by the polymerase chain reaction
    - Quantitation by spectrophotometry
    - Quantitation by gel electrophoresis
    - Restriction fragment length polymorphism analysis
    - Southern blotting

Result.

Isolated DNA is estimated by making use of diphenylamine method and are separated using agarose gel electrophoresis.

Viva questions

How might you optimize the purity of DNA

Why must you handle DNA gently in this extraction procedure?

What are the importance of DNA isolation?

What are DNA. Mention its types?

What are the principles of DNA isolation?

Mention uses of alcohol in DNA isolation.

What is the need of cell lysis in DNA isolation?

What are the action of lysozyme in DNA isolation?

How Acetate purify DNA during DNA isolation?

What are the chemicals needed for DNA isolation?

Spotters: EDTA, Lysozyme, SDS, Sodium acetate, Tris

118. Isolation of chromosomal DNA from Goat Liver

Aim

To isolate genomic DNA from goat liver

Principle

DNA can be isolated from cells and tissues by high salt or phenol extraction. Here, chromatin and proteins are dissociated by treatment with SDS. The proteins are denatured by phenyl chloroform treatment. It becomes insoluble and can be prepared by different types of chemicals.

Materials required

Ethanol, Saline EDTA-pH-8.0 (0.9% NaCl and 0.01 M EDTA), 10% SDS, 80% phenol, 95% ethanol, liver tissue, conical flask, chloroform, iso amyl alcohol etc.,

Procedure

- Homogenize 2.5g of liver tissue in 25mL of saline EDTA and transferred to a 250mL conical flask.
- Add 2.5mL of 10% SDS and 2.5mL of 80% phenol and shaken well for 10 minutes.
- Centrifuge the mixture at 10000 rpm for 10 minutes and separate the aqueous layer and transfer to fresh centrifuge tubes and add equal volume of chloroform, isoamyl alcohol (24 : 1) to interphase and phenol phase and shaken for 25 minutes.
- Centrifuge at 10000 rpm for 10 minutes.
- Collect the aqueous phase.
- Add equal volume of 80% phenol and again centrifuge at 10000 rpm for 10 minutes.
- Add 95% ice cold ethanol and shake the flask gently.
- Centifuge at 15,000 rpm for 15 minutes
- Collect the DNA as a white pellet.

Result

By the addition of ice-cold ethanol, DNA strands are obtained as a white mass or turbidity.

Spotters

EDTA, SDS, Phenol, Alcohol

Viva questions

What is the role of phenol in DNA isolation?

How SDS removes lipid-containing parts from the cell?

Indicate the uses of alcohol in DNA isolation

119. Isolation of chromosomal DNA from Human Peripheral Blood

Aim

To isolate chromosomal DNA from human blood

Background information

Peripheral blood is obtained from the circulation remote from the heart; the blood in the systemic circulation. Peripheral blood cells are the cellular components of blood, consisting of red blood cells, white blood cells, and platelets, which are found within the circulating pool of blood and not sequestered within the lymphatic system, spleen, liver, or bone marrow.

Materials required

10x RBC Lysis Buffer

Ammonium chloride	-89.9g
Potassium carbonate	-10.0g
0.5 M EDTA	- 2.0mL

Dissolve the above in approximately 800mL double distilled water and adjust pH to 7.3 and make up to 1 liter.

Nucleic Acid Lysis Buffer

TRIS Base (10 mM)	- 1.21g
NaCl (400mM)	- 23.4g
Na_2EDTA (2 mM)	- 0.75g
SDS (0.7%)	- 7.0g
Distilled water	- 1000mL

Proteinase-K - Dilute to 10mG/mL by adding 10mL of double distilled water containing 10% glycerol.

Saturated NaCl Solution - Add approximately 350 to 400 g of NaCl to 1 liter of double distilled water

Other Reagents Needed

100% Ethanol

70% Ethanol

IX TE Buffer (10mM Tris pH 8 & 1mm EDTA)

Procedure

- Collect 1mL peripheral blood and Transfer contents to 10mL polypropylene conical centrifuge tube.
- Bring volume to 10mL with RBC Lysis Buffer.
- Let stand at room temperature for 10 to 15 minutes.
- Centrifuge at 1500 rpm for 10 minutes in a 4°C centrifuge.
- Carefully decant supernatant.
- Add 1.5mL of Nucleic Acid Lysis Buffer and gently vortex.
- Add 100µL of Proteinase-K and pulse vortex until the pellet is loose and dissociated.
- Incubate the sample at 37°C for 48 hours.
- Add 0.5mL of saturated NaCl solution and gently, but completely, mix.
- Let the sample stand at 4°C for 10 minutes.
- Centrifuge at 4°C for 10 minutes at 2500rpm.
- Take fresh centrifuge tube add 4mL of ice-cold 100% ethanol (EtOH).
- Very carefully transfer the supernatant to tube containing the EtOH. Avoid collecting any of the precipitated protein.

- Allow the sample to stand upright at room temperature until the emergence of the precipitated DNA. This will have the appearance of a translucent white "slime" that is almost neutrally buoyant.
- Use a clean plastic disposable inoculation loop to lift the precipitated DNA from the 10mL tube and transfer to the 1.5mL micro centrifuge tube.
- Using the same inoculation loop, gently press out most of the remaining ethylalcohol from the DNA pellet.
- Decant/remove the ethylalcohol from the bottom of the micro centrifuge tube containing the DNA.
- Wash the DNA pellet with 1mL of ice-cold 70% EtOH.
- Pellet in a micro centrifuge for 2 minutes at 15000rpm.
- Decant the supernatant.
- Carefully remove any remaining ethylalcohol from the DNA tube.
- Allow pellet to air dry for 10 to 15 minutes.
- Depending on the size of the pellet, add 300 to 400µL of TE buffer to the pellet.
- Allow sample to dissolve at room temperature for the remainder of the day, and then place in a refrigerator overnight.
- If pellet is still not dissolved, place at 37 to 55°C for one hour.
- Quantify DNA by taking an OD260 reading or diphenylamine method or agarose gel electrophoresis.

Observation and result

White mass of DNA is observed and is subjected to analysis

Spotters

RBC lysis buffer, Nucleic acid lisis buffer, proteinase, sodium chloride, alcohol.

Viva questions

What are the major principles involved in DNA isolation?

What is the end use of isolated DNA?

120. Isolation of chromosomal DNA from plants

Aim

To isolate genomic DNA from plant materials

Background information

The search for a more efficient means of extracting DNA of both higher quality and yield has lead to the development of a variety of protocols, however the fundamentals of DNA extraction remains the same. DNA must be purified from cellular material in a manner that prevents degradation. Because of this, even crude extraction procedures can still be adopted to prepare a sufficient amount of DNA to allow for multiple end uses. DNA extraction from plant tissue can vary depending on the material used. Essentially any mechanical means of breaking down the cell wall and membranes to allow access to nuclear material, without its degradation is required. For this, usually an initial grinding stage with liquid nitrogen is employed to break down cell wall material and allow access to DNA while harmful cellular enzymes and chemicals remain inactivated. Once the tissue has been sufficiently ground, it can then be resuspended in a suitable buffer, such as CTAB. In order to purify DNA, insoluble particulates are removed through centrifugation while soluble proteins and other material are separated through mixing with chloroform and centrifugation. DNA must then be precipitated from the aqueous phase and washed thoroughly to remove contaminating salts. The purified DNA is then resuspended and stored in TE buffer or sterile distilled water. This method has been shown to give intact genomic DNA from plant tissue. To check the quality of the extracted DNA, a sample is run on an agarose gel, stained with ethidium bromide, and visualised under UV light.

Materials required

CTAB buffer, Microfuge tubes, Mortar and Pestle, Liquid Nitrogen, Microfuge, Absolute Ethanol (ice cold), 70 % Ethanol (ice cold), 7.5 M Ammonium Acetate, water bath, Chloroform:Iso Amyl Alcohol (24:1), Water (sterile), RNase water (10µG/mL).

CTAB buffer

CTAB (Hexadecyl trimethyl-ammonium bromide)	- 2.0 g
1 M Tries pH 8.0	- 10.0mL
0.5 M Na₂EDTA pH 8.0	- 4.0mL
5 M NaCl	- 28.0mL
Distilled water	- 40.0mL
PVP 40 (Polyvinyl pyrrolidone)	– 1g

Adjust all to pH 5.0 with HCL and make up to 100mL with distilled water.

Procedure

- Grind 200mG of plant tissue to a fine paste in approximately 500µL of CTAB buffer.
- Transfer CTAB/plant extract mixture to a microfuge tube.
- Incubate the CTAB/plant extract mixture for about 15 min at 55°C in a water bath.
- After incubation, spin the CTAB/plant extract mixture at 10000rpm for 5 min to spin down cell debris. Transfer the supernatant to clean microfuge tubes.
- To each tube add 250µL of Chloroform : Iso Amyl Alcohol (24:1) and mix the solution by inversion. After mixing, spin the tubes at 13000 rpm for 1 min.
- Transfer the upper aqueous phase only (contains the DNA) to a clean microfuge tube.
- Add 50µL of 7.5 M Ammonium Acetate followed by 500µL of ice-cold absolute ethanol.
- Invert the tubes slowly several times to precipitate the DNA. Generally the DNA can be seen to precipitate out of solution (Alternatively the tubes can be placed for 1 hr at -20°C after the addition of ethanol to precipitate the DNA).
- Following precipitation, the DNA can be pipetted off by slowly rotating/spinning a tip in the cold solution. The precipitated DNA sticks to the pipette and visible as a clear thick precipitate. To wash the DNA, transfer the precipitate into a microfuge tube containing 500µL of ice cold 70% ethanol and slowly invert the tube (alternatively the precipitate can be isolated by spinning the tube at 13000 rpm for a minute to form a pellet. Remove the supernatant and wash the DNA pellet by adding two changes of ice cold 70% ethanol).
- After the wash, spin the DNA into a pellet by centrifuging at 13000 rpm for 1 min.
- Remove all the supernatant and allow the DNA pellet to dry (approximately 15 min-Do not allow the DNA to over dry or it will be hard to re-dissolve).

- Resuspend the DNA in sterile DNase free RNase water (approximately 50-400μL H_2O; the amount of water needed to dissolve the DNA can vary, depending on how much is isolated). RNaseA (10μG/mL) can be added to the water prior to dissolving the DNA to remove any RNA in the preparation.

- After resuspension, incubate the DNA at 65°C for 20 min to destroy any DNases that may be present and store at 4°C.

- Agarose gel electrophoresis of the DNA will show the integrity of the DNA, while spectrophotometry will give an indication of the concentration and cleanliness.

Observation

White mass of DNA is isolated & separated using agarose gel electrophoresis.

Spotters

CTAB, Iso amyl alcohol, chloroform.

Viva questions

What is the role of centrifugation in DNA isolation?

What are the roles of CTAB in DNA extraction?

121. Isolation of RNA from Human Blood

Aim

To isolate RNA from human blood

Background information

RNA is found in the nucleus and cytoplasm of cells; it plays an important role in protein synthesis and other chemical activities of the cell. The structure of RNA is similar to that of DNA. There are several classes of RNA. They are mRNA, tRNA and rRNA. Messenger RNA (mRNA) is the RNA that carries information from DNA to the ribosome, the sites of protein synthesis (translation) in the cell. The most prominent examples of non-coding RNAs are transfer RNA (tRNA) and ribosomal RNA (rRNA), both of which are involved in the process of translation. There are also non-coding RNAs involved in gene regulation, RNA processing and other roles. Certain RNAs are able to catalyse chemical reactions such as cutting and ligating other RNA molecules and the catalysis of peptide bond formation in the ribosome; these are known as ribozymes. Severo Ochoa won the 1959 Nobel Prize in Medicine after he discovered how RNA is synthesized.

RNA extraction is the purification of RNA from biological samples. This procedure is complicated by the ubiquitous presence of ribonuclease enzymes in cells and tissues, which can rapidly degrade RNA. Several methods are used in molecular biology to isolate RNA from samples, the most common of these is Guanidinium thiocyanate-phenol-chloroform extraction. This method often uses a proprietary formulation of this reagent called Trizol. Trizol is a combination of phenol and Guanidinium thiocyanate. Guanidinium thiocyanate denatures proteins, including RNases, and separates rRNA from ribosomes, while phenol, isopropanol and water are solvents with poor miscibility. In the presence of chloroform or BCP (bromochloropropane), these solvents separate entirely into two phases that are recognized by their colour: a clear, upper aqueous phase (containing the nucleic acids) and a bright pink lower phase (containing the proteins dissolved in phenol and the lipids dissolved in chloroform). Other denaturing chemicals such as 2-mercaptoethanol and sarcosine may also be used.

Materials required

Polypropelene centrifuge tubes, centrifuge, phosphate buffered saline, TE buffer (See Page 334) Trizol, Chloroform, isopropanol etc.,

10x RBC Lysis Buffer

Ammonium chloride	-89.9 g
Potassium carbonate	-10.0 g
0.5 M EDTA	- 2.0mL

Dissolve the above in approximately 800mL double distilled water and adjust pH to 7.3. and make up to 1 liter.

Procedure

- Collect 1mL of blood and transfer content of tube into a 10mL polypropylene conical centrifuge tube.
- Bring volume to 5mL with RBC Lysis Buffer, mix gently.
- Let stand at room temperature for 10 to 15 minutes or at 4°C for 20 to 30 minutes.
- Pellet cells at 1500 rpm for 10 minutes in a 4°C centrifuge.
- Carefully decant supernatant.
- Gently resuspend the pellet in 0.1mL of RBC Lysis Buffer and transfer to a 1.5mL micro centrifuge tube. Let stand at 4°C for 2 to 5 minutes (RBC Lysis).
- Centrifuge for 2 minutes by centrifuging at 4°C in a microfuge at 3000 rpm. Carefully aspirate the supernatant (If the resulting pellet is still red, repeat the RBC lysis as needed).
- Resuspend the pellet in 0.1mL of ice-cold PBS.
- Centrifuge for 2 minutes by centrifuging at 4°C in a microfuge at 3000 rpm. Carefully aspirate the supernatant.
- Resuspend pellet in 100µL ice-cold PBS, add 0.1mL Trizol and shake vigorously for 1min and wait 5 min at RT. Samples can be stored at -80°C at this step.
- Add 200µL Chloroform per tube, shake vigorously by hand for 15 sec, wait 3 min.
- Spin 15 min at full speed at 4°C.
- Transfer colorless phase into new 1.5mL tube. Avoid touching the interphase (there sits the DNA). Add 500µL isopropanol, wait 10 min at RT.
- Spin 10 min at full speed at 4°C.
- Wash pellet once with 1mL 75% ethanol.
- Spin 10 min at full speed at 4°C.
- Remove supernatant completely, let the pellet dry for 5 min at room temperature (tube stays open)
- Redissolve pellet in 25µL water.
- Take 1µL, dilute 1:100 in TE, measure UV absorbance 260/280 nm or estimate RNA by orcinol method or detect using electrophoresis.

Observation and results

RNA pellet may be noted and is subjected for estimation

Spotters

RNA (mRNA, tRNA) structure, PBS

Viva questions

What is the importance of RNA?
How do you detect RNA in solution?

122. Isolation of Plasmid DNA (Alkaline Lysis Method)

Aim

To isolate plasmid DNA from the given culture.

Principle

Plasmids are extra chromosomal covalently closed, autonomously replicating DNA elements, present mostly in bacteria. They are known to carry gene specifying resistance to antibiotics and also several other selectable marker genes. Certain Plasmids are present high copy number in a cell (relaxed type) and others are found in low copies (stringent Plasmids). Certain Plasmids could be amplified in copy number by challenging the host cell with high concentration of antibiotics. Plasmids are widely using as a vector to carry gene of interest between different organism. Plasmids are the corner stone in molecular biology without which extensive work in recombinant DNA technology could not have been done. Isolation of Plasmids from host cell involves washing of cells, breaking open the cell wall and the membrane and removal of unwanted proteins, chromosomal DNA and cell wall particles. Large-scale isolation procedure and mini preparation protocols are available in plenty.

Materials Required

Solution A:

23mM trisHcl	-30.3mG
50mM glucose	-90mG
Lysozyme	-100mG
Water	-10mL

Solution B

0.2 M sodium hydroxide	-0.8g
1%SDS	-1g
Water	-100mL

Solution C

3M sodium acetate (pH 4.8)	-24.6g
Water	-1000mL

Adjust pH with glacial acetic acid and make the volume
Solution D

50mM trisHcl	-0.6g
100mM sodium acetate	-8.2g
Water	-100mL

Isoamylalcohol -3 methyl 1 butanol $(CH_3)_2 CHCH_2CH_2OH$.

Ethanol- CH_3CH_2OH-DNA gets precipitated when treated with ethanol.

Saline citrate -   Preserve DNA

Isopropyl alcohol - Denatures ethyl alcohol

Sodium acetate - The DNA gets stabilized in this for several months.

Procedure

- Transfer 1mL of an overnight culture in to an eppendoff tube.

- Sediment the cells by centrifuging at 5000 rpm for 10 minutes. Drain off excess fluid.

- Resuspend the cells in 100 μL solution A. Incubate on ice for 30 minutes.

- Add 200μL of freshly prepared solution B. Vortex briefly and keep on ice for 5 minutes. The cells will lyse immediately and the solutions become viscous.

- Add 150μL of solution C. Vortex briefly and keep on ice for 60 minutes. The bulk of chromosomal DNA and cell materials will precipitate into a white viscous clump.

- Cell material present along with chromosomal DNA can be separated by means of centrifugation at 5000rpm for 10 minutes.

- Transfer this supernatent to fresh eppendoff tube and add 1.5mL 100% alcohol and incubate for 30 minutes. Centrifuge at 15,000rpm for 10 minutes. Collect plasmid DNA as pellet.

Observation and Result

Plasmid DNA pellet is observed and is subjected to estimation and separation.

Viva questions

How do you preserve DNA/ Plasmid?
What are the difference between plasmid & chromosomal DNA?
Mention different uses of chemicals in plasmid DNA isolation.

123. Restriction digestion of DNA

Aim

To digest the given DNA sample with the chosen Restriction Endonuclease and check the fragments.

Principle

One of the basic requirements for the cloning technique is to open up the target DNA. This can be done by mechanical means such as sonication etc., but these physical means are less preferred as they would yield DNA fragments with unknown ends. Hence in cloning procedures restriction procedures are used. Among three restriction endonucleases, type II are preferred owing to their specificity in restriction digestion sequence.

In this experiment, DNA with 48,58bp is digested with Hind III restriction endonuclease, which is derived from *Haemophillus influenzae*. This enzyme recognizes AAGCTT base sequence in both strands and nicks in-between A and A in both strands. A Hind III digested l DNA yielding 8 fragments.

Materials required

Conical flask, Eppendoff tubes, Micropipettes, Vortex mixture, Electrophoretic apparatus, Agarose gel, Lamda DNA, Lambda DNA Hind III digest, HindIII, 10x Assay buffer, Double distilled water, 0.5M EDTA, Gel loading buffer, Ethidium bromide, TAE buffer. (Refer Page 345).

Assay buffer (500mm KCl, 100mm Tris Hcl & 15 mm mgcl$_2$)

Procedure

In eppendoff tube the following components are added in the same order at the specific concentration

DNA	-10μL
Double distilled water	-7μL
10x buffer	-2μL
Hind III	-1μL
Final volume	-20μL

- Incubate at 37 ° C for one hour
- Stop the reaction by adding 0.5M EDTA (pH-8) to the final concentration of 10mM.
- Add 5μL of tracking dye and run electrophoresis on 0.7% agarose gel.

Observation Result And Discussion

Type II restriction enzyme HinD III is used to cut DNA. It produced 4 bands, when it is separated through agarose gel electrophoresis.

Viva questions

Define restriction enzyme.

What are the types of restriction enzyme?

Why type II restriction enzyme is much important than others?

Expand Hind III, Bam H1.

What are the common properties of plasmid DNA?

Mention importance of lambda DNA, pBR 322, pUC 18?

Expand pBR and pUC.

What is single digestion and double digestion?

Spotters: Plasmid picture, Hind III, Bam H1 or any restriction enzyme

124. Principles and Applications of Agarose Gel Electrophoresis

Aim

To know the principles and applications of agarose gel electrophoresis

To separate nucleic acids from the crude extract.

Principle

Electrophoresis is a migration of charged particles under the influence of an electric field. Electrophoresis is a Greek word, which means born by electricity. Alexander Reuss made the first electrophoresis observation in 1807. Movement or velocity of molecule in electrophoresis can be expressed as,

$$V = \mu \times E$$

V= velocity of the molecule

μ= Electrophoretic mobility

E= electrical field strength.

Velocity of the molecule in electrophoresis is directly proportional to its mobility and electrical field strength.

Electrophoretic mobility of a molecule in electrophoresis is depend on charge, pore size, buffer, pH, ion strength, temperature of the medium and shape of the molecule.

In addition, movement of a molecule in electrophoresis is also affected by Electro endosmosis. Cations (+) present in electrophoretic media and on surface cause a bulk liquid flow towards cathode. This opposite movement of fluid is some times called as electroendosmosis.

Application of gel

The most popular method to separate, identify and purify nucleic acid fragments is electrophoresis through agarose gel. This technique is simple, rapid and capable of dissolving fragments that cannot be done by other means like density gradient centrifugation. DNA or RNA fragments separated during electrophoresis process can be located in the gel directely by staining. Ethidium bromide, an intercalating fluoresent dye binds with DNA, when are examined under UV transilluminator, give fluoresent bands. By this method, DNA fragments whose concentration in gel , as little as few nanograms can be detected.

The mobility of DNA in gel depends on sevaral parameters. They are, Size of the DNA molecule, Concentration of the gel, Configuration of the molecule, temperature and Electrical parameters.

Characters of agarose gel

Agarose is one of the electrophoresis solid support. Is is a purified product from agar agar. It is a polysaccharide of repeating beta galacto pyranose and 3,6-anhydro α, L galacto pyranose residues. The impurities such as sulphate, methoxyl, pyruvate and carboxyl groups are minimised to a greater extent described to have very high gel strength and medium or low electro endosmosis. Agarose dissolves in water on boiling and form a gel when cooling. The fact that the agarose gel is easy to prepare, nontoxic, optically clear, chemically inert and has large pores. It fulfils virtually the most of the requirements of a good supporting media for electrophoresis.

Materials Required

Sample: Nucleic acid

Requirement: Electrophoretic apparatus, Agarose, Gel loading buffer(TAE buffer 50x)

TAE buffer : (Electrophoresis running buffer)

Tris	-	242gM
Glacial acetic acid	-	57.1mL
0.5M EDTA (pH -8)	-	100mL

Make up the volume to 1 lit using distilled water . If TBE, replace glacial acetic with boric acid.

Gel tracking dye composition:

1X TAE buffer	-	10mL
Glycerol	-	3mL
Bromothymol blue (0.025%)	-	25mL

Ethidium bromide:

Stock	-	100μG/mL
Working concentration	-	200μg/mL

Ethidium bromide is prepared in sterile distilled water and stored in dark place. It is highly carcinogenic. Handle carefully.

UV transilluminator.

Procedure

- The nucleic acid is prepared from the given culture / Plant tissue / animal cells.

- At the same time, 0.7% agarose gel is prepared.

- It is prepared as follows; 280mG of agarose powder is weighed and put in a 100mL of dry flask and Add 40mL of 1x TAE buffer. Heated the slurry in a boiling water bath until the agarose dissolves & the solution becomes clear.

- Allow the solution to 50^{0}C and Add 0.2 μg / mL of Ethidium Bromide.

- Seal the open sides of the gel platforms with cellotapes and placed it on a leveled table.

- Pour the gel solution to the platform and placed the well forming comb in the slot.

- Left the assembly undisturbed at room temperature for 30-45min to set.
- Carefully taken out the comb and removed the cellotape.
- Place the gel platform on the bed of the electrophoresis tank. Pour the running buffer to cover the gel to a depth of about 1mm.
- Take 20µL DNA sample and add 20µL gel loading dye.
- Load about 10.mL sample into wells using gel loading tips . Because of the density of the gel-loading buffer, the samples settle down into the well.
- Connect the Electrophoretic apparatus with power pack. Then started to run at constant voltage mode. (Continued running till the bromothymol blue is about 0.5 cm close to the end of the gel.)
- After running, Disconnect the apparatus and examined nucleic acid bands through UV Trans illuminator.

Observation and result

DNA and Plasmid crude isolates are separated and detected using ethidium bromide staining. Only one band is noted on gel under UV trans illuminator.

Viva questions

Mention properties of Agarose.

What is electrophoresis?

What are the principles of electrophoresis?

Mention different types of electrophoresis.

What are the uses of ethidium Bromide DNA separation?

How Ethydium bromide binds to DNA? Mention its principle.

Have you used agarose or agar in gel electrophoresis of DNA?

Why you are using gel loading dye in DNA gel electrophoresis?

What are the factors associated with nucleic acid mobility in electrophoresis?

What are the purposes of using buffer in electrophoresis unit?

Spotters: Agarose, TAE, Ethidium Bromide, Electrophoresis unit

125. Elution of DNA

Aim

To retrieve and purify any specific DNA fragment from an agarose gel slice; the expected yield is from 50%–75% of the amount in the gel slice.

To isolate specific bands or regions of agarose-separated DNA for use in subsequent experiments and/or procedures.

Background information

There are many methods for eluting DNA from a piece of agarose. They are electroelution, DEAE cellulose method, and optimized freeze-squeeze (OFS) method. OFS method has several advantages over these others. First, it is not as confused as the others, which is desirable when you are working with small amounts of DNA or where ethidium bromide is used. Second, it is very simple and fast to perform. Third, the yields of DNA are excellent. When small fragments are eluted (less than 5 kb) from 80-95% can be recovered. Even lambda DNA (at 50 kb) can be recovered in yields up to 50%. Fourth, the DNA is excellent shape after precipitation. With some methods of elution, there is a significant amount of degradation of the DNA. With this method, even lambda-sized pieces can be obtained with little or no apparent damage.

Materials required

pBR325 DNA (500 ng/d), 10X Assay buffer (Ref. Page 343), EcoRI, pGEM3Z DNA (500 ng), DNA, Yeast tRNA (as a carrier) - 10 mg/ml, 95% Ethanol, 80% Ethanol

Elution Buffer

0.5 M sodium acetate (pH 7.0)

1 mM EDTA (pH 8.0)

0.1X TE:

1 mM Tris (pH 8.0)

0.1 mM EDTA (pH 8.0)

Procedure

Restriction digestion - Refer Experiment No 123

Restriction, separation, Elution and liagtion are a processs of cloning experiment. Digest 1pg of pBR325, and 1-2 pg of each DNA that is to be ligated to the pBR325, each separately with EcoRI as follows:

I. 2 μL pBR325 DNA (500 ng/d)

    6 μL H20

    1 μL 10X Assay buffer

    1 μL EcoRI

II. 2 μL pGEM3Z DNA (500 ng/d)

    6 μL H20

    1 μL 10X Assay buffer

    1 μL EcoRI

III. 8 μL of DNA + H20

    1 μL 10X Assay buffer

    1 μL EcoRI

Generally, a 0.8% Agarose gel will provide sufficient separation for most digested fragments. Increase agarose to 1.2% to isolate small fragments of 100 to 500 base pairs, decrease agarose to 0.6% for fragments larger than 8 KB.

Separation : **Separate** restricted DNA and Plasmid using agarose gel electrophoresis (Ref. expt. 124)

Elution

●   Take a picture of the gel.

- Carefully cut around the band (trying not to scratch the tray beneath the gel). Also, cut around the DNA that will be eluted from the other lanes. The gel pieces should be the width of the lane and no more than about a centimeter wide in other direction. [If you want to test the difference in ligation and transformation efficiency between larger fragments and smaller fragments, cut some of the lanes in halves (or smaller pieces) according to molecular weight.]

- Carefully transfer the gel pieces into separate 1.5mL microfuge tubes using flat spatulas and/or forceps (don't use fine forceps or you will damage the gel slices). Label the tubes accordingly.

- Add 1.5mL elution buffer until the level of the buffer is a few millimeters above the level of the gel slice. Heat in a 65°C water bath until the agarose melts (about 5 minutes).

- Fast-freeze by placing in a -70°C freezer for 10 minutes.

- Immediately (i.e., before the solution can thaw) centrifuge for 10 minutes.

- Transfer the supernatant into a new tube.

- Add 0.8mL fresh elution buffer to the pellet.

- Heat in a 65°C water bath until the pellet melts (about 5 minutes).

- Fast-freeze by placing in a -70°C freezer for 10 minutes.

- Immediately (i.e., before the solution can thaw) centrifuge for 10 minutes.

- Pool the supernatants with the supernatant from previous steps (discard the tube containing the pellet).

- Add an equal volume of 1-butanol to the supernatant fraction and mix thoroughly. Then, place the tube onto the Shaker for 15 minutes (this will remove the ethidium bromide from the DNA). Discard the top (butanol) phase and repeat with new 1-butanol one or two more times.

- Add 50µG of yeast tRNA and mix thoroughly.

- Add 2.5 volumes of cold 95% ethanol and mix gently. Allow to precipitate at -70°C for 30 minutes or more. Overnight is best.

- Centrifuge for 15 minutes.

- Decant off and discard the supernatant and add 200µL of cold 80% ethanol to the pellet. Mix until the pellet is dislodged from the bottom of the tube.

- Centrifuge for 5 minutes. Decant off and discard the supernatant.

- Dry the pellet in the Speed-Vac.

- Rehydrate the DNA pellets in 20µL of 0.1X TE.

- If there is any remaining debris in the tube, spin for 30 seconds and transfer the supernatant into a new microfuge tube (either 1.5mL or 0.5mL).

- To confirm the recovery of the DNA, run 1 of each sample on a standard gel (0.6-0.7%) and calculate the percent recovered.

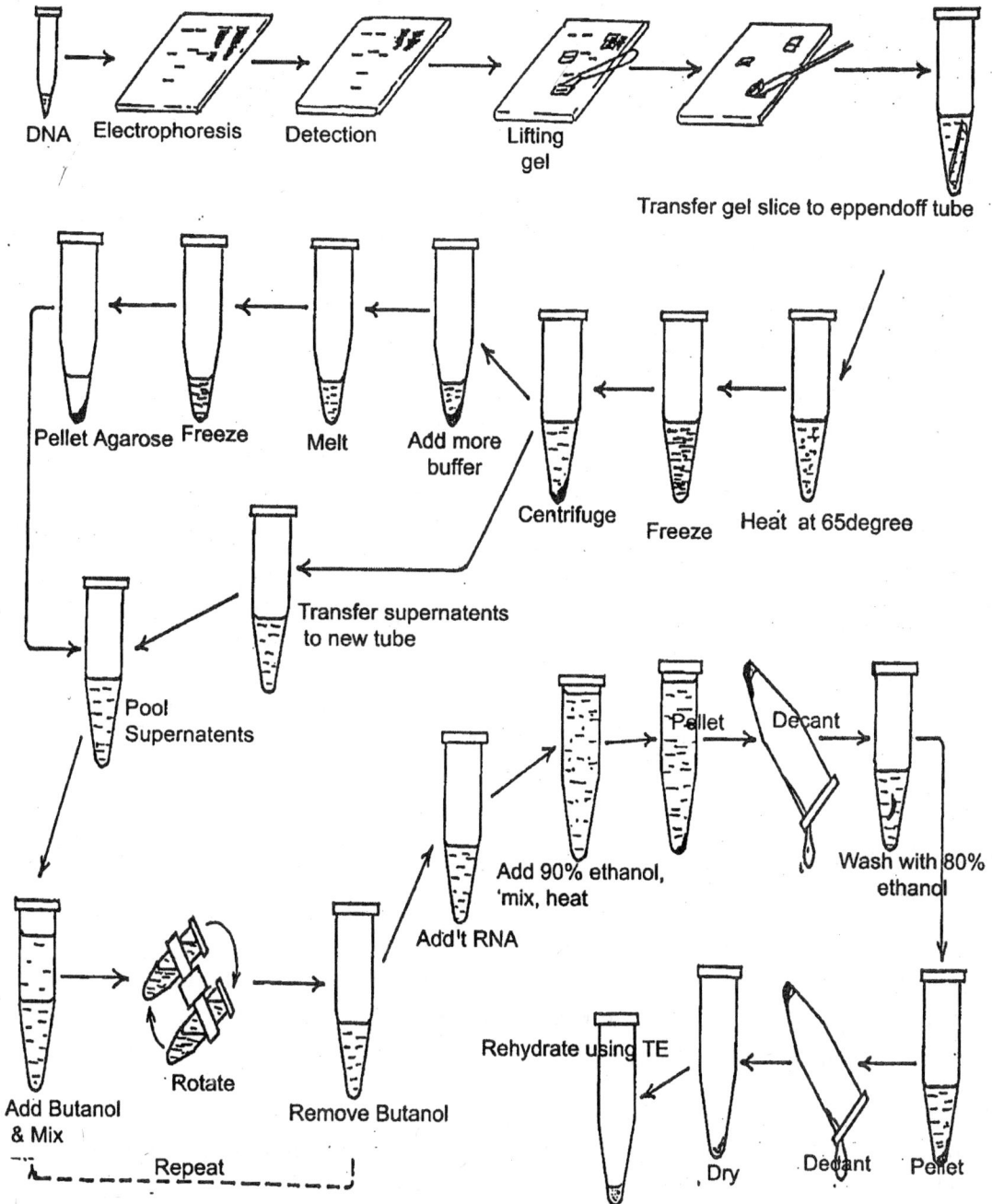

Fig 125.1 – Elution of DNA

Observation and results

DNA of interest available as a pellet.

Spotters

TAE, Agarose, Restriction enzyme, chloroform.

Viva questions

How do you cut plasmid DNA?

What is restriction endonuclease?

How do you purify DNA from gel?

126. Ligation of Insert DNA to Vector DNA

Aim

To ligate target DNA into the vector.

Background information

DNA cloning requires the DNA sequence of interest to be inserted in a vector DNA molecule. For this, both the vector as well as insert DNA is prepared by digestion with compatible restriction enzymes, so that the ends produced during digestion is complementary in both. When setting up ligation, it is important to consider the permutations that can occur and bias the relative concentration of DNA accordingly. Usually a 5- to 10-fold excess of insert over the vector DNA is the norm. This ensures that enough ligated product will be produced in the right orientation.

Materials required

Vector digest, Insert DNA, T4 DNA ligase, Ligation buffer (50mM Tris-HCI, 10 mM MgCI2, 20 mM DTT, 1 mM ATP, 50/mG/mL), Nuclease-free BSA, (Bovine Serum Albumin.) pH7.4

Procedure

Set up ligation in 0.5mL microfuge tubes as follows:

- ☐ Vector digest (DH5./L).   -   10μL
- ☐ Insert DNA.   -   20μL
- ☐ Ligation buffer.   -   60μL
- ☐ Ligase.   -   10μL

- • Mix well by flicking the tube.
- • Spin briefly in a microfuge to push all the liquid to the bottom of the tube. Incubate at 16°C overnight.
- • Stop the reaction by placing it at 70°C for 10 minutes.
- • Run an aliquot on a minigel and verify.

Observation

Run aliquots of ligated DNA side by side with unligated DNA to minimize and observe the difference. Being circular ligated plasmid DNA will tend to run faster than unligated plasmid DNA.

Spotters

Ligation buffer, ligase, DNA vector / plasmid.

Viva questions

Define ligation and ligase

What are the importances of ligation?

127. Polymerase Chain Reaction

Aim

To amplify the given sample of DNA using PCR.

Principle

Polymerase chain reaction (PCR) is a very simple method for *in vitro* DNA amplification using Taq polymerase. This technique involves DNA synthesis in 3 simple steps.

Step 1. Denaturation of the template into single strands.

Step 2. Annealing of primers to the template.

Step 3. Extension of new DNA.

Materials required

Millique water or autoclaved double-distilled water, sterile microfuge (0.2mL), 10 X Taq polymerase assay buffer with $MgCl_2$, or NTP mix solution, template DNA, forward and reverse primers, Taq DNA polymerase enzyme, sterile mineral oil, and a PCR machine.

1. *DNA template:* Between 1 and 5ng of cloned DNA or between 40 and 100ng of genomic DNA should be used per reaction. It is convenient to dilute template stocks to an appropriate concentration, e.g., 5ng/mL in dH_2O for cloned DNA.

2. *Primers:* Primers should be prepared by butanol extraction and resuspended in dH_2O at 100ng/mL. Each primer should be used at ~100ng per reaction.

3. *Buffer:* Buffer should be prepared as a (10X stock. 10X PCR buffer: 100 mM Tris. HCl pH 8.3, 500mM KCl, 15mM $MgCl_2$. This buffer can be prepared containing 0.1% gelatin).

4. *Taq DNA polymerase:* Taq should be used at 2.5U per reaction.

5. *Magnesium:* Extra magnesium can be added to the PCR reaction. If using the buffer above, a final $Mg2+$ concentration of 1.5 mM will be obtained. If necessary, magnesium can be titrated to obtain an optimal concentration. Suggested concentrations for this would be 1.5, 3.0, 4.5, 6.0 and 10 mM. Magnesium can be prepared as $MgCl_2$ at 25 mM and autoclaved. Increasing the magnesium concentration has the same effect as lowering the annealing temperature.

6. *Nucleotides:* dNTPs should be prepared from 100-mM commercial stocks as a 10X stock at 2 mM each dNTP. This is most easily done by adding 2mL of each dNTP to 92mL $dH2O$ in an eppendoff.

7. *Water:* Water should be autoclaved and used solely for PCR. Milli-Q water is fine for PCR or "water for injection" if the distilled water is in doubt. It can be aliquotted into 1mL volumes and kept separate from DNA and other sources of contamination. Each aliquot should be discarded following a single use.

8. *Paraffin oil:* In some instruments, paraffin oil must be added to prevent evaporation of the sample.

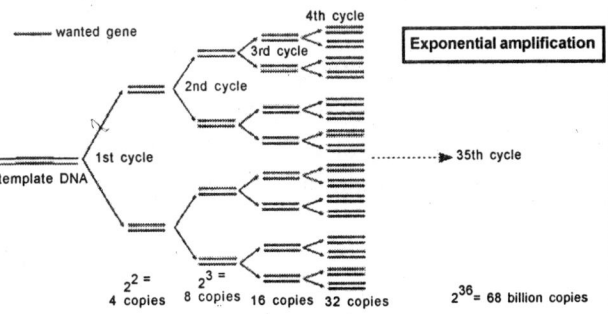

Fig. 127.1 - PCR - Amplification

Procedure

- Add 38µL of sterile millique water (or autoclaved double distilled water) to a sterile eppendoff tubes.
- Add 5µL of 10 X Taq polymerase assay buffer with $MgCl_2$ to the microfuge.
- Add 3µL of 2.5 mm dNTP mixed solution to the eppendoff tube.
- Add 1µL of control template DNA.
- Add 1 mol each of forward and reverse primers.
- Add 1–2 units (0.5–0.7µL) of Taq DNA polymerase.
- Gently mix.
- Layer the reaction mixture with 50 µL of mineral oil to avoid evaporation.
- Carry out the amplification using the following reaction conditions:
  - Initial denaturation at 94°C for 1 min.
  - Denaturation at 94°C for 30 sec.
  - Annealing at 48°C for 30 sec.
  - Extension at 72°C for 1 min.
  - Final extension at 72°C for 2 min.

Result

.The DNA will be amplified.

Spotters

PCR picture, PCR machine, Taq polymerase, Ligase.

Viva questions

What are the principles of DNA amplification?

Who invented PCR?

What is primer?

128. Southern Blotting

Aim

To blot and confirm the availability of known or unknown DNA.

To know the presence or absence of a particular fragment in genomic DNA

Background information

E. D. Southern first developed this method in 1975. The advent of Southern blotting technique was a turning point in the field of molecular biology. It involves the capillary transfer of DNA fragments from an agarose gel to various types of membranes. Restriction Fragment Length Polymorphisms can be analyzed using the technique, wherein DNA fragments are separated on agarose gels denatured in situ and transferred onto membranes for analysis.

Materials required

Denaturation solution: 1.5 M NaCl, and 0.5 M NaOH,

Neutralization solution: 1.5 M NaCl,; 0.5 M Tris-Cl (pH 7.5), and 1 mM EDTA (pH 8.0),

20xSSPE preparation

Take 600mL Water in conical flask

Add 175.3g sodium chloride, 27.6g sodium phosphate monobasic and 9.4g EDTA

Add NaOH to pH 7.4 (~27mL/liter of 10N NaOH)

Add H_2O to bring final volume to 1 Liter and sterilize at 121^0C for 20 minutes

Depurinization solution: 0.25 N HCl

Nylon or nitrocellulose membrane

Prehybridization buffer (per 1mL)

20 x SSPE	0.3mL
Dry milk	5mG
10% SDS	50µL
Denatured carrier DNA	10µL (100mG/mL)
ddH2O	0.64mL

Hybridization buffer

Denature multi-prime labeled probe ($1 \times 108 \sim 1 \times 10^9$cpm/ µG) in boiling water bath for 5min and cool on ice-water bath. Add the probe to the prehybridization buffer.

Procedure

- Select the target DNA.

- Digest the DNA using required restriction enzyme.

- Electrophorese the restricted DNA using agarose gel.

- After agarose gel electrophoresis, photograph the gel and soak it in 0.25 N HCl for 15 minutes at room temperature, with gentle shaking (Depurination).

- Decant the acid solution and denature the DNA by soaking the gel in several volumes of denaturation solution for 30 minutes at room temperature, with constant shaking.

- Neutralize the gel by shaking in several volumes of neutralization solution for 30 minutes at room temperature, with shaking.

- Wrap a piece of Whatman 3-mm paper around a glass plate. Place the wrapped support on a large plastic tray with the ends of the 3-mm paper dipping into the 20 X SSPE solutions in tray.

- Invert the gel and place it on a damp 3-mm paper on the support. Make sure that there are no air bubbles between the 3-mm paper and the gel.

- Cut a piece of nylon membrane slightly bigger than the gel. Use gloves and forceps to handle the membrane.

- Float the membrane on 20X SSPE until it wets completely.

- Place the wet nylon membrane on top of the gel. Remove all the air bubbles that are trapped between the gel and tile membrane.

- Wet 2 pieces of Whatman 3-mm paper, cut to exactly the same size as the gel in 10X SSPE, and place them on top of the membrane. Again remove the air bubbles.
- Cut a stack of coarse filter paper just smaller than the gel size. Keep on top of the Whatman filter papers.
- Put a glass plate on the top and place (about 1 kg) on it to exert pressure.
- Allow the transfer of DNA to proceed for about 12–24 hours.
- Remove the stack of coarse filter papers and the 3-mm paper above the gel.
- Turn over the dehydrated gel and membrane and lay them gel side up on a dry sheet of 3-mm paper. Mark the position of the wells on the membrane with a soft pencil.
- Peel off the gel. The transfer can be checked by restaining the gel. If the transfer is complete, no DNA should be retained on the gel.
- Soak the membrane in 6X SSPE at room temperature for a few minutes.
- Allow excess fluid to drain off from the membrane and set it to dry at room temperature on a sheet of 3-mm paper.
- Place the dried filter between 2 sheets of 3-mm paper.
- Fix the DNA on the membrane by baking for 2 hours at 80°C under a vacuum or cross linking on a UV transilluminator for a few minutes.
- Wrap the membrane with Plastic wrap or keep it in an envelope made up of Whatman No. 1 filter paper and store.

Prehybridization

- Add 30μl of prehybridization buffer per 1cm2 of the membrane. Incubate for 1hr at 65°C.

Hybridization

- Drain excess fluid from the membrane and apply 20μL of hybridization buffer per 1cm2.
- Incubate for at least 12hr at 65°C.
- Wash the membrane in the following solutions.
  - □ 1x SSPE/0.05% SDS at room temperature for 15 min 2 changes
  - □ 1x SSPE/0.05% SDS at 65°C for 15 min 2 changes
- Remove most of the liquid from the membrane by placing on a pad of paper towels.
- Wrap the membrane with Plastic Wrap and expose to a X-ray film (Kodak XAR-2) at -70°C using a intensifying screen.

Observation

Restain the gel in ethidium bromide 5mG/mL for 45 minutes and view on a UV transilluminator after proper washings. There should not be any DNA on the gel, as the entire DNA should have been transferred to the membrane. There will be only one band in the lane. In the case of genomic DNA, a continuous smear should be visible, as digestion will result in many pieces of varying sizes.

Spotters

Southern blot setup / picture

Viva questions

What is the purpose of doing Southern blot?
How DNA from gel is transferred to membrane

129. Northern Blotting

Aim

To study gene expression by the detection of RNA (or isolated mRNA) in a sample.

Background information

Northern blot analysis allows the detection and quantification of specific RNA species from a particular cell type. Isolated RNA is electrophoresed through an agarose / formaldehyde gel which separates the RNA species by size. The faster migrating RNA fragments are the smallest, however, the distance of migration is not linear and rather it is inversely proportional to the size of RNA molecule. When RNA has separated following electrophoresis, it is stained with ethidium bromide and visualised using ultra violet light. For gels of total RNA the 28S and 18S ribosomal subunits are visible and act as convenient size markers (approx 4.8 and 1.9kb, respectively). To probe for a specific mRNA species by northern blot, it is first necessary to transfer the RNA from the agarose/formaldehyde gel to a nylon membrane. RNA is detected by hybridization using a labelled probe. The probe is a DNA or RNA molecule which is chemically or radioactively labeled.

Materials required

Stock Solutions

10X MOPS

>0.2M MOPS (42g)
>
>50mM anhydrous sodium acetate (4.1g)
>
>10mM EDTA (20mL of 0.5 M)
>
>pH to 6.5 and bring to a total volume of 1L with DEPC-treated water

RNA Sample Loading Buffer

>50mL formamide
>
>18mL formaldehyde (37%)
>
>12mL DEPC water
>
>10mL of 10X MOPS 3

10X Tracking Dye

>0.1% Bromophenol blue
>
>0.1% Xylene cyanol
>
>Dissolve in DEPC water

20X SSPE- refer page 353

TE Buffer refer page 334

Procedure

Gel Electrophoresis

- Prepare formaldehyde-agarose gel. Add 65mL of DEPC-treated water to 1.08 g of agarose and microwave until agarose dissolves completely. Allow solution to cool to 60°C, and then add 9mL of 10X MOPS and 16mL of 37% formaldehyde. Swirl to mix and pour into gel box (9 x 11 cm).

- Transfer 0.5 - 2mG of total RNA to a new tube and dry samples by speed vacuum (it is not necessary to dry).

- Resuspend dried samples in 18mL of loading buffer. Add 2mL of 10X tracking dye, 0.05mL of EtBr, and 1mL of glycerol.
- Heat RNA samples to 65°C for 10 minutes, cool on ice for ~1 minute and then do a quick spin down of the samples.
- Prepare 1XMOPS running buffer (50mL of 10X MOPS and 450mL of DW water).
- Place gel in gel box and submerge in running buffer.
- Load RNA samples onto gel and run at 30-50 V until bromophenol blue (fastest migrating of the two tracking dye bands) migrates ~ 60-75% of the total distance of the gel.

Transfer RNA from gel to nylon membrane

- Rinse gel in Distilled water 6 times, 5 minutes each. Then rinse once for 5 minutes in 20X SSPE.
- Cut membrane so that it is the exact size of the gel. Rinse membrane once in Distilled water (DW) then soak in 20X SSPE for 5 minutes.
- Assemble transfer apparatus.
- Cut a wick that is the exact size the gel. Cover the platform of the gel box with the wick so that there is an even amount of the wick in each of the wells. Fill the wells with 10X SSPE.
- Add parafilm to the sides of the gel box so that the solution does not evaporate during the transfer.
- Flip gel over and remove any air bubbles that are trapped underneath of it.
- Place the membrane on top of the gel. Try to position correctly so that you do not have to adjust the membrane at all as RNA transfers immediately. Again remove any air bubbles.
- Place 3 pieces of Whatman paper that are larger than the membrane and that have been pre-soaked in 2X SSPE on top of the membrane.
- Then sack ~25-50 paper towels on top if the Whatman paper. Lastly place a heavy object on top of the paper towels.
- Transfer for 16-20 hrs.
- After the transfer, mark the blot with a pencil. To do this, carefully remove the paper towels and the Whatman paper so as not to disturb the gel or the membrane. Flip the membrane and gel over and trace the wells with a pencil.
- Wash membrane in 20X SSPE for 30 minutes, then soak in 2X SSPE for 5 minutes. Wrap the membrane in plastic wrap and cross-link by UV.
- Stain blot with methylene blue by successively washing the blot in 2X SSPE for 5 minutes; 1N acetic acid for 5 minutes; 0.04% methylene blue in 0.5 M sodium acetate (pH 5.2) for 5 minutes; rinse in DW until most of the membrane is destained except for the ribosomal bands. The blot may be wrapped and stored at -80°C at this point, desiccated at 4°C for months or probed immediately.

Northern Probe Preparation

- Begin to prepare probe template by making desired DNA fragment by PCR and/or restriction digest of larger fragment. Isolate fragment by gel purification and gene clean treatment. Fragments can be many different sizes although fragments that contain several hundred base pairs often work best.
- Use 25-50ng of DNA in 1X TE. Boil for 10 minutes, quickly chill on ice and then spin down.
- After the 5-15 minute incubation remove unincorporated labeled nucleotides.
- Test % incorporation by spotting 1mL of the probe onto a DE-81 Whatman filter circles.
- Repeat this and wash this one with 0.5M phosphate buffer and count.

Hybridization

- Prehybridize the blot in 5-10mL of hybridization buffer per 11 X 14 cm membrane at 42°C in Northern oven for 30 minutes or longer.
- Add 50mL of salmon sperm and then boil for 10 minutes chill on ice, and add the whole probe to the prehybridized blot. Incubate at 65-70°C for 16-24 hrs.
- Remove hybridization solution and wash blot:
  - □ Twice in 6X SSPE/0.5% SDS for 15 minutes at RT.
  - □ Twice in 1X SSPE/0.5% SDS for 10 minutes at 37°C.
  - □ Once in 0.1X SSPE/0.1% SDS for 30 minutes at 65°C.
- Wrap blot in plastic wrap and expose to film and/or phosphoimager.

Spotters

Northern blot setup

Viva questions

How RNA samples are separated

130. Mutagenesis

Aim

To demonstrate the effect of spontaneous and UV induced mutation.

Principle

Mutation is a sudden and predictable change in the genetic material. It is a natural as any metabolic process and occurs spontaneously at a low frequency. We do not know for certain how spontaneous mutation arise in nature. It has been observed that the process of DNA replication is somewhat error prone, while most replicative errors are corrected then and there or soon afterwards a few of them escape and are manifested as spontaneous mutation.

Treatment of cells with some chemical and physical agents increases the frequency of mutation. Such agents are useful in the laboratory to generate mutations which inturn have contributed to the development of genetics.

130a. Spontaneous mutation

In this experiment, Ampicillin is used as a spontaneous mutation inducer. Environmental factors play an important role in this type of mutation. During this experiment sensitive type organisms are converted into resistant type spontaneously.

Materials required

Nutrient agar deeps, Wooden spacer, Sterile petri plates, 1% Ampicillin, Isopropyl alcohol, L-rod, *Escherichia coli*

Procedure

- Prepare two nutrient agar deeps and maintain them in liquid state.
- Place the wooden spacer under one edge of empty sterile petri plate.
- Cool one of the melted deep to approximately 45° C

- Pour the content to the plate. Be sure that the medium covers the entire bottom surface of the plate. When the agar has solidified completely, remove the wooden spacer.
- Cool the second melted deep to 45 °C
- Add 0.1 mL of 1% Ampicillin to the agar deep. Rotate the deep gently to mix agar and streptomycin.
- When the agar in the plate has solidified, pour the contents of the 2nd deep carefully over the top. Remember that the wooden spacer should be removed before the 2nd deep is poured.
- When the contents are solidified, label the high and low ampicillin concentration area of the plate.
- Place the glass spreader in the beaker containing 95% isopropyl alcohol.
- Using aseptic technique, pipette 0.2mL of E.coli broth on the surface of the gradient plate.
- Remove the spreader from the beaker and gently shake off excess alcohol. While holding the spreader down and away from your body, quickly pass it through the flame of the Bunsen burner.
- Use the glass spreader to spread E.coli over the surface of gradient plate. Return the spreader to the beaker containing alcohol.
- Invert and incubate the plates at 37^0 C for 48 hours.
- Observe the plates in the high concentration area for any Ampicillin resistant mutants. Count number of colonies and record the results.
- Select well-isolated colonies from mid area and streak throughout the plate by using nicrome wire loop.
- Return the plate to the incubator for an additional 2 days.
- Examine the plate again to note the effect of streaking on resistant colonies.

130b. Isolation of UV induced mutants of *E.coli*

Materials required

Escherichia coli, Centrifuge tubes, micro centrifuge, saline, Luria Bertani Medium (LB), Petriplates, diluents, test tubes, pipettes, UV chamber etc.

Procedure

- Prepare mid log culture of *E. coli* KL 96.
- Spin the culture and washed with saline in order to remove LB medium.
- Serially dilute up to 10^{-7}.
- Plate $10^{-5}, 10^{-6}$ and 10^{-7} on LB agar for Total Viable Count (TVC).
- Plate e 10^{-1} and 10^{-2} dilution on LB agar with streptomycin for the isolation of spontaneous mutant.
- Plate $10^{-3}, 10^{-3}$ and 10^{-4} diluted culture on LB with ampicillin plate and expose to UV for different time durations.
- Incubate 37°C for 24hours and observe the results are recorded.
- The frequency of spontaneous mutation and induced mutation are calculated.

130c. Chemical Induced Mutation
EMS mutagenisis of *E.coli*

Aim:

To isolate chemically induced mutants of *Escherichia coli*.

Principle:

Treatment of cells with some chemical mutagens, increase the frequency of mutation. Such agents are useful in the laboratory to generate mutation which inturn have contributed to the development of genetics. In this experiment, Ethylmethane sulphonate (EMS) is used to induce mutation. It belongs to the class of mutagen called alkylating agents. Treatment with alkylating agents results in the addition of alkylgroups to the ring of nitrogens as well as oxygens of purines and pyrimidines of the DNA. They also leads to the formation of phosphodiesters in the nucleic acids. The base pairing properties of such alkylated bases are different from normal bases. This leads to the introduction of a wrong base in first cycle of replication. In the second cycle, the mutation actually gets fixed and adenine gets incorportated instead of guanine. The net result is the transistionals repalcement of a GC base pair by AT base pair.

Resistance to drugs may be generally developed to drugs in the following ways. Prevention of entry of an antibiotic into the cell due to mutation in cellwall or cell membrane component. Modification of antibiotic binding sites by mutation.

Materials required

Escherichia coli, eppendoff micro centrifuge, saline, LB medium, Petriplates, diluents, test tubes, pipettes, EMS etc.

Procedure

- Prepare mid log culture of *Escherichia coli* KL 16/96 in 1:50 ratio in LB.
- Spin culture in 1mL eppendoff tubes at 10,000 rpm for 10minutes. Wash twice with sterile saline.
- Resuspend the culture in saline in 4 eppondoff tubes.
- Dilute the content from 1st tube upto 10^{-8} using sterile saline.
- Spread $10^{-6}, 10^{-7}, 10^{-8}$ diluted sample on air dried LB agar(TVC).
- Plate undiluted inoculum from the 2nd eppendoff tube on LB with ampicillin plates(TSM).
- Add EMS (50mG/mL) to the 3rd and 4th tubes and Incubate at 37°C for 20 minutes.
- Spin, wash thrice the EMS tube with saline.
- Resuspend in 10mL LB.
- Incubate at 37°C for overnight.
- Serial dilute upto 10^{-6} with saline.
- Spread 0.1mL of sample from $10^{-4}, 10^{-5}$ and 10^{-6} on LB ampicillin plate. Incubate at 37°C for 24 hours(IM).
- Observe growth and calculate frequency of induced mutation

Frequency calculation

Frequency of spontaneous mutation = number of colonies on antibiotics plates/ Total viable count X 100

Frequency of UV mutation = number of colonies on UV induced plates/ Total viable count X 100

Frequency of Chemical mutation = number of colonies on chemical treated cultures/ Total viable count X 100

Observation and result

Spontaneous mutation ability of the test organism is assessed by making use of an inducer ampicillin. Continuous exposure of organism to ampicillin may produce resistant strains. If you isolate ampicillin resistant colonies indicates that spontaneous mutation. Frequency of spontaneous mutatiom may very low.

UV light has its own ability to penetrate cells and cause Thyamine dimer. Rate of UV mutation is checked by exposing organism to UV on plain and antibiotics containing plates. Frequency of UV mutagenesis is high when compared to spontaneous mutation.

Ames test is one of the most important method used to assess mutagenecity of the organisms. When organism is exposed to mutagenic chemicals like EMS, organisms may change its character. Sometimes sensitive bacteria is converted to resistant. Frequency of chemical mutagenesis is high and also depends on the nature of chemicals.

Viva questions

Define mutation.

Mention different types of mutation.

Define mutagen, mutagenesis.

What is Thymine dimer?

Give two examples for physical and chemical mutagenic agent.

What is repair mechanism?

Explain SOS, Recombinant repair?

What is photo reactivation?

How mutation is lethal to bacterial cell?

How do you check mutagenicity of chemical agent?

What is Ames test?

Spotters: Ames test, EMS, NTG, UV, Repair photo

131. Isolation of Protoplast and sphaeroplast from bacteria
131 a. Protoplast isolation

Aim

To isolate protoplast from the given culture.

Principle

A protoplast is a plant, bacterial or fungal cell without any cell wall, which is removed either mechanical or enzymatic means. *Protoplast* refers to that unit of biology which is composed of a cell's nucleus and the surrounding protoplasmic materials. During and subsequent digestion of the cell wall, the protoplast becomes very sensitive to osmotic stress. This means cell wall digestion and protoplast storage must be done in an isotonic solution to prevent rupture of the plasma membrane.

The strength and rigidity of most bacterial cellwall resides in Murine component, which may be demaged or destroyed by specific enzyme (lyzozyme). This leads to the formation of osomotically sensitive cell. The surrounding medium is generally hypotonic or hypertonic which results in the lysis of the cell. Lysis can be prevented by adding 0.3 -0.8M sucrose and also by certain salts. So, osmotically sensitive cells remain intact as protoplast. The structural variation in the Murine substrate leads to differences in the sensitivity. Osmotic sensitive cells may also be generated by interaction with cellwall inhibiting antibiotic Eg: penicillin. In the osmotically stressed environment, osmotic sensitive spheres are formed from rod shaped gram positive and gram negative bacteria which can be monitored by light microscopic procedure.

Materials required

Gram positive cells, sucrose, lysozyme

Procedure

- Select Rapidly growing midlog phase gram-positive culture.
- Wash Cultures twice in a buffer of pH 6-8
- Resuspend Washed cultures in buffer containing hypertonic sucrose 0.2 - 1M and lysozyme 0.5mG-1.5mG.
- Incubate this reaction mixture for 30minutes at room temperature.
- This treatment should result in complete protoplast formation (to prevent protoplast lysis Add EDTA.)
- Stain osmotically sensitive sphere shaped protoplast by methylene blue & observed under light microscope.

131 b. Spheroplast Isolation

Aim

To isolate Spheroplast from the given culture.

Principle

Partial Cell wall containing cells are called Spheroplast. It is prepared from gram negative bacteria. All gram negative cells have murine structure that is sensitive to lysozyme however since outer membrane of gram negative bacteria is impermeable to lysozyme. The integrity of outer membrane must be compromised before lysozyme treatment. This can be done either by SDS treatment or by tris hydrochloride EDTA treatment.

Materials required

Gram negative cells, Hydrochloric Acid, Sucrose, EDTA, Lysozyme

Procedure

- Take the midlog phase culture of gram negative bacteria in eppendoff tube and washed twice with 10 mM Tris Hcl at 4°C
- Resuspend the pellets 30mM Tris Hcl containing 20% sucrose.
- Allow the resuspended reaction mixture for 5 min and spin at 3000 rpm for 5 min.
- Resuspend the pellets in 1.5mG/mL of lysozyme and 10mM EDTA.
- Incubate this reaction mixture at room temperature for 30-60 min.
- Observe the spheroplast under light microscope.

Observation

Structural variations are observed in both the procedures. When the treated culture is compared with untreated culture morphological variation is observed.

Result

Spheroplasts are isolated from gram negative cells and protoplaste are from gram positive cells.

Viva questions

Define protoplasts and spheroplasts.
Differentiate protoplast from spheroplasts
How do you obtain protoplast?
Which part of the bacterial cell is susceptible to lysozyme?
How do you maintain protoplast in the environment?
What are the uses of protoplast?

Spotters : Lysozyme, picture of protoplast and sphaeroplast.

132. Transformation

Aim

To transform *Escherichia coli* DH5α with the chosen plasmid and to calculate transformation frequency.

Principle

The bacterial transformation is a process in which a recipient cells acquire DNA molecule from the surrounding medium. Transformation begins with the uptake of DNA fragment and the uptake is generally enhanced when the cells are in competent state, the state at which, competent factors are elaborated. In an experimental condition, the recipient can be made competent by incubating it with calcium chloride for the prescribed time. The process of transformation terminates with the recombinant exchange of the donor DNA and its expression can be verified by using appropriate plating technique.

pUC18: These are high copy number *Escherichia coli* cloning vector. pUC18 is double stranded circular DNA with 2686 base pairs. They have Ampicillin resistant gene marker. pUC means plasmid University of California.

IPTG: It is an inducer in cloning studies to allow maximum expression of genes cloned in expression vectors. It helps in stimulating the production of beta galactosidase enzyme. It is a lactose analog, which binds and inhibits the Lac repressor and thereby strongly induces beta galactosidase production.

Xgal: X gal is a chromogenic substrate of beta galactosidase enzyme. It is widely used in cloning experiments for checking the presence of Lac operon. In enables easy detection of vectors, which carry the beta galactosidase gene. It is basically used in detection of the recombinant bacteriophages/vector/ bacteria (white) and parental vector (blue) when plated on medium containing X gal and IPTG.

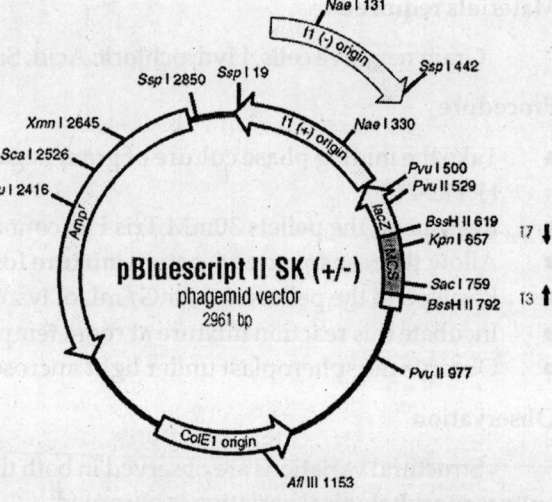

Fig. 132 : Structure of pBluescript

Materials Required

Escherichia coli DH5α: rec⁻, F⁻, nal^r, Plasmid DNA: pUC 18/ plasmid Bluescript, Conical flask, Petriplates, Pipettes, Vortex mixer, Eppendoff tubes, LB medium, LB Ampicillin with Xgal and IPTG, 0.5M calcium chloride (ice cold)

Xgal (5-bromo-4 –chloro-3-indolyl-beta – D-galactoside): Dissolve Xgal in dimethyl formamide to make a 20mG/mL solution. Cover the container with aluminium foil to prevent damage by light. Store at-20° C

IPTG: (Iso Propyl Thio Beta-D-Galactoside):Make a solution of IPTG by dissolving 2g of IPTGin 8mL of distilled water. Adjust volume to 10mL, filter sterilize and store at –20°C

Procedure

Competent cell preparation

- Inoculate 20mL of LB medium with 200mL of overnight culture of *Escherichia coli* DH5α (1:100).
- Grow at 37°C with aeration till OD 590=0.2.
- Add 1.5mL of culture into the prechilled microfuge tube.
- Spin at 4000 rpm for 5 minutes at 4°C. Discard supernatant completely.
- Resuspend the pellet in 0.5mL ice cold 0.5M calcium chloride. Incubate at 0° C for 35 minutes.

- Centrifuge at 3000rpm for 5minutes at 4 °C.
- Resuspend the pellet in150μL of ice cold calcium chloride solution. Incubate at 0 ° C for 1 hour.
- Now competent cells are ready. This is used for the transformation procedure.

Transformation

- Take competent cells in three microfuge tubes.
- Add 5μL DNA to the first tube, add 1μL DNA to the second tube and add double distilled water to the remaining tube.
- Incubate all tubes at 0°C for one hour.
- Remove tubes from the ice and immediately perform Heat shock at 42°C for two minutes.
- Add 500μL of LB to all tubes and incubate at 37 ° C for 1-2 hours with out aeration.
- Centrifuge at 3000rpm for 5 minutes.
- Drain off most of the liquids leaving behind approximately100μL, resuspend the pellet and plate on LB Ampicillin with X gal and IPTG.
- Incubate all plates at 37 ° C for 24 hours and observe the results.
- From the observed results calculate the frequency of transformation.

Frequency calculation

$$\text{Transformation frequency} = \frac{\text{No. of blue colonies}}{\text{Total No. of white colonies}}$$

Percentage of transformation = frequency x 100

Result and discussion

White and blue colonies are noted on Xgal and IPTG containing plates. Blue colour colonies indictes that the transformation is complete. Frequency of transformation may vary from one process to other.

Viva questions

Define transformation.

Who discovered transformation?

List few naturally competent bacteria.

What is competency?

How do you make non competent cells into a competent cells?

Which chemical is used to create competency in bacteria?

Mention few plasmids having Lac Operon.

What is blue white selection?

Define alpha complementation?

What are the role of Xgal, and IPTG in pUC8 transformation?

Explain about plasmid bluescript.

Spotters : Xgal, IPTG, pUC18/ Bluescript, *E.coli* DH5α and Calcium chloride

133. Transduction -Generalized

Aim

To transduce *Escherichia coli* strain AB1157 for Arg+ and check to Co- Transduction frequency with his+and pro+

Principle

Transduction is a general process by which genes from one bacterium (donor) can be transferred in to another (recipient)through an intermediate vector which is a bacteriophage. The transferred donor gene can replace the corresponding gene from the recipient by recombination and the resulting recombinant (transductant) can be selected by appropriate means.

When the P1 phage infects, the donor *E.coli* (KL96/16), the injected phage DNA replicates several times resulting in a pool of phage DNA, the structural components of phage such as the head, tail , tail fibres etc.. are synthesized, the phage DNA is packed in the head, other structures are added on and finally the infected cell lyses releasing a group of primary phages. During this process, the host DNA also degraded into fragments of various sizes. During the process of assembly of the phage fragments of the host DNA which are the same size as phage DNA get wrongly packed into the phage heads and are released as the cell lyses. These breakaged phages are normal as far as infection is concerned, since infection is determined by the structures of tail and tail fibres etc, but they cannot produce progeny phage since they carry a fragment of *E.coli* DNA instead of P1 DNA. Since any fragments of the *E.coli* chromosome can be packed into the P1 phage head as long as it is of right size any gene can be transduce by P1 phage. Hence P1 is called a general transducing phage. The size of the P1 DNA is approximately 1/50 of *E.coli* DNA. There fore the transduction and co transduction frequency is related to the distance between the markers. F (co transduction frequency)$=(1-d/L)3$ where d is the distance between the markers(in minutes) and L is the maximum DNA that could be accomodated into the P1 phage head, usually taken to be two minutes. The above formula called Wu's formula has been used in deducting linkage between markers/genes.

Materials Required

Culture :Donor- *P1 Lysate*, Recipient - *E.coli* AB1157
Glasswares : Petriplates , Pipettes , L-rod, Conical flask , Eppendoff tubes
Media : LB media, Minimal medium
Stock solutions : Streptomycin , Calcium chloride, Sodium citrate, Aminoacids , Vitamin B1, Magnesium sulphate

Procedure

- Prepare P1 lysate and overnight recipient
- Centrifuge the culture at 5000rpm for 10 minutes.
- Resuspend pellet in 1mL saline
- Serially dilute donor lysate up to 10^{-3}
- Add 0.1 mL to recipient to 0.2mL calcium chloride
- Mix well- keep 37^0 C for 15 minutes.
- Add 0.1 mL of 1M sodium citrate(chelating agent)
- Spin wash the culture with saline once
- Resuspend in 0.2mL saline
- Spread on selective minimal medium
- Spread on appropriate selective plate (LB with rif, kan)

- Patch on co transductants
- From the observation calculate co transduction frequency.

Observation and result

Note presence or absence of growth on LB selective and minimal medium. Colonies grown on LB selective medium is patched on selective minimal medium to know co transductants. Presence of growth in both medium indicates P1 lysate carries DNA of donor to recepient.

Viva questions

Define transduction and transductants.
What are the nature of P1 Phage?
How do you perform transduction?
How do you calculate transduction frequency?
Who discovered transduction?
Name the experiment to demonstrate DNA as a genetic materials through phage.

Spotters: Transduction picture.

134. Conjugation –Interupted

Aim

To compare conjugation frequencies with distances between the markers by gradient mating using an Hfr donor.

Principle

In a Hfr X F- mating , chromosome transfer proceeds unidirectional commencing from the given point of origin which is determined by the site and orientation of the integration of the F plasmid. Since DNA transfer has a tendency to break off spontaneously (unlike the mating pairs) there is a gradient of transfer of markers, while most of the recipient cells will receive markers located close to the origin of transfer only a few will receive, one's located at the terminus. Thus the number of recombinants obtained for a marker when an F- is crossed with a given Hfr will be inversely proportional to the distance of the marker from the origin of transfer. This principle has been extremely useful in genetic mapping. In this experiment, chromosomal transfer between the mated cultures is artificially interrupted by agitation and the transfer gradient is recorded.

Materials required:

Cultures used: Donor – *Escherichia coli* Hfr str^s / tet^r / Kan^s,
Recipient – *E. coli* CSH57 str^r / tet^s / Kan^r, ile, met⁻, arg⁻, ieu⁻

Glasswares: Conical flask, screw cap tubes, test tubes, petri plates, pipettes, vortex mixer.
Media: LB broth, minimal medium.
Stock solutions: Amino acids, streptomycin, Vitamin B1, saline.

Procedure

- Prepare Donor and recipient, overnight culture in LB (don't shake)
- Subculture – 1:50 LB and incubate 2 – 2 ½ hours (dont shake).
- Mix – 4.5mL R + 0.5mL D (9:1).

- Incubate at 37⁰ C without shaking.
- Interrupt at different time till 100 minutes.
- Take 0.1mL culture in Sterile stoppered tube and vortex for 5 minutes
- Dilute Upto 10^{-5} with saline and plate 10^{-3}, 10^{-4} in selective plates (minimal agar with all required Amino acids except one).
- Incubate at 37⁰ C for 24 hours.
- Patch on other selective plates for Co-conjugants.

Observation and result

Experiment of interrupted conjugation is performed at regular interval. Diiferent time growth is noted on different minimal medium with or with out aminoacids. Different time interval related growth indicates conjugation and passage of different gene at different time interval through conjugation canol.

Viva questions

Who discovered conjugation?
Define conjugation, F pili, Hfr.
Have you construct genetic map through conjugation?
Name donor bacterium and its characters.

Spotters: Picture of conjugation.

135. Ampicillin selection of auxotrophs

Aim

To enrich auxotrophic mutants from the mutagenised *E.coli* culture and isolate them.

Principle

Ampicillin is a derivative of penicillin. It is a bactericidal agent and kills growing cells by interfering with the cell wall synthesis. This provide an selection technique for enriching auxotrophs from the population. In a minimal medium, among the population, prototrophs alone would grow and hence the addition of ampicillin would lyses the growing cells. As auxotrophs cannot grow in minimal media, they escape death due to ampicillin. Some times extensive cell lysis of the prototrophs cell leads to cross feeding of auxotrophs, killing them also. This problem can be circumvented if a hypertonic medium with sucrose/glucose and Mg2+ is used. This converts growing cells in to protoplasts and hence they donot lyse.

Materials required

NTG/EMS treated culture of *E.coli* KL 96/16, Glucose minimal medium, LB medium, Ampicillin (1g/100mL), Saline, Glucose 40%, E. coli CSH57 etc.,

Procedure

- Dilute overnight culture 1:25 in 5mL glucose minimal medium
- Aerate at 37 ° C for 90-120 minutes.
- Add ampicillin 100µG/mL-kills all growing cells.
- Aerate till complete lysis.
- Spin 10,000 rpm for 10 minutes. The pellets thus obtained are auxotrophs, few prototrophs and dead cell debris.

- Resuspend the pellet in LB and incubate overnight
- Dilute 10^{-7} with sterile saline.
- Plate 10^{-5}, 10^{-6} on LB plates (spread plating)
- Patch at least 40-50 CFU on LB+ minimal medium with sterile toothpicks.
- Incubate overnight at 37 ° C

Calculate auxotroph frequency.

Auxotroph frequency =number of auxotrophs/no patched.

Viva questions

What is auxotrophs and prototrophs?

What are the characters of auxotrophs?

Is auxotroph grows on minimal medium?

On what basis ampicillin selects auxotrophs.

Spotters: Ampicillin, picture of auxotrophic mutant isolation.

Virology

136. Isolation of Coliphage from Sewage

Aim

    To isolate virulent phage from sewage

Background information

    Phages are viruses that infects bacteria. Coli phage infects intestinal bacteria like *Escherichia coli*. Sewage is a rich source of coli phages, because sewage contains faecal matter and is rich in organic matter. Faecal bacteria grow enormously by utilizing organic matter present in sewage. Isolating phage from sewage is not an easy process. It requires stepwise careful Isolation and enrichment process.

Materials required

    Overnight culture of *Escherichia coli* and fresh sewage collected in screw-capped bottles, filteration unit, test tubes, centrifuge, conical flask, sewage.

Media :   Nutrient Broth and Agar

Procedure

Enrichment of sewage sample

- Add 5mL of nutrient broth and 5mL of the *E. coli* broth culture to 45 mL of the raw sewage sample available in 250mL Conical flask aseptically (Handle the raw sewage with caution).

- Incubate the flask for 24 hours at 37°C.

Filtration and seeding

- Centrifuge the enriched phage sample at 2500 rpm for 20 minutes.
- Decant the supernatant into a 125mL flask.
- Filter the supernatant through a sterile membrane filter apparatus to collect the bacteria-free, phage-containing filtrate in the vacuum flask.
- Prepare hard nutrient agar and poured in to sterile Petri plates and allowed to solidify.
- Prepare soft agar in test tubes of 5 mL quantities and maintained in liquid condition.
- Inoculate 0.1mL of the *E. coli* culture to all the molten soft-agar tubes using a sterile 1mL pipette.
- Add 1 to 5 drops of the Sewage filtrate to the labelled molten soft-agar tubes using a sterile Pasteur pipette and mix properly.
- Pour properly mixed soft agar into the appropriately labeled hard agar plate.
- Allow soft agar media to harden.
- Incubate all plates in an inverted position for 24hours at 37°C and observe plates after incubation.

Observation and Result

    Clear lytic areas are seen on the plate. *E. coli* has grown in to a lawn. Clear lytic area indicates the presence of phages

138. Determining Bacteriophage Titers

Aim

To describe a bacteriophage.
To develop techniques for cultivating bacteriophages.
To determine a bacteriophage titer.

Background Information

.Bacteriophages can be isolated from different environments. Since they grow and reproduce within bacteria, one would expect to find them wherever a large population of bacteria is present. For example, large numbers of *E. coli* grow in the intestinal tract of warm-blooded animals. Therefore, animal manure and untreated sewage are excellent sources of coliphages. Concentration of bacteriophages specific for a particular host may be relatively low in natural environment, the first step in the isolation procedure is an enrichment step. When the sample is incubated with a population of the proper host, phages specific for that bacterium will greatly multiply in number. The phages then are much easier to isolate since they are present in greater numbers. Membrane filtration serves

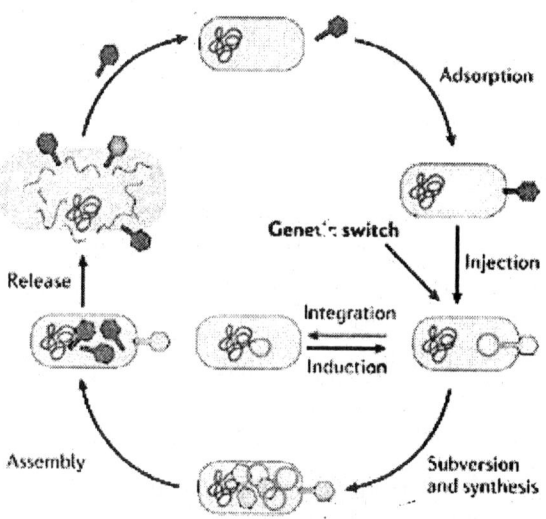

Fig 116.1: Life cycle of Phage

to remove cell debris and most bacteria. Any bacteria that may remain in the enriched culture can be killed and lysed by treatment with chloroform. The filtrate containing bacterial viruses may now be stored in the refrigerator for months. Individual viruses in the filtrate can be isolated by mixing a small amount of filtrate with a young culture of the host bacterium and then spreading the mixture out on the surface of a petri plate containing nutrient agar. This is called the double-layered culture technique. In practice, the viruses and bacteria are mixed with a dilute agar medium (the top agar) and then poured in a thin layer on the surface of harder bottom, or base agar. When the top agar solidifies, the viruses and bacteria are immobilized. Whenever a virus particle is present in the agar, it will infect an adjacent bacterial cell, reproduce, and lyse its host cell. The virus particle will then give rise to millions of virions, and a clear area of lysed bacteria will develop in the bacterial lawn. This clear area is called a plaque. Ideally, each virus will produce one plaque containing enormous numbers of its progeny. Samples of each plaque can then be removed and used to culture large quantities of a single type of virus for further study. Because each plaque arises from a single virus particle, a count of the number of plaques will enable one to calculate the concentration of viruses in the original undiluted sample.

Materials required

Flask of raw sewage, centrifuge, 0.22 and 0.45 μm membrane filters, filter apparatus, aluminum foil, 500-mL flask, graduated cylinder, 1 tube broth, Concentrated broth , *Escherichia coli* , 24-hour broth culture, incubator, Bunsen burner, chloroform, sterile screw-cap tubes, sterile saline (0.85% NaCl), petri plates, Hard agar, water bath, thermometer, wax pencil.

Procedure

Enrichment

- Obtain about 50 mL of raw sewage. Centrifuge it for 10 minutes using clinical centrifuge.

- Pass the supernatant through a 0.22 μm membrane filter to remove bacterial contaminants.

● Add 20 mL of the supernatant to a 500-mL flask containing 20 mL of sterile, twofold concentrated broth.

● Inoculate the mixture with 1 mL of an overnight (10^9 cells per milliliter) *E. coli* culture . Incubate for 24 hours at 35°C.

● Inoculate a Tube-broth culture tube with 1 mL of *E. coli* and incubate it at 35°C overnight or for 24 hours. This will serve as a stock culture.

Isolation of phages

● Filter the Phage enriched sewage through another 0.45 μm membrane filter . Transfer 8.0-mL portions of the filtrate into sterile, screw-cap tubes .

● Add 0.2 mL of chloroform to each screw–cap tube with a sterile pipette. Mix thoroughly.

● The virus stock can be used immediately or kept in the refrigerator until it can be analyzed.

● Prepare a serial dilution of the enriched bacteriophage sample. Withdraw a sample and transfer an aliquot to the next tube and mix properly . With a new pipette, transfer an aliquot to the next tube in the series (Use a new, sterile pipette for each transfer).

● After all dilutions have been prepared, add 2 drops of the overnight *E. coli* culture to the melted, cooled 10^{-4} to 10^{-8} dilution tubes of soft agar. Keep the tubes in the 48° to 50°C water bath as much of the time as possible during this process.

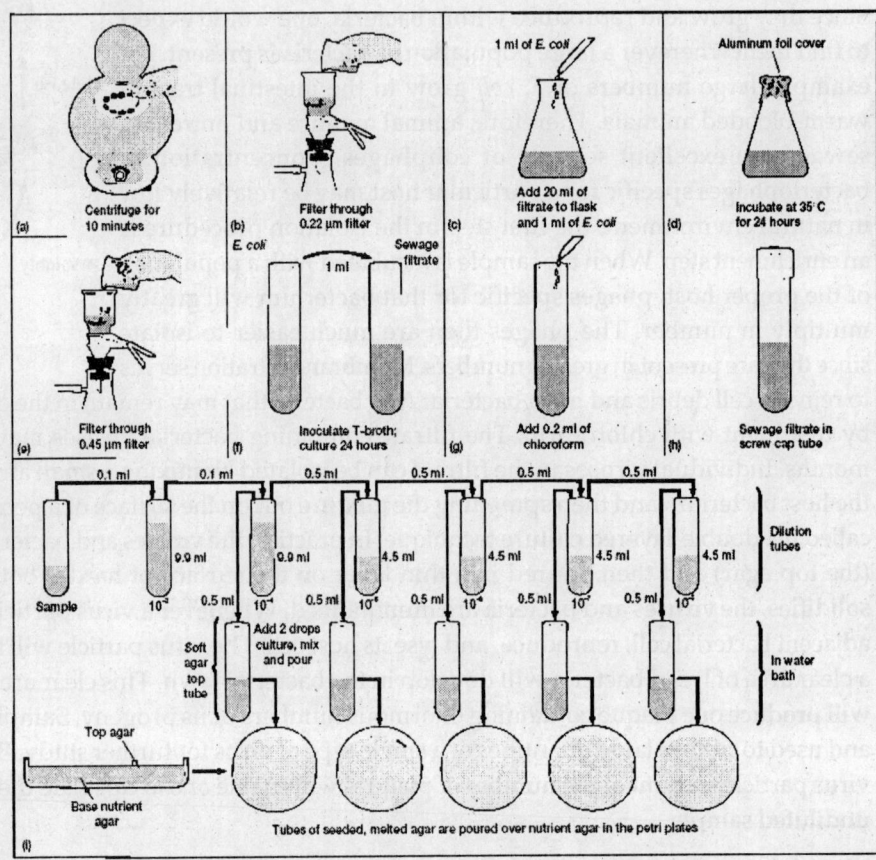

Fig 116.2 : Steps of Phage isolation and Titration

6. Transfer 0.5 mL of 10^{-4} dilution to a 45°C soft agar top tube. Mix quickly and thoroughly, and pour the soft agar aseptically into a petri plate containing sterile bottom agar. Immediately spread the top agar over the surface of the base nutrient agar by tilting the plate. Set the plate aside to harden. Repeat this procedure with each of the other four dilutions.

7. Incubate the plates in an inverted position at 35°C for 8 to 24 hours.

Observation

Examine the plates carefully and, using a Quebec colony counter, count the number of plaques on each plate.

Use the plate(s) with the most favorable number of plaques (25 to 250) to determine the number of coliphages in 1 mL of the original enriched sample. This is done by dividing the plaque number by the dilution factor as shown by the following example:

Plaque count = number of plaques/0.5X dilution

Viva questions

What is meant by a plaque-forming unit?

What are coliphages?

Why is enrichment of the sewage necessary for the isolation of coliphages?

Describe the similarities between the plaque technique in this exercise and the standard plate count for bacteria.

What effect does chloroform have on viruses? On bacteria?

Why are two different size filters used in this experiment?

Who coined the term phages?

Which is the host for phages?

What is the need of filtration in this experiment?

How do you detect phage growth on agar medium?

Spotter: Phage grown Petri plate with PFU

138. Cultivation of viruses in embryonated egg

Aim

To cultivate viruses using embryonated eggs.

Background information

Woodruff and Good Pasteur (1931) used fertilized chicken egg for viral cultivation. This is a simpler technique than animal inoculation. Usually eggs will not interfere with virus multiplication due to the absence of immune response. Suitable cells for the growth of viruses are available in embryo and its membrane, which may facilitate the growth of viruses.

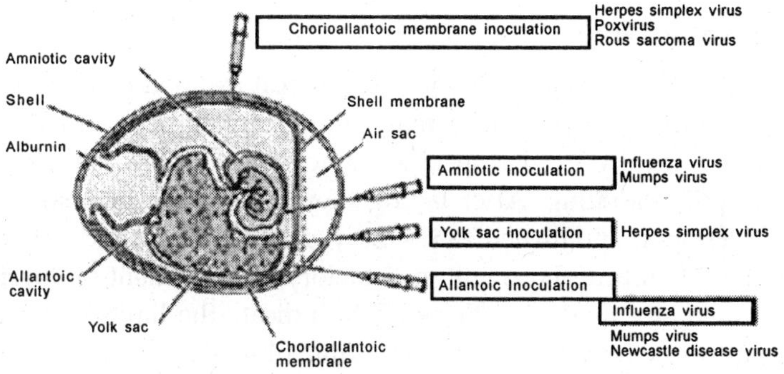

Fig 138.1 Site of specific virus for cultivation.

Materials Required

Egg holders, candling lamp, hole puncture, Syringes, gauze, pencils, gloves, sterile forceps, Pasteur pipette with bulbs, screw caped sterile vials, egg, melted paraffin wax and 70% ethanol.

Procedure

● Disinfect the egg shell using iodine or alcohol.

● Drill egg shell using hole puncture.

● Inoculate the Specimen in the embryonated egg through appropriate route as described in figure 138.1.

● After 2-5 days post injection, recognize viral growth in the egg by death of embryo, pocks or haemagglutination.

Result

Death of the embryo or formation of typical pocks (Pock assay), Haemagglutination or lesions on the membranes of the egg are results of the viral growth. After growth viruses are identified with the help of serological techniques. Eg. Poxviruses produce pock or lesions; Influenza virus produce haemagglutination.

Viva Questions :

What is the purpose of cultivating viruses on embryonated egg?
Mention different sites of egg used for virus cultivation.
What is CAM?
How do you cultivate Herpes simplex virus in embryonated egg?
How do you detect virus growth in embryonated egg?
What is Pock assay?
Define Haemagglutination.

Spotter:

Picture of embryonated egg.

139. Chick embryo fibroblast culture technique for Virus Cultivation

Aim

To cultivate viruses using chick embryo fibroblast technique.

Background information

The development of routine cell culture methods has reduced the importance of eggs but they are still valuable for the isolation of many important viruses and for the production of vaccines. Fertile eggs must be obtained ideally from a specific pathogen free flock, should be clean, preferably unwashed and pale shelled to simplify candling. After laying they have to be incubated for 10 days at 37° C with 40-70% humidity and good aeration and turned twice daily. After 6 days they are candled, infertile and dead eggs are discarded. On the day of culture those with satisfactory development of chorioallantioic blood vessels and showing embryonic movement are marked with pencil to indicate the limits of the air sac. Fibroblast cells obtained from chick embryo are cultivated for virus detection through observing cytopathic effect.

Materials required

Embryonated eggs preferably 10-12 days old.
Phosphate buffer saline (pH 7.2).
0.25% trypsin in PBS (TVG).
Growth medium (MEM, supplemented with 10% bovine serum)

Media preparation for cell culture - Refer experiment 176.

TVG (Trypsin Versene Glucose) - Refer experiment 177.

Procedure

- Candle and select 10-11 day old eggs.
- Place the egg in an egg cup, air sac upwards and wipe clean with spirit.
- Break the shell with the sharp end of a sterile forceps, and lift the membrane. With a bent forceps pick up the embryo and place it in a petri dish containing PBS.

- Dissect the embryo in the dish, remove and discard the head, limbs and viscera. Pick up the fibroblastic tissue and transfer into a wide neck bottle containing PBS.

- Mince the tissue finely with scissors, and wash minced tissue several times in PBS to remove blood cells and debris.

- Transfer tissue to transfusion bottle containing sterile silicone covered magnet and 50mL of 0.25 % trypsin solution and stopper securely.

- Trypsinize on magnetic stirrer unit 37° C for 30 mins : avoid frothing of contents.

- The tissue will disintegrate, forming a turbid suspension of cells. Filter the suspension through sterile gauze and centrifuge filtrate for 10min at 1000 rev/min.

- Discard supernatant and resuspend cells in 100 mL growth medium.

- Centrifuge once again and resuspend the cells in fresh medium.

- Dilute 0.9mL suspension with 0.1mL trypan blue solution and count cells in haemocytometer.

- Adjust concentration to 1 10 cells / mL growth medium and Pour into Tissue culture flask.

- Incubate at 37° C until monolayer is formed (2-3 days).

- When cells have formed a monolayer, remove growth medium, inoculate virus, add maintenance medium (MEM, Eagles base with 1-2% bovine serum) and incubate.

Observation and results

Monolayer of cells are formed. Cytopathic effect may be observed if monolayer is inoculated with virus.

Viva questions

What is chick embryo fibroblast?
How do you cultivate fibroblast cells?
Define monolayer.
What is cytopathic effect?
Define primary cells, continuous cells, cell strains, cell lines.
Name the medium used for the cultivation of cells.
How do you detect virus growth in cell culture system?
What are the major components of cell culture medium?
Why phenol red is used in cell culture medium?

Spotters: Structure of monolayer.

General Biochemistry

CHAPTER 11

140. Preparation of Buffers

Aim

To prepare buffer of required pH.

To study the nature of Buffers

Principle

A buffer solution is one that resists pH change on addition of small amount acid or alkali. Buffer solutions are used in many biochemical experiments, where the pH needs to be accurately controlled. A pH meter measures the electrical potential developed by a pair of electrode dipping into a solution for the measurement of pH and the electrode system. Sensitive to change H^+ activity of the solution in chosen. This electrode system consists of a sequence of an electrode whose potential varies with the pH of the solution.

Preparation of Acetate Buffer

Materials Required

A. Sodium Acetate (0.2M) – 1.64g of sodium acetate dissolved in 100mL of water.

B. Acetic Acid (0.2M) - 1.15mL of glacial acetic acid made up to 100mL with water.

Hydrochloric acid (0.1mL/l)

pH meter

Procedure

Calibrate the pH meter using standard buffer of pH – 4.0, 7.0 and 9.0.

Wash the electrodes with distilled water, then measure the pH using 0.2 molar buffers.

Mix X mL of A and Y mL of B solutions to a total of 50 mL as described in table and check the pH of the solution. Standard pH values of solution is given in table 140.1.

Table : 140.1- Acetate Buffer of different pH

X/A	Y/B	pH
46.3	03.7	3.6
44	06	3.8
41	09	4.0
36.8	13.2	4.2
30.5	19.5	4.4
25.5	24.5	4.6
20	30	4.8
14.8	35.2	5.0
10.5	39.5	5.2
08.8	41.2	5.4
04.8	45.2	5.6

Preparation of Phosphate buffer

Stock solution A: 2M monobasic sodium phosphate, monohydrate (276 g/L).

Stock solution B: 2M dibasic sodium phosphate (284 g/L).

Mixing an appropriate volume (mL) of A and B as shown in the table below and diluting to a total volume to 200 mL. This will yield 1M Phosphate buffer.

Table 140.2 : Phosphate buffer of different pH

A	B	pH
90.0	10.0	5.9
87.7	12.3	6.0
85.5	15.0	6.1
81.5	19.5	6.2
77.5	22.5	6.3
73.5	26.5	6.4
68.5	31.5	6.5
62.5	37.5	6.6
56.5	43.5	6.7
51.0	49.0	6.8
45.0	55.0	6.9
39.0	61.0	7.0
33.0	67.0	7.1
28.0	72.0	7.2
23.0	77.0	7.3
19.0	81.0	7.4
16.0	84.0	7.5
13.0	87.0	7.6
10.5	89.5	7.7
8.5	91.5	7.8

Result

Buffer solution is used for various biochemical, chemical and other reactions to maintain pH.

Viva questions

Define Buffer

What are the important properties of buffer?

Name any one buffer available in human body.

How do you prepare buffer?

141. pKa Value Determination

Aim

To determine the pKa value of an acid by titration method.

Principle

pKa means - log (Ka) where Ka is the ionization constant for the partially ionized acid, and the log is also base 10. pK_a, the symbol for Acid dissociation constant (pK for short). The negative logarithm of the acid dissociation constant, Ka. Just like the pH, the pKa explains that, the acid or basic properties of a substance. The value of pK_a indicates the strength of an acid: the larger the value the weaker the acid. In aqueous solution, simple acids are partially dissociated to an appreciable extent in the pH range $pK_a \pm 2$. The actual extent of the dissociation can be calculated if the acid concentration and pH are known.

$$pKa = -Log_{10}(Ka)$$

A knowledge of pK_a value is essential for understanding the behaviour of acids and bases in solution. For example, many compounds used for medication are weak acids or bases, so a knowledge of pK_a and log p values is essential for an understanding how the compound enters (or does not enter) the blood stream. Other applications include aquatic chemistry, chemical oceanography, buffer solutions, acid-base homeostasis and certain kinds of enzyme kinetics, such as Michaelis–Menten kinetics, which involve a pre-equilibrium step. Also, knowledge of pK_a values is a prerequisite for a quantitative understanding of the interaction between acids or bases and metal ions to form complexes in solution.

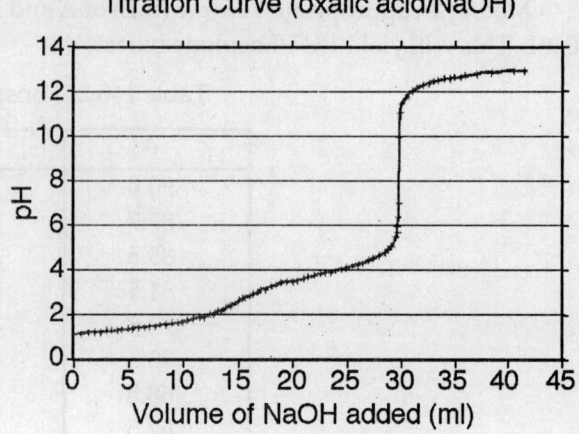

Fig 141 : 1 - Titration curve

pKa <2 means strong acid
pKa >2 but <7 means weak acid
pKa >7 but <10 means weak base
pKa >10 means strong base

pK_a values are commonly determined by means of titrations, in a medium of high ionic strength and at constant temperature. A typical procedure would be as follows. A solution of the compound in the medium is acidified with a strong acid to the point where the compound is fully protonated. The solution is then titrated with a strong base until all the protons have been removed. At each point in the titration pH is measured using a pH meter. The equilibrium constants are found by fitting calculated pH values to the observed values, using the method of least squares.

The total volume of added strong base should be small compared to the initial volume of to keep the ionic strength nearly constant. This will ensure that pK_a remains invariant during the titration.

A calculated titration curve for oxalic acid is shown in Fig. 141.1. Oxalic acid has pK_a values of 1.27 and 4.27. Therefore the buffer regions will be centered at about pH 1.3 and pH 4.3. The buffer regions carry the information necessary to get the pK_a values as the concentrations of acid and conjugate base change along a buffer region.

Between the two buffer regions there is an end-point, or equivalence point, where the pH rises by about two units. This end-point is not sharp and is typical of a diprotic acid whose buffer regions overlap by a small amount: $pK_{a2} - pK_{a1}$ is about three in this example. (If the difference in pK values were about two or less, the end-point would not be noticeable.) The second end-point begins at about pH 6.3 and is sharp. This indicates that all the protons have been removed. When this is so, the solution is not buffered and the pH rises steeply on addition of a small amount of strong base. However, the pH does not continue to rise indefinitely. A new buffer region begins at about pH 11 ($pK_w - 3$), which is where self-ionization of water becomes important.

Materials Required

0.1N acetic acid, 0.1N Sodium hydroxide , pH meter, Beaker, Glass rod, pH buffer (4,7,9).

Tissue paper

Procedure

- Prepare 20mL of 0.1N acetic acid and pour into a beaker.
- Dip the electrode of a pH meter and measure the pH.
- Now add exactly 0.5mL of 0.1N NaOH solution.
- Mix well with glass rod and measure the pH.
- Repeat the above steps till the pH of the solution is above 10.
- Plot the value in a graph sheet taking the volume of NaOH added in the X axis and pH in the Y axis.
- Connect all the point; this is called as the titration curve.
- *From the titration curve calculate pKa value*

Table 141.2: pKa Value Determination

S. No.	Volume of acid (mL)	Volume of NaOH added(mL)	pH	pKa Value
1		0.5		
2	Total 10mL of 0.1N acid	1.0		
3		1.5		
4		2.0		
5		2.5		

Table 141.1: pKa Value of different power

Effective pH range	pKa 25°C	Buffer
1.2−2.6	1.97	Maleate (pK1)
1.7−2.9	2.15	Phosphate (pK1)
2.2−3.6	2.35	Glycine (pK1)
2.2−6.5	3.13	Citrate (pK1)
3.0−4.5	3.75	Formate
3.0−6.2	4.76	Citrate (pK2)
3.2−5.2	4.21	Succinate (pK1)
3.6−5.6	4.76	Acetate
5.0−7.4	6.27	Cacodylate
5.5−6.5	5.64	Succinate (pK2)
5.5−6.7	6.1	MES
5.5−7.2	6.4	Citrate (pK3)
5.5−7.2	6.24	Maleate (pK2)
5.8−7.2	6.46	Bis-Tris
5.8−8.0	7.2	Phosphate (pK2)
6.0−12.0	9.5	Ethanolamine
6.0−8.0	6.35	Carbonate (pK1)
6.1−7.5	6.78	ACES
6.1−7.5	6.76	PIPES
6.5−7.9	7.14	MOPS
6.8−8.2	7.48	HEPES
7.4−8.8	8.05	Tricine
7.5−9.0	8.06	Tris
8.5−10.2	9.23	Borate
9.5−11.1	10.33	Carbonate (pK2)
9.7−11.1	10.4	CAPS

Result

pKa value of given acid / base is _____

Viva questions

Define pKa, pKb.
How do you determine pKa value?
Define Normality.
What are the purposes of doing this experiment?
Mention few important principles of this experiment.

142. Beer- Lambert's Law Verification

Aim

To demonstrate Beer – Lambert's law with the help of a standard graph.

Principle

The absorption of light by a substance or solution can be quantified with the help of two basic laws.

Beer Law: When a beam of monochromatic light enters an absorbing medium, the intensity of light coming out decreases exponentially with the increase in the concentration of light absorbing constituent in the medium.

$$A \alpha C$$

Lamberts law: This law states that, under similar condition, that the intensity of light coming out decreases exponentially with the increase in the length of the medium through which light passes.

$$A \alpha L$$

Measurement of light depends on both laws, it is popularly known as Beer Lambert's Law

$$A \alpha C x L$$

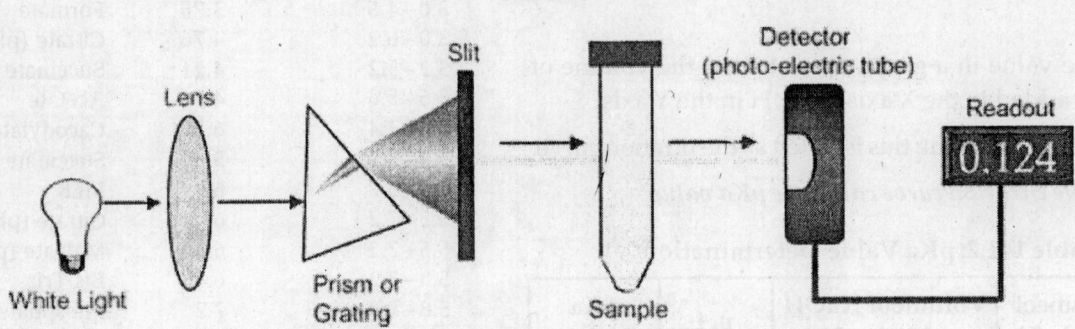

Fig. 142.1 - Light path in Spectro photometer

Materials required

Colorimeter with a series of filter or Spectrophotometer

Copper sulphate : 5mG/mL concentration

Potassium dichromate : 1mG/mL concentration

An 'unknown' mixture of two dyes.

Procedure

- Prepare copper sulphate solution and potassium dichromate separately in 100mL of distilled water.

- Take a series of clean tube and number them in duplicates.

- Pipette out the $CuSO_4$ and potassium dichromate separately in test tubes as described in table No. 143.1 to prepare standard graph.

Table 142.1- Preparation procedure

S. No	Name of the solution	Tube No						
		1	2	3	4	5	6	7
Copper sulphate standard graph								
1	Copper sulphate in mL	0.0	0.5	1.0	1.5	2.0	2.5	3.0
	Distilled water	5.0	4.5	4.0	3.5	3.0	2.5	2.0
Potassium dichromate standard graph								
2	Potassium dichromate in mL	0.0	0.5	1.0	1.5	2.0	2.5	3.0
	Distilled water	5.0	4.5	4.0	3.5	3.0	2.5	2.0

- Mix the solution well and switch on the instrument (Colorimeter or Spectrophotometer) and allow it to set warmed it for 15 – 20 minutes.

- Take the OD value of $CuSO_4$ at 620nm and potassium dichromate at 440nm and recorded.

- Draw a standard graph by taking concentration of $CuSO_4$ / $K_2Cr_2O_7$ (mG/mL) in X-axis and the OD value in Y-axis.

- Concentration of an unknown solution can be determined using standard graph.

Table 142.2: Standard Graph – Copper sulphate

S. No	Copper sulphate (1mG/mL) in mL	Distilled water (H_2O)in mL	Concentration of $CuSO_4$ in mG	OD Value
1	0.0	5.0	0.00	
2	0.5	4.5	0.50	
3	1.0	4.0	1.00	
4	1.5	3.5	1.50	
5	2.0	3.0	2.00	
6	2.5	2.5	2.50	
7	3.0	2.0	3.00	

Table 142.3: Standard Graph – Potassium di chromate

S. No	$K_2Cr_2O_7$ (2mG/mL) in mL	Distilled water (H_2O)in mL	Concentration of $K_2Cr_2O_7$ in mG	OD Value
1	0.0	5.0	0.00	
2	0.5	4.5	0.50	
3	1.0	4.0	1.00	
4	1.5	3.5	1.50	
5	2.0	3.0	2.00	
6	2.5	2.5	2.50	
7	3.0	2.0	6.00	

Observation and result

Different colours at different concentrations showed different OD value, which proved beer lamberts law.

Viva questions

Define Beers and Lambert's law.

What is the principles of Beers and Lamberts Law?

Name the instruments works under Beers Lamberts law.

143. Qualitative Estimation of carbohydrates

Aim

To analyse the availability of carbohydrates.

Background information

Carbohydrates are distributed in living tissues. They are made from carbon, hydrogen and oxygen. Carbohydrates are divided into three main classes namely Monosaccharides, oligosaccharides / disaccharides and polysaccharides. Carbohydrates are a source of energy. Monosaccharides are the simplest carbohydrates and are often called single sugars. They can be classified according to the number of carbon atoms in a molecule. They are n = 3 - trioses, e.g. glyceraldehydes; n = 5 -pentoses, e.g. ribose and deoxyribose and n = 6 -hexoses, e.g. fructose, glucose and galactose. Glucose is the most important carbohydrate fuel in human cells. Two glucose molecules react to form the dissacharide maltose. Starch and cellulose are polysaccharides made up of glucose units. Galactose molecules look very similar to glucose molecules. They can also exist in α and β forms. Galactose reacts with glucose to make the dissacharide lactose. Galactose cannot play the same part in respiration as glucose. Fructose, glucose and galactose are all hexoses. Fructose reacts with glucose to make the dissacharide sucrose. A glycosidic bond forms and holds the two monosaccharide units together. The three most important disaccharides are sucrose, lactose and maltose. Monosaccharides can undergo a series of condensation reactions, adding one unit after another to the chain until very large molecules (polysaccharides) are formed. This is called condensation polymerization. Starch is often produced in plants as a way of storing energy. It exists in two forms: amylose and amylopectin. Glycogen is amylopectin with very short distances between the branching side-chains. Cellulose is a third polymer made from glucose. But this time it's made from α-glucose molecules and the polymer molecules are 'straight'.

Materials Required

Anthrone reagent – Refer experiment 147 (Page 390)

Fehling's A and B solution

A. Dissolve 34.65g cupric sulphate in water and makeupto 500mL

B. Dissolve 125g Potassium hydroxide and 173g potassium sodium tartarate (Rochelle salt) in water and make upto 500mL

Molisch's reagent: 5 % α naphthal in alcohol, i.e., 5g of α naphthal dissolved in 100mL of ethanol.

Iodine solution: 0.005% in 3% KI, i.e., 3g of KI dissolved in 100mL water and then 5mg of iodine is dissolved.

Benedict's solution: 17.3g of sodium citrate and 10g of sodium carbonate are dissolved in 75mL of water. 1.73g of $CuSO_4.5H_2O$ is dissolved in 20mL of water. Mix the $CuSO_4$ solution with alkaline citrate with constant stirring, finally the whole volume is made up to 100mL with water.

Barfoed's reagent: 13.3g of copper acetate in 200mL of water and add 2mL of glacial acetic acid.

Concentrated HCl

Concentrated H_2SO_4

Osazone Reagent

Dissolve Phenyl hydrazine hydrochloride and Sodium acetate in the distilled water in the ratio of 1 : 2

Acetic acid

Bial's Reagent: Dissolve 3g orcinol in 500mL concentrated HCl, add 2.5mL of a 10% solution of ferric chloride hexahydrate, and dilute to one liter with water; this is approximately 6M HCl. The reagent is stable for months, but its yellow colour gradually darkens and some precipitate forms; this doesn't seem to affect its reactivity.

Seliwanoff's Reagent: Dissolve 1g resorcinol in 330mL concentrated HCl, dilute to one liter (approx. 4 M HCl final). This reagent seems to be stable for more than a year, though we usually make less than the recipe specifies.

Principle

Molisch's test: Con. H_2SO_4 dehydrates carbohydrates to form furfural and its derivatives. This product combines with sulphonated α naphthal to give purple colour.

Iodine test: Iodine forms a coloured absorption complex with polysaccharides due to the formation of micellae aggregate. Iodine will form a polysaccharide inclusion complex.

Benedict's test: Carbohydrates with a potential aldehyde or ketone group have reducing property when placed in an alkaline solution. Cupric ions present in the solution will be reduced to cuprous ion. This will give a red coloured precipitate. Moreover, this test is more specific for reducing sugars.

Barfoed' test: Barfoed's reagent is weakly acidic and it is only reduced by monosaccharides. Prolonged boiling may hydrolyze the disaccharide to give false positive test.

Bial's test: When pentose is heated with con.HCl, furfural, which condenses with orcinol in the presence of ferric ion to give a blue green colour.

Seliwanoff's test: Ketoses are dehydrated more rapidly than aldose to give a furfural derivatives, which then condenses with resorcinol to form a red colour complex.

Osazone test: Compounds containing aldehyde and keto groups form crystalline osazone with phenyl hydrazine hydrochloride. Osazone crystals have characteristic shape and melting point which helps in the identification of reducing sugar.

Procedure

Perform the following qualitative tests using unknown carbohydrates.

S.No	Experiment Name & Procedure	Observation	Inference
1.	**Test For Solubility** a) Water b) Acid c) Alkali d) Alcohol	Mono and di saccharides are highly soluble in water. Polysaccharides are soluble in acid or alkali	This confirms the presence of carbohydrates other than polysaccharides. This confirms the presence of polysaccharides.
2.	**Molisch's Test -** Add 2 drops of Molisch reagent to 2mL of the sugar solution and mix thoroughly and pour 5mL concentrated sulphuric acid along the sides of the test tube.	A purple ring is formed at the junction of two layers, which spreads on standing.	This shows the presence of carbohydrate.
3.	**Anthrone Test -** To 2mL of test solution add 1mL Anthrone reagent.	Blue green complex formed	This shows the presence of aldehyde and ketone group.
4.	**Benedict's Test -** To 8 drops of test solution add 5mL of Benedict's solution and heated to boiling.	Orange red precipitate obtained. No characteristic colour change.	Presence of reducing sugar. Absence of reducing sugar.

5.	Fehling's Test - To 5mL of test solution add equal volume of Fehling's A and B solution and heated to boiling.	A reddish brown precipitate formed	This shows the presence of reducing sugar.
6.	Barfoed's Test - To 5mL of test solution add 5mL of Barfoed's reagent and heated to boiling.	Brick red precipitate is Obtained at the bottom of test tube.	Presence of reducing monosaccharide
		No characteristic colour change.	Absence of reducing monosaccharide.
7.	Selivanoff's Test - To 2mL of Selivanoff's reagent add 3 drops of test solution and heated to boiling.	Cherry red colour Obtained.	Presence of fructose.
		No characteristic colour change.	Absence of fructose.
8.	Iodine Test - Add 2 drops of iodine to 1mL of the test solution.	Deep blue colour	Presence of polysaccharide.
		Dark brown colour	Prescence of polysaccharide (Glycogen).
		No characteristic colour change.	Absence of polysaccharide.
9.	Osazone Test - Take 1mL osazare reagent in test tube. To this add 5mL of test solution and acidified with 2 drops of glacial acetic acid and heated in a boiling water bath for 15 minutes	Yellow colour precipitate formed. The following crystals maybe observed under microscope	This shows the presence of aldehyde and ketone group
		a. Needle shaped crystals	Presence of Glucose
		b. Needle shaped crystals	Presence of Fructose
		c. Palm leaf shaped crystals	Presence of Galactose
		d. Powder buff shaped crystals	Presence of Lactose
		e. Flower petal shaped crystals	Presence of Maltose is confirmed
10.	Bials Test - To 5mL Bials reagent add 2-3mL of test solution and worm gently and cool under tap water.	Blue green colour obtained.	Prescence of pentose sugar.
		No characteristic colour change.	Absence of pentose sugar.

Result

The given sample contains — — — — — — — — — — — — carbohydrate.

144. Qualitative Test for Proteins

Aim

To identify the protein present in the given sample solution

Background information

Proteins are about 50% of the dry weight of most cells and are the most structurally complex macromolecules. Each type of protein has its own unique structure and function. Proteins are polymers of about 20 amino acids (the monomer). Amino acids are built from a central carbon bonded to four *different* groups. They are hydrogen (–H), amino group (–NH$_2$), carboxyl group (–COOH), and some side chain symbolized by "R". To form protein, the amino acids are linked by dehydration synthesis to form peptide bonds. The chain of amino acids is also known as a polypeptide. Some proteins contain only one polypeptide chain while others, such as haemoglobin, contain several polypeptide chains all twisted together.

Procedure

S. No.	Experiment	Observation	Inference
1)	**Solubility:** a) Water b) Dilute NaOH solution	Colloidal solution formed. Partially soluble.	Presence of protein. Presence of protein.
2)	**Precipitation by neutral salt solution:** To 1mL of the substance add equal volume of a saturated solution of Ammonium sulphate.	White precipitate formed. White precipitate is formed.	Presence of Globulin. Presence of Albumin.
3)	**Precipitation by heavy Metals -** To 1mL of the sample add equal volume of 5% Mercuric nitrate.	White precipitate formed.	Presence of protein.
4)	**Precipitation by alcohol -** To 1mL of the substance add equal volume of alcohol.	White precipitate formed.	Presence of protein.
5)	**Heat coagulation -** About 1mL of the substance is taken in clean test tube and heated.	Cloudy white precipitate formed by coagulation.	Presence of protein.
6)	**Biuret test -** To 1mL of the substance add few drops of Biuret reagent.	Purple colour formed.	Presence of protein.
7)	**Ninhydrin test -** To 1mL of the test solution add few drops of Ninhydrin reagent and heat for 2 minutes.	A purple colour obtained.	Presence of amino acid in the protein.
8)	**Xanthoprotic test -** To 1mL of test solution add few drops of conc. nitric acid and heat it. Cool it. Then add few drops of 40% NaOH.	Yellow colour formed after the addition of conc. Nitric acid and this turns red on the addition of NaOH.	Presence of aromatic Amino acid in the Protein.

9)	**Pauly's test** - To 1mL of test solution add few drops of 1% sulphanilic acid and Cool it in an ice bath. Then add 1mL of 5% $NaNO_2$ and 1mL of 1% Na_2CO_3.	Deep blue colour dye is obtained.	Presence of Tyrosine and histidine units in protein.
10)	**Millon's test** - To 1mL of test solution add Millon's reagent and heat it for few minutes.	Red colour obtained.	Presence of phenolic group containing aminoacid (tyrosine) in the protein.
11)	**Morner's test** - To 1mL of the test solution add Millons Reagent and heat it in a boiling water bath.	Green colour obtained.	Presence of Tyrosine in the protein.
12)	**Folin's phenol test** - To 1mL of the test solution add equal volume of Folin's reagent followed by the addition of 1% of Na_2CO_3.	Blue colour obtained.	Presence of Tyrosine in the protein.
13)	**Aldehyde test** - To 1mL of the test solution add 2-3 drops of 1% HCHO and then carefully add few drops of conc. H_2SO_4 along the sides of the test tube.	A violet colour ring formed at the junction of the two layers.	Presence of Tryptophan in the protein.
14)	**Ehrlisch's test** - To 1mL of the test solution add few drops of Ehrlisch's reagent and heat it in a boiling water bath.	Pinkish red colour obtained.	Presence of Tryptophan in the protein.
15)	**Sakaguchi's test** - To 2mL of test solution add few drops of alpha- naphthol in alcohol followed by the addition of 1mL of 20% NaOH and a few drops of Bromine water.	Red colour obtained.	Presence of Arginine in the protein.
16)	**Sulphur test** - To 1mL of test solution add few drops of 45% NaOH and boil it for 2 minutes cool it, then add lead acetate.	Dirty black precipitate obtained.	Presence of Cysteine in the protein.
17)	**Sodium nitroprusside test** - To 2mL of test solution add few drops of 20% NaOH .Then add 1mL of sodium – nitroprusside followed by the addition of 1.5mL of 1% Glycine.Boil it for few minutes. Then add 1mL of 6N HCl.	Reddish purple colour obtained.	Presence of Methionine in the protein.
18)	**Molisch's test** - To 1mL of the substance add few drops of Molisch's reagent then add Conc.sulphuric acid along the sides of the test tubes.	Violet colour ring formed at the junction of two layers.	Presence of Carbohydrate unit in the protein.

Results:

The given protein sample contain which contains the following, Arginine, Tyrosine, Tryptophan, Cysteine, Methionine.

146. Qualitative Test for Amino Acids

Aim

To identify the amino acid present in the given sample solution

Principle

Amino acids are basic units of proteins. There are 21 amino acids, which occur, commonly in biological systems. Their reaction varies with the nature of -R- groups. In the Ninhydrin test amino acids react with mild oxidizing agents (Ninhydrin) at 70°C to form NH_3, CO_2 and aldehyde of amino acids. In the second step reduced Ninhydrin reacts with oxidized Ninhydrin in the presence of ammonia (NH_3) forming a blue-coloured products. There are specific test for aromatic amino acids and sulphur containing amino acids.

Materials required

Millon's Reagent: Dissolve 15g of Mercuric Sulphate in 100mL of 15% of Sulphuric acid.

Sulphanilic Acid: 1g of Sulphanilic Acid in 100mL of 10% HCl (1% solution).

Sodium Nitrate(5%): Dissolve 5g of $NaNO_2$ in 100mL of water.

Sodium Carbonate: (1%)- Dissolve 1g of Na_2CO_3 in 100mL of water (1% solution)

Ehrlisch's Reagent: Dissolve 10g of p-dimethyl amino benzaldehyde in 100mL of 10% HCl.

α-Naphthol: Dissolve 1g of α-Naphthol in 100mL of alcohol.

Sodium hydroxide (40%): Dissolve 40g of NaOH 100mL of water (40% solution)

Bromine Water: Few drops of Bromine in 100mL of water.

Lead Acetate(1%): Dissolve 1g of lead dissolved in 100mL of water.

Sodium hydroxide (1%): Dissolve 1g of NaOH in 100 mL of water. (1% solution).

Con.Sulphuric acid

Glacial acetic acid

Principle

Ninhydrin Test: Ninhydrin is a powerful oxidising agent reacts with amino-acids,between pH 4-8 to give a purple colour complex.Ninhydrin reagent is reduced to hydrindantin during reaction with a-amino-acids.The amino acid in turn is converted into an aldehyde. Ammonia&Carbon dioxide are evolved.Hydrindantin and ammonia interact with another molecule of ninhydrin to form Ruhemann's purple coloured complex.

Xanthoproteic Test: Amino acid containing aromatic chains will form Xanthoproteic acid when it is treated with Con.HNO_3 Salts of these derivatives are orange in colour when treated with alkali.

Pauly's Test: Diazotised sulphanilic acid couples with amino phenol and immidazole to form a coloured azo compound in cold condition.

Millon's Test: Phenolic amino acid on treatment with Millon's reagent gives red colour. Mercuric sulphate forms a coloured compound with hydroxyl group of amino acid (Tyrosine).

Morner's Test: Amino acid containing aromatic hydroxyl group reacts with this reagent to give green colour. This test is to specify for amino acid containing aromatic hydroxyl group.(tyrosine)

Folin's Test: Amino acid containing aromatic ring reacts with this reagent to give blue colour.

Hopkin's Cole Test: This reaction is answered by tryptophan. This reaction is due to the prsence of indole group in tryptophan.

Ehrlisch Test: Indole group containing amino acid reacts with this reagent to give purple colour or pinkish red coloured complex.

Sakaguchi Test: This reaction is specific for guanidino group of Arginine or protein containing Arginine.

Sulphur Test: Amino acids containing the thiol or sulphydryl group reacts with sodium plumbate to form a dark grey or black precipitate which is insoluble in dil.HCl.

Sodium Nitroprusside (Bollin's) Test: Amino acids containing the free thiol group $(S-H)$ (due to cysteine) yield a red colour, with sodium nitroprusside in an ammoniacal environment. Cystine which contains disulphide linkage $(S-S)$ may be reduced to cysteine using reducing agent such as sodium cyanide, sodium brohydride or sodium bisulphate which then yields a positive result.

S. No	Experiment	Observation	Inference
1.	**Ninhydrin Test -** To 2mL of the test solution add 2mL of Ninhydrin reagent and boil for 5 minutes.	Blue / Purple colour formation	Presence of á Amino acids
2.	**Xanthoprotein Test -** To 2mL of the test solution add few drops of concentrated Nitric acid and then add a few drops of dilute sodium hydroxide	Yellow Colour formed after the addition of con. HNO_3 and this turns to red colour while NaOH is added	Presence of Aromatic amino acid.
		No characteristic colour change	Absence of aromatic amino acid.
3.	**Millon's Test -** To few drops of the test solution add a few drops Mercuric Sulphate followed by the addition of Sodium nitrite. Then add a few drops of 5% $NaNO_2$.	Red colour is obtained	Presence of phenolic group containing amino acid. Presence of Tyrosine
		No characteristic red colour	Absence of phenolic group containing amino acid.
4.	**Hopkin's-Cole Test -** To 2mL of Glyoxylic acid add 2mL of test solution and mixed well. Then carefully add 2mL of concentrated sulphuric acid through the sides of the test tube	Ring is formed at the junction of two layer	Presence of Tryptophan
5.	**Pauly's Test -** Mix 1mL of sulphanilic acid to 2mL of the test solution and cool it in ice. Add 1mL of 5% sodium nitrite solution. After 5minutes add 5mL of 1% sodium carbonate solution	Deep red colour dye is obtained	Presence of Histidine and Tyrosine.
		No characteristic coloured dye	Absence of Histidine, Tyrosine and Tryptophan.

6.	**Morner's Test -** To few drops of the test solution add a few drops of Morner's reagent and heat the solution in a boiling water bath.	Green colour is formed.	Presence of Tyrosine.
		No characteristic colour change.	Absence of Tyrosine.
7.	**Ehrlich's Test -** To 1mL of the Ehrlich's reagent, 1mL of test solution is added	Red colour is developed due to the presence of Indole ring in the Tryptophan	Presence of Tryptophan
8.	**Folin's Phenol Test -** To 2mL of the test solution add equal mL of Folin's Phenol reagent and then add 1% Na_2CO_3	Blue colour is obtained.	Presence of Tyrosine.
		No characteristic colour change	Absence of Tyrosine.
9.	**Aldehyde Test -** To few drops of the test solution add 1mL of 1% HCHO and then add 1mL of con.H_2SO_4	A violet colour ring is formed at the junction of two layers.	Presence of Tryptophan.
		No characteristic colour change.	Absence of Tryptophan.
10.	**Hopkin's Cole Test -** To few drops of the test solution add 1mL of glyoxallic acid and then add con.H_2SO_4 carefully along the sides of the test tube.	A violet colour ring formed at the junction of two layers.	Presence of Tryptophan.
		No characteristic colour change.	Absence of Tryptophan
11.	**Ehrisch's Test:** To 2mL of the test solution add equal volumes of ehrlish's reagent and heat the solution in a boiling water bath for a few minutes.	Pinkish red colour obtained.	Presence of Tryptophan.
		No characteristic colour change	Absence of Tryptophan
12.	**Sakaguchi's Test -** 3mL of test solution is mixed with 1mL of 40% sodium hydroxide solution and add 2 drops of α – napthol then a few drops of bromine water is added	Red colour obtained	Presence of Arginine.
		No characteristic colour change	Absence of Arginine.
13.	**Sodium Nitroprusside Test -** To 2mL of test solution add 1mL of 20% NaOH followed by the addition of sodium nitroprusside and 1mL of glycine.Now heat the mixture.Cool it.Then add 6N HCl slowly in drops through the sides of test tube.	Redddish purple colour is obtained.	Presence of Methionine.
		No characteristic colour change.	Absence of Methionine.
14.	**Sulphur Test -** To few drops of test solution add equal volumes of 45%NaOH and then heat for 2 min in boiling water bath.Cool it. Then add 5mL of lead acetate solution.	Dirty coloured black precipitate obtained.	Presence of Cysteine.
		No characteristic change	Absence of Cysteine.

Result

The given sample contain — — — — — — — — — — — — —aminoacid.

146. Quantitative estimation for Lipids

Aim

To analyze the for the presence of lipids

Background information

Lipids are a broad group of naturally-occurring molecules which includes fats, oils, waxes, phospholipids, steroids (like cholesterol), and some other related compounds. Fats and oils are made from two kinds of molecules, which include glycerol and three fatty acids joined by dehydration synthesis. Since there are three fatty acids attached, these are known as triglycerides. The terms saturated, mono-unsaturated, and poly-unsaturated refer to the number of hydrogens attached to the hydrocarbon tails of the fatty acids as compared to the number of double bonds between carbon atoms in the tail. Triglycerides contain the maximum possible amount of hydrogens, these would be called saturated fats. The hydrocarbon chains in these fatty acids are, thus, fairly straight and can pack closely together, making these fats solid at room temperature. Oils, mostly from plant sources, have some double bonds between some of the carbons in the hydrocarbon tail, causing bends or "kinks" in the shape of the molecules. Because some of the carbons share double bonds, they're not bonded to as many hydrogens as they could if they weren't double bonded to each other. Therefore these oils are called unsaturated fats. Because of the kinks in the hydrocarbon tails, unsaturated fats can't pack as closely together, making them liquid at room temperature. Many people have heard that the unsaturated fats are "healthier" than the saturated ones. Hydrogenated vegetable oil (as in shortening and commercial peanut butters where a solid consistency is sought) started out as "good" unsaturated oil. However, this commercial product has had all the double bonds artificially broken and hydrogens artificially added to turn it into saturated fat that bears no resemblance to the original oil from which it came.

Phospholipids are made from glycerol, two fatty acids, and (in place of the third fatty acid) a phosphate group with some other molecule attached to its other end. The hydrocarbon tails of the fatty acids are still hydrophobic, but the phosphate group end of the molecule is hydrophilic because of the oxygens with all of their pairs of unshared electrons. This means that phospholipids are soluble in both water and oil.

An emulsifying agent is a substance which is soluble in both oil and water, thus enabling the two to mix. A "famous" phospholipid is lecithin which is found in egg yolk and soybeans. Lecithin is used to emulsify the lipids and hold them in the water as an emulsion.

Cholesterol is not a "bad guy!" Our body make about 2 g of cholesterol per day, and that makes up about 85% of blood cholesterol, while only about 15% comes from dietary sources. Cholesterol is the precursor to our sex hormones and Vitamin D. Vitamin D is formed by the action of UV light in sunlight on cholesterol molecules that have 'risen" to near the surface of the skin.

Lipoproteins are clusters of proteins and lipids all tangled up together. These act as a means of carrying lipids, including cholesterol, around in our blood. There are two main categories of lipoproteins distinguished by how compact/dense they are. LDL or low-density lipoprotein is the "bad guy," being associated with deposition of 'cholesterol" on the walls of someone's arteries. HDL or high-density lipoprotein is the "good guy," being associated with carrying "cholesterol" out of the blood system.

Materials Required

Ethanol, Chloroform, bi salts solution and detergents, Potassium bi sulfate, 10% alcoholic sodium hydroxide, Alcoholic bromine solution, Acetic anhydride, Sulphuric acid

S. No	Experiment	Observation	Inference
1.	**Solubility Test** The solubility of the substance is conducted with the following solvents		
a)	Water	Insoluble	Presence of Lipids.
b)	Sodium Hydroxide	Insoluble	Presence of Lipids.
c)	Alcohol	Insoluble	Presence of Lipids.
d)	Benzene	Soluble	Presence of Lipids.
e)	Chloroform	Soluble	Presence of Lipids.
f)	Ether	Soluble	Presence of Lipids.
2.	**Emulsification Test :** The sample is emulsified with 5mL of water 5mL of bile salts solution and detergents	Temporary emulsion on vigorous shaking Highly stable emulsion	The water do not have the tendency to reduce the surface tension of water but the bi salts and detergents can break the large fat into small droplets and can reduce the surface tension of oil gently
3.	**Acrolein Test :** To a pinch of potassium bi sulfate in a dry test tube add 4 drops of sample and heated	Pungent smelling fumes	Acrolein is evolved which has the pungent smell. All fats answer this test.
4.	**Saponification Test :** To 5mL of the sample added 2.5mL of ethanol and 10mL of 10% alcoholic sodium hydroxide. It is shaken well and placed in the boiling water bath for 15 minutes. Then it is made up to 20mL with water and divided into four equal parts and added		
	a) Concentrated Hydrochloric acid	A white precipitate	The insoluble fatty acids are precipitated.
	b) Standard Saline	Pale white layer on the surface	
	c) 3drops of calcium chloride solution	A white precipitate	
	d) 3drops of magnesium chloride solution	A white precipitate	
5.	**Test for Un saturation :** 3drops of the sample and 3mL of ethanol are mixed well. Then added alcoholic bromine solution, until bromine imparts its colour	Colourless at first and gradually turned into yellow Deep green colour	Reserce of Lipids.

| 6. | **Test for Cholesterol**

a) **Libermann-Burchard Test :** 2mL of sample added 2mL of chloroform and 10drops of acetic anhydride mixed well and the concentrated sulphuric acid was added along the sides of the test tubes

b) **Salkowski Test :** To 2mL of sample add 2mL of chloroform then added equal volume of concentrated sulfuric acid. | Two layers appeared brown layer and low yellow fluorescent layer | This indicates the presence of Cholesterol.

This confirms the presence of Cholesterol. |

Procedure

Result

The given sample contain — — — — — — — — — — — — — lipid.

147. Estimation of Carbohydrate by Anthrone Method

Aim

To estimate the amount of carbohydrate present in the given sample

Principle

This method is used to estimate total carbohydrate present in the sample. The anthrone reaction is the basis of rapid and convenient method for the determination of hexoses and pentoses, either free or present in polysaccharides. Carbohydrates are dehydrated by concentrated sulphuric acid to form furfural (Hexose) or 5 – hydroxymethyl furfurol (Pentose). Furfural or hydoxy methyl furfurol condenses with anthrone gives rise to a green coloured complex which was measured colourimetrically at 620 - 640nm.

Materials Required

Anthrone reagent (0.2%)

Dissolve 0.2g of anthrone in 5 mL of ethanol. Add slowly 75% of sulphuric acid till the mark reaches 100mL in standard measuring flask.

Stock standard (1000µg/mL)

Dissolve 100mG of glucose in 100mL of distilled water

Working standard

Makeup 10 mL of stock standard to 100mL. It gives 100µG/mL concentration.

Unknown sample

Other materials :

Spectrophoto meter, Aluminium foil, Water bath, Test tubes, Standard measuring flask,

Cuvette, Micropipette, Pipette.

Procedure

Standard graph preparation

- Prepare various concentration of the working standard solution in a series of test tube from 0.1mL to 1mL (10µG to 100µG).
- Make up the volume to 1mL with distilled water.
- Keep the tubes in an ice bath and slowly add 5 mL of the cold anthrone reagent and mix properly.
- Close the tubes with aluminium foil and place it in a boiling water bath for 10 min.
- Cool the tubes and measure OD at 620 nm.
- Blank should be prepared as per previous steps without adding test or standard solution.
- Plot the graph and calculate the carbohydrate content of the sample given.

Testing unknown solution

1mL of test solution is taken in test tube.
Follow steps as like standard graph.
Calculate concentration of carbohydrate using standard graph.

Table 147.1:Estimation of Carbohydrate

S. No	Volume of working standard in mL	Volume of water in (mL)	Concentration of working sample (µG / mL)	Volume of anthrone in mL	OD at 620nm
1	0.1	0.9	10	5	
2	0.2	0.8	20	5	
3	0.3	0.7	30	5	
4	0.4	0.6	40	5	
5	0.5	0.5	50	5	
6	0.6	0.4	60	5	
7	0.7	0.3	70	5	
8	0.8	0.2	80	5	
9	0.9	0.1	90	5	
10	1.0	0.0	100	5	
Test Sample 1mL		0.0	Unknown	5	

Observation

Green colour formation is noted and meadured OD at 620nm

Result

The given test sample contains — — — — — — — — — — — — — — —mG of glucose per 100mL.

Viva questions

What is the principle of carbohydrate estimation by anthrone method?
How do you prepare Anthrone reagent?
What is the purpose of using H_2SO_4 in this experiment?
Name the intermediate compound produced during Carbohydrate estimation through Anthrone method.

Spotters: Anthrone.

148. Estimation of Reducing Sugar by DNS Method

Aim

To estimate reducing sugar content of test sample.

Principle

Reducing sugar was analysed by dinitrosalicylicacid (DNS) method (Miller *et al.,* 1959). It is a simple, sensitive and adoptable method. Reagents reacts with reducing sugar produces dark yellow colour to light brown colour.

Materials required

Test tubes, conical flask, cuvette, spectrophotometer, DNS reagent, test sample

Preparation of DNS reagent

Sodium hydroxide	1gm
Phenol	2mL
Sodium potasium tartarate	20gm
Sodium corbonate	0.05gm
3,5-dinitro salicilicacid	1gm

All these ingredient are added to the 100mL distilled water in this sequence.

Procedure

Preparation of standard graph

- Prepare an aqueous solution of glucose at a concentration of 1mG / mL .

- To a series of 10 test tubes, add a glucose stock solution corresponding to the required sugar concentration (0.1-1mL).

- Make up the volume to 3mL using double distilled water (Use distilled water as a blank).

- Add 2mL of DNS and heated in boiling water bath at 80°C for 15 minutes and cooled.

- Read the absorbency at 580nm.

- Plot the values on a graph.

Analysis of reducing sugar from sample

- Take 5 mL of sample aseptically and centrifuged at 5000RPM for 10minutes.

- Add 1mL of supernatent to a test tube and make up the volume to 3mL using double distilled water(Use distilled water as a blank).

- Add 2mL of DNS and heated in boiling water bath at 80°C for 15 minutes and cooled.

- Read the absorbency at 580nm.

- The concentration of reducing sugar/mL is determined using the standard graph.

Observation and result

Dark yellow colour is noted on the test sample which indicates the presence of reducing sugar.

149. Estimation of reducing sugars by Benedict's Test

Aim

To estimate the amount of glucose present in the given unknown sample by Benedict's method.

Principle

Benedict's quantitative reagent is the modified form of qualitative reagent. It consists of cupric sulphate, sodium carbonate and sodium citrate, potassium thiocyanate, and potassium ferrocyanide.

The alkali present in the Benedict's reagent analyses the sugar, thereby causing them to be a strong reducing agent. Ferrocyanide serves to dissolve the copper hydroxide while thiocyanate helps to convert the red cuprous oxide to white crystals of cuprous thiocyanate, which gives the clear end point.

Materials required

(i) Benedict's quantitative reagent (BQR) - Cupric Sulfate - 1-2% . Sodium Carbonate - 6-7%.

Sodium Citrate, 16-17% . Potassium Ferrocyanide, trihydrate <1%. Potassium Thiocyanate , 10-11%. Water - 100mL.

(ii)Anhydrous sodium carbonate

(iii)Working standard glucose solution

(iv)Porcelain beads.

Test tubes, beaker, burette, pipette etc.,

Procedure

Titration I: Standardisation of Benedict's Qualitative Reagent

- Accurately pipette out 5mL of Benedict's quantitative reagent into a clean conical flask.
- Add two spatula full of 2g of sodium carbonate into the conical flask.
- Also add few pieces of porcelain beads in order to avoid bumping.
- Heat the contents t to temperature approximately 60-70°C.
- Titrate the contents against the standard glucose solution with regular shaking until the blue colour disappeared.
- Chalky white precipitate Appearance indicates the end point.
- Repeat the titrations for concordant values.

Titration II: Estimation of Glucose

- Makeup the given unknown sample solution to 100mL with distilled water in a standard flask.
- Shake well to get uniform concentration.
- Fill the burette with this unknown solution and titrate against Benedict's quantitative reagent available in a beaker.
- Chalky white precipitate Appearance indicates the end point.
- Repeat the titrations for concordant values.

Result

The amount of glucose present in 100mLof the given solution _____mG

Table 149.1- Titration I : Standardisation of Benedict's Quantitative reagent
Std Glucose Vs Benedict's Quantitative reagent   Indicator : Self

| S.No. | Contents in conical Flask   (mL) | Burette reading | | Concordant Value (mL) |
		Initial	Final	
1.				
2.				
3.				

Table 149.2 -Titration II : Estimation of Glucose
Standard Benedict's Quantitative reagent Vs Unknown Glucose Indicator : Self

| S.No. | Contents in conical Flask   (mL) | Burette reading | | Concordant Value (mL) |
		Initial	Final	
1.				
2.				
3.				

Calculation

100mL of the unknown solution contains = $\dfrac{\text{Standard value} \times 100}{\text{unknown value}}$

100mL of Sample contain is _____ glucose.

150. Estimation of Reducing Sugar by Nelson - Somogyi's Method

Aim

To estimate reducing sugar by Nelson - Somogyi's Method.

Principle

This is one of the most widely used methods for the estimation of reducing sugar. Reducing sugar reduce Copper sulphate in the reagent to red orange cuprous oxide. The cuprous oxide on reaction with arsenomolybdate produces bluish green coloured complex. Molybdic acid is also converted to molybdenum.

Materials Required

Alkaline copper tartarate

A. Dissolve 2.5g anhydrous sodium carbonate, 2g sodium bicarbonate, 2.5 g sodium potassium tartarate and 20g anhydrous sodium sulphate in 80mL water and make upto 100mL.

B. Dissolve 15g copper sulphate in a small volume of distilled water. Add one drop of sulphuric acid and make up to 100mL

Mix 4mL solution B and 96mL Solution A

Arsenomolybdate reagent

Dissolve 2.5g ammonium molybdate in 45mL water. Add 2.5mL Sulphuric acid and mix well. Then add 25mL Disodium hydrogen arsenate (Dissolve 0.3g in 25mL of water). Mix well and incubate at 37°C for 24 – 48 hours.

Standard glucose solution

Dissolve 100mG in 100mL of water.

Procedure

- Pipette out 0.2 to 1mL of standard glucose solution into a different test tube makeup the volume to 2mL with distilled water.
- Add 1mL of alkaline copper tartarate reagent to each tube.
- Place the tube in boiling water bath for 10 minutes.
- Cool the tubes and add 1mL of Arsenomolybdate reagent.
- Make up the volume to 10mL with distilled water.
- Read absorbance at 620nm after 10 minutes.
- Carry out a blank under the same condition using 2mL distilled water instead of sugar soluton.

Result

The given unknown sample contains .... mG/% of sugar.

151. Estimation of sugar by Folin Wu method

Aim

To estimate glucose concentration from serum or unknown solutions.

Principle

This method is based on that glucose is heated with an alkaline copper solution the glucose produces a precipitate of cuprous oxide, which inturn is dissolved by and reduces phospho molybdic solution to a blue colour, which is compared calorimetrically at 440nm. This method is mainly used for blood glucose detection.

Materials required

Sodium tungstate

Dissolve 10g of sodium tungstate in distilled water and make to 100mL.

Sulphuric acid

Dilute 2mL of concentrated sulphuric acid to 100mL with distilled water.

Alkaline copper tartarate solution

Dissolve 20g of anhydrous sodium carbonate in 200mL distilled water, followed by 3.75g of tartaric acid. Dissolve and add 2.25g copper sulphate. Make the volume to 500mL with distilled water.

Phospho molybdic reagent

Dissolve 17.5g of molybdic acid and 2.5g sodium tungstate in 100mL of 10% sodium hydroxide solution, add 100mL of distilled water. Boil for 30 to 40 minutes to expel all ammonia present in molybdic acid. Add 62.5mL phosphoric acid and make up to 250mL with distilled water.

Glucose stock standard solution

Dissolve 1000mG in 100 mL of water.

Working standard

Dilute 1mL of stock standard with 9mL of distilled water.

Procedure

Preparation of protein free filtrate

Add 3.5mL of distilled water and 1mL of blood followed by 0.2mL of sodium tungstate in a 10mL of centrifuge tube. Mix and add 0.2mL of sulphuric acid. Mix well, stand for 5minutes and centrifuge at 3000rpm for 5 minutes.

Glucose estimation

- Take 2mL of protein free filtrate / unknown sugar solution in a Folin Wu sugar tube.

- Add 2mL alkaline copper reagent, mix well and place in a boiling water bath for 8 minutes.

- Remove the tube from water bath and cool in a beaker of cold water for 2-3 minutes.

- Add 2mL of phospho molybdic acid reagent and let stand for few minutes until the cuprous oxide has completely dissolved.

- Dilute to 12.5mL mark with distilled water.

- Mix well and read OD at 440nm in spectrophotometer.

- Similarly run black using 2mL of distilled water in place of protein free blood filtrate.

- For standard graph, prepare various concentration of glucose (10 -100mG/0.1 – 1mL) in a test tube and make upto 2mL and follow as like unknown procedure.

Result

The given sample contains – – – –mG of glucose.

152. Estimation of Protein by Lowry's Method

Aim

To estimate the amount of protein present in the given sample.

Principle

Protein reacts with the Folin- Ciocalteau reagent to give a coloured complex. Tyrosine and tryptophan residues of protein reduce sodium tungstate and sodium molybdate anions in folin reagent which when combines with Copper of copper sulphate gives blue coloured complex (Hetero polymolybdenum and tungsten blue). The copper atom present in copper sulphate complexed with nitrogen atom of the peptide bond of protein during reaction time that is also a reason for blue/purple colour formation. The intensity of colour depends on the amount of these aromatic amino acids present and will thus vary for different protein.

Materials Required

Solution1: Alkaline sodium carbonate solution

Take 2 g of sodium hydroxide in 400mL of double distilled water. Mix well and then add 10g of anhydrous sodium carbonate. Shake well and make up to 500mL using distilled water.

Solution 2 : Copper sulphate Solution

Dissolve 1 g of copper sulphate in 50mL of distilled water

Solution 3 : Sodium potassium tararate solution

Dissolve 1g of sodium potassium tartarate in 50 mL of water

Solution 4: Mixed reagent

Add 0.5 mL of solution 2 with 0.5mL of solution 3. To this mixture add 99 mL of solution 1. follow the same order as describes here and prepare the solution fresh.

Solution 5: Folin-Ciocalteau reagent

Dilute the commercial reagent with an equal volume of distilled water on the day of use (This is a solution of sodium tungstate and sodium molybdate in phosphoric and hydrochloric acids)

Solution 6: Standard protein -Bovine Serum Albumin

Dissolve 10mG of BSA in 10 mL of double distilled water

Solution 7 : Working standard

Makeup 1 mL of stock standard to 10mL. It gives 100µG/mL concentration.

Other materials

Aluminium foil, Water bath, Test tubes, Standard measuring flask, Cuvette, Micropipette, Pipette.

Procedure

- Pipette out various concentration of working standard solution into a series of test tubes and made up the volume to 0.2 mL with distilled water (10μL to 100μL).
- To each test tube add 1 mL of the mixed reagent and mix thoroughly and allow to stand at room temperature for 10 min or longer.
- Add 0.3mL of diluted Folin-Ciocolteau reagent rapidly and mix properly.
- Incubate all tubes for 60 minutes.
- Measure OD of the standard and test solution at 660nm and plot the standard graph.
- Run the blank.
- The test protein sample is performed as like the standard solution and calculate the amount of protein present in the given sample.

Table 152.1: Estimation of Protein-Lowry's Method

S. No	Volume of Standard μL	Volume of water μL	Conc. of working sample	Mixed reagent (mL)	Folin's Reagent(mL)	OD-value (660 nm)
1	10	190	10 μG	1	0.3	
2	20	180	20 μG	1	0.3	
3	30	170	30 μG	1	0.3	
4	40	160	40 μG	1	0.3	
5	50	150	50 μG	1	0.3	
6	60	140	60 μG	1	0.3	
7	70	130	70 μG	1	0.3	
8	80	120	80 μG	1	0.3	
9	90	110	90 μG	1	0.3	
10	100	100	100 μG	1	0.3	
Test sample 200 μL			Unknown	1	0.3	
Blank 200μL Water			Nil	1	0.3	000

Observation

Blue colour is noted and read using spectrophotometer

Result

Concentration of protein present in the given sample is $-------\mu G/mL$

Viva questions

What are the major components of Folin reagent?
How do you extract protein from bacterial cell?
Mention about the principle of Folin?
List out reagents used in protein estimation?

153. Estimation of Protein by Biuret test

Aim

To perform the estimation of protein by Biuret method.

Principle

Biuret method is the simplest method for protein estimation. This method is sensitive to the amino acid composition of the protein. Its sensitivity is moderately constant from protein to protein and because of its simple procedure and quick result, it is used to estimate protein in crude extract over a large range of concentration. This method can also be used to monitor the concentration of protein during purification.

This assay is based on copper ions binding to peptide bonds of protein under alkaline conditions to give a violet or purple colour. The intensity of the charge transfer absorption bond resulting from the Cu-protein complex is linearly proportional to the mass of protein present in the solution. The chromophore or light-absorbing center seems to be a complex between the peptide backbone and cupric ions.

Materials Required

Biuret reagent

Dissolve 1.5gm of CuSO4 and 4.5gms of Na-K tartrate in 250mL 0.2 N NaOH solution. Add 2.5gms of KI and make up the volume to 500mL with 0.2 N NaOH.

0.2 N NaOH.

Protein standard

Bovine serum albumin at a concentration of 1mG/mL in distilled water is used as a stock solution.

Procedure

- Pipette out standard protein solution into a series of tubes (0.0, 0.2, ..., 1mL) and make up the total volume to 4mL by adding water (Use 1mL of Unknown sample).
- The blank tube will have only 4mL of water.
- Add 6mL of biuret reagent to each tube and mix well.
- Keep the tubes at 37°C for 10 minutes during which a purple colour will develop.
- Measure the optical density of each tube at 520nm (green filter).
- Draw the standard graph to the known concentration of a protein and calculate unknown / test sample protein concentrations.

Result

The given sample contains .... mG of protein.

154. Estimation of proteins by Bradford methods

Aim

To estimate concentration of protein by Bradford method

Background information

A simple procedure for the determination of protein concentration in solutions is the Bradford protein assay which was described first by Bradford (Bradford *et al.*, 1976). An estimation of protein concentration is essential to be done rapidly and accurately in many fields of protein study. The Bradford assay has become the preferred method for quantifying protein in many laboratories. This technique is simpler, faster, and more sensitive than the Lowry method. Furthermore, when compared with the Lowry method, it is subject to less interference by common reagents and nonprotein components of biological samples. The Bradford assay relies on the binding of the dye Coomassie Blue G-250 to protein. The quantity of protein can be estimated by determining the amount of dye in the blue ionic form. This is usually achieved by measuring the absorbance of the solution at 595 nm. The dye appears to bind most readily to arginyl and lysyl residues of proteins.

Materials required

Bradford reagent

The assay reagent is made by dissolving 100mG of Coomassie Brillient Blue G250 in 50 mL of 95% ethanol. The solution is then mixed with 100mL of 85% phosphoric acid and made up to 1 L with distilled water. The reagent should be filtered through Whatman no. 1 filter paper and then stored in an amber bottle at room temperature.

Protein standard

Bovine serum albumin at a concentration of 1 mG/mL in distilled water is used as a stock solution.

Quartz (silica) spectrophotometer cuvettes should not be used, as the dye binds to this material. Traces of dye bound to glassware or plastic can be removed by rinsing with methanol or detergent solution.

Procedure

- Pipette 0.1mL to 1mL of protein standard in a series of test tubes, which contains 10 to 100μG of protein and made up to 1mL using distilled water.

- Use one mL of distilled water as the reagent blank.

- Take 0.1 mL of unknown sample and made up to 1mL using distilled water.

- Add 5 mL of bradford reagent to each tube and mix well by inversion or gentle vortex mixing. Avoid foaming.

- Measure the Absorbance at 595nm of the samples and standards against the reagent blank between 2 min and 1 h after mixing.

- Prepare standard curve using standard values.

Result

The given sample contains .... mG/mL of protein.

155. Determination of acid number of an edible oil

Aim

To determine the acid number of the given edible oil.

Principle

The acid number is defined as the number of milligram of KOH required to neutralize the free fatty acid present in one gram of oil or fat. Fat may become rancid during the storage for a long time. Fat or oil are hydrolysed by micro organisms with the formation of free fatty acids. The amount of free fatty acid present in the oil is the indicator of the age and quality of that oil. Thus the high acid number will indicate that the oil is old and rancid.

Materials required

(i) Oxalic acid (0.1N)

(ii) KOH

(iii) Fat solvent (Ethanol and ether in 1:1 ratio)

(iv) Phenolphthalein

Procedure

Titration I: Standardisation of KOH

- Pipette out 10mL of the standard oxalic acid (0.1N) into a clean conical flask.
- Add 2 drops of phenolphthalein indicator and titrate against KOH taken in the burette till the appearance of permanent pale pink colour.
- Repeat the titration for concordant values.

Titration II: Determination of Acid number

- Weigh around 1g of the oil and transfer into a clean conical flask.
- Add 20mL of lipid solvent to dissolve the oil and shake well.
- Add a few drops of phenolphthalein indicator and titrate against standardized KOH taken in the burette.
- Permanent pale pink colour formation indicates the end point.
- Repeat the titration for concordant values.

Titration III: Blank titration

- Pipette out 20mL of lipid solvent into a clean conical flask.
- Add 2 drops of phenolphthalein indicator and titrate it against KOH taken in the burette.
- Permanent pale pink colour formation indicates the end point.
- Repeat the titration for concordant values.

Result

Acid number of given edible oil is _____ mG

Table 155.1-Titration I - Standardisation of KOH

Standard oxalic acid Vs KOH   Indicator : Phenolphthalein

S.No.	Volume of unknown oxalic acid (mL)	Burette reading		Concordant Value (mL)
		Initial (mL)	Final (mL)	
1.				
2.				
3.				

Calculation:

Volume of oxalic acid, V_1 =   mL

Normality of oxalic acid, N_1 =   N

Volume of KOH, V_2 =   mL

Normality of KOH, N_2 =   N

$$V_1 \times N_1 = V_2 \times N_2$$

Table 155.2-Titration II - Determination of acid number

Standard KOH Vs Oil   Indicator : Phenolphthalein

S.No.	Volume of lipid solvent (mL)	Burette reading		Concordant Value (mL)
		Initial	Final	
1.				
2.				
3.				

Volume of KOH consumed of oil = Test value – Blank value =   mL

Table 155.3- Titration III - Blank titration Determination of acid number

Standard KOH Vs lipid solvent   Indicator : Phenolphthalein

S.No.	Contents in conical Flask (mL)	Burette reading		Concordant Value (mL)
		Initial	Final	
1.				
2.				
3.				

Acid number = $\dfrac{\text{Volume of KOH} \times \text{Volume of KOH consumed} \times \text{Equivalent weight of KOH} \times 1000}{\text{Weight of oil} \times 1000}$

156. Determination of Saponification number of an edible oil

Aim

To determine the saponification number of the given edible oil.

Principle

Saponification value is defined as the number of milligram of KOH required to neutralise the fatty acid resulting in the complete hydrolysis of 1g of oil or fat. It gives an indication of the nature of the fatty acid present in the fat. On refluxing the fat or oil with alkali, the ester of glycerol is hydrolysed into glycerol and potassium salt of free fatty acid. If the length of the free fatty acid chain is longer, the acid is lesser in the utilization of KOH is less and vice-versa. A weighed amount of fat is saponified with known amount of alcoholic KOH, excess alkali is back titrated with standardized acid and the saponification value of the oil is determined.

Materials required

(i) Alcoholic KOH 0.5N

(ii) Hydrochloric acid 0.5N

(iii) Sodium carbonate 0.5N

(iv) Phenolphthalein

(v) Methyl orange

Burette, pipette, conical flask, test sample, beaker etc.,

Procedure

Titration I: Standardisation of Hydrochloric acid

- Pipette out 10mL of standard sodium carbonate into a clean conical flask.
- Add 2 drops of methyl orange indicator and titrate it against HCl taken in the burette.
- Change of yellow to red colour indicates end point.
- Repeat the titration for concordant values.

Titration II: Determination of saponification value

- Weigh around 1g of oil and transfer into a clean conical flask.
- Add 5mL of lipid solvent and 25mL of alcoholic KOH and heat in the water bath for about 30 minutes.
- Add two drops of phenolphthalein indicator and titrate it against standardised HCl taken in the burette.
- Disappearance of pink colour indicates end point.
- Repeat the titration for concordant values.

Blank titration:

- Pipette out 20mL of alcoholic KOH
- Add 5mL of lipid solvent, in a clean conical flask.
- Add 2 drops of phenolphthalein indicator and titrate against HCl taken in the burette.
- Disappearance of pink colour indicates end point.
- Repeat the titration for concordant values.

Result

The saponification number of the given edible oil is _____ mG

Table 156.1- Titration I -Standardisation of hydrochloric acid
Standard Sodium carbonate Vs HCl   Indicator : Methyl orange

S.No.	Volume of sodium carbonate (mL)	Burette reading		Concordant Value (mL)
		Initial	Final	
1.				
2.				
3.				

Calculation

Volume of sodium carbonate, V_1 =   mL

Normality of sodium carbonate, N_1 =   N

Volume of HCl, V_2 =   mL

Normality of HCl, N_2 =   N

$$V_1 \times N_1 = V_2 \times N_2$$

Table 156.2- Titration II - Determination of saponification value

Oil+Lipid solvent+KOH Vs HCl   Indicator : Phenolphthalein

S.No.	Contents of conical flask (mL)	Burette reading		Concordant Value (mL)	Volume of HCl (mL)
		Initial	Final		
1.					
2.					
3.					

$$\text{Saponification} = \frac{\text{Volume of KOH} \times \text{Equivalent weight} \times \text{Normality}}{2.542 \times 1000}$$

Table 156.3 - Titration III Blank titration

Lipid solvent+KOH Vs HCl   Indicator : Phenolphthalein

S.No.	Contents of conical flask (mL)	Burette reading		Concordant Value (mL)
		Initial	Final	
1.				
2.				
3.				

157. Determination of iodine number of an edible oil

Aim

To determine the iodine number of the given oil by Hanu's method.

Principle

Iodine number is defined as the number of grams of iodine taken up by 100g of oil or fat. In this case, addition reaction takes place across the double bonds of unsaturated fatty acids present in the fat by the addition of a halogen, such as iodine. Thus, the iodine number gives the indication of the degree of unsaturation of fats. Iodine value is directly proportional to the degree of unsaturation. Determination of iodine number is used for the assessment of its purity. In Hanu's method, the oil is treated with Hanu's reagent. (Iodine bromide in chloroform) for a period of time. The unreacted iodine is titrated against standardized thiosulphate solution.

Materials Required

(i) Sodium thiosulphate 0.1N

(ii) Potassium dichromate 0.1N

(iii) Potassium iodide 10%

(iv) Hanu's solution(With the aid of heat 13.2g of iodine is dissolved in 1litre of glacial acetic acid and to this, 3mL of bromine water is added and mixed thoroughly.)

(v) Hydrochloric acid – 20%

(vi) Starch : Indicator

Procedure

Titration I: Standardisation of sodium thiosulphate

● Pipette out 10mL of standard (0.1N) potassium dichromate in a clean conical flask.

● Add 10mL of 10% potassium iodide and 5 mL of 20% hydrochloric acid followed by 75mL of water. Tritrate this solution against thiosulphate solution taken in the burette till the formation of pale yellow colour.

● Then add a few drops of starch indicator and titrated with thio sulphate solution till the blue colour disappears.

● Repeat the titrations for concordant values.

Titration II: Determination of iodine number

● Weigh 1g of the oil and transferred into a clean conical flask and incubate for about 30 minutes.

● Add 10mL of 10% potassium iodide followed by 80mL of water.

● Titrate the liberated iodine with standardized thiosulphate till the formation of pale yellow colour.

● Then add a few drops of starch indicator and continue the titration till the disappearance of the blue colour (Mix the contents present in the flask thoroughly while the process of titration . A duplicate is also conducted by the same method. The blank titration is also performed without the oil).

Result

Iodine Number of the given edible oil is _____g.

Table 157.1- Titration I - Standardisation of sodium thiosulphate
Indicator : Starch

| S.No. | Contents of conical flask (mL) | Burette reading | | Concordant Value (mL) |
		Initial	Final	
1.				
2.				
3.				

Calculation

Volume of potassium dichromate, V_1　　=　　mL
Normality of potassium dichromate, N_1 =　　N
Volume of thiocyanate, V_2　　　=　　mL
Normality of thiocyanate, N_2　　　=　　N

$$V_1 \times N_1 = V_2 \times N_2$$

Table 157.2-Titration II- Determination of iodine number

Indicator : Starch

S.No.	Contents of conical flask (mL)	Burette reading		Concordant Value (mL)
		Initial	Final	
1.				
2.				
3.				

Volume of iodine not consumed by oil = Volume of Hanu's solution that reacted with sodium thiosulphate .

158. Estimation of DNA by Diphenylamine Method

Aim

To estimate the amount of DNA present in the sample.

Principle

When DNA is treated with diphenylamine under acid conditions, a blue compound is formed with a sharp absorption maximum at 595 nm. This reaction is given by 2-Deoxypentoses in general and is not specific for DNA (Adenine and guanine). In acid solution, the straight chain form of a deoxy pentose is converted to the highly reactive α-hydroxylevulinic acid which reacts with diphenylamine to give a blue complex .

Materials Required

DNA standard solution

5 mG of DNA as weighted accurately and make up to 25 mL with 5 mM sodium hydroxide.

Diphenylamine reagent

Dissolve 0.5g of pure diphenylamine in 48.7mL of glacial acetic acid. Add slowly 2.5 mL of concentrated sulphuric acid. Stir well and store for future use.

Other materials

Boiling water bath, Spectrophotometer, Aluminium foil, Water bath, Test tubes,

Standard measuring flask, Cuvette, Micropipette, Pipette

Procedure

- Pipette out different aliquots of standard DNA solution in the range of 0.05,0.1mL, 0.15 mL .....0.5mL with 0.05mL interval).

- Make content of each tube to 1 mL using distilled water.
- To the aliquots add 5 mL of diphenylamine reagent.
- Close the test tubes with aluminium foil and keep it firm by rubber bands.
- Heat on a boiling water bath for 10 min, cool and read the OD value at 595 nm.
- Read the test and standards against water blank.

Note

The graph is drawn and amount of DNA in the given unknown solution is calculated.

Perform estimation of unknown DNA as per previous procedure using 0.2mL sample./

Table 158.1 : Estimation of DNA

S. No	Volume of standard solution in (mL)	Volume of water (mL)	Conc. Of DNA in working sample(μg)	Volume of diphenylamine reagent(mL)	Incubation	OD at 595nm
01	0.05	0.95	10			
02	0.10	0.90	20			
03	0.15	0.85	30			
04	0.20	0.80	40			
05	0.25	0.75	50	5 mL	Boiling water bath for 10 min	
06	0.30	0.70	60			
07	0.3.5	0.65	70			
08	0.40	0.60	80			
09	0.45	0.55	90			
10	0.50	0.50	100			
Unknown 0.2 mL		0.8 mL	Unknown			

Observation

Blue colour formation is observed

Result

The amount of DNA present in the given sample is   uG/mL.

159. Estimation of RNA by Orcinol Method

Aim

To estimate the RNA from the given sample.

Principle

This is a general reaction for pentoses. Ribose Moieties of RNA form furfural when it is heated with concentrated hydrochloric acid. Orcinol reacts with the furfural in the presence of ferric chloride as a catalyst to give a brilliant green colour. Purine nucleotides only give any significant reaction.

Materials Required

Standard RNA solution

Dissolve 5 mG of RNA in 50 mL of Distilled water.

Orcinol solution

Dissolve 1 g of orcinol in 5 mL ethanol taken in a 100mL volumetric flask. Make up the content of the flask to 100mL using distilled water.

Concentrated hydrochloric acid

Ferric chloride solution (10%)

Dissolve 10g of ferric chloride in 100mL distilled water

Orcinol Reagent

Transfer 10mL of 10% ferric chloride solution to 390mL of conc. Hydrochloric acid. Mix this solution to 100 mL of orcinol solution. Continuously stir the mixture while adding and store it for future use.

Procedure

- Different aliquots of standard RNA solution is taken and make up to 3mL with distilled water (10µG to 100µG).

- Add 3mL of orcinol reagent to all tubes.

- Heat them on a boiling water bath for 10 minutes.

- Observe for the development of colour.

- After cooling them optical dencity is measured at 665 against blank.

- Plot a graph between OD and the amount of RNA and from this standard curve.

- Blank is prepared by using 3 mL of distilled water and 3 mL of orcinol and follow steps 3, 4 and 5.

- 2 mL of unknown sample is taken and made upto 3 mL and 3mL of orcinol.

Observation and Result

The amount of RNA present in the given sample is   /mL.

Table 159.1 : Estimation of RNA

S. No	Volume of standard solution in (mL)	Volume of water (mL)	Conc. Of RNA in working solution (µg/mL)	Volume of Orcinol reagent	Incubation	OD value 595nm
01	0.1	2.9	10			
02	0.2	2.8	20			
03	0.3	2.7	30			
04	0.4	2.6	40			
05	0.5	2.5	50			
06	0.6	2.4	60	3 mL	Boiling water bath 10 min	
07	0.7	2.3	70			
08	0.8	2.2	80			
09	0.9	2.1	90			
10	1.0	2.0	100			
11	Unknown 2mL	1.0	Unknown			

160. Estimation of alcohol

Aim

To estimate alcohol content of the given sample.

Principle

Ethanol content of the fermentation medium is estimated through chromic acid method

This method was developed by Caputi *et.al.*, in 1968. Assay of alcohol depends on the reaction between acid and alcohol. In this experiment potassium dichromate act as an indicator. During the reaction six-valent potassium dichromate is converted into three-valent potassium dichromate. Sulfuric acid acts as an oxidative agent. During the reaction orange colour potassium dichromate is converted into greenish black component.

Materials required

Alcohol distillation unit, heating mandle, beaker, chromic acid (Ref Appendix), water bath, spectrophotometer etc.

Procedure

Preparation of alcohol standard graph

- Prepare different concentration of alcohol in double distilled water (1-10%).
- Starting with 1% , add 1mL of the alcoholic solution to 24mL of distilled water available in conical flask.
- Pour 25 mL of sample to distillation flask.
- Distill the contents .
- Collect 10- 15 mL of distillate in a beaker containing 25 mL of 3.4 % chromic acid.
- Make up the volume to 50mL using double distilled water and mixed thoroughly
- Heat the contents up to 80°C for 15 minutes
- Read the absorbency at 580 nm.
- Plot the values on a graph and prepare standard graph

Analysis of culture filtrate for alcohol content

- Aseptically withdraw 10 mL of culture filtrate from the fermentation medium
- Centrifuge the sample at 10,000 rpm for 10 minutes.
- Add 1mL of sample to 24 mL of distilled water .
- Distill the contents .
- Collect 10- 15 mL of distillate in a beaker containing 25 mL of 3.4 % chromic acid.
- Make up the volume to 50mL using double distilled water and mixed thoroughly
- Heat the contents up to 80°C for 15 minutes
- Read the absorbency at 580 nm.
- Plot the values on a graph and prepare standard graph
- Alcohol content is determined using alcohol standard graph

Observation and result

Greenish to black colour is noted.

161. Separation of amino acids by paper chromatography.

Aim

To identify the amino acid present in the sample by paper chromatography technique.

Principle

Amino acid in a given mixture or sample aliquot are separated on the basis of difference in the solubility and hence differential partioning coefficient in a binary solvent system. The amino acid with higher solubility in stationary phase slowly as compare to those with higher solubility in the mobile phases. The separated amino acids are detected by spraying the air dried chromatogram with ninhydrin agent. All the amino acid give purple or bluish colour or reaction with ninhydrin except proline and hydroxy proline which give a yellow coloured product. The reactions leading to the formation of purple complexes as given us.

Ninhydrin + amino acid $\longrightarrow$ hydrindantin

Ninhydrin + Aminoacid + Hydrindantin $\longrightarrow$ purple coloured product

Materials required

What man NO.1 filter paper sheet
Micropipette/ micro syringe
Hair drier
Sprayer
Oven set at 105°c
Chromatographic chamber saturated with water vapour

Developing Solvent

Prepare butanol, acetic acid and water in the ratio of 4:1:5 in a separating funnel and mix it thoroughly.

Ninhydrin spray reagent

Prepare fresh by dissolving 0.2 g ninhydrin in 100mL acetone.

Standard Aminoacid

Prepare solutions of standard amino acids such as methionine, trypthophan, alanine, glycine, etc., (1mG/mL in10% iso-propanol).

A sample containing mixture of unknown amino acids.

Procedure

- Take what man NO.1 filter paper sheet with 10cm length and 5cm width.
- Draw a line one or 2cm above the base of the filter paper.
- Put small circular marks along the base line in such a way that the distance from the edge of the paper and the first spot and the distance between the adjacent spots is not less than 2.5cm.
- About 20μL of sample is loaded using capillary tube at the center of spotted drawing.
- Diameter of the spotted material should be as small as possible and if required.
- The applied solution is dried prior to loading additional volume.

- Fill chromatographic chamber with sufficient volume of the mobile phase and the chamber has been earlier saturated with vapours.
- Now place the filter paper erect in a container filled with organic mobile phase.
- Tightly close the container.
- Leave the container undisturbed until the solvent system traverse the entire length of the paper.
- Remove the chromatogram from the chamber and air dry it.
- Spray the paper with ninhydrin reagent and lit it again at room temperature prior to transferring it to an oven at 105°C for 5 – 10 minutes. Locate the position of amino acids as bluish or purple coloured spots on the chromatogram.
- Calculate the Rf value of standard amino acids as well as those in the given mixture or sample as follows.

  Rf = Distance travelled by unknown amino acid / Distance traveled by the   solvent system.
- Identify the amino acids in the mixture or sample by comparing Rf values with those of applied standard amino acids.

Result

The amino acid present in the amino acid sample are Valine and Threonine.

162. Estimation of aminoacid by Ninhydrin method

Aim

To estimate free aminoacids from a test sample by ninhydrin method

Principle

Ninhydrin is one of a powerful oxidizing agent, decarboxylates the alpha aminoacids and yields an intensely coloured bluish product which is measured calorimetrically.

Nin hydrin+Aminoacid→Hydrindandin+Ammonia

Hydrindandin+Ammonia → Purple coloured product

Materials required

Ninhydrin: it is prepared by mixing solution A and B.

Solution A – Dissolve 0.8g stannous chloride in 500mL of 0.2M citrate buffer

Solution B- dissolve 20g of ninhydrin in 500mL of 2 methoxiethanol.

Diluent- mix equal volume of water and n propanol

Test tube, standard measuring flask, water bath, spectrophoto meter, 80% ethanol, conical flask.

Stock aminoacid: Dissolve 5mG of leucine in 50mL of Distilled water in a flask

Working standard: take 10mL stock and dilute to 100mL

Procedure

Standard graph

- Prepare working standard in a series of test tubes. Concentration of standard ranges from 10µG to100 µG (0.1mL to1mL).
- Add one mL ninhydrin solution.
- Make up the volume to 2 mL with distilled water
- Heat the tube in a boiling water bath for 20 minutes.
- Add 5mL of diluent and mix the content.
- Read the intensity of the colour in spectrophotometer / calorimeter at 570nm after 15 minutes
- Use 0.1mL of 80% ethanol along with other reagent as blank.

Test

- Add one mL of ninhydrin to the 0.1mL of test sample.
- Make up the volume to 2 mL with distilled water
- Heat the tube in a boiling water bath for 20 minutes
- Add 5mL of diluent and mix the content.
- Read the intensity of the colour in spectrophotometer / calorimeter at 570nm after 15 minutes
- Use 0.1mL of 80% ethanol along with other reagent as blank.

Observation

Development of purple colour is noted

Result

Draw standard graph and find quality of free aminoacid present in the sample.

163. Separation of lipids by Thin Layer Chromatography

Aim

To identify lipids through TLC method

Background informations

Thin layer chromatography (TLC) consists of a thin layer adsorbent such as silica gel, alumina or cellulose on a flat carrier like a glass plate, a thick aluminum foil, or a plastic sheet. This layer of adsorbent acts as a stationary phase. This method is widely used in lipid analysis or is the standard method in organic chemistry for qualitative analysis of organic reactions. The adsorbent like silica has hydroxyl groups which act as interacting groups. The sample partitions between the mobile and the stationary phase. Individual components in the sample will interact with the stationary phase based on charge, solubility and adsorption. The components could then be visualised by iodine vapors or fluorescent dyes. The retention factor or the Rf value is a characteristic of the substance. This is a constant for a

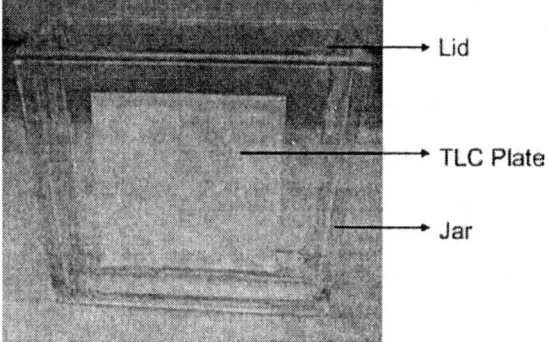

Fig 163.1: Thin Layer chromatography chamber and TLC plate.

particular substance for that specific solvent and plate system. The Rf value is the ratio of the distance moved by the compound to that moved by the solvent.

Materials required

TLC plate, Mobile phase solvent, Glass jar

Protocol

- Add 30g silica gel G in stoppered flask containing 60mL distilled water (1:2).
- Make slurry by stirring for 1-2 minutes and pour into the applicator positioned on the head glass plate.
- Coat the slurry over the glass plates at a thickness of 0.25mm for chemical analysis by moving the applicator at a uniform speed from one end to the other. Leave the plates to dry at room temperature for 15-30minutes.
- Heat the plates in an oven at 100-120 ° C for 1-2 hours to remove the moisture and to activate the adsorbent on the plate.
- Leave 2.5cm from one end of the glass plate and atleast an equal distance from the edges.
- Spot the sample and the respective standards onto the plate.
- Pour the appropriate developing solvent (toluene: Ethylacetate: formic acid (6:3:1))into a glass jar at least one hr before use. This is to saturate the jar with the running solvent vapors.
- Dip the plate in the running solvent just below the sample load.
- Allow the solvent to run due to capillary action till it reaches nearly the end of the plate (Fig 164.2).
- Remove the plate from the jar and let it dry.
- Spray Iodine vapour for visualisation of the compound.
- Measure the distance of the solvent and the compound travelled to obtain the Rf values.

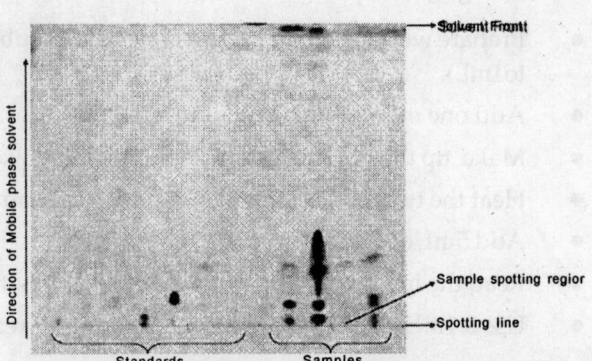

Fig163.2 Thin Layer Chromatography. An example of a lipid containing sample developed and stained with Iodine vapors.

Observation

Different spots are noted.

Result

Spots are compared with standard and identified

164. Separation of plant pigments by Column chromatography.

Aim

To separate the pigments present in the given sample by column chromatography.

Back Ground Information

In column chromatography, separation is achieved by passage of the sample through vertically fixed tubular glass or poly propylene column which is packed with an appropriate chromatography media. Usually commercially available column have a porous sintered plate fused at their base, which prevents the stationary phase from flowing out of the column. This sintered base is positioned as near the base as possible in order to minimize the dead space to reduce the chances of post column mixing of the separated compounds. Alternatively, a simple glass burette with a plug of glass wool at the base can be used as a column. At the base can be used as a column. At the base there is small capillary tubing through which the effluent from the column flows into the test tubes in which fractions are collected. At the top the column a solvent reservoir with a delivery system is fitted. Column chromatographic techniques have been classified on the basis of the nature of the interactions occurring between ultimately results in their separation. Various types of column chromatography are described.

Introduction

Adsorption is a phenomenon in which compounds are held onto the surfaces of a solid adsorbent, having specific adsorption sites, through weak non-ionic interactions such as Vander wall's. Compounds bind with varying strengths and hence can selectively be adsorbed. For good resolution, selection of right type of the adsorbent and the elutent or mobile phase is essential. Some of the commonly used absorbants include charcoal, silica, alumina, hydroxyl apatite etc., Elutant influences quality of separation since polarity of the mobile phase influences the adsorption considerably. Non-polar solvents favour maximum adsorption, which decreases with increase in polarity of the solvent.

Polar solvents are preferred for the substances having polar or hydrophilic groups.

Non polar solvents for substances having hydrophobic or non polar groups.

Example, alcoholic solvent for OH group containing substances; with carbonyl groups and hydrocarbons such as toluene or hexane for non polar substances. For gradient elution, mixture of the polar and non polar solvents of different ratios can be used to obtain eluent of varying polarities.

Chemicals and other materials

Silica gel 60 (Merck), Petroleum ether, Acetone, NaCl, $CaCO_3$, Na_2SO_4, Fresh leaves

Apparatus and glass wares

Glass chromatography column with a porous membrane at the bottom and a stopcock at the outlet, 5 measuring cylinder 25 mL, Beaker 100 mL, Beaker 600 mL, 9 Erlenmeyer flask, Mortar & pestle , Glass rod, Cork ring, Swan-neck lamp

Procedure

Extraction of the leaf pigments

- Using a pestle; fresh leaves are grinded in a mortar containing 22 mL of acetone, 3 mL of petroleum ether and a spatula tip-full of $CaCO_3$. The pigment extract is filtered.

- The filtrate is poured into a separation funnel and is mixed with 20 mL of petroleum ether and 20 mL of 10% aqueous NaCl solution.

- The separating funnel is shaken carefully. When the layers have separated the lower layer is allowed to drain into a beaker. This phase is thrown away.

- The upper layer is washed 3-4 times with 5 mL of distilled water.

- Afterwards the extract is placed in an Erlenmeyer flask and is dried with about 4 spatula tips of Na_2SO_4. The liquid is carefully decanted into an Erlenmeyer flask.

Eluting solvent (mobile phase)

Mixture of petroleum ether and acetone (7:3)

Silica gel slurry

- Using a beaker of an Appropriate size, a slurry of silica gel and eluting solvent is prepared.

Packing of the column

- A uniform well-consolidated packing of the column is critical to the success of this chromatographic seperation.
- A clean, dry column is aligned in a vertical position.
- A beaker is placed under the column outlet.
- The column is slowly and evenly filled about two-thirds full with silica gel slurry.
- The stop cock is opened to allow liquid to drain into the beaker.
- Pouring the slurry down a glass rod held against the wall of the column will minimize bubbling and turbulence.
- The side of the chromatographic tube is gently tapped with a cork ring during the packing process, to make the silica gel compact.

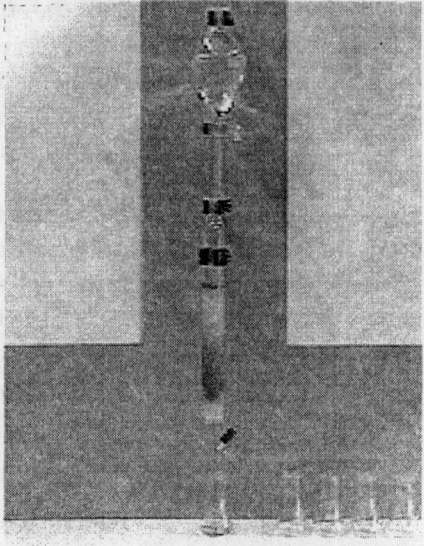

Fig 164.1 : Column chromatography

- Meanwhile the stop cock is opened to allow the excess eluting solvent to run out.
- Using a powder funnel a small amount of sand is carefully added to the top of the silica gel column to prevent it from being disturbed when fresh solvent eluent is added.
- The solvent level is allowed to drop to 1 mm above sand.
- The bottom outlet of the separation column is closed. It is very important not to allow the column to run dry.

Experimental procedure

- Using a volumetric pipette 20 mL of the leaf extract is added directly (or carefully down the side of the column) to the sand layer.
- Then the mobile phase is drained continuously to the top of the column by aid of a separation funnel.
- The bottom outlet of the column is opened.
- The eluent flows down through the column.
- The column, with the adsorbent and the sample, is 'developed': As the eluent passes down the column, the components of the mixture begin to move down the column.
- The separated zones 'flow out' of the column, where the elutes are collected in Erlenmeyers.
- The flasks are changed as the eluete changes colour.
- Using a swan-neck lamp a bright beam of light is directed at the leaf extract and at the samples eluted from chromatography column.
- Leaf extract and the samples containing chlorophyll or pheophytin produce a reddish glow. This phenomenon is known as fluorescence.

Observations

The mobile phase slowly flows down through the silica gel column by gravity leaving behind zones of colour - the chromatogram. The theory of column chromatography is analogous to that of thin-layer chromatography. The different components in the sample mixture pass through the column at different rates due to differences in their partitioning behaviour between the mobile liquid phase and the stationary phase.

Leaf pigments	Colour
Carotenes	golden
Pheophytin	olive green
Chlorophyll a	blue green
Chlorophyll b	yellow green
Lutein	yellow
Xanthophylls	yellow

Result

Yellow, yellow green , olive green components are separated and they may be xanthophils and chlorophils.

165. Determination of the effect of pH on the Activity of human salivary α - amylase

Aim

To determine the effect of pH on salivary amylase activity

Principle

α - amylase catalyses the hydrolysis of α-1-4 linkage of starch and produces reducing sugars. Sugar reduces 3,5 Dinitro salicylic acid into 3 amino –5 nitro salicylic acid, an orange-red complex. Read the OD at 540nm. Enzymes are active over a limited pH range only and a plot of activity against pH usually produces a bell-shaped curve. The pH value of maximum activity is known as optimum pH and is characteristic of the enzyme. The variation of activity with pH is due to the change in the state of ionization of the enzyme protein for other compounds of the reaction mixture.

Materials required

DNS reagent (Refer page 391 & 392), 1% starch (Substrate): 1gm of starch dissolved in buffer of different pH; Saliva (1:20 dilute), Phosphate or acetate Buffer (Refer experiment No. 140 Page 374).

Procedure

- Arrange 7 test tubes in a rack.
- Add 0.5 mL of buffer to the first tube and 0.5mL of substrate g pH7 (blank). Add 0.5 mL of Saliva to remaining 6 tubes.
- Add 0.5 mL of substrate of pH values of 4.0, 5.0, 5.5, 6.0, 7.0, and 8.0 to the respective test tube.
- Incubate all the test tubes for exactly 20 minutes at room temperature.
- Add 1mL of DNS reagent to each test tube and keep all tubes in a boiling water bath for exactly 5minutes.
- Then add 10mL of distilled H_2O to each tube and read OD at 540 nm.
- Plot the graph by taking different pH values along the x-axis and activity on y-axis.

Result

The optimum pH of human salivary α-amylase is _____ mL/min.

166. Determining the effect of temperature on the activity of human salivary α-amylase

Aim

To determine the effect of temperature on salivary amylase activity

Principle

α - amylase catalyses the hydrolysis of α-1.4 linkage of starch and produces reducing sugars. The liberated reducing sugars add an orange-red colour complex. The effect of temperature on an enzyme-catalyzed reaction indicates the structural changes in the enzyme. Molecules must possess a certain energy of attraction before they can react and the enzyme functions as a catalyst lowering the energy of attraction. Energy of an enzyme-catalyzed reaction can be determined by measuring the minimum velocity at different temperature. The energy is more active at optimum temperature. Below this temperature, the enzyme activity decreases and above this temperature, the enzyme becomes denatured or loses the structure required for catalytic activity.

Reagents

DNS reagent (Refer Page 391 & 392), 1% starch, Phosphate buffer pH4 (Refer page 375), Saliva (1:20 dilute)

Procedure

- Arrange 6 clean and dry test tubes in a test tube rack.
- Pipette out 0.5mL of saliva to first five tubes and add 0.5mL of buffer to 6th tube (blank).
- Add 0.5mL of substrate to each tube.
- Incubate all tubes for 20 minutes at respective temperatures (13°C, 25°C, 36°C, 50°C and 60°C).
- Add 1mL of DNS reagent to each test tube and keep all test tubes in a boiling water bath for exactly 5 minutes.
- Add 10 mL of distilled water to each tube and read the OD at 540 nm.
- Plot the graph by taking temperature on the *x*-axis and activity on the *y*-axis.

Result

The optimum temperature of the human salivary α-amylases is — — — — —.

167. Demonstrating the Presence of Catalase

Aim

To assess the availability of Catalase in tissues and other biomaterials.

Background Information

Catalase is an enzyme found in many animal tissues such as meat and liver, and many plant tissues, such as stems of seedlings. Catalase is found in the organelle peroxisomes and microbodies in a cell. In industry, it is used to generate oxygen to convert latex to foam rubber. The presence of catalase is important because it can decompose hydrogen peroxide, which is a byproduct of certain cell oxidations and is very toxic. Catalase can eliminate the hydrogen peroxide immediately. It is the fastest-acting enzyme known.

Principle

The evolution of gas should be observed when catalase is placed into hydrogen peroxide. The hydrogen peroxide is decomposed into water.

Materials required

Mortar & pestle, Animal tissue, hydrogen peroxide

Procedure

- Grind 10gms of fresh biomaterials in 10mL of distilled water in mortar with a pestle.
- Filter the extract.
- Dilute the filtrate by 100% with distilled water.
- Add a drop of the filtrate to 5mL of hydrogen peroxide.
- Observe for the evolution of gas.

Observation

Bubbles noted.

Plant Tissue Culture

Introduction

Tissue culture refers to the growth and maintenance of a plant in nutrient medium under *in vitro* condition. The term "plant tissue culture" is used for culturing of unorganized tissues or callus. The methodology of tissue culture consists of separation of the cells, tissues, and organs of a plant called "explants", and growing them aseptically on a nutrient medium under controlled conditions of temperature and light. The explants give rise to an unorganized, proliferative mass of undifferentiated cells called callus, which later produces shoots. An important contribution made by this technique is the revelation of a unique capacity of plant cells that is the cellular totipotency, which means that all living cells in a plant body can potentially give rise to a whole plant. Plant tissue culture technology can be divided into 5 classes based on the type of materials used.

(*i*) **Callus culture** - Culture of callus on agar medium produced from explants.

(*ii*) **Cell culture** - Culture of cell in liquid media, usually aerated by agitation.

(*iii*) **Organ culture** - Aseptic culture of embryos, anthers, roots, shoot and ovaries etc.

(*iv*) **Meristem culture** - Aseptic culture of shoots meristem or explant tissue in nutrient media.

(*v*) **Protoplast culture** - The aseptic isolation and culture of plant protoplast from cultured cell or plant tissue.

168. Preparation of media for plant tissue culture

Aim

To prepare specific and nutritional media for plant tissue culture

To understand selective requirements of plant tissue culture

Background information

The composition of the growth medium is designed to sustain the plant cells, encourage cell division and control development of either an undifferentiated cell mass, or particular plant organs. The concentration of the growth regulators in the medium, namely auxin and cytokinin, seems to be the critical factor for determining whether a tissue culture is initiated, and how it subsequently develops. The first medium formulations used for plant culture work are based on experience of microorganisms. Today, the most commonly used culture media are based on following components:

Macroelements — N, P, K, Ca, Mg and S.

Microelements — Fe, Cu, Mn, Co, Mo, BI, Zn, Cl Al, Ni and Si.

Carbon source — Sucrose, glucose, fructose, or sorbitol.

Organic compounds (Vitamins) — thiamine, niacin, pyridoxine, biotin, folic acid, ascorbic acid, tocopherol

Myo-inositol or casein hydrolysate

Complex organics — Coconut milk and water, yeast extract, fruit juices, or pulps.

Plant growth regulators — Auxins, cytokinins, Gibberellins, abscisic acid

Gelling agents — Agar, agarose, gellan gum.

Other components — MES, activated charcoal, antibiotics, fungicides.

One of the most successful media is the MS medium, devised by Murashige and Skoog (1962), based on the constitution of tobacco plants. The choice or formulation of the media basically depends on the requirements of the cultivated explant and species. Other medium used in plant tissue culture are LM medium (Linsmaier and Skoog, 1965), White's medium (White, 1963) - culture of tomato roots , Gamborg's B5 medium (Gamborg *et al.,* 1968) - devised for soybean callus culture, SH medium (Schenk and Hildebrandt, 1972) - callus culture of both monocotyledons and dicotyledons, Nitsch's medium (Nitsch and Nitsch, 1969) - anther culture, KM medium (Kao and Michayluck, 1975) - grow cells and protoplasts, Chu (N6) is defined to improve the formation, growth, and differentiation of pollen in rice.

Table 168.1 Composition of commonly used tissue culture media in molar concentration

Compounds	MS	LM	Gamborg's	Nitsch's	KM	CHU (N6)	SH
KNO_3	18.79 mM	18.79 mM	24.73 mM	9.40 mM	18.79 mM	27.99 mM	24.73 mM
NH_4NO_3	20.61 mM	20.61 mM	–	9.00 mM	7.70 mM	–	–
$(NH_4)_2SO_4$	–	–	1.01 mM	–	–	3.50 mM	–
KH_2PO_4	1.26 mM	1.26 mM	–	0.50mM	1.25mM	2.94mM	–
NaH_2PO_4	–	–	1.09 mM	–	–	–	2.61mM
$CaCl_2$	2.99 mM	2.99 mM	1.02 mM	1.50mM	4.08mM	1.13mM	1.36mM
$MgSO_4 7H_2O$	1.50 mM	1.50 mM	1.01 mM	0.75 mM	1.22 mM	0.75 mM	1.62 mM
$CoCl_2 6H_2O$	0.11 mM	0.11 mM	0.11 mM		0.11 mM		0.42 mM
$CuSO_4 5H_2O$	0.10 mM	0.10 mM	0.10 mM	0.10 mM	0.10 mM		0.80 mM
FeNa EDTA	0.10 mM	0.10 mM	0.10 mM	0.10 mM	0.10 mM	0.10 mM	53.94 mM
H_3BO_3	0.10 mM	0.10 mM	38.52 mM	0.16 mM	48.52 mM	˹.88 mM	80.86 mM
KI	5.00 mM	5.00 mM	4.52 mM		4.52 mM	4.˻ ꞁ mM	6.02 mM
$MnCl_2 H_2O$	0.10 mM	0.10 mM	59.16 mM	0.11 mM	59.17 mM	19.70 mM	59.17 mM
$Na_2MoO_4 2H_2O$	1.03 mM	1.03 mM	1.03 mM	1.03 mM	1.03 mM		0.41 mM
$ZnSO_4 7H_2O$	29.91 mM	29.91 mM	6.96 mM	34.78 mM	6.96 mM	5.22 mM	3.48 mM
Glycine	26.64 mM	–	–	26.64 mM	–	26.64 mM	
Nicotinic acid	4.06 mM	–	8.12 mM	40.62 mM	–	4.06 mM	40.61 mM
Pyridoxin-HCl	2.43 mM	–	4.86 mM	2.43 mM	–	2.43 mM	2.43 mM
Thiamine-HCl	0.30 mM	1.19 mM	29.65 mM	1.48 mM	–	2.96 mM	14.82 mM
Myo-inositol	0.56 mM	0.56 mM	0.56 mM	0.56 mM	–	–	5.55 mM
KCL	–	–	–	–	4.02 mM	–	–
Folic acid	–	–	–	1.13 mM	–	–	–
Biotin	–	–	–	0.21 mM	–	–	–

pH - Usual range of 4.5 to 6.0

Materials required

Balance, autoclave, hot air oven, magnetic stirrer, refrigerator, heater, pH meter, distillation unit, spirit lamp, culture bottles, conical flasks, beakers, measuring cylinders, screw cap bottles etc.

Procedure

The best-suited media for tissue culture is MS Media. It is prepared by the following procedure.

- Take one-liter conical flask and prepare stock solutions separately (Table 168.2).
- Add 100mL Stock A (major elements), 1mL Stock B (minor elements), 10mL Stock C (ironic elements) and 1mL Stock D (vitamin source).
- Boil the solution for few minutes and made up to 1000mL.
- Add 30g sucrose and 8g agar agar (add coconut milk if needed).
- Add required volume of Indole acetic acid-IAA (The known quantities of auxin are first dissolved in 5 mL of NaOH or KOH and the final volume is made up by adding distilled water) and 6-Benzyl amino purine-BAP (The required quantities of cytokinins are well dissolved in 5 mL of 0.1 N HCl and the final volume is made by water).
- Check the pH of the medium and adjust to 5.6 to 5.8.
- Dispense 25mL of the media into culture bottles.
- Autoclave the media at 121°C for 15 minutes.
- Allow the media to solidify and inoculate explants using aseptic technique.

Table 168. 2: Composition of Stock Solutions

S. No	Composition	mg/liter
Stock A		
1.	Ammonium nitrate (NH_4NO_3)	1650.00
2.	Potassium nitrate (KNO_3)	1900.00
3.	Magnesium sulfate ($MgSO_4, 7H_2O$)	370
4.	Potassium dihydrogen phosphate (KH_2PO_4)	170
5.	Calcium chloride ($CaCl_2, 7H_2O$)	440
Stock B		
1.	Boric acid (H_3BO_3)	6.200
2.	Manganese sulfate ($MnSO_4, 4H_2O$)	2.300
3.	Zinc sulfate ($ZnSO_4, 7H_2O$)	8.600
4.	Potassium iodide (KI)	0.830
5.	Sodium molybdate ($Na_2MoO_4, 5H_2O$)	0.250
6.	Cobalt chloride ($CoCl_2, 6H_2O$)	0.250
7.	Cupric sulfate ($CuSO_4, 5H_2O$)	0.025
Stock C		
1.	Disodium ethylene diamino tetra acetate (Na_2EDTA)	37.3
2.	Ferric sulfate ($FeSO_4, 2H_2O$)	27.8

Stock D

1.	Glycine	2.00
2.	Nicotinic acid	0.50
3.	Thiamine hydrochloride	0.50
4.	Pyridoxine hydrochloride	0.50

Observation

Solidified medium is prepared and stored.

Spotters

MS medium

Viva questions

Why are cytokinins added in tissue culture medium?

Name any two vitamins used in tissue culture medium.

How do you sterilize tissue culture medium?

169. Sterilization, inoculation and incubation of explants

Aim

To prepare sterile explant material.

To inoculate plant tissue aseptically.

To incubate tissue on sterile and specific environment.

Background information

The starting point for all tissue culture is plant tissue, called an explant. It can be initiated from any part of a plant—root, stem, petiole, leaf, or flower— although the success of any one of these varies between species. It is essential that the surface of the explant is sterilized to remove all microbial contamination. Plant cell division is slow when compared to the growth of bacteria and fungi, and even minor contaminants will easily overgrow the plant tissue culture. The explant is then incubated on a sterile nutrient medium to initiate the tissue culture. The composition of the growth medium is designed to sustain the plant cells, encourage cell division, and control development of either an undifferentiated cell mass, or particular plant organs.

Materials required

Explant, saturated chlorine, 10% hypochlorite, 0.1% mercuric chloride, Laminar flow chamber, alcohol, forceps

Procedure

Sterilization of Plant Material

- Select explants from healthy plants.

- Wash throughly by keeping them under running tap water for an hour.

- After washing, treat the material with freshly prepared saturated chlorine water for 2 minutes or 10% hypochlorite bleach solution for 5 minutes, gently agitate once or twice during this time.

- Wash free of bleach by immersing the explant in 4 successive beakers of sterile distilled water, leaving them for 2–3 minutes in each.

- Place the material in freshly prepared 0.1% mercuric chloride solution for 1 minute.

- Wash free of mercury by immersing the explant in 4 successive beakers of sterile distilled water, leaving them for 2–3 minutes in each.

Inoculation

- Transfer the surface-sterilized explants to an inoculation chamber where maintain aseptic conditions.

- Disinfect the chamber with ethanol and subjected to UV radiation for 20 minutes.

- Clean the outer surfaces of the culture bottles with ethanol before placing them in the chamber.

- Sterilize forceps by dipping them in ethanol and holding them into the spirit lamp.

- With the help of the flamed forceps, inoculate the explants onto the media.

- Flame the bottleneck and replace the caps tightly.

Incubation of Cultures

- Transfer the culture bottles to the incubator.

- Maintain the temperature inside the culture room at around 24±2°C.

- Expose the culture to 16 hours of light and 8 hours of darkness (Fluorescent tubes are used as light source).

- Allow the cultures to grow and periodically observe the media. Carryout Subculturing once in 6 weeks.

Observation and Assessment of Tissue Culture Development

Incubate the explants for 4–6 weeks, and inspect at weekly or biweekly intervals. The growth of obvious bacterial or fungal colonies indicates contamination. The development of dark brown tissue cultures can also be a consequence of contamination.

Viva questions

What is the role of hypochlorite in explant sterilization

List out chemicals used in explant sterilization.

Mention the role of light and dark in explant incubation

170. Isolation of protoplasts - Plant

Aim

To isolate protoplast from the given plant material.

To cultivate protoplast.

Background information

Protoplasts are cell wall removed cells. It is usually isolated by digestion with enzymes. Cellulase enzymes digest the cellulose in plant cell wall while pectinase enzymes break down the pectin holding cells together. Once the cell wall has been removed, the resulting protoplast is spherical in shape. Digestion is usually carried out after incubation in an isotonic solution (a solution of higher concentration than the cell contents that causes the cells to plasmolyze). This makes the cell walls easier to digest. Debris is filtered and/or centrifuged out of the suspension and the protoplasts are then centrifuged to form a pellet. On resuspension, the protoplasts can be cultured on media that induce cell division and differentiation. A large number of plants can be regenerated from a single experiment—a gram of potato leaf tissue can produce more than a million protoplasts, for example. Protoplasts can be isolated from a range of plant tissues: leaves, stems, roots, flowers, anthers, and even pollen. Protoplasts are used in a number of ways for research and plant improvement. They can be treated in a variety of ways (electroporation, incubation with bacteria, heat shock, high pH treatment) to induce them to take up DNA. The protoplasts can then be cultured and plants regenerated. In this way, genetically engineered plants can be produced more easily than is possible using intact cells/plants. Plants from distantly related or unrelated species are unable to reproduce sexually, as their genomes/modes of reproduction, etc. are incompatible. Protoplasts from unrelated species can be fused to produce plants combining desirable characteristics such as disease resistance, good flavour and cold tolerance. Fusion is carried out by application of an electric current or by treatment with chemicals such as polyethylene glycol (PEG). Fusion products can be selected for on media containing antibiotics or herbicides. These can then be induced to form shoots and roots and hybrid plants can be tested for desirable characteristics.

Materials required

Plant leaf, scalpel or sharp knife, Forceps, tile, glass petri dish, 10 cm3 syringe, 1 cm3 syringe, 13% sorbitol solution, Viscozyme enzyme, Ficoll, Cellulase enzyme, dropper, small filter funnel, 60-mm gauze square (approximately 12 cm × 12 cm), Tape, Centrifuge tube, Slide and cover slip, A centrifuge, high-power microscope and incubator.

Table 170.1 - Composition of reagents.

Chemical	Composition							
	Solution A (Digestion medium)		Solution B (Wash medium)		Solution C		Solution D	
	mM	mG	mM	mG	mM	mG	mM	mG
D Sorbitol	500	4560	500	9110	-	-	100	900
Sucrose	-	-	-	-	500	8560	400	6800
CaCl₂	1	7.35	1	14.7	1	7.40	1	7.40
MES-KOH	5	49	5	98	5	98	5	98
Cellulase	2%	1000	-	-	-	-	-	-
Macerozyme R100	0.3%	15000	-	-	-	-	-	-
Distilled water	50mL	100mL	100mL	100mL				
pH	5.5	6	6	6				

Procedure

Method for isolating large numbers of metabolically competent protoplasts from leaves of monocotyledons (grasses), dicotyledons (such as spinach and sunflower), or from hypocotyl tissue.

- Prepare leaf slices of monocots and dicots by cutting the leaves with a sharp razor blade into segments of 0.5–1 mm in size. In the case of dicots, the epidermis can be scraped off before cutting by rubbing with fine carborundum powder or with a fine nylon brush.

- Incubate the leaf slices or pieces in a 19-cm-diameter dish containing the digestion medium for 3 hours at 25°C, covered with a plastic film. It may be advantageous to replace the digestion medium at intervals of 1 hour, as the enzymes might become inactivated by substances released from broken cells.

- After completion of incubation, discard the digestion medium.

- Wash plant tissue 3 times by shaking gently with 20mL wash medium (Solution B).

- After each wash, collect the tissue by pouring through a tea strainer (0.5- to 1-mm pore size) and filter the combined washes through nylon mesh (100–200 mm pore size) to remove vascular tissue and undigested material.

- Collect the protoplasts by centrifuging the combined filtered washes for 3 minutes at 1500rpm and aspirate the supernatant and discard (This crude protoplast preparation also contains some cells and chloroplasts and it is important to purify the protoplasts to remove these contaminants. This can be done with solutions of sucrose and sorbitol of different densities).

- Resuspend the protoplast pellet in 40mL of Solution C and divide this suspension into two 100mL/10mL centrifuge tubes.

- To each tube, slowly add 5mL/0.5mL of Solution D and then overlay this with 5mL/0.5mL of wash medium (Solution B) to make a 3-step gradient.

- Centrifuge at 4500rpm for 5 minutes.

- The protoplasts now collect as a band at the interface between the 2 top layers. Carefully remove them with a Pasteur pipette

- Examine the protoplasts using a light microscope.

- Add 10%–20% Ficoll to increase the percentage of the floating protoplasts and centrifuge at 3000rpm for 5 minutes.

- Aspirate top layer and the purified protoplasts can be concentrated by diluting with 10mL of Solution B.

Observation

Spherical shaped protoplasts are isolated and cultivated using MS medium and also subject for protoplast fusion.

Spotters

Protoplast.

Viva questions

What are the chemicals involved in protoplast isolation?

What are the purposes of protoplast isolation?

171. Protoplast Fusion (Somatic Hybridization)

Aim

To fuse protoplast.

To perform protoplast fusion.

Materials required

Microcentrifuge, glass slide, cover slip, Glass dropper, fusion mix, protoplast suspension, microscope.

Making the Fusion Mix

PEG (12 mL of 50% solution)

HEPES buffer 0.9 g (Refer Page 470)

10 mL water pH 8.0

Procedure

Chemical Protoplast Fusion Protocol

- Mix 2 droplets of protoplasts from 2 genetically different strains, along with a droplet of PEG (polyethylene glycol) in a test tube.

- Flood the protoplasts with baking soda dissolved in basic growing mix.

- After 20 minutes, wash with basic growing mix and centrifuge in the salad spinner centrifuge.

- Transfer the fused protoplasts onto callus culture medium.

Electrical Protoplast Fusion Protocol

- Place 2 droplets of protoplasts from 2 genetically different strains, between 2 electrodes.

- Apply 10 volts per millimeter of electrode separation for 1 minute.

- Apply a 10- to 20-msec pulse at 100 volts per millimeter. This will require building an electrical pulse apparatus.

- Wash with basic growing mix and centrifuge in the salad spinner centrifuge.

- Transfer the fused protoplasts onto callus culture medium.

Observation

Fused cells are noted. Cells are transferred to MS medium for cultivation.

Viva questions

What are the uses of protoplast fusion?

What is PEG? Mention the role of PEG in protoplast fusiopn.

172. Suspension Culture

Aim

To perform individual cell culture in suspension.

Background information

Plant cell suspension cultures are mostly used for the biochemical investigation of cell physiology, growth, metabolism, and for large- or medium-scale production of secondary metabolites. For such purposes, normally suspension cultures are used which are propagated in Erlenmeyer flasks on a shaker and are maintained by regular subculturing after short intervals (usually 1 or 2 weeks). Long-term conservation of suspension cultures is usually successful by cryopreservation. A simple procedure is described here to maintain suspended plant cell cultures for medium terms. With this method, suspension cultures of *Agrostis tenuis, Nicotiana tabacum, Nicotiana chinensis, Oryza sativa,* and *Solanum marginatum*, could be maintained viable under reduced temperatures for more than 4 months without transfer to fresh medium. The suspension cultures are kept without shaking at 10°C (in dark or in dim light at about 50 lux) in screw-cap plastic bottles (tissue culture flasks with membranes) that permitted sterile air to pass through easily.

Isolation of single cells from intact plant organs

Leaf tissue is the most suitable material for the isolation of single cells. Isolation of mesophyll cells / individual cells in the laboratory can be achieved by either mechanical method or enzymatic method.

Mechanical Method

Materials required

Fresh leaves of *Calystegia sepium*, MS medium, 90 percent ethonal, 7% calcium hypochlorite, Scalpel, Potter-Elvehjem glass homogenizer tube, Sterile metal Tyler filters (38 µm and 61 µm mesh diameters), Centrifuge (low-speed), Culture tubes / vials, Sterile distilled water.

Procedure

- Immerse the leaves rapidly in 95% ethyl alcohol.
- Rinse the leaves in filter sterilized 7% solution of calcium hypochlorite for 15 minutes.
- Wash the leaves in sterile distilled water 2-3 times.
- Cut the leaves into small pieces (0.5 – 1 cm^2) with a sterile scalpel.
- Transfer 1-5g of leaves into a homogenizer.
- Add 10mL of MS medium to the tube.
- Homogenize the leaves.
- Filter the homogenate through two layers of sterile filter, with mesh diameters of 61µm (upper) and 38 µm (lower filter).
- Centrifuge the filtrate at 2000rpm for 10minutes to remove fine debris.
- Discard the supernatant.
- Suspend the sediment consisting of free cells, in a volume of the MS liquid medium sufficient to achieve the required density.
- Inoculate the free cells into the liquid medium for culturing.
- Incubate the vials at 26°C in the dark or light.

Observation and Results

Free mesophyll cells would sediment in the centrifuge tubes, during centrifugation, which could be used for culturing on a suitable medium.

By enzymatic method

Large scale enzymatic isolation of metabolically active mesophyll cells by pectinase has been practiced for several herbaceous species.

Materials Required

Tobacco leaves (collected either 1-2 hours after sunrise or from dark pretreated plants which are 60 to 80 days old), MS liquid medium, Sterile enzyme solution 80mL (0.5% macerozyme + 0.8% mannitol+ 1% potassium dextran sulphate), 70% ethanol, 3% sodium hypochloride, SDS, Sterile distilled water, Culture vials , Fine forceps, Scalpel, Vaccum pump, Reciprocating shaker (stoke 4-5cm at the speed of 120 cycles/min), Spirit lamp/Bunsen burner .

Procedure

- Wash the youngest fully expanded tobacco leaves in running tap water and then with a mild detergent (0.05% SDS).

- Rinse the leaves with 70% ethanol for 30 seconds and later with sterile distilled water.

- Sterile the leaves in 30% solution of sodium hypochloride for 30 minutes.

- Rinse the leaves in sterile distilled water 3-4 times to remove the disinfectant completely.

- Using sterile forceps, peel off the lower epidermis.

- Cut the peeled leaves into pieces of 4cm2 with sterile scalpel.

- Transfer 2g of peeled leaf pieces into flask containing 20% filter sterilized enzyme solution composed of 0.5% macrozyme, 0.8% mannitol and 1% potassium dextran sulphate.

- Evacuate the flasks with a vacuum pump for a few Seconds to infiltrate the enzyme into the leaf pieces.

- Incubate the flasks for 2 hours at 25°C, changing enzyme solution every 30 minutes, on a reciprocating shaker with a stroke of 4-5cm at the speed of 120 rpm.

- Wash the cells with culture medium twice.

Observation and result

Incubated flasks will contain predominantly palisade cells, which could be used for culturing in a nutrient medium.

Single cell culture

Materials required

Free cells, MS liquid medium (containing 0.6% agar), Sterile petriplates , Parafilm, Inverted micro scope.

Procedure

- Suspend the free cells in the MS liquid medium and filter the cell suspension through fine gauze.

- Dissolve MS solid medium and allow it to cool to 35-40°C

- Mix the cell suspension and molted MS agar medium in equal proportion (50:50).

- Shake well for even distribution of cells throughout the medium.

- Pour the medium containing cells (approximately 10mL in each) in Petri plates to form a thin layer.

- Seal the culture Petri plate.

- Incubate the culture plates at 25°C in the dark for 3-4 weeks.

Observation and results

- Observe the plates before incubation under an inverted microscope for single cells and may be marked with a wax marking pencil on the outside of the plate to ensure the isolation of pure single cell clones.

- Incubated plates may be observed for the development of colonies on the agar surface.

- Colonies / calluses will be observed on the agar surface after 3-4 weeks incubation of the cultured plates.

173. Regeneration of plants using callus culture

Aim

To regenerate new plants from explant.

To regenerate plants from callus.

Background information

Tissue culture involves several stages of plant growth, callus formation, shooting, roots, and flowering. It starts with sterilizing a piece of plant tissue.

Materials required

MS medium and other essentials.

Procedure

Sterilizing Plant Materials

Refer Experiment 169.

Callus Formation Protocol

- Prepare a batch of basic media without added coconut milk or malt extract.

- Follow the sterilization steps for the medium, instruments, and the chamber.

- Organize the cultures, sterile media, sterilized tools, and sterile paper towels, and sterile water at one end of the chamber. At the other end of the chamber, organize a small paper bag for trash, a jar of bleach solution, and a spot for freshly inoculated cultures. The idea is for materials to always move in the same direction. This will help keep you from getting confused.

- Sterilize the plant tissue (refer experiment no 169).

- Take a sterilized piece of tissue from the jar with a pair of forceps (do not touch the plant material with your hands). Working on a dampened sterile paper towel, use the scalpel or a razor blade to cut the tissue sample into 2- to 3-cm-long pieces.

- Put 1 piece of the tissue into each container (it is important to have only 1 shoot per container at this stage so that if the shoot is contaminated it cannot spread to the others). Shut the lids of the containers.

- Store jars at room temperature away from direct sunlight. Callus will start to become visible after about 7 days post-initiation.

- Friable type II callus should be separated from more organized callus and/ or watery unorganized callus 2–3 weeks after initiation.

- Friable type II callus should be visually selected at each subsequent transfer to maintain an optimal phenotype.

- Callus should be transferred to fresh medium at 2- to 4-week intervals, depending on growth rate. Switching to different types of media also helps maintain vigor.

- Callus can be maintained at room temperature in the dark.

Shoot Multiplication Protocol

- Prepare a batch of media containing 5% to 10% coconut milk.

- Follow the sterilization steps for the medium, instruments, and chamber.

- Organize the cultures, sterile media, sterilized tools, sterile paper towels, and sterile water at one end of the chamber. At the other end of the chamber organize a small paper bag for trash, a jar of bleach solution, and a spot for freshly inoculated cultures. The idea is for materials to always move in the same direction. This will help keep you from getting confused.

- With a pair of forceps, remove a culture from its container. Moisten the sterile paper with some sterile water. It is important to do all the manipulation on a damp paper towel, as these plants are very soft and can desiccate readily.

- Cut stems off the culture and transfer to new jars. At this stage, up to 5 stems may be put inside each jar.

- Store cultures as explained in the previous stage.

Root Formation Protocol

Once you have established enough shoots, let them grow to at least 2 cm before beginning the rooting process.

- Prepare a batch of media containing malt extract.

- Follow the sterilization steps for the medium, instruments, and chamber.

- Organize the cultures, sterile media, sterilized tools, sterile paper towels, and sterile water at one end of the chamber. At the other end of the chamber, organize a small paper bag for trash, a jar of bleach solution, and a spot for freshly inoculated cultures. The idea is for materials to always move in the same direction. This will help keep you from getting confused.

- With a pair of forceps, remove a stem from its container. Wash all of the media off the culture and transfer to malt media. (Malt contains auxins, which promote root formation.)

- Up to 5 shoots may be put in each culture vessel. Store containers in their usual place as before. Roots should form within 2 to 4 weeks.

Acclimatization Protocol

- Fill plastic "vegetable" bags with a potting mix that contains no fertilizer.

- Autoclave for 15 minutes in the pressure cooker.

- When cool, inoculate with mycorrhizae.

- Remove the rooted plants from agar medium using a pair of forceps.

- Wash off the agar thoroughly from the roots using lukewarm water.

- Poke a hole in the middle of the potting mix, using a sterile instrument, gently insert the roots in that hole.

- Dampen the potting mix with basic nutrient mix.

- Spray the foliage with a hand spray containing sterile water.

- Keep these bags inside larger plastic containers with a glass cover, out of direct sunlight. Gradually remove the glass cover, but watch for signs of desiccation and if needed, use the hand spray to spray water on the foliage. Gradually increase the light intensity for the plants also.

- When the roots are well established and the plants are acclimatized (this should take about 4–6 weeks), they can be given fertilizer and be treated like any other plant.

Observation

New plant will emerge from a callus

174. Anther/Ovule Culture Protocol

Aim

To cultivate new plant from anther or ovum.

Materials required

Immature flower buds, refrigerator, culture tube, ethanol, sodium hypochlorite, glove box, MS medium semisolid, MS medium solid.

Procedure

- Collect immature flower buds from plants grown either in the field, the greenhouse, or *in vitro*.

- Preculture the flower buds in dry test tubes in the refrigerator for 2 days.

- Dip the flower buds in 70% ethanol for 30 seconds, and then surface sterilize with 0.5%–1.0% sodium hypochlorite for 20 min.

- Rinse the flower buds with sterile distilled water 3 times, and aseptically excise the anthers and/or ovules using a scalpel and a needle.

- Culture the anthers/ovules on semisolid nutrient medium.

- Incubate the cultures under complete darkness at room temperature.

- Once calli or embryos are initiated, transfer the cultures to daylight.

- Culture the developing embryoids on standard propagation medium.

Observation

New plant will regenerated from anther / ovule.

Animal Cell Culture

Introduction

Cell culture has become one of the major tools used in the life sciences today. **Tissue Culture** is the general term for the removal of cells, tissues or organs from an animal or plant and their subsequent placement into an artificial environment conducive to growth. This environment usually consists of a suitable glass or plastic culture vessel containing a liquid or semisolid medium that supplies the nutrients essential for survival and growth. The culture of whole organs or intact organ fragments with the intent of studying their continued function or development is called **Organ Culture**. When the cells are removed from the organ fragments prior to, or during cultivation, thus disrupting their normal relationships with neighbouring cells, it is called **Cell Culture**.

A culture started from cells, tissues, or organs taken directly from an animal / organism and before the first subculture are called **Primary Culture**. There are two basic methods for doing this. First, for **Explant Cultures**, small pieces of tissue are attached to a glass or treated plastic culture vessel and bathed in culture medium. Subculturing of a primary culture gives cell lines. If the cell line dies after several subcultures are called **finite cell line**. However if it continues to grow indefinately are called **continuous cell line**.

Different cell types which can be grown in culture includes connective tissue elements such as fibroblasts, skeletal tissue (bone and cartilage), skeletal, cardiac and smooth muscle, epithelial tissue (liver, lung, breast, skin, bladder and kidney), neural cells (glial cells and neurons, although neurons do not proliferate *in vitro*), endocrine cells (adrenal, pituitary, pancreatic islet cells), melanocytes and many different types of tumor cells. The development of these tissue culture techniques owes much to two major branches of medical research: cancer research and virology

The development of animal cell culture can be traced back to the work of Ross Harrison in 1907 on cell entrapment and growth from explants of frog embryo tissue. The cell growth that he observed in clotted lymph fluid in a depression slide is often regarded as the foundation of animal cell culture as a science. In his technique ('the hanging drop') the isolated tissue was suspended on the underside of a coverslip which was sealed over a depression in a microscope slide.

Applications of cell culture system

Cell cultures provide a good model system for studying 1) basic cell biology and biochemistry, 2) the interactions between disease-causing agents and cells, 3) the effects of drugs on cells, 4) the process and triggers for aging, and 5) nutritional studies. Other uses include Toxicity Testing, Cancer Research, Virology, Cell-Based Manufacturing, Genetic Counseling, Genetic Engineering, Gene Therapy, Drug Screening and Development

175. Washing and sterilization of Glassware for animal cell culture

Aim

To clean and sterilize soiled glassware's.

Background information

All apparatus and liquids that come in contact with cultures must be sterilized. The choice of method depends largely on the stability of the item at higher temperature. Heat resistant materials are sterilized by autoclaving or by using hot air oven. Irradiation, filtration are used to sterilize heat labile materials. Sterilization procedures are designed not just to kill replicating microbes but also to eliminate the more resistant spores.

Materials required

Disinfectant, Detergent, Soaking bath, baskets, aluminium foil, oven, autoclave etc.,

Required glassware's of particular practical.

Procedure

Washing of glasswares

- Collect all required glasswares for the particular practical.
- Clean the outside surface of glassware with Vim and inside with only Teepol and scrubbed with a clean brush, which is only meant for brushing glassware.
- Wash in tap water and leave in 5% Teepol solution overnight.
- Next morning wash in tap water at least 20 times and leave in 10% HCl overnight.
- Next day wash in tap water and rinse in 2 changes of demineralised distilled water at least 10 times in each, leave in third bucket of demineralised distilled water overnight.
- Take out next day, dry , pack and sterilize in hot air oven

Packing and sterilization

Pipettes

Wrap the pipette with brown paper and sterilize in a hot air oven at 160°C for two hours.

Petridishes

Wrap the Petri dishes in brown paper and tie with twine and sterilize in a hot air oven at 160°C for two hours.

Culture & media storage bottles, measuring cylinders and beakers

Cover mouth with aluminum foil, over which brown paper is tied with twine at the neck and sterilize in a hot oven at 160°C. Plastic measuring cylinders and beakers are autoclaved at 121°C for 30min.

Plastic centrifuge tubes, Eppendoff tubes, screw cap vials & tubes, :

Arrange neatly the following items in a plastic or glass beaker and cover the mouth with aluminum foil and over that wrap brown paper tied with twine at the neck. Sterilize by autoclaving at 121°C for 30min.

Coverslips

Coverslips are put into a Petri dish, which is covered with brown paper and tied with twine. Sterilize in a hot air oven at 160°C for two hours.

Filter Apparatus

Wrap filter apparatus first with aluminum foil and then with brown paper, tie it with twine tightly. Sterilize by autoclaving at 121° C for 30min.

Screw cap

Place screw caps in glass petriplates with open side down. Wrap the petriplates containing caps in steam permeable nylon paper. Autoclave for 20minutes at 121°C

- After proper sterilization switch off oven / autoclave and allow it to cool.

- Use glassware's within 24 – 48 hours.

Spotters

Hot air oven, autoclave.

Viva questions

What are the differences between hot air oven and autoclave?

What is the need of cleaning of soiled glassware's?

What are the principles of autoclaving?

Why autoclaving temperature is set at 121°C?

176. Preparation of Media for Animal Cell Culture

Aim

To prepare specific and active media for animal cell culture

Background information

The growing interest in products from animal cells has caused an extensive research effort for the development of media for cell cultivation. The basic components in the media used for cultivation of animal cells vary depending upon the character of the cells, and the cultivation method. Basic components consist of an energy source, nitrogen source, vitamins, fats, fatty acids and fat soluble components, inorganic salts, nucleic acid, antibiotics, oxygen, pH buffering systems, hormones, growth factors, serum. Extensive efforts are directed toward developing serum-free protein media or chemically defined media (e.g., MEM — minimum essential media).

Basic Components in Media

1. Energy sources — Glucose, fructose.

2. Nitrogen sources — amino acids.

3. Vitamins: mainly water-soluble vitamins — B and C.

4. Fat and fat-soluble components: fatty acids, cholesterols.

5. Inorganic salts: Na+, K+, Ca_2+, Mg_2+

6. Nucleic acid precursors

7. Antibiotics.

8. pH and buffering systems.

9. Oxygen.

10. Hormones and growth factors.

Box 176.1 - Hank's Buffered / Balanced Salt Solution (HBSS)

0.137 M NaCl, 5.4 mM KCl, 0.25 mM Na_2HPO_4, 0.44 mM KH_2PO_4, 1.3 mM $CaCl_2$, 1.0 mM $MgSO_4$, 4.2 mM $NaHCO_3$

Dulbecco's Modified Eagle's Medium
Component description (mg/l)

Calcium chloride - 200, Ferric nitrate $9H_2O$ - 0.1, Potassium chloride - 400, Magnesium sulfate - 97.67, Sodium chloride- 6400, L Arginine - 84, L Cystine - 62.57, Glycine -30, L Histidine - 42 , L Isoleucine - 104.8, L Leucine -104.8, L Lysine - 146.2, L Methionine - 30, L Phenylalanine -66, L Serine - 42, L Threonine - 95.2, L Tryptophan - 16, L Tyrosine - 103.79, L Valine - 93.6, Calcium D Pantothenate - 4, Choline chloride - 4, Folic acid - 4, Myoinositol - 7, Niacinamide - 4, Pyridoxine hcl - 4, Riboflavin - 0.4, Thiamine hcl - 4, D Glucose - 4500, Phenol red - 15.9, Sodium pyruvate - 110, Sodium bicarbonate -3700

Water for Animal Cell Media

Water used for culture media should be pyrogen-free. It is highly recommended to use fresh ultrapure water.

Purity of Chemicals, Stability, and Shelf Life

Chemicals of the highest purity are required for preparation of media. Commercial chemicals, although pure, inevitably contain traces of contaminants. Some of the traces may be toxic (like Hg). With regard to stability of media ingredients, inorganic chemicals are indefinitely stable. Vitamins are the least stable. Hormones, several antibiotics, and growth factors are recommended to be stored frozen (–20°C) or refrigerated (0°C–4°C).

Several ingredients used in animal cell culture media are known for their instability, e.g., ascorbic acid and glutamine. Most factors affect the shelf life of media, among them are the following: Natural decay rates of unstable compounds, pH, moisture, storage temperature, access of oxygen, and an exposure to near-ultraviolet, day light, or inflorescence light. Most media should be stored at 31°C and in a dark place. Storage of media by freezing may cause loss of some purely soluble ingredients. Powdered media may be stored for several years.

Sera in Animal Cell Media

Sera is the most important and most problematic component in animal cell media. During more than 3 decays, sera has been an essential medium component with the following functions:

1. Provides nutrients. 2. Provides proteins that solubilize essential nutrients that do not dissolve readily. 3. Binds essential nutrients that are toxic when present in excessive amounts and releasing slowly in a controlled manner. 4. Provides hormones and growth factors. 5. Modulates the physical and chemical properties of the medium (viscosity, rate of diffusion) — protect cells in agitated culture. 6. Has a pH-buffering function.

Despite these advantages, there are several problems associated with the use of serum for cell cultures.

1. Serum is the most expensive component. 2. Being highly viscous, sera slows down the sterilization by filtration of the media. 3. From time to time, there is a shortage in supply of sera. 4. Possible availability of contaminants. For example, Mycoplasma, viruses. 5. Availability of serum in media increases the complicity of the downstream processing of the desired biological media.

Materials required

Eagles medium, Hanks balanced Salt solutions, conical flask, double distilled water, pH meter, Balance etc.,

Procedure

Media preparation for cell culture

Dehydrated Tissue Culture Media

1.Take 900mL of triple distilled water.

2.Add the contents of one unit vial of dehydrated media to the water at room temperature with stirring until dissolved.

3.Rinse the vial with a small amount of triple distilled water to remove traces of powder and add to the above solution.

4.Add 2.2 grams of sodium bicarbonate.

5.Adjust the pH if required between 7.1 to 7.4 using 1N HC1 or 1N NaOH or by bubbling carbon dioxide. Note that pH tends to rise during filtration and hence adjust it 0.2 to 0.3 units below the final desired pH.

6.Make up final volume to 1000mL with triple distilled water.

Sterilization of tissue culture Media

Sterilize the media by filtering through sterile membrane filter (sterilized by autoclaving at 121°C for 15 min) of 0.22 micron or less porosity using positive pressure to minimise loss of carbon dioxide.

Antibiotics

The following antibiotics can be aseptically added to one litre of media :

1. Amphotericin B.   2.5 mG
2. Gentamycin   1.0 mL (50mG/mL Solution)
3. Benzyl Penicillin   10000 units
4. Streptomycin   100 mG

Sterility check

Add 0.5 - 1.0mL of filtered media to a tube containing sterile thioglycolate broth and incubate at 37° C for 48 hours. If the broth is clear after 48 hours the media is sterile.

Spotters

Antibiotics,BSS, Bovine serum, Fetal calf serum

Viva questions

Define media? How is cell culture media different from bacteriological media?

What are the major uses of serum in media?

How do you check sterility of medium?

Why is sterilization technique used to sterilize cell culture medium?

177. Preparation of TVG Buffer

Aim

To prepare TVG buffer for tissue culture work.

Background information

Successful of tissue culture / cell culture depends on good buffer system. TVG buffer is a good buffer which is used to maintain isotonic environment and also resist any pH change.

Materials required

Conical flask, pH meter and the following stock solutions

10x PBS (Phosphate buffered Saline)

NaCl	80.00g
KCl	02.00g
$Na_2H PO_4$	14.42g
$KH_2 PO_4$	02.00g
Distilled Water	1 litre

2% Trypsin

Trypsin	2.00g
Distilled Water	100mL

Stir the above solution on a magnetic stirrer for 4h at 4°C. Sterilize by filtering through sterile membrane filter of 0.22μm pore size. A sterility check can be done before using the solution.

0.2 % Versene

EDTA 200mG

Distilled Water   100mL

Sterilize by autoclaving at 15lbs & 121°C for 15 minutes.

10 % Glucose

Glucose   10.00g

Distilled Water   100mL

Sterilize by autoclaving at 15lbs & 121°C for 15 minutes.

1 % Phenol Red

Phenol Red   1.00g

Distilled Water   100mL

Procedure

- Prepare 840mL of 1X PBS and to this add 1.0 mL of 1% phenol red (indicator). Sterilize by autoclaving at 121°C for 15 minutes.

- Cool this sterile solution and then add 50 mL 2% Trypsin, 100mL 0.2% Versene and 5mL 10% Glucose.

- Do a sterility test before using this TVG.

Result: TVG buffer is prepared.

178. Aseptic Technique and Good Cell Culture Practice

Aim

To ensure all cell culture procedures are performed to a standard that will prevent contamination from bacteria, fungi and mycoplasma and cross contamination with other cell lines.

Materials required

Dettol/ Lysol solution (2.5g/l) , 1% formaldehyde based disinfectant, 70% ethanol in water

Equipment

Personal protective equipment (sterile gloves, laboratory coat, safety visor)

Microbiological safety cabinet at appropriate containment level.

Procedure

- Sanitize the cabinet using 70% ethanol before commencing work.

- Sanitize gloves by washing them in 70% ethanol and allowing to air dry for 30 seconds before commencing work.

- Put all materials and equipment into the cabinet prior to starting work after sanitize the exterior surfaces with 70% ethanol.

- Whilst working do not contaminate gloves by touching anything outside the cabinet (especially face and hair). If gloves become contaminated re-sanitize with 70% ethanol before proceeding.

- Discard gloves after handling contaminated cultures and at the end of all cell culture procedures.

- Equipment in the cabinet or that which will be taken into the cabinet during cell culture procedures (media bottles, pipette tip boxes, pipette aids) should be wiped with tissue soaked with 70% ethanol prior to use.

- Movement within and immediately outside the cabinet must not be rapid. Slow movement will allow the air within the cabinet to circulate properly.

- Speech, sneezing and coughing must be directed away from the cabinet so as not to disrupt the airflow.

- After completing work disinfect all equipment and material before removing from the cabinet. Spray the work surfaces inside the cabinet with 70% ethanol and wipe dry with tissue. Dispose of tissue by autoclaving.

- Put Cell culture discard materials in the cabinet for a minimum of two hours (preferably overnight) prior to discarding down the sink with copious amounts of water.

- Periodically clean the cabinet surfaces with a disinfectant or fumigate the cabinet according to the manufacturers instructions.

Spotters

Laminar air flow, ethanol, hypo chlorite.

Viva questions

What is aseptic technique?

How do you clean laminar airflow?

What are the methods adopted to maintain aseptic technique?

179. Primary cell Culture and maintenance of cell lines

Aim

To isolate primary cell from tissue.

To maintain primary cells.

Background information

Cell and organ cultures are used to maintain living animal cells and groups of cells outside the body (*in vitro*). With separate, living cell cultures, it is possible to see and study the behavior of animal cells in greater detail than when they are in the animal (*in vivo*). Cells grown and cultured for study have been taken from a wide variety of species, such as human, monkey, mice, dog, cat, frog, insect, fish, and many others. The cultures have come from a number of organs — heart, lungs, liver, kidney, blood, skin, etc. In cancer research, it is common practice to grow cells from normal and cancerous tissues to compare their properties.

Primary cells are prepared directly from animals and can be subcultured only once or twice. These are widely used as the best culture system because they support the widest range of viruses. E.g. Chick embryo fibroblast cells, Monkey Kidney cells.

Materials required

Curved dissecting forceps, sterile culture tube, sterile Petri dish, sterile pipettes, sterile culture flasks, sterile medium tube, hanks balanced salt solution, Incubator, Compound microscope, Safety goggles, Lab aprons, Pre-Lab preparation, Embryonated eggs preferably 10-12days old, Phosphate buffer saline (pH 7.2), 0.25% trypsin in PBS. Growth medium (MEM supplemented with 10% bovine serum), filtration unit, silicone/téflonCoated magnet, solution bottles.

Procedure

Refer Experiment No. 139 of virology

Spotters

Monolayer growth of chick embryo fibroblast.

180. Trypsinizing and subculturing cells from a monolayer

Aim

To trypsinize monolayer cells for subculturing

Background information

A primary culture is grown to confluency in a 60mm petri plate or 25-cm^2 tissue culture flask containing 5mL tissue culture medium. Cells are dispersed by trypsin treatment and then reseeded into secondary cultures. The process of removing cells from the primary culture and transferring them to secondary cultures constitutes a passage, or subculture.

Materials required

Primary cultures of cells, HBSS (Hanks Balanced Salt Solution) without Ca^{2+} and MG^{2+}, Trypsin/EDTA solution, Complete medium with serum with 10% to 15% (v/v) FBS, Sterile Pasteur pipettes, 37°C incubator, Tissue culture plasticware or glassware, including pipettes and flasks, CO$_2$ incubator.

Procedure

- Remove all medium from primary culture with a sterile Pasteur pipette. Wash the adhering cell monolayer once or twice with a small volume of HBSS without Ca^{2+} and Mg^{2+} (Use a buffered salt solution that is Ca2+ and Mg^{2+} free to wash cells. Ca^{2+} and Mg^{2+} in the salt solution can cause cells to stick together).

- Add enough trypsin/EDTA solution to culture to cover adhering cell layer.

- Place plate on a 37°C warming tray 1 to 2 min. Tap the bottom of the plate on the countertop to dislodge cells.

- Check culture with an inverted microscope to be sure that cells are rounded up and detached from the surface. If cells are not sufficiently detached, return plate to warming tray for an additional minute or 2.

- Add 2mL of complete medium. Draw cell suspension into a Pasteur pipette and rinse cell layer 2 or 3-times to dissociate cells and dislodge any remaining adherent cells. As soon as cells are detached, add serum or medium containing serum to inhibit further trypsin activity that might damage cells. If cultures are to be split 13 or 14 rather than 12 , add sufficient medium such that 1mL of cell suspension can be transferred into each fresh culture vessel.

- Add an equal volume of cell suspension to fresh plates or flasks that have been appropriately labeled. Alternatively, cells can be counted using a haemocytometer and diluted to the desired density so a specific number of cells can be added to each culture vessel. A final concentration of ~5×10^4 cells/mL is appropriate for most subcultures.

- Add 4mL fresh medium to each new culture. Incubate in a humidified 37°C, 5% CO_2 incubator.

- Feed cultures after 3 or 4 days by removing old medium and adding fresh 37°C medium.

Observation

Individual cells will observed and may subcultured

181. Subculture of Adherent Cell Lines

Aim

To subculture adherent cell lines for further use and storage.

Background information

Adherent cell lines will grow *in vitro* until they have covered the surface area available or the medium is depleted of nutrients. At this point the cell lines should be sub-cultured in order to prevent the culture dying. To subculture the cells they need to be brought into suspension. The degree of adhesion varies from cell line to cell line but in the majority of cases proteases, e.g. trypsin, are used to release the cells from the flask. However, this may not be appropriate for some lines where exposure to proteases is harmful or where the enzymes used remove membrane markers/receptors of interest. In these cases cells should be brought into suspension into a small volume of medium mechanically with the aid of cell scrapers.

Materials required

Media– pre-warmed to 37°C , 70% ethanol in water, PBS without Ca^{2+}/MG^{2+}, 25% trypsin/EDTA in HBSS, without Ca^{2+}/MG^{2+}, Trypsin , Soybean trypsin Inhibitor

Equipment

Personal protective equipment (sterile gloves, Laboratory coat, safety visor), Waterbath set to appropriate temperature, Microbiological safety cabinet at appropriate containment level, CO_2 incubator , Pre-labeled flasks , Marker Pen , Pipettes , Ampule Rack, Tissue

Procedure

- View cultures using an inverted microscope to assess the degree of confluency and confirm the absence of bacterial and fungal contaminants.

- Remove spent medium.

- Wash the cell monolayer with PBS without Ca^{2+}/MG^{2+} using a volume equivalent to half the volume of culture medium. Repeat this wash step if the cells are known to adhere strongly.

- Pipette trypsin/EDTA onto the washed cell monolayer using 1mL/25cm^2 of surface area. Rotate flask to cover the monolayer with trypsin. Decant the excess trypsin.

- Return flask to the incubator and leave for 2-10 minutes.

- Examine the cells using an inverted microscope to ensure that all the cells are detached and floating. The side of the flasks may be gently tapped to release any remaining attached cells.

- Resuspend the cells in a small volume of fresh serum-containing medium to inactivate the trypsin. Remove 100-200mL and perform a cell count (count cells using haemocytometer) .

- Transfer the required number of cells to a new-labeled flask containing pre-warmed medium.

- Incubate as appropriate for the cell line.

- Repeat this process as demanded by the growth characteristics of the cell line.

Observation

Individual cells will observed and may subcultured.

182. Subculture of Semi-Adherent Cell Lines

Aim

To subculture semi adherent cell lines for further use and storage.

Background information

Some cultures grow as a mixed population (e.g. B95-8 - marmoset) where a proportion of cells do not attach to the tissue culture flask and remain in suspension. Therefore to maintain this heterogeneity both the attached cells and the cells in suspension must be subcultured.

Materials required

Media– pre-warmed to 37°C, 70% ethanol in water, PBS without Ca^{2+}/MG^{2+}, 25% trypsin/EDTA in HBSS, without Ca^{2+}/MG^{2+}, Trypsin, Soybean trypsin Inhibitor.

Equipment

Personal protective equipment (sterile gloves, Laboratory coat, safety visor), Water bath set to appropriate temperature, Microbiological safety cabinet at appropriate containment level, CO_2 incubator, Pre-labeled flasks, Marker Pen, Pipettes, Ampule Rack, Tissue

Procedure

- View cultures using an inverted phase contrast microscope to assess the degree of confluency and confirm the absence of bacterial and fungal contaminants. Give the flask a gentle knock first, this may dislodge the cells from the flask and remove the need for a trypsinisation step with the subsequent loss of some cells due to the washings.

- Decant spent medium into a sterile centrifuge tube and retain. .

- Wash any remaining attached cells with PBS without Ca^{2+}/MG^{2+} using 1-2mL for each 25cm² of surface area. Retain the washings.

- Pipette trypsin/EDTA onto the washed cell monolayer using 1mL/25cm² of surface area. Rotate flask to cover the monolayer with trypsin. Decant the excess trypsin.

- Return flask to incubator and leave for 2-10 minutes.

- Examine the cells using an inverted microscope to ensure that all the cells are detached and floating. The side of the flasks may be gently tapped to release any remaining attached cells.

- Transfer the cells into the centrifuge tube containing the retained spent medium and cells.

- Centrifuge the remaining cell suspension at 3000rpm for 5 minutes. Also centrifuge the washings from Number 3 above if they contain significant numbers of cells.

- Decant the supernatants and resuspend the cell pellets in a small volume (10-20mL) of fresh culture medium. Pool the cell suspensions. Count the cells.

- Pipette the required number of cells to a new-labeled flask and dilute to the required volume using fresh medium.

- Repeat this process every 2-3 days as necessary.

Observation

Trypsinised free/individual cells are observed under microscopy. This could be used for further processing.

183. Subculture of Suspension Cell Lines

Aim

To subculture Suspension cell lines for further use and storage.

Background information

In general terms cultures derived from blood (e.g. lymphocytes) grow in suspension. Cells may grow as single cells or in clumps (e.g. EBV transformed lymphoblastoid cell lines). For these types of lines subculture by dilution is relatively easy. But for lines that grow in clumps it may be necessary to bring the cells into a single cell suspension by centrifugation and resuspension by pipetting in a smaller volume before counting.

Materials required

Media– pre-warmed to 37°C, 70% ethanol in water, PBS without Ca^{2+}/MG^{2+}, 25% trypsin/EDTA in HBSS, without Ca^{2+}/MG^{2+}, Trypsin, Soybean trypsin Inhibitor

Equipment

Personal protective equipment (sterile gloves, Laboratory coat, safety visor), Waterbath set to appropriate temperature, Microbiological safety cabinet at appropriate containment level, CO_2 incubator, Pre-labeled flasks, Marker Pen, Pipettes, Ampule Rack, Tissue etc.,

Procedure

- View cultures using an inverted phase contrast microscope. Cells growing in exponential growth phase should be bright, round and refractile. Hybridomas may be very sticky and require a gentle knock to the flask to detach the cells. EBV transformed cells can grow in very large clumps that are very difficult to count and the center of the large clumps may be non-viable.

- Do not centrifuge to subculture unless the pH of the medium is acidic (phenol red = yellow) which indicates the cells have overgrown and may not recover. If this is so, centrifuge at 2000rpm for 5 minutes, re-seed at a slightly higher cell density and add 10- 20% of conditioned medium (supernatant) to the fresh media.

● Take a small sample of the cells from the cell suspension (100-200mL). Count cells using haemocytometer. Calculate cells/mL and re-seed the desired number of cells into freshly prepared flasks without centrifugation just by diluting the cells.

● Repeat this every 2-3 days.

Observation

Individual cells will grown as suspension.

184. Cell Viability Test by Trypan Blue Exclusion

Aim

To check viability of cell lines.

Background information

Viable cells are impermeable to tryphan blue, naphthalene black. This procedure is used to determine the number of viable cells present in the cell culture. A non-viable cell will have a blue cytoplasm; a viable cell will have a clear cytoplasm.

Materials required

Phosphate-buffered saline or serum-free complete culture medium, 0.4% trypan blue solution, Binocular microscope, Haemacytometer etc.,

Procedure

● Centrifuge 1mL cell suspension at 1000rpm for 5 min.

● Resuspend the cell pellet in 1mL PBS or serum-free complete culture medium (*Serum proteins stain with trypan blue and can produce misleading results. Determinations must be made in serum-free solution*).

● Mix 1 part of trypan blue solution and 1 part cell suspension.

● Take clean haemocytometer and fix the cover slip in place.

● Load the counting chamber of the haemocytometer.

● Using a binocular microscope, count the unstained (viable) and stained (dead) cells separately in a haemacytometer. Count all cells within each of the four corner squares

● Calculate the percentage of viable cells as follows:

$$\text{Number of viable cells} = \frac{\text{Viable cells}}{\text{Total number of cells (dead and viable)}} \times 100$$

Observation

Maximum number of stained cells are noted.

Spotters

Tryphan blue, stained viable monolayer cells

185. Assay of cell viability by dye uptake

Aim

To assess cell viability using dye uptake mechanism

Principle

Viable cells takeup diacetyl fluorescein and hydrolyse it to fluorescein, to which the cell membrane of live cells is impermeable. Live cells fluoresce green and dead cells do not. Non viable cells are stained with propidium iodide.

Materials required

Cell suspension, Fluorescein di acetate in $10\mu G/mL$, in HBSS. Propidium iodide 500 $\mu G/mL$, Flurescent microscope etc.,

Procedure

- Prepare cell suspension at a high concentration.

- Add a fluoresent dye mixture at a proportion of 1:10 to give a final concentration of $1\mu G/mL$ Fluorescein di acetate and $50\mu G/mL$ Propidium iodide.

- Incubate the cells at 37°C for 10 minutes.

- Place a drop of cells in microscope slide, place a cover slip and examine the cells by fluorescent microscopy.

Observation

Green and brown coloured cells are noted

186. Cell Fusion/Hybridoma Production Protocol

Aim

To hybridize myeloma and spleen cells.

To understand hybridoma technology.

To produce monoclonal antibody.

Background information

In 1975, Kohler and Milstein developed a procedure to fuse myeloma cells with B lymphocyte cells from the spleen of the immunized animal. These fused cells retained the ever-living characteristics of the myeloma cells and the spleen cells. To produce the hybridoma, as discovered by Kohler and Milstein (1975), a malignant tumor cell called a myeloma and a B-lymphocyte cell are brought together and treated with series of sine waves to align the cells for electrofusion or chemical treatment.

The hybrid cell is screened on the basis of the ability to grow on a specific medium in which neither the pure spleen cells nor the pure myeloma can grow. The hybrid cell will possess the property of the immortal character of the tumor cell and the specific antibody production. The hybridoma and its clones can be injected into animals to induce antibody-secreting myelomas, or they can be grown in mass culture to produce specific antibody.

Materials required

Mice (6-10 weeks old), myeloma cell line, Antigen, adjuvants (Freund's complete and incomplete) Hanks Balanced salt solution,

Cell fusion medium

Complete cell growth medium

10% Fetal Bovine Serum

Penicillin-Streptomycin 1 X

Sodium pyruvate, 110 mG/L

HAT Medium

Complete cell growth medium

Hypoxanthine 5 mM

Aminopterin 2 mM

Thymidine 0.8 mM

HT Medium

Complete cell growth medium

Hypoxanthine 5 mM

Thymidine 0.8 mM

Cytospin materials, Wheaton Glass Staining Dishes, Slide Cover Glass, Microscope slides, Pipette tips, Glycerin or microscope oil, Lens paper, Thermo Shandon Paper Inserts, PBS with 5% BSA, Microscope, Inverted microscope with long focal length objectives, Upright microscope.

Other supplies

BALB/c female mice, pipettes - 10mL and 25mL, tissue culture flasks, 96 well tissue culture plates (about 1 per fusion, up to 67/spleen), autoclaved sets of forceps and scissors, autoclaved screen for spleen cell dispersion, 5cc syringe (plunger used to disperse cells on screen), 1cc syringe, 18g & 25g (1/2 inch) needles, T-150 tissue culture plates, 15 & 50mL sterile conical tubes.

Procedure

Immunization

- Immunize mouse three times (d0, d14, d21) i.p. with protein of interest and 100µL adjuvant (total volume 200mL). Use 1-100mG of protein (The protein amount for the first immunization is twice the amount of all subsequent immunizations).

- Bleed mouse before each immunization for serum collection (~100mL).

- Perform mouse serum ELISA after d21 sampling. The titer from day 0 to day 21should increase by 100-1000 fold.

- Perform booster injections with antigen (no adjuvant, add 100mL 1xPBS instead) three times three days in a row (d28, d29, d30).

- Perform fusion on d31

Preparation of Myeloma cells

- Grow myeloma cells in complete culture medium to log phase prior to the day of the fusion procedure

- Centrifuge cells once and count cells.

- Dilute the cells to 3.5×10^5 cells / mL.

Spleen cell collection

- Euthanize mouse via cervical dislocation.

- Place entire mouse in a beaker containing ~200mL of 80% Betadine, 70% ethanol.

- Remove spleen using aseptic techniques *(use 3 sets of tools (scissors, forceps), one each for skin, IP sheath, spleen)*

- Transfer spleen to Petri dish containing 5mL Hybridization Serum free medium (Hyb SFM)+ 10% Faetal calf serum (FCS) *(for transport only – not necessary if removing spleen in same area where fusion will be done)*

- In hood, move spleen to new Petri dish in 1mL Hyb-SFM+10% FCS.

- Trim fat and connective tissue, and then cut spleen into small pieces. *(cut spleen into 5 sections longitudinally, then cut each section in half)*

- Using two sterile watchmaker's forceps, secure a piece of spleen with one forceps while "milking" cells from the piece into the medium. *(Place capsule pieces aside in a pile in the petri dish).*

- Transfer cells to a 50mL tube, through several (~4) washes with 2-3mL medium *(Also wash capsule sections. Wash "main" spleen cell collection 4 or 5 times, and capsule collection 2 or 3 times. Transfer all material, including chunks and capsules, to 50mL tube)*

- Pipette cell suspension a few times, then let sit (~1min) until larger tissue pieces have fallen to the bottom of the tube.

- Collect upper cell suspension and place in new 50mL tube. Centrifuge at 900-1000rpm for 5min.

- Pour off supernatant.

- *Resuspend spleen cells in 20mL HYB-SFM + 10% FBS*

- *Count spleen cells (both undiluted and 1:10)*

Fusion

- Mix myeloma and spleen cells.

- Centrifuge mixed cells 900-1000rpm 5 min.

- *Wash cells with 25mL Hyb-SFM medium (no additives) and centrifuge(just do one wash only; do not resuspend)*

- *Loosen pellet by finger-flicking. Aim for a slurry of cells; do not want chunks or pelleted cells.*

- Slowly add 1.5mL Poly Ethylene glycol (PEG) per 3×10^8 mixed cells. *(Do at room temperature. Dispense PEG along sides of tube. After dispensing PEG, mix by swirling tube.)*

- Incubate for 1 minute at 37°C

- Add very slowly (slower than cells over Ficoll) a total of 20mL Hyb-SFM. (use two 10mL pipettes). 1mL in first minute; 3mL in second minute; *(Dispense as close to dropwise as possible)* and 16mL in third minute

- Centrifuge

- Calculate total amount of HAT Fusion medium necessary for plating. Use tissue culture treated 24 well plates, 10^6 total cells/well. For each well, calculate 2mL of medium

- Add required number of cells in two 25mL of medium. Pour 2mL of medium with cells in each tissue culture wells.

- Put all but one flask into incubator to maintain temperature while plating.

- Wrap plates in plastic Wrap, three to a stack, place in incubator (37°C, 5% CO2)

Clone Testing

- After 10-14 days when clones are visible by eye and medium in some wells just begins to turn yellowish, test all wells by ELISA.

- Pick individual clones from ELISA positive wells. Transfer to round bottom, cell-treated 96 well plates, 1 clone/well 150μL medium/well Use 30μL to pick clones

- When 96-well clones are just visible by eye (usually 3 days later), test by ELISA.

- Test supernatants for IgG (or other fusion protein tag) and the protein of interest in parallel.

- For clones that recognize the protein of interest and not the IgG or fusion protein tag, transfer to 24 well plates – 1mL/well

- Transfer to 6well plates – 3-4mL/well. Collect the supernatants for additional testing depending on the protein: e.g. fusions for CD markers or surface proteins should be tested by flow cytometry. Monoclonal antibodies to an IgG isotype should be tested against various isotypes, etc to identify clones of highest interest.

- When well-grown, fix an aliquot of cells for clonality testing by flow cytometry, freeze an aliquot, and collect supernatant for mouse isotype ELISA

- After an additional 2 weeks in HAT (4 weeks total), wean cells into HT medium.

- After 2 weeks in HT medium, wean cells into Hyb+10%FCS

- Wean to Hyb-SFM for bulk culture for purification.

Observation

Myeloma and spleen cells are isolated and fused.

Fused cells are grown in HAT medium.

Cloned cells are grown in tissue culture larger wells.

Assay of specific antibodies are done.

Spotters

Hybridoma technology photo, spleen cells, cancer cell line, Spleen.

Genetics

187. Lifecycle of *Drosophila melanogaster*

Aim

To understand the nature and lifecycle of test fly *Drosophila melanogaster*.
To maintain *Drosophila* in laboratory.

Background information

Drosophila melanogaster is a fruit fly, a little insect about 3mm long, accumulates around spoiled fruit. It is one of the most valuable organisms in biological research, particularly in genetics and developmental biology. Drosophila has been used as a model organism for research for almost a century, and today, several thousand scientists are working on many different aspects of the fruit fly. Drosophila has four pairs of chromosomes: the X/Y sex chromosomes and the autosomes 2, 3, and 4. The fourth chromosome is quite tiny and rarely heard from. The size of the genome is about 165 million bases and estimated 14,000 genes. Some of the reasons for the popularity of fruit fly are; the flies are small and easily reared in the laboratory & they have à short life cycle. A new generation of adult flies can be produced every two weeks. The giant ("polytene") chromosome is present in the salivary glands of the mature larvae.

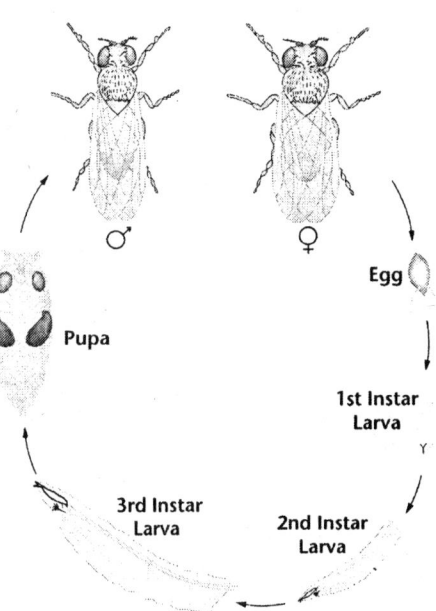

Fig. 187.1 – Lifecycle of *Drosophila melanogaster*

Life cycle

Drosophila melanogaster is a common fruit fly used as a test system and has contributed to the establishment of the basic principles of heredity. It is also called the "Cinderella of Genetics". *Drosophila melanogaster* is a dipterous, holometabolous insect. It has a characteristic larval stage preceded by the egg and succeeded by the pupalstage.

Egg

Egg is about 0.5mm in length, ovoid in shape, and white. Extending from the anterior dorsal surface, there is a pair of egg filaments. The terminal portion of these filaments are flattened into spoonlike floats. This floats keep the egg from sinking into the semi-liquid medium.

Larva

The larva hatches out from the egg within a day. It is white, segmented, and wormlike. The head is narrow and has black mouth parts (jaw hooks). The larva undergoes 2 moults, so that the larval phase consists of 3 instars. After this stage, the larva crawls out of the medium and finally attaches to the inner drier surface of the bottle. This culminates in pupation.

Pupa

Soon after the formation of the "pupal horn" from the anterior spiracle, the larval body is shortened and the skin becomes hardened and pigmented. The pupa is considered a reorganization stage. During this process, most of the adult structures are developed from the imaginal disc. A fully transformed adult fly emerges out through the anterior end of the pupal case. At the times of eclosion, the fly is greatly elongated and light in colour, with wings yet to be unfolded. Immediately after this, the wings unfold and the body gradually turns dark and brown. After 6 hours of emergence, the adult fly attains the ability to participate in reproduction.

Adult

The body is divided into head, thorax, and abdomen. The head has a pair of compound eyes and a pair of antennae. The thorax is divided into 3 segments — prothorax, mesothorax, and metathorax, each with a pair of legs. The mesothorax has a pair of wings and the metathorax has a pair of halters. The abdomen is segmented in 4 or 5 sections in males and 6 or 7 in females. The abdominal tip in males is darkly pigmented.

188. Culturing Techniques and Handling of Flies

Aim

To cultivate *Drosophila melanogaster* in laboratory condition.

Background information

Drosophila, like other animals, requires an optimum temperature for its survival, growth, and breeding (20°–25°C). The temperature around and above 31°C makes the flies sterile and reduces the oviposition; it may also result in death. At lower temperatures, the life cycle is prolonged and the viability may be impaired. The routinely used food media for the maintenance of *Drosophila* is "cream of wheat agar" medium.

Materials required

The ingredients of cream wheat medium are as follows:

Distilled water	– 1000mL
Wheat flour (rava/ sooji)	– 100g
Jaggery	– 100g
Agar agar	– 10g
Propionic acid	– 7.5mL
Yeast granules.	

Procedure

Take a clean vessel and boil 1000mL of water. Then add 100 gm of jaggery and stir well. To this add 10g of agar agar, which acts as a solidifying agent. Once it boils, add 100 gm of sooji. Then add 7.5mL of propionic acid, which acts as an antimicrobial agent. By constant stirring, the medium becomes a viscous fluid. Transfer the hot mixture into the culture bottle. Allow the bottles to cool, add yeast and plug with cotton.

Handling of Flies

The flies should be handled with a fine painting brush. In the process of handling the flies, care should be taken to avoid damage. The flies should be discarded after observation.

Etherization

When flies have to be analyzed, either for routine observation or for experiments, they are anaesthetized to make them inactive. The procedure is to transfer flies from the media bottle to another empty wide-mouthed bottle, referred to as an etherizer. The mouth of this bottle is to be covered with a stopper sprayed with ether.

Sexing

Adult flies are 2–3 mm long, while females are slightly larger than males. The males carry a sex comb on the first tarsal segment of the first leg. Males can also be identified by the presence of black pigmentation at the tip of the rounded abdomen. The tip of the female's abdomen is pointed and nonpigmented. After the separation of the 2 sexes, the unwanted flies should be discarded immediately into a bowl of detergent water.

Table 188.1 - Differentiation between Male and Female Drosophila

S. No	Characters	Male	Female
1.	Body size	small	large
2.	Dorsal side of abdomen	3 separate dark bands	5 separate dark bands
3.	Abdominal tip pigmentation	present	absent
4.	Abdominal tip shape	round	pointed
5.	Sex comb in foreleg	present	absent

Isolation of Virgins

In many experiments with *Drosophila*, it is essential that the sperm of a particular genotype (male) is used for fertilization of a particular female. To ensure this, it is often essential to isolate virgin females. The females can store and utilize the sperms from 1 insemination for a large part of the reproductive life. Females that have any chance of being nonvirgins should not be used for crosses. For ensuring virginity, females are removed before 6 hrs of their emergence and males are removed from the culture bottle before 12 hrs of emergence.

Making and Conducting Crosses

To make crosses between different strains 1–10 virgins from the first strain are mated in a culture bottle with the corresponding number of males from other strains. The reciprocal mating of the 2 strains is also done. As soon as the cross is made, the bottle is marked with the nature of the cross and the date of crossing. If the larva does not appear after 5–7 days, then the culture is discarded. If the culture is successful, then the parents are discarded and the already-laid eggs are allowed to develop into adults.

Analysis of the Progeny

The aim is to understand the pattern of inheritance of a character from parents to offspring and to subsequent generations. Therefore, each progeny (F1, F2, and test cross) has to be carefully analyzed and classified according to the phenotype and sex of each individual. Utmost care must be taken to record the number of flies in each category. From each experiment bottle, the counting must be restricted to the first 7 days from the third day of eclosion. A minimum of 200 flies must be analyzed from each of the F1, F2, and test cross progenies.

189. Mounting of genitalia in *Drosophila melanogaster*

Aim

To mount the flies to look various parts of genetalia.

Background information

The genital plate is located in the abdominal region of the male and female flies, but in the males the genital plate is more prominent and used as a copulatory pad. It is also called the epandrium. The genital plate is horseshoe-shaped, and it is bent in the posterior region. It is divided into 2 parts, the heel and the toe. Inside the arch, a pair of anal plates and a pair of primary claspersis are present. On the primary claspers, 6–19 dark spines, or bristles are present, which are very thick. Spine number is species-specific. The main function of the genital plate is to hold the female to transfer the sperm into her genital organ during copulation.

Materials required

Male flies, 1N HCl, Creosote solution, Cavity slides, Glycerine, Cover slips

Procedure

- Remove the last abdominal segment of the male *Drosophila melanogaster*.

- Transfer the segment into 1N HCl taken in a cavity slide and allow it to sit for 15 minutes.

- Blot out the HCl, use 2 or 3 drops of creosote solution, and allow it to sit for about 20 minutes.

- Remove the pellicle organ and clean the genital plate.

- Transfer the genital plate onto a clean plain slide and mount the genital plate with glycerine.

Observation

Dark region will be noted.

190. Mounting of the sex comb in *Drosophila melanogaster*

Aim

To mount sex comb to differentiate male and female flies

Background information

The sex comb is a specialized structure present exclusively in the forelegs of male flies. Location, size, and structure vary from species to species. An adult *Drosophila* has 3 pairs of legs: Forelegs, Midlegs, and Hindlegs.

In adult males, the forelegs have a comblike structure with chitinized black teeth called the sex comb. It is present in the first tarsal segment of the forelegs of the males. It is absent in the females. The sex comb helps the male hold the female during copulation or mating.

Materials required

Glass slides, Cover slip, Needles, Male flies, Glycerin, Dissecting microscope

Procedure

- Etherize the flies and separate the males.

- Separate the forelegs using needles under the dissecting microscope.

- Put a drop of glycerin on the forelegs and place the cover slip on top.

- Search and observe the sex comb on the first tarsal segment.

Observation

Black colour spot is noted on forlegs of Drosophila.

Result

Sex comp is present in male flies

191. Monohybrid experiments in *Drosophila melanogaster*

Aim

To perform experiment to prove mendels mono hybrid experiment

Background information

A monohybrid cross is a cross between parents who are heterozygous at one locus. Monohybrid inheritance is the inheritance of single character. The different forms of the characteristics are usually controlled by different alleles of the same gene. For example a monohybrid cross between two pure breeding plants, one with yellow seeds and one with green seeds, would be expected to produce an F1 genereation with only yellow seeds because the allele for yellow seeds is dominant to that of green. A monohybrid experiment compares only one trait. The simplest form of a cross is a **monohybrid cross**, which analyses a single trait and its associated variations. During gamete formation, the members of a pair of alleles are duplicated and then segregated from one cell into four separate gametes so that each contains only one member of the pair (**Law of Segregation**).

Materials required

Wild body *Drosophila melanogaster*, Ebony body *Drosophila melanogaster*, Bottles with standard medium, Anaesthetic ether, Etherizer, Re-etherizer, Needles, Brushes, Yeast granules, Glass plate

Procedure

- Select wild type and ebony type flies.

- Place male and female flies in fresh media containing petriplates (PI - Day 1) and allowed to cross.

- Maintain flies in the plates and observe the plates after 6-8 days for the presence of larvae. This is considered as F1 generation.

- Discard adult flies.

- Determine sex and other characters of F1 Generation (F1 larvae emerge as fly on 14th – 20th days). In general all F1 flies are identical phenotypically and heterozygous genotypically.

- Collect F1 males and females (5 each) and add them to a new petriplate with fresh media. Allow them for crossing (PII D1).

- Wait for 7 days (28th day) and clear adult flies and look for larvae.

- Allow larvae to hatch. F2 offspring emerge on 31st - 40th day. Determine eye colour, sex and other characters

- Tabulate the results and determine the phenotypic nature.

Cross Diagram

P1   Wild-type body (EE) **X** ebony body (ee) [homozygous parents]

↓

F1   Wild-type body (Ee) [heterozygous offspring]

Crossing F1 Male & F1Female

P2   Wild-type body Male (Ee) X Wild-type body Female (Ee)

↓

F2   Phenotype ratio 3 wild-type: 1 ebony body
Genotype ratio 1 EE : 2 Ee : 1 ee

Result

Results of this experiment proved mendels monohybrid ratio of inheritance.

192. Dihybrid experiments in *Drosophila melanogaster*

Aim

To prove mendels dihybrid experiment using Drosophila

Background information

A dihybrid cross, in which two characteristics are observed, F1 generation only expressed the dominant phenotypes. In F2 generation, both dominant and recessive traits are expressed and four phenotype categories were noticed with the ratio of 9:3:3:1. This cross lead to law of independent assortment, which states that each pair of alleles segregate independenly of other pairs of alleles during gametogenesis.

Materials required

Wild body normal wing drosophila, Ebony body vestigial wing drosophila, Bottles with standard medium, Anaesthetic ether, Etherizer, Re-etherizer, Needles, Brushes, Yeast granules, Glass plate.

Procedure

- Select Wild body normal wing Drosophila male and Ebony body vestigial wing Drosophila female.

- Place male and female flies in fresh media containing petriplates (PI - Day 1) and allowed to cross.

- Maintain flies in the plates and observe the plates after 6-8 days for the presence of larvae. This is considered as F1 generation.

- Discard adult flies.

- Determine sex and other characters of F1 Generation (F1 larvae emerge as fly on 14th – 20th days). In general all F1 flies are identical phenotypically and heterozygous genotypically.

- Collect F1 males and females (5 each) and add them to a new petriplate with fresh media. Allow them for crossing (PII D1).

- Wait for 7 days (28th day) and clear adult flies and look for larvae.

- Allow larvae to hatch. F2 offspring emerge on 31st - 40th day. Determine eye colour, sex and other characters

- Tabulate the results and determine the phenotypic nature.

Cross Diagram

Dihybrid crosses involve manipulation and analysis of two traits controlled by pairs of alleles at different loci, where the loci for ebony body colour and vestigial wing are on separate autosomes. Therefore the genotypes and gametes are the same for male and female.

P1   Wild body normal wing (EEWW) **X** Ebony body vestigial wing(eeww)

$$\downarrow$$

F1   Wild body normal wing (EeWw) [heterozygous offspring]

Crossing F1 Male & F1Female

P2   Wild body normal wing (EeWw) X Wild body normal wing (EeWw)

$$\downarrow$$

F2   Phenotype ratio 9 Wild body normal wing : 3 Wild body Vestigial wing :
3 Ebony body normal wing : Ebony body Vestigial wing

In a dihybrid cross, each of the F1 parents can produce four different gamete types, so there are 16 (= 4 x 4) possible offspring combinations. Because the two traits show complete dominance and separate independently of each other (**Law of Independent Assortment**), the expected genotypic and phenotypic ratios from an analysis of these 16 possibilities can be calculated.

Genotype –	1 EEWW	- Wild body normal wing
	2 EEWw	- Wild body normal wing
	2 EeWW	- Wild body normal wing
	4 EeWw	- Wild body normal wing
	1 EEww	- Wild body vestigial wing
	2 Eeww	- Wild body vestigial wing
	1 eeWW	- Ebony body vestigial wing
	2 eeWw	- Ebony body vestigial wing
	1 eeww	- Ebony body vestigial wing

Genotype Ratio - 1:2:1:2:4:2:1:2:1

These ratios can be derived from the results of a dihybrid ratio. A basic principle of probability theory is that the probability of two independent events occurring together is equal to the *product* of the two independent probabilities. Mendel's work on peas was done before the discovery of chromosomes, and his **Law of Independent Assortment** postulated that each trait would segregate independently of every other.

193. Demonstration of the law of independent assortment

Aim

To demonstrate mendels law of independent assortment using dihybrid experiment.

Background information

Mendel's second law is known as the law of independent assortment, which states that 2 different sets of genes assort independently of each other during the formation of gametes through meiosis. The cross conducted taking 2 contrasting pairs of characteristics is known as the dihybrid cross and it produces 9:3:3:1 in the F2 generation. In *Drosophila,* this was stated by Morgan. In this experiment, pairs of contrasting characters, such as sepia-eye and vestigial-eye mutants were taken to study whether inheritance patterns follow the Mendelian laws or not. Vestigial wing is characterized by reduced wings and balancers and the sepia-eye mutant is characterized by brown eyes.

Materials required

Wild body normal wing Drosophila, Ebony body vestigial wing Drosophila, Bottles with standard medium, Anaesthetic ether, Etherizer, Re-etherizer, Needles, Brushes, Yeast granules, Glass plate

Procedure

- Select Wild body normal wing Drosophila male and Ebony body vestigial wing Drosophila female.

- Place male and female flies in fresh media containing petriplates (PI - Day 1) and allowed to cross.

- Maintain flies in the plates and observe the plates after 6-8 days for the presence of larvae. This is considered as F1 generation.

- Discard adult flies.

- Determine sex and other characters of F1 Generation (F1 larvae emerge as fly on 14th – 20th days). In general all F1 flies are identical phenotypically and heterozygous genotypically.

- Collect F1 males and females (5 each) and add them to a new petriplate with fresh media. Allow them for crossing (PII D1).

- Wait for 7 days (28th day) and clear adult flies and look for larvae.

- Allow larvae to hatch. F2 offspring emerge on 31st - 40th day. Determine eye colour, sex and other characters

- Tabulate the results and determine the phenotypic nature.

Cross Diagram

Dihybrid crosses involve manipulation and analysis of two traits controlled by pairs of alleles at different loci, where the loci for ebony body colour and vestigial wing are on separate autosomes. Therefore the genotypes and gametes are the same for male and female.

P1   Wild body normal wing (EEWW) X Ebony body vestigial wing(eeww)

↓

F1   Wild body normal wing (EeWw) [heterozygous offspring]

Crossing F1 Male & F1Female

P2   Wild body normal wing (EeWw) X Wild body normal wing (EeWw)

↓

F2   Phenotype ratio 9 Wild body normal wing : 3 Wild body Vestigial wing : 3 Ebony body normal wing : Ebony body Vestigial wing

In a dihybrid cross, each of the F1 parents can produce four different gamete types, so there are 16 (= 4 x 4) possible offspring combinations. Because the two traits show complete dominance and separate independently of each other (**Law of Independent Assortment**), the expected genotypic and phenotypic ratios from an analysis of these 16 possibilities can be calculated.

Genotype –	1 EEWW	- Wild body normal wing
	2 EEWw	- Wild body normal wing
	2 EeWW	- Wild body normal wing
	4 EeWw	- Wild body normal wing
	1 EEww	- Wild body vestigial wing
	2 Eeww	- Wild body vestigial wing
	1 eeWW	- Ebony body vestigial wing
	2 eeWw	- Ebony body vestigial wing
	1 eeww	- Ebony body vestigial wing

Genotype Ratio - 1:2:1:2:4:2:1:2:1

These ratios can be derived from the results of a dihybrid ratio. A basic principle of probability theory is that the probability of two independent events occurring together is equal to the *product* of the two independent probabilities. Mendel's work on peas was done before the discovery of chromosomes, and his **Law of Independent Assortment** postulated that each trait would segregate independently of every other.

194. Demonstration of law of segregation

Aim

To demonstrate mendels law of segregation using monohybrid experiment.

Background information

Heredity, or the inheritance of parental character, offsprings has long been the subject of a great deal of experimental work in biology. Gregor Mendel, an Austin monk, carried out an extensive series of experiments on the common edible pea (*Pisum sativum*) to find out their inheritance patterns. The law of segregation is one of the laws proposed by Mendel, which states that the genes or alleles present in F1 will not blend or contaminate or influence one another; rather, they segregate in the same pure form that they arrived from the parent. The members of an allele pair separate from each other without influencing each other, when an individual forms haploid germ cells.

Materials required

Wild wing *Drosophila melanogaster*, Vestigial-wing *Drosophila melanogaster*, Bottles with standard medium, Anaesthetic ether, Etherizer, Re-etherizer, Needles, Brushes, Yeast granules, Glass plate

Procedure

- Cultivate *Drosophila melanogaster* normal and vestigial-winged mutant flies in standard media bottles separately.

- Place male and female flies in fresh media containing petriplates (PI - Day 1) and allowed to cross.

- Maintain flies in the plates and observe the plates after 6-8 days for the presence of larvae. This is considered as F1 generation.

- Discard adult flies.

- Determine sex and other characters of F1 Generation (F1 larvae emerge as fly on 14th – 20th days) (In general all F1 flies are identical phenotypically and heterozygous genotypically).

- Collect F1 males and females (5 each) and add them to a new petriplate with fresh media. Allow them for crossing (PII D1).

- Wait for 7 days (28th day) and clear adult flies and look for larvae.

- Allow larvae to hatch. F2 offspring emerge on 31st - 40th day. Determine eye colour, sex and other characters

- Tabulate the results and determine the phenotypic nature.

Cross Diagram

P1   Wild Normal Wing(WW) **X** Mutant Vestigial wing(ww) [homozygous parents]

↓

F1   Wild Normal Wing (Ww) [heterozygous offspring]

Crossing F1 Male & F1Female

P2   Wild Normal Wing Male (Ww) X Wild Normal Wing Female (Ww)

↓

F2   Phenotype ratio 3 Wild Normal Wing: 1 Mutant Vestigial wing
Genotype ratio 1 WW : 2 Ww : 1 ww

Observation

Phenotype ratio 3 Wild Normal Wing: 1 Mutant Vestigial wing
Genotype ratio 1 WW : 2 Ww : 1 ww

195. Determination of Phenomenon of Segregation – Artificial - Probability

Aim

To determine law of segregation through artificial mechanical process using probability analysis.

Materials required

Two boxes, 100 yellow coloured balls, 100 green coloured balls.

Procedure

- Count 50 yellow balls and 50 green balls.

- Put 50 yellow balls & 50 green balls in box A and mix thoroughly

- Repeat the same procedure for box B using green balls (You have now had 100 balls in each box of both colours in equal numbers).

- Now without looking, withdraw one ball each from each of the boxes and record the colour pairs, continue until the boxes are empty and you have 100 pairs.

- Add up the number of three combinations Viz Yellow and yellow; yellow and green, green and green.

- Find out combinations approach 1:2:1 ratio, assuming that yellow ball represents round seed (Y) (dominant) and the green ball represents wrinkled seed (y) (recessive).

Explanation

The boxes represent the plant and the balls represent the gametes carrying different alleles. The random selection of pairs corresponds to random fusion of male and female gemetes. The pairs of balls thus represents zygotic combinations. Since each box contains equal number of yellow and green balls, then there is an equal chance at each random selection that the combination will be any one of the following.

Yellow from box A with yellow from box B = YY

Yellow from box A with green from box B = Yy

Green from box A with yellow from box B = Yy

Green from box A with green from box B = yy

Spotters

Viva questions

196. Determination of Phenomenon of independent assortment – Artificial - Probability

Aim

To determine law of independent assortment through artificial mechanical process using probability analysis.

Materials required

Two boxes, four types of colourded balls viz., red, green, blue and yellow (eighty each), paper, pencil etc.,

Procedure

- Count 40 balls of each colour (red, green, blue and yellow).

- Put them in box A and mix thoroughly

- Repeat the same procedure for box B (You have now 160 balls in each box of four colour in equal numbers).

- Now without looking, withdraw one ball each from each of the boxes and record the colour pairs, continue until the boxes are empty and you have 160 pairs.

- Calculate the ratio assuming that both boxes represent the two plants and the balls, the gametes carrying different alleles.

Explanation

Each box contains equal numbers of four types of balls representing gametes. If the two plants croses where phenotypically round seeded and seeds yellow coloured with genotype RrYy, then the four gametes would be RY, Ry, rY and ry. Let them represented as follows

RY is represented by Red ball

Ry is represented by blue ball

rY is represented by yellow ball

ry is represented by green ball

Find out the phenotype using these indicators and whether the ration approaches 9:3:3:1

Round yellow (RRYY)

Round green (RRyy)

Wringle Yellow (rrYY)

Wringle green (rryy)

Red from Box A with red from box B

Red from Box A with blue from box B

Red from Box A with yellow from box B

Red from Box A with green from box B

Blue from Box A with red from box B

Blue from Box A with blue from box B

Blue from Box A with yellow from box B

Blue from Box A with green from box B

Yellow from Box A with red from box B

Yellow from Box A with blue from box B

Yellow from Box A with yellow from box B

Yellow from Box A with green from box B

Green from Box A with red from box B

Green from Box A with blue from box B

Green from Box A with yellow from box B

Green from Box A with green from box B

Cell Biology

197. Mitosis in onion root

Aim

To study different phases of mitosis.

Background information

Cell cycle has four phases; they are G1 (Cells metabolically active, organelles begins to increase in number), S (replication of DNA), G2 (Synthesis of proteins; final preparation for cell division) and M (Mitosis). Mitosis is also called somatic cell division or equatorial division. The process of cell division, whereby chromosomes are duplicated and distributed equally to the daughter cells, is called mitosis. It helps to maintain the constant chromosome number in all cells of the body. Phases of mitosis are Interphase, Prophase, Metaphase, Anaphase, Telophase and Cytokinesis.

Materials required

Fresh grown onion root tip, 5-10mL distilled water, 5mL 6M HCl, 1mL Feulgen reagent, 5mL 45% acetic acid, dropper pipettes, beaker, slide, coverslip, a pencil with eraser to squash the slide, microscope, Carnoy's solution (1 glacial acetic acid: 3 Absolute alcohol).

Feulgen Solution (Schiff Reagent)

Fuchsin, Basic	-1g
Water	- 200mL
Potassium metabisulphite	- 2g
Hydrochloric acid. Pure	- 2mL
Decolourising charcoal	- 0.5g

Boil water and add fuchsin, when dissolved cool to about 50°C and add metabisulphite, dissolve and allow to cool to room temperature. Add acid, plug flask with cotton and leave overnight. Add charcoal, shake and filter. The solution should now be colourless.

Procedure

- Take an onion. Cut off any old root growth. Place the onion in a beaker (50mL) of water (root portion should under water. To do this, push toothpicks into the side of the onion which extend outward and hold it on the rim of the cup. New roots should grow within two days).

- Cut off 0.5-1 cm of growth at the root tip.

- Transfer the root immediately to Carnoy's solution and incubate for 24 hours and store roots in 70% ethanol in a refrigerator. This stops cell division.

- After obtaining the root tip, pour off the fixative and replace it with 2-5mL distilled water. Solutions may be poured into a beaker or down the drain.

- After 1 minute, remove the water with a pipette and add 2-5mL 6M HCl.

- After 3 minutes, carefully remove the acid and wash tissue off with distilled water. Agitate the vial for 1-2 minutes. Discard the water.

- Transfer the tissue to a vial containing 1-2mL Feulgen reagent. After 20 minutes, transfer the tissue to a vial containing 5mL 45% acetic acid using forceps.

- Place 1-2 drops of acetic acid onto a microscope slide and transfer the tissue to the drop. Using dissecting pins and razor blades tease and macerate the tissue into tiny pieces.

- Place a coverslip over the macerated tissue trying not to get air bubbles under the coverslip. Press down firmly onto the coverslip with a small cork or pencil eraser to spread the cells in a very thin layer. Push down in a perpendicular direction and the coverslip should not break.

- Once the slide has been prepared, observe it and draw all the different views of cells present under high power.

Observations

Observe different stages of mitosis and draw various stages.

Record the number of cells having different stages of mitosis and calculate mitotic index. **Mitotic index** is a measure for the proliferation status of a cell population. It is defined as the ratio between the number of cells in mitosis and the total number of cells.

Possible observation comments

Interphase

Interphase is also called the resting stage. This is a transitional phase between the successive mitotic divisions.

1. Replication of DNA takes place.

2. The volume of the nucleus increases.

3. The chromosomes are thinly coiled.

Observation

Prophase

1. Each chromosome consists of chromatids united by a centromere.

2. Spindle formation is initiated.

3. The chromosomes shorten, thicken, and become stainable.

4. The nuclear membrane and nucleolus start disappearing.

Metaphase

1. Disappearance of the nucleolus and nuclear membrane.

2. Chromosomes are at their maximum condensed state.

3. Spindle formation is complete.

4. The chromosomes align in the equatorial position of the spindle and form the equatorial plate that is at a right angle to the spindle axis.

5. The centromeres are arranged exactly at the equatorial plate and the arms are directed toward the poles.

Anaphase

1. The centromere of the chromosomes divides and the 2 chromatids of each pair separate.

2. Sister chromatids start moving toward the opposite poles due to the contraction of chromosomal fibers.

3. The daughter chromosomes assume "V" or "J" shapes.

Telophase

1. It is the reverse of prophase.

2. The chromosomes aggregate at the poles.

3. The spindle starts disappearing.

4. The new nuclear membrane starts to reappear around each set of chromosomes.

5. The nucleolus gets reorganized.

Cytokinesis

A cell plate is formed by the formation of phragnoplast from the Golgi complex. Later the primary and secondary wall layers are deposited. Finally, the cells are divided into 2 daughter cells. The cytoplasm gets divided into 2 parts.

Table 197.1-mitosis result report

Stage	Number of cells
Inter phase	
Prophase	
Meta phase	
Anaphase	
Telophase	
Total number of dividing and normal cells	

Spotters

Different stages of cell division, Feulgen reagent, Carnoy's solution

Viva questions

Why root tip is taken to study mitosis?

Define mitosis, mitotic index.

What are the different stages of cell division?

Define cell cycle, cytokinensis

198. Meiosis in flower buds of *Allium cepa* (Onion)

Aim

To understand meiotic cell division in sexual part of the plant

Background information

Meiosis a process of reductional division in which the number of chromosomes per cell is cut in half. In animals, meiosis always results in the formation of gametes, while in other organisms it can give rise to spores. In other words, it is defined as a form of cell division happening in sexually reproducing organisms by which two consecutive nuclear divisions (meiosis I and meiosis II) occur without the chromosomal replication in between, leading to the production of four haploid gametes (sex cells), each containing one of every pair of homologous chromosomes.

Materials required

Onion flower, Carnoy's fluid (1 glacial acetic acid: 3 Absolute alcohol), Aceto-carmine stain, Glass slides, Cover slips, blotting paper.

Aceto-Carmine stain

Carmine	0.5g
Glacial acetic acid	45mL
Water	55mL

Place carmine and water in a 200mL flask, bring to boil, add acetic acid, plug flask with cotton wool and boil again; cool and filter.

Procedure

- Select unopened flower buds from the influorescence of Onion.
- Fix the flower bud in Carnoy's fluid.
- Take a preserved flower bud and place it on a glass slide.
- Separate the anthers and discard other parts of the bud.
- Add 1 or 2 drops of acetocarmine stain and squash the anthers.
- Allow the material to stain for 5 minutes.
- Place a cover slip and tap it gently.
- Warm it slightly over the flame of a spirit lamp.
- Place a piece of blotting paper on the cover slip and apply uniform pressure using thumb.
- Observe the slide under the microscope to differentiate different meiotic stages.

Observation

Different stages of meiosis are noted based on following descriptions.

Interphase

Before under going meiosis-I, each cell will remain in an interphase, during which the genetic materials are duplicated due to active DNA replication.

Prophase-I

In the first meiotic division, production in the chromosome number occurs without separation of chromatids. Prophase is the longest phase and has 5 stages.

Leptotene

Chromosomes appear as long threadlike structure interwoven together. Chromosomes display a beaded appearance and are called chromomeres. Ends of chromosomes are drawn toward nuclear membrane near the centriole. In some plants, chromosomes may form synthetic knots.

Zygotene

The homologous chromosomes pair with one another, gene by gene, over the entire length of the chromosomes. The pairing of the homologous chromosomes is called synapsis. Each pair of homologous chromosomes is known as bivalent.

Pachytene

Each paired chromosomes become shorter and thicker than in earlier substages and splits into 2 sister chromatids except at the region of the centromere. As a result of the longitudinal division of each homologous chromosome into 2 chromatids, there are 4 group of chromatids in the nucleus parallel to each other, called tetrads.

Diplotene

During the diplotene stage, chiasmata appear to move towards the ends of the synapsed chromosomes in the process of terminalization. Repulsion of homologous chiasmata are very clear in pachytene because of the increased condensation of the chromosomes.

Diakinesis

The chromosomes begin to coil, and so become shorter and thicker. Terminalization is completed. The nucleolus detaches from the nucleolar organizer and disappears completely. The nuclei envelope starts to degenerate and spindle formation is well underway.

Metaphase-I

The bivalents orient themselves at random on the equatorial plate. The centromere of each chromosome of a terminalized tetrad is directed toward the opposite poles. The chromosomal microtubular spindle fibers remain attached, with the centromeres and homologous chromosomes ready to separate.

Anaphase-I

It is characterized by the separation of whole chromosomes of each homologous pair (tetrad), so that each pole of the dividing cell receives either a paternal or maternal longitudinally double chromosome of each tetrad. This ensures a change in chromosome number from diploid to monoploid or haploid in the resultant reorganized daughter nuclei.

Telophase-I

The chromosomes may persist for a time in the condensed state, the nucleolus and nuclear membrane may be reconstituted, and cytokinesis may also occur to produce 2 haploid cells.

Metaphase-II

Metaphase-II is of very short duration. The chromosomes rearrange in the equatorial plate. The centromere lies in the equator, while the arms are directed toward the poles. The centromeres divide and separate into 2 daughter chromosomes.

Anaphase-II

Daughter chromosomes start migrating toward the opposite poles and the movement is brought about by the action of spindle fibers.

Telophase-II

The chromosomes uncoil after reaching the opposite poles and become less distinct. The nuclear membrane and nucleolus reappear, resulting in the formation of 4 daughter nuclei, which are haploid.

Cytokinesis

This separates each nucleus from the others. The cell wall is formed and 4 haploid cells are produced.

Spotters

Different stages of meiosis.

Viva questions

Define meiosis

What is the need of meiosis in animals and plants?

Is meiosis occurs in prokaryotic cells.

199. Meiosis in Grasshopper Testis (*Poecilocerus pictus*)

Aim

To understand meiotic cell division in animals.

Background information

Refer previous experiment - Page 462.

Materials required

Grasshopper testis, Carnoy's fluid, Aceto-carmine stain, Glass slides, Cover slips, blotting paper.

Composition of Carnoy's fluid & Aceto-carmine stain - refer previous experiment - Page 462.

Procedure

- One or two testes of the grasshopper are removed and fixed in Carnoy's fluid.

- Transfer testes to 10% alcohol and stored after 2-14 hours.

- The testes are placed on a glass slide.

- Apply 1 to 2 drops of acetocarmine stain.

- With a sharp blade, cut the teste lobes into minute pieces and kept for 10 minutes.

- Gently cover the preparation with a coverslip, taking care so that air bubbles are not formed.

- Warm the slide gently and place it between 2 folds of filter paper.

- Press the material with the tip of the finger and remove the excess stain, which comes out on the sides of the coverslip.

- Observe the slide under the microscope.

Observation, Spotters and Viva questions

Refer previous experiment - Page 462, 463, 464.

200. Barr Body staining from buccal epithelial cells

Aim

To study the Barr body from the smear of Buccal epithelial cells (female).

Background information

A Barr body is nothing but an inactivated (heterochromatinized) X chromosome. It was first observed by Murray Barr in 1949. It is found only in female cells, because in those 1 X chromosome is enough for metabolic activity. It is absent in male somatic cells, because there only 1 X chromosome is present, which is in an active state.

Materials required

Buccal epithelial cells, Giemsa stain, Carnoy's fixative, Slides, Cover slip, Microscope, etc.

Procedure

- Gently rub the inside of the cheek with a flat rounded piece of wood and transfer the scraping over a clean glass slide.

- Prepare a thin and uniform film of cells on the slide and air-dry.

- Keep air-dried smear in Carnoy's fixative for 30–35 minutes.

- Pour the Giemsa stain and allowed to stand for 20–25 minutes.

- Wash the slide with distilled water to remove the excess stain.

- Air-dry the smear and observed under the microscope.

Observations

Violet-Barr bodies are observed inside a pink nucleus.

Spotters

Structure of barr body.

Viva questions

What is barr body?

Why the name barr body is given to that inclusion of human cell?

Why female buccal cells are taken to stain barr body?

201. Normal Human Karyotyping

Aim

To study the chromosomal sets (Karyotype) of a normal human.

Background informations

Karyotyping is based on the size and position of chromosomes and centromeres, respectively. It was first developed by Albert Levan in 1960. Based on the centromeric position that is on the length of arms of chromosomes, he divided chromosomes as:

1, 2, 3, 16, 19, and 20 - Metacentric

4–12, 17, 18, and X - Submetacentric

13–15, 21, 22, and Y - Telocentric

Later, Pataii classified the chromosomes into different families (Groups):

Group A: 1-3 Chromosomes-Metacentric; longer than the all other chromosomes

Group B: 4 and 5 Chromosomes-Submetacentric

Group C: 6-12 and X Chromosomes-Submetacentric

Group D: 13-15 Chromosomes-Acrocentric

Group E: 16-18 - Chromosomes-16: Metacentric, 17 and 18: Submetacentric

Group F: 19 and 20 Chromosomes-Metacentric, comparatively smaller

Group G: 21, 22 and Y Chromosomes-Acrocentric and the smallest in size

The chromosomes of groups D and G have secondary constrictions.

Principle

Karyotyping is a valuable research tool used to determine the chromosome complement within cultured cells. It is important to keep in mind that karyotypes evolve with continued culture. Because of this evolution, it is important for the interpretation of biochemical or other data, that the karyotype of a specific subline be determined. Numerous different technical procedures have been reported that produce banding patterns on metaphase chromosomes. A band is defined as the part of a chromosome that is clearly distinguishable from its adjacent segments by appearing darker or lighter. The chromosomes are visualized as consisting of a continuous series of light and dark bands. A G staining method resulting in G-bands uses a Giemsa or Leishman dye mixture as the staining agent.

Materials required

Fresh venous blood, Heparinized syringes, Eagle's spinner modified media with PHA, Culture flasks, Tissue culture grade incubator, 10 mg/mL Colcemid, Clinical centrifuge and tubes, 0.075M KCl, Absolute methanol and glacial acetic acid (3:1 mixture, prepared fresh), Dry ice, Slides, cover slips and permount, Alkaline solution for G-banding, Saline-citrate for G-banding, Ethanol (70% and 95% (v/v)), Giemsa stain.

Procedure

- Draw 5mL of venous blood into a sterile syringe containing 0.5mL of sodium heparin (1000 units/mL). The blood may be collected in a heparinized vacutainer, and transferred to a syringe.

- Bend a clean, covered 18-gauge needle to a 45° angle and place it on the syringe. Invert the syringe (needle pointing up, plunger down), and stand it on end for 1½ to 2 hours at room temperature. During this time the erythrocytes settle by gravity, leaving approximately 4mL of leukocyte-rich plasma on the top, and a white buffy coat of leukocytes in the middle.

- Carefully tip the syringe (do not invert) and slowly expel the leukocyte-rich plasma and the fluffy coat into a sterile tissue culture flask containing 8mL of Eagle's spinner modified media supplemented with 0.1mL of phytohemaglutin (PHA).

- Incubate the culture for 66–72 hours at 37°C. Gently agitate the culture once or twice daily during the incubation period.

- Add 0.1mL of colcemid (10mg/mL) to the culture flasks and incubate for an additional 2 hours.

- Transfer the colcemid-treated cells to a 15-mL centrifuge tube and centrifuge at 1500rpm for 10 minutes.

- Aspirate and discard all but retain 0.5mL of the supernatant. Gently tap the bottom of the centrifuge tube to resuspend the cells in the remaining 0.5mL of culture media.

- Add 10mL of 0.075 M KCl, dropwise at first, and then with gentle agitation to the centrifuge tube. Gently mix with each drop. Start timing the next step immediately with the first drop of KCl.

- Let the cells stand exactly 6 minutes in the hypotonic KCl. The hypotonic solution should not be in contact with the cells in excess of 15 minutes from the time it is added.

- Centrifuge the cells at 1500rpm for 6 minutes. Aspirate the KCl and discard all but retain 0.5mL of the supernatant. Gently resuspend the cells in this small volume of fluid.

- Add 10mL freshly prepared fixative, dropwise at first and then with gentle agitation. Gentle and continuous agitation is important at this step to prevent clumping of the cells.

- Allow the cells to stand in fixative at room temperature for 30 minutes.

- Centrifuge at 1500rpm for 5 minutes and remove all but retain 0.5mL of supernatant. Resuspend the cells in fresh fixative.

- Wash the cells twice more in 10mL volumes of fixative. Add the fixative slowly, recentrifuge, and aspirate the fixative as previously directed. The fixed, pelleted cells may be stored for several weeks at 4°C.

- Resuspend the pellet of cells in just enough fixative to cause a slightly turbid appearance.

- Prop a piece of dry ice against the side of a styrofoam container and lace a clean slide onto the dry ice to chill the slide.

- Remove the slides from the dry ice and allow them to air dry. Perform the desired banding and/or staining procedures. Preparation of chromosomes for karyotype analysis can be performed in a number of ways, and each will yield differing pieces of information. The chromosomes may be stained with aceto-orcein, feulgen, or a basophilic dye such as toluidine blue or methylene blue if only the general morphology is desired. If more detail is desired, the chromosomes can be treated with various enzymes in combination with stains to yield banding patterns on each chromosome. These techniques have become common place and will yield far more diagnostic information than giemsa stain alone (the most commonly used process). A band is an area of a chromosome that is clearly distinct from its neighboring area, but may be lighter or darker than its neighboring region. The standard methods of banding are the Q, G, R, and C banding techniques.

G-banding Procedure

- Treat fixed and flamed slides in alkaline solution, room temperature for 30 seconds. Rinse in saline-citrate solution, 3 changes for 5–10 minutes each. Incubate in saline-citrate solution, 65°C for 60–72 hours. Treat with 3 changes of 70% ethanol and 3 changes of 95% ethanol (3 minutes) each.

- Air dry.

- Stain in buffered Giemsa for 5 minutes.

- Rinse briefly in distilled water.

- Air dry and mount.

- Photograph appropriate spreads and produce 8 × 10 high contrast photographs of your chromosome spreads.

- Cut each chromosome from the photograph and arrange the chromosomes according to size and the position of the centromere.

- Tape or glue each chromosome to the form supplied for this purpose.

- In the construction of the karyotype, the autosomes are numbered 1 to 22, in descending order of length. The sex chromosomes are referred to as X and Y. The symbols p and q are used to designate, respectively, the short and long arms of each chromosome.

- A description of the karyotype should be recorded on the karyotype sheet. First record the number of chromosomes, including the sex chromosomes, followed by a comma (,). The sex chromosome constitution is given next. Any structural rearrangements and additional or missing chromosomes are listed next. Other information such as the cell line number, the date karyotype is prepared, the specimen type, and the technologist should also be recorded on the karyotype sheet.

Observation

Different size and shape chromosomes may be observed and photographed.

Spotters

Karyotype pattern.

Viva questions

What is karyotyping and karyotype.

Mention the importance of karyotyping.

202. Preparation of Polytene Chromosomes

Aim

To prepare salivary gland chromosomes in *Drosophila melanogaster*.

Background information

Larval stages of *Drosophila* salivary gland contain large, multistranded polytene chromosomes. **Polytene** chromosomes are produced by repeated replication during synapsis without separation into daughter nuclei. Edouard-Gérard Balbiani, in 1881, observed salivary gland chromosomes in *Chironomous* larva. Theophilus Painter discovered the same in *Drosophila melanogaster*. The polytene chromosomes are the largest chromosomes available for cytological studies. These chromosomes are clearly seen in the third instar larva of *Drosophila melanogaster*. The salivary gland chromosomes undergo somatic pairing and endoduplication without separation. This multistranded chromosome contains 1024 chromosomal fibrils. When stained, chromosomes shows bands and interbands. Along the length, there are bulged regions called Balbiani rings, or puffs, which are the sites of genetic action.

Materials required

Dissecting microscope, compound microscope, Third instar larva of Drosophila / Larva of chironomous, 1N HCl, Physiological saline (0.9% NaCl), Aceto orcein, 45% acetic acid, Nail polish or wax for sealing, Slides and cover slips, scalpels, insect pin, 2 teasing needles

Aceto-orcein staining solution (1%)

Orcein	- 1g
Glacial acetic acid	- 55mL
Double distilled water	- 100mL

Pour 55mL boiling glacial acetic acid over 1g orcein powder. Cool the solution, add 45mL of distilled water and filter. Prepare fresh before use.

Procedure

● Select a large larva of *Drosophila melanogaster*.

● Using the stereomicroscope, dissect the larva by placing one teasing needle on the posterior aspect of the larva and the other needle at the anterior end, near the black mouth parts.

● Carefully pull outward with the anterior needle (There are two transparent salivary glands located anteriorly in the larva. The glands are characterized by a granular, bead-like appearance. A narrow, white ribbon of fat surrounds the glands).

● Discard all parts of the larva except the salivary glands.

● Place 2 drops of aceto-orcein stain on the salivary glands, and let it stand for 10 minutes.

● Place a cover slip over the glands, and using thumb and a paper towel, push down on the slide (The pressure applied will squash the glands, rupture the nuclear membrane and free the chromosomes).

● Using a compound microscope, observe the slide under low and high magnification.

Observation

White mass of salivary gland is observed and subjected for staining.

Result

Giant chromosomes of salivary gland is observed.

Spotters

Larva of Drosophila, structure of giant chromosome.

Viva questions

What is giant chromosome?

How is giant chromosomes formed

203. Isolation of Chloroplasts from Spinach Leaves

Aim

To isolate chloroplast from spinach leaves

Background information

Chloroplasts are specialized organelles found in all higher plant cells. These organelles contain the plant cell's chlorophyll, hence provide the green colour. They have a double outer membrane. The thylakoids and grana (singular = granum) are present in chloroplast where photosynthesis takes place.

Materials required

Solutions

Spinach leaves (fresh) suspension solution

Sorbitol pH 7.6, adjust with NaOH	0.33 M
$MgCl_2$	1 mM
HEPES (4-(2-hydroxyethyl)-1-piperazineethanesulfonic acid)	50 mM
EDTA	2 mM

Grinding Solution

Sorbitol pH 7.6, adjust with NaOH	0.33 M
$MgCl_2$	4 mM
Ascorbic acid (Vitamin C)	2 mM
Sodium pyrophosphate	10 mM
NaCl	0.35 M

Other Chemicals

Sodium hydroxide, Sodium pyrophosphate, Sodium chloride, Spinach leaves (fresh), Magnesium chloride, Ascorbic acid, Sorbitol, HEPES, muslin cloth, Hydrochloric acid

EDTA.

Mortar and pestle, knife, centrifuge.

Procedure

- Prepare an ice bath and precool all glassware to be used (including a mortar and pestle).

- Select several fresh spinach leaves. Remove the large veins by tearing from the leaves. Weigh out 4g of deveined leaf tissue.

- Chop the tissue as fine as possible with a knife and chopping board.

- Add the tissue to an ice-cold mortar containing 15mL of grinding solution and grind the tissue to a paste.

- Filter the ground up tissue solution through double-layered muslin cloth into a beaker, and squeeze the tissue pulp to recover all of the liquid suspension.

- Transfer the green suspension to a cold 50mL centrifuge tube and centrifuge for 1 minute at 1000rpm at 4°C to pellet the unbroken cells and cell fragments.

- Decant the supernatant into a clean centrifuge tube and centrifuge again for 7 minutes at 3000rpm to pellet the chloroplasts. Decant and discard the supernatant.

- Resuspend the chloroplasts in 5mL of cold suspension solution (or 0.35 M NaCl). Use a cold glass-stirring rod to gently disrupt the packed pellet.

- Enclose the tube in aluminum foil and place at 0°C to 4°C.

- Using a haemacytometer, determine the number of chloroplasts per mL of suspension media.

Observations

Individual chloroplast cells are observed and counted.

Spotters

Chloroplast structure

Viva questions

What is chloroplast?

What are the uses of chloroplast?

Is an animal and bacterial cells have chloroplast

Which part of the chloroplast is active?

X. Appendix A - Culture Media

Acetobacter Agar (Mannitol) (pH-7.4)

It is used for isolation of Acetobacter species.

Peptic digest of animal tissue	-3g
Yeast extract	-5g
Mannitol	-25g
Agar	-15g
Distilled water	-1000mL

Actinomycetes isolation medium (pH-8.1)

Sodium casionate	-2g
L-Asparagine	-01g
Sodium propionate	-4g
Dipotassium phosphate	-0.5g
Magnesium phosphate	-0.1g
Ferrous sulphate	-0.001g
Agar	-15g
Distilled water	-1000mL

Alkaline Peptone Water (pH-8.8)

Peptone	-5g
Sodium chloride	-5g
Distilled water	-100mL

Amies Transport medium (pH-7.2)

Charcoal neutral	-10g
Sodium chloride	-3g
Sodium hydrogen	
Phosphate	-1.15g
KH_2PO_4	-0.2g
Potassium chloride	-0.2g
Sodium thioglycollate	-1g
Calcium chloride	-0.1g
Magnesium chloride	-0.1g
Agar	-4g
Distilled water	-1000mL

Anaerobic CNA Agar

Casein enzymatic hydrolysate	-12g
Peptic digest of animal tissue	-5g
Yeast extract	-3g
Beef extract	-3g
Corn starch	-1g
Dextrose	-1g
Sodium chloride	-5g
Dithiothreitol (DTE)	-0.10g
L-cysteine hydrochloride	-0.50g
Vitamin K1	-0.01g
Hemin	-0.01g

Colistin	-0.01g
Nalidixic acid	-0.01g
Agar	-13.50g
Distilled water	-1000mL

Ashby medium (pH-7)

Mannitol	-20g
Dipotassium hydrogen phosphate	-0.2g
Magnesium sulphate	-0.2g
Sodium chloride	-0.2g
Dipotassium sulphate	-0.1g
Calcium carbonate	-5g
Agar agar	-20g
Distilled water	-1000mL

Azatobacter Agar (Mannitol –pH-8.3)

Dipotassium phosphate	-1g
Magnesium sulphate	-0.20g
Sodium chloride	-0.20g
Ferrous sulphate	-trace
Soil extract	-5g
Mannitol	-20g
Agar	-15g
Distilled water	-1000mL

Azide Dextrose Broth (pH – 7.2)

Peptone special	-15g
Beef extract	-4.50g
Dextrose	-7.50g
Sodium chloride	-7.50g
Sodium azide	-0.20g
Distilled water	-1000mL

Azospirillum medium

Maleic acid	-5g
Dipotassium posphate	-0.5g
Ferrous sulphate	-0.5g
Magnesium sulphate	-0.2g
Manganous sulphate	-0.01g
Sodium chloride	-0.1g
Bromothymol blue	-0.002g
Sodium molybdate	-0.002g
Calcium chloride	-0.02g
Agar agar	-1.75g
Distilled water	-1000mL
Potassium hydroxide	-4g

Add Potassium hydroxide separately.

Bacillus Cereus Agar (pH - 7.2 ± 0.2)

Peptic digest of animal tissue	-1g
Mannitol	-10g
Sodium chloride	-2g
Magnesium sulphate	-0.1g
Disodium phosphate	-2.5g
Monosodium phosphate	-0.25g
Sodium pyruvate	-10g
Bromothymol blue	-0.12g
Agar	-15g
Polymyxin B	-1vial
Egg yolk emulsion	-25mL
Distilled water	-1000mL

Bile Esculin Agar Medium (pH 7)

Peptone	-5g
Beef extract	-3g
Oxgall (bile)	-40g
Esculin	-1g
Ferric citrate	-0.5g
Agar	-15g
Distilled water	-1000 mL

Bismuth Sulfite Agar (pH - 7.7 ± 0.2)

Peptic digest of animal tissue	-10 g
Beef extract	- 5 g
Dextrose	- 5 g
Disodium phosphate	- 4 g
Ferrous Sulfite	- 0.3g
Bismuth Sulfite agar	- 8 g
Brilliant green	-0.025g
Agar	-20 g
Distilled water	-1000mL

Blood Agar (pH 7.2 - 7.6)

Peptone	-5g
Yeast extract	-2g
Sodium chloride	-5g
Agar	-15g
Distilled water	-1000mL
Blood	-50mL

Bordet Gengou Agar Base

Potato, Infusion	-125 g
Sodium Chloride	-5.5 g
Agar	-20.0 g

Suspend ingredients in 1 L of purified water containing 10 g of glycerol.

BPL Agar for Streptococci (pH 6.8 ± 0.2)

Meat peptone	-7g

Sodium chloride	-5g
Lactose	-15g
Phenol red	-0.04g
Brillient green	-0.005g
Agar	-13g
Distilled water	-1000 mL

Brain-Heart Infusion Agar (pH-7.4)

Calf brains, infusion	- 200.0 g
Beef hearts, infusion from	-250.0 g
Proteose peptone	-10.0 g
Dextrose	-2.0 g
Sodium chloride	-5.0 g
Disodium phosphate	- 2.5 g
Agar	-15.0 g
Distilled water	-1000 mL

Brewer's Anaerobic Agar (pH 7.2)

Bacto tryptone	- 5.0 g
Proteose peptone	-10.0 g
Bacto yeast extract.	- 5.0 g
Bacto dextrose	-10.0 g
Sodium chloride	-5.0 g
Agar	-20 g
Sodium thioglycollate	-2 g
Sodium formaldehyde sulfoxylate	-1 g
Resazurin	-0.002 g
Distilled water	-1000 mL

Brilliant Green Bile Lactose (2%) Broth

Peptone	-10.0 g
Oxgall	-20.0 g
Lactose	-10.0 g
Brilliant green	-0.0133 g
Distilled water	-1000 mL

CLED Agar

Pancreatic Digest of Gelatin	-4.0 g
Pancreatic Digest of Casein	-4.0 g
Beef Extract	-3.0 g
Lactose	-10.0 g
L-Cystine	-128.0 mG
Bromthymol Blue	-0.02 g
Agar	-15.0 g
Distilled water	-1000 mL

Cellulose degradation Media

Sodium nitrate	-2g
K_2HPO_4	-1g
$MgSo_4$	-0.5g
KCL	-0.5g

Carboxy methyl cellulose	-5g
Peptone	-2g
Agar	-20g
Distilled water	-1000mL

Cetrimide Agar

Peptone	–20g
Potassium sulphate	-10g
Magnesium chloride	-1.4g
Cetyl methylammonium	
Bromide	-0.3g
Agar	–15g
Distilled water	-1000mL
pH	-7-7.4

Chocolate Agar

Prepare blood agar base and sterilize. Then add defibrinated blood, heat the medium in a 80°C water bath until it becomes brown in colour. This takes about 10-15 minutes.

Chu's No. 11 Medium, Modified (pH 7.5 ± 0.2)

$NaNO_3$	-1.5g
$MgSO_4 \cdot 7H_2O$	-0.08g
$Na_2SiO_3 \cdot 9H_2O$	-0.06g
$CaCl_2 \cdot 2H_2O$.	-0.04g
$K_2HPO_4 \cdot 3H_2O$	-0.04g
Na_2CO_3	-0.02g
Citric acid	-6.0mG
Ferric ammonium citrate	-6.0mG
EDTA	-1.0mG
Seawater	-999.0mL
Trace metal solution A5 with cobalt 1.0mL	

Trace Metal Solution A5 with Cobalt:

H_3BO_3.	- 2.86g
$MnCl_2 \cdot 4H_2O$	-1.81g
$Na_2MoO_4 \cdot 2H_2O$	-0.39g
$ZnSO_4 \cdot 7H_2O$	-0.222g
$CuSO_4 \cdot H_2O$	-0.079g
$Co(NO_3)_2 \cdot 6H_2O$	-0.049g

Preparation of Trace Metal Solution A5 with Cobalt:
Add components to distilled/deionized water and bring volume to 1.0L. Mix thoroughly.

Preparation of Medium: Add components to seawater and bring volume to 1.0L. Mix thoroughly. Gently heat and bring to boiling. Distribute into tubes or flasks. Autoclave for 15 min at 15 psi pressure–121°C.

CIN Agar Base (Yersinia Selective Agar Base)

Pancreatic Digest of Gelatin	-10.0 g
Peptic Digest of Animal Tissue	-5.0 g
Beef Extract.	-5.0 g
Yeast Extract	-2.0 g
Mannitol	-20.0 g
Sodium Pyruvate	-2.0 g
Sodium Chloride	-1.0 g
Magnesium Sulfate	-1.0 mG
Sodium Deoxycholate	-0.5 g
Irgasan	-4.0 mG
Agar	-12.0 g
Crystal Violet	-1.0 mG
Neutral Red	- 0.03 g

Yersinia Antimicrobial Supplement CN
Formula Per 10 mL

Cefsulodin	-4.0 mG
Novobiocin	-2.5 mG

Crystal Violet Blood Agar

Add 1mL of 0.02% aqueous solution of crystal violet to every 100mL of sterile blood agar.

Cooked Meat Medium

Beef Heart	-98.0 g
Proteose Peptone	-20.0 g
Dextrose	-2.0 g
Sodium Chloride	-5.0 g
Distilled water	-1000 mL

Czapek Dox Agar

Sodium nitrate	-3g
Dipotassium hydrogen phosphate	-1g
Magnesium sulphate	-0.5g
Potassium chloride	-0.5g
Ferrous sulphate	-0.01g
Sucrose	-30g
Agar agar	-15g
Distilled water	-1000mL

Czapek Mineral salt agar medium

Sodium nitrate	- 2g
K_2HPO_4	-1g
$MgSO_4$	-0.5g
KCL	-0.5g
Carboxymethyl celluloe (CMC)	-5g
Peptone	-2g
Agar	-20g

Dissolve agar in 400 mL of water; Dissolve $MgSO_4$, KCl and peptone, $NaNo_3$ in 200 mL of water; Dissolve K_2HPO_4 in 100 mL of water; Dissolve CMC in 200 mL of water with heat and mix; Mix all the solution and made upto 1000 mL

Deoxyribonuclease (DNase Test) Agar (pH 7.3)

Deoxyribonucleic acid	-2.0 g
Phytone peptone	-5.0 g
Sodium chloride	-5.0 g
Trypticase	-15.0 g
Agar	-15.0 g
Distilled water	-1,000.0 mL

Dorset Egg Medium (pH 7.2 - 7.4)

Nutrient broth	-20mL
Whole fresh egg	-80mL

Endo Agar (pH 7.5)

Peptone	-10.0 g
Lactose	-10.0 g
Dipotassium phosphate	-3.5 g
Sodium sulfite	-2.5 g
Basic fuchsin	-0.4 g
Agar	-15.0 g
Distilled water	-1000 mL

Eosin-Methylene Blue (EMB) Agar (pH 7.2)

Peptone	-10.0 g
Lactose	-5.0 g
Sucrose	-5.0 g
Dipotassium phosphate	-2.0 g
Agar	-13.5 g
Eosin Y	-0.4 g
Methylene blue	-0.06 g
Distilled water	-1000 mL

Eugon Agar (pH 7.0)

Tryptose	-15.0 g
Soytone	-5.0 g
Dextrose	-5.0 g
L-cystine	-0.2 g
Sodium chloride	-4.0 g
Sodium sulfite.	-0.2 g
Agar	-15.0 g
Distilled water	-1000 mL

Fermentation medium (pH 7)

Glucose/sucrose/fructose	-20%
Yeast extract	-10g
Potassium di hydrogen phosphate	-2g
Malt extract	-5g

Distilled water	-1000mL

Gram Negative Broth (pH 7 ± 0.2)

Tryptose	- 20g
Dextrose	- 1g
Mannitol	- 2g
Sodium citrate	- 5g
Sodium deoxycholate	- 0.5g
Dipotassium phosphate	- 4g
Monopotassium phosphate	- 1.5g
Sodium chloride	- 5g
Distilled water	-1000mL

Growth media (pH 7) for alcohol formentation

Glucose	-20g
Yeast extract	-10g
Potassium di hydrogen phosphate	-2g
Magnesium sulphate	-5g
Distilled water	-1000mL

Hektoen enteric agar (pH 7.5 ± 0.2)

Protease peptone	-12g
Yeast extract	- 3g
Lactose	-12g
Sucrose	-12g
Salicin	- 2g
Bile salt mixture	- 9g
Sodium Chloride	- 5g
Sodium thiosulphate	- 5g
Ferric ammonium citrate	-1.5g
Acid fuschin	- 0.1g
Agar	- 15g
Distilled water	-1000mL
Bromothymol blue	- 0.065

Jensens medium

Sucrose	-20g
Dipotassium posphate	-1g
Ferrous sulphate	-0.1g
Magnesium sulphate	-0.2g
Sodium chloride	-0.5g
Sodium molybdate	-0.005g
Casein carbonate	-2g
Agar	-15g
Distilled water	-1000mL

KF Streptococcus Agar (pH 7.2)

Protease Peptone	-3 10.0 g
Yeast extract	-10.0 g
Sodium chloride	-5.0 g

Sodium glycerophosphate	-10.0 g
Maltose	-20.0 g
Lactose	-1.0 g
Sodium azide	-0.4 g
Bromocresol purple	-0.015 g
Agar	-20.0 g
Distilled water	-1,000.0 mL

Kenknight and Mundiers Medium

Dextrose	-1g
KH_2PO_4	-0.1g
Sodium nitrate	-0.1g
Potassium chloride	-0.1g
Magnecium sulphate	-0.1g
Distilled water	-1000mL

Kanamycin Blood Agar

Prepare 1.5g kanamycin in 100mL of water. Add 1mL of this solution to every 100mL of blood agar.

Lauryl Tryptose Broth (pH 6.8)

Tryptose	-20.0 g
Lactose	-5.0 g
Potassium phosphate, dibasic	-2.75 g
Potassium phosphate, monobasic	-2.75 g
Sodium chloride	-5.0 g
Sodium lauryl sulfate	-0.1 g
Distilled water	-1000 mL

Levinthols medium (pH-7.8)

Protease peptone no. 3	– 20g
NaCl	–6g
KNO_3	-1g

Tris(hydroxymethyl)aminomethane-0.02 M.

The medium was boiled, filtered, and add 0.01% $Na_2S_2O_4$ added before autoclaving. Just before use, filter sterilized DPN (1g/mL) is added. Glucose (0.5%, w/v, autoclaved separately) is added where indicated. Hemin stock solution is prepared by adding 2.5 mG of hemin to 1 mL of 0.2 M KOH in 47.5% ethanol, and diluting to 5 mL with sterile water.

Loeffler Serum Medium (pH 7.4)

Tryptose	-10g
Dextrose	–5g
Sodium chloride	–5g
Horse serum	–30mL
Distilled water	-1000mL

Löwenstein–Jensen Medium

Asparagine	-3.6 g
Monopotassium phosphate	-2.4 g
Magnesium sulfate	-0.24 g
Magnesium citrate	-0.6 g
Potato flour	- 30.0 g
Malachite green	- 0.4 g
Distilled water	- 600.0 mL

Mannitol Salt Agar (pH 7.4)

Beef extract	-1.0 g
Peptone	-10.0 g
Sodium chloride	-75.0 g
D–Mannitol.	-10.0 g
Agar	-15.0 g
Phenol red	-0.025 g
Distilled water	-1000 mL

M-Endo Broth (pH 7.5)

Yeast extract.	-6.0 g
Thiotone peptone	-20.0 g
Lactose.	-25.0 g
Dipotassium phosphate	- 7.0 g
Sodium sulfite	-2.5 g
Basic fuchsin	-1.0 g
Distilled water	-1000 mL

Note: Heat until boiling but do not autoclave.

M-FC Broth (pH 7.4)

Biosate peptone or tryptose	-10.0 g
Polypeptone peptone or protease peptone-	5.0 g
Yeast extract	-3.0 g
Sodium chloride	-5.0 g
Lactose	-12.5 g
Bile salts	-1.5 g
Aniline blue.	-0.1 g
Distilled water	-1000 mL

Note: Add 10 mL of rosolic acid (1% in 0.2 N sodium hydroxide). Heat to boiling with gentle agitation. Do not autoclave.

Mac Conkey agar (pH 7.1)

Bacto peptone	-17g
Peptone	-3g
Lactose	-10g
Bile salt mixture	-1.5g
Sodium chloride	-5g
Agar	-13.5g
Neutral red	-0.03g

Crystal Violet — -0.001g

Distilled water — -1000mL

Modified Tinsdale Medium

Protease peptone — -2g

Sodium chloride — -0.5g

Serum — -10mL

Sodium hydroxide0.1mol/l — -6mL

L-Cystine 4g/l — -6mL

Potassium tellurite-10g/l — -3mL

Sodium thiosulphate 25g/l — -1.7mL

Agar agar — –2g

Make up to 100mL with Distilled water

Mueller Hinton Agar (pH 7.3 $\pm$ 0.2)

Beef infusion — -300g

Casein acid hydrolysate — -17g

Starch — -1.5g

Agar — -17g

Distilled water — -1000mL

Neomycin Blood Agar

Prepare stock solution

of neomycin by dissolving 0.5 g neomycin sulphate in 5mL sterile water. From this prepare a working solution by mixing 2 mL of stock solution with 6mL of sterile water. Add 1mL of working solution to 250mL of blood agar.

New York City agar medium

10% Lysed horse blood — - 100mL

Yeast extract — - 30g

Vancomycin — -2mG/l

Colistin — -7.5mG/l

Amphotericin — -1mG/l

Trimethoprim — -3mG/l

Nutrient Agar (pH 7.0)

Peptone — -5.0 g

Beef extract — -3.0 g

Sodium Chloride — -5.0g

Agar agar — -15g

Distilled water — -1000 mL

Nutrient Broth (pH 7.0)

Peptone — -5.0 g

Beef extract — -3.0 g

Sodium Chloride — -5.0g

Distilled water — -1,000.0 mL

Plate Count Agar (Standard Methods Agar, Tryptone Glucose Yeast Agar; pH 7.0)

Tryptone — -5.0 g

Yeast extract — -2.5 g

Dextrose (glucose) — -1.0 g

Agar. — -15.0 g

Distilled water — -1000 mL

Presence-Absence Broth (P-A Broth)

Pancreatic digest of casein . — -10.0 g

Lactose — -7.5 g

Pancreatic digest of gelatin — -5.0 g

Beef extract — -3.0 g

Sodium chloride — -2.5 g

K_2HPO_4 — -1.375 g

KH_2PO_4. — -1.375 g

Sodium lauryl sulfate. — -0.05 g

Bromcresol purple. — -8.5 mG

Distilled water — -1000mL

Potato Dextrose Agar (pH 5.6)

Potatoes, infusion from — -200.0 g

Dextrose — -20.0 g

Agar — -15.0 g

Distilled water

Pringsheims broth (Pringsheims, 1964)

KNO_3 — -0.02%

$MgSO_4 7H_2O$ — - 0.001%

$(NH_4)_2HPO_4$ — -0.002%

$Cacl_2 6H_2O$ — -0.0005%

$FeCl_2$ — - 0.00005%

Rose Bengal Chloromphenicol Agar (pH 7.2)

Mycological peptone — -5g

Dextrose — -10g

Monopotassium phosphate — -1g

Magnesium sulphate — -0.5g

Rose bengal — -0.05

Chloramphenicol — -0.1g

Agar — -15g

Distilled water — -1000mL

Sabouraud (Dextrose) Agar (pH 5.6)

Peptone — -10.0 g

Dextrose — -40.0 g

Agar. — -15.0 g

Distilled water — -1000mL

Salmonella –Shigella Agar (pH 7 $\pm$ 0.2)

Peptic digest of animal tissue — -5g

Protease peptone — -5g

Beef extract — -5g

Lactose — -10g

Bile salt mixture — -8.5g

Sodium citrate — -10g

Sodium thiosulphate — -8.5g

Ferric citrate — -1g

Brilliant green — -0.00033

Neutral red — -0.025

Agar — -15g

Distilled water — -1000mL

Soft Agar (pH 7.0)

Nutrient broth — -13.g

Agar — -0.75g

Starch casein nitrate agar (pH 7)

Soluble starch — -10g

Casein	-0.3g
Potassium nitrate	-2g
Sodium chloride	-2g
K_2HPO_4	-2g
Magnecium sulphate	-0.05g
Calcium carbonate	-0.02g
Ferrous sulphate	-0.01g
Agar	-15g
Distilled water	-1000mL

TCBS Agar

Yeast Extract	-5.0 g
Protease Peptone No. 3	-10.0 g
Sodium Citrate	-10.0 g
Sodium Thiosulfate	-10.0 g
Oxgall	-8.0 g
Saccharose	-20.0 g
Sodium Chloride	-10.0 g
Ferric Ammonium Citrate	-1.0 g
Bromthymol Blue	-0.04 g
Thymol Blue	-0.04 g
Agar	-15.0 g
Distilled water	-1000 mL

Thayer-Martin Modified Medium (pH 7.0)

Bacto GC medium base	-36.0 g
Haemoglobin	-10.0 g
Bacto supplement B or VX	-10.0 mL
Bacto antimicrobic vial CNVT	-10.0 mL
Distilled water	-1000mL

Thioglycollate Broth (pH 7.1)

Peptone	-15.0 g
Yeast extract	-5.0 g
Dextrose	-5.0 g
L-cystine	- 0.75 g
Thioglycollic acid	- 0.5 g
Agar	- 0.75 g
Sodium chloride	-2.5 g
Resazurin	-0.001 g
Distilled water	-1000mL

Todd-Hewitt Broth (pH 7.8)

Beef heart, infusion	-500.0 g
Neopeptone	-20.0 g
Dextrose	-2.0 g
Sodium chloride	-2.0 g
Disodium phosphate	-0.4 g
Sodium carbonate	-2.5 g
Distilled water	-1000mL

Trypticase (Tryptic) Soy Agar (pH 7.3)

Trypticase (tryptone)	-15.0 g
Phytone (soytone)	-5.0 g
Sodium chloride	-5.0 g
Agar	-15.0 g
Distilled water	-1,000.0 mL

V-8 Juice Agar

Agar	-15.0g
CaCO	-2.0g
V-8 canned vegetable juice	-200mL

Violet Red Bile Agar (pH 7.4)

Yeast extract	- 3.0 g
Peptone	-7.0 g
Bile salts no. 3	-1.5 g
Lactose	-10.0 g
Sodium chloride	-5.0 g
Agar	-15.0 g
Neutral red	-0.03 g
Crystal violet	-0.002 g
Distilled water	-1000mL

Vogel-Johnson Agar (pH 7.2)

Tryptone	-10.0 g
Yeast extract	-5.0 g
Mannitol	-10.0 g
Dipotassium phosphate	-5.0 g
Lithium chloride	-5.0 g
Glycine	-10.0 g
Agar	-15.0 g
Phenol red	-0.025 g
Distilled water	-1000mL

Xylose Lysine Decarboxylase (pH 7.4+0.2)

Yeast extract	- 3g
L – lysine	- 5g
Lactose	- 7.5g
Sucrose	- 7.5g
Xylose	- 3.5g
Sodium chloride	- 5g
Sodium deoxycholate	- 2.5 g
Sodium thiosulphate	- 6.8g
Ferric Ammonium citrate	- 0.8g
Phenol red	- 0.08g
Distilled water	- 1000mL

YM Agar

Yeast extract	-3.0 g
Malt extract	-3.0 g
Peptone	-5.0 g
Dextrose	-10.0 g
Agar.	-20.0 g
Distilled water	-1000mL

Yeast extract mannitol agar (pH 6.8+0.2)

Yeast extract	-1g
Calcium carbonate	-1g
Sodium chloride	-0.1g
Magnesium sulphate	-0.2g
Mannitol	-10g
Distilled water	-1000mL
Agar	-15g
Congo red	-2.5 mL
(1% solution)	

X. Appendix B - Staining Reagents

Gram's staining reagent
Crystal violet
Solution A

Crystal violet	-2g
Ethyl alcohol	-20 mL

Solution B

Ammonium oxalate	-0.8g
Distilled water	-80 mL

Solution A is mixed with Solution B

Gram's iodine

Iodine	-1g
Potassium iodide	-2g
Distilled water	-300 mL

Decolourizer

Ethanol (95 %)	-100mL

Safranine

Safranine	-0.5g
Distilled water	-100 mL

Simple staining
Methylene blue

Methylene blue	-0.5g
20 %KOH	-0.1mL
Ethanol	-30mL

Carbol fuschin

Basic fuschin	-10g
Ethanol	-100mL
Phenol	-50g

make upto one liter using Distilled water

Negative staining
Nigrosin

Nigrosin	-0.5 g
Distilled water	-100mL

Indian ink
Capsule Stainng
Solution A

10% carbolfuchsin in alcohol	-5mL
Distilled water	-95mL

Solution B
20% copper sulphate solution

Spore staining
Malachite green

Malachite green	-5g
Distilled water	-100mL

Safranine

Safranin	-0.5g
Distilled water	-100mL

Alberts staining
Toludine blue- malachite green stain

Toludine blue	-0.15g
Malachite green	-0.20g
Glacial acetic acid	-1mL
Ethanol	-2mL
Distilled water	-100mL

Albert's iodine

Potassium iodide	-1.5g
Iodine	-1g
Distilled water	-150mL

Flagella staining
Mordant solution

Saturated aqueous solution of picric acid	-5mL
Distilled water	-15mL
Tannic acid	-1g
Ferrous sulphate	-1.5g

Silver nitrate reagent

Dissolve 0.5g of silver nitrate in 25mL of distilled water. Slowly add ammonium hydroxide drop by drop with a pipette until the solution turns cloudy. Continue to add ammonium hydroxide until the solution turns nearly clear. If too much of ammonium hydroxide is added, the bacterium will not stain properly.

Fontana staining
Fixative

Acetic acid	-1mL
Formalin	-2mL
Distilled water	-100mL

Mordant

Phenol	-1g
Tannic acid	-5g
Distilled water	-100mL

Ammoniacal silver nitrate solution

Sol A : Silver nitrate 0.5g in 100mL distilled water

Sol B : 5mL of concentrated ammonia in 45mL of distilled water

To 90 mL of solution A 35mL of solution B is mixed dropwise till the white precipitate formed redissolves to give a faint opalescent solution

Wayson's stain

Basic fuschin	-0.20g
Methylene blue	-075g
Ethanol 95%	-20mL
Phenol 50g/1	-200mL

Kinyoun Acid-Fast Stain

Kinyoun Carbolfuchsin

Basic fuchsin	-4 g
95% alcohol.	-20 mL
Phenol crystals	-8 g
Distilled water	-100 mL

Acid-alcohol

Concentrated hydrochloric acid	-3 mL
95% ethyl alcohol.	-97 mL

Methylene Blue Counterstain

Methylene blue	-0.3 g
Distilled water.	-100 mL

Ziehl-Neelsen Acid-Fast Stain

Solution A: Dissolve 0.3 g of basic fuchsin (90% dye content) in 10 mL of 95% ethyl alcohol.
Solution B: Dissolve 5 g of phenol in 95 mL of distilled water.

Mix solutions A and B. Note: Add either 1 drop of Tergitol No. 4 per 30 mL of carbolfuchsin or 2

drops of Triton X-100 per 100 mL of stain for use in the heatless method. Tergitol No. 4 and Triton X act as detergents, emulsifiers, and wetting agents.

Acid-alcohol, 3%

Concentrated hydrochloric acid	-3 mL
95% alcohol	-97 mL

Methylene Blue

Lacto phenol Cotton blue stain

Phenol crystal	-20 g
Lactic acid	-20 mL
Glycerol	-40 mL
Distilled water	-20 mL

Dissolve the ingredients by heating the container in a hot water bath. Add 0.05 g cotton blue.

Giemsa stain composition

Giemsa stain	-0.75 g
Glycerol	-25mL
Methanol	-75mL

Giemsa and glycerol are mixed and grind to make paste using mortar and pestle. To this add methanol and stir. This mixture is poured in a dark bottle. Incubate it at 37°C for 24 hours. Dilute 1:10 in buffered water when it is used for staining.

X. Appendix C - Biochemical Test Media and Reagents

Indole Test

Peptone Water

Peptone	-1g
Sodium chloride	-0.5g
Distilled water	-100 mL
pH	-7.4

Kovac's Indole Reagent

Para dimethyl amino benzoldehyde	-2g
Iso amyl alcohol	-30 mL
Concentrated Hcl	-10 mL

Methyl Red Test

MR-VP broth

Peptone	-0.5g
Glucose	-0.5g
Dipotassium hydrogen phosphate	-0.5g
Distilled water	-100 mL
pH	-7.4 -7.6

Methyl Red Solution

Methyl red	-0.05g
Ethanol	-28 mL
Distilled water	-22 mL

Voges Proskauver Test

MR-VP broth

Peptone	-0.5g
Glucose	-0.5g
Dipotassium hydrogen phosphate	-0.5g
Distilled water	-100 mL
pH	-7.4 -7.6

α–Napthol

α napthol	-5g
Ethyl alcohol	-100mL

Potassium Hydroxide

Potassium hydroxide	-40g
Distilled water	-100mL

Citrate Utilization Test

Simmons Citrate Agar

Magnesium sulphate	-0.2g
Ammonium dihydrogen phosphate	-1g
Dipotassium phosphate	-1g
Sodium citrate	-2g
Sodium chloride	-5g
Bromothymol blue	-0.08g
Agar agar	-15g

Distilled water	-1000 mL
pH	-6.8 –7

Catalase Test

3 % Hydrogen peroxide

Triple Sugar Iron Test

Triple Sugar Iron Agar

Peptic digest of animal tissue	-10g
Casein enzyme hydrolysate	-10g
Yeast extract	-3g
Beef extract	-3g
Lactose	-10g
Saccharose	-10g
Dextrose	-1g
Ferrous sulphate	-0.2
Sodium chloride	-5g
Sodium thiosulphate	-0.3g
Phenol red	-0.024g
Agar agar	-15g
Distilled water	-1000 mL
pH	-7.4

Nitrate reduction test

Nitrate Broth

Peptone	-5g
Beef extract	-3g
Potassium nitrate	-1g
Distilled water	-1000 mL
pH	-6.8 –7.2

Sulphanilic Acid

Sulphanilic acid	-0.16g
Glacial acetic acid	-5.7 mL
Distilled water	-14.3 mL

Alpha Napthalamine Reagent

Alpha napthalamine	-0.1g
Glacial acetic acid	-5.7 mL
Distilled water	-14.3 mL

Zinc Powder

Urease Test

Urea

Urea Agar Base

Peptic digest of animal tissue	-1g
Dextrose	-1g
Sodium chloride	-5g
Mono potassium phosphate	-2g
Urea	-20g

Phenol red	-0.012
Distilled water	-1000 mL
pH	-6.8 -7

Oxidative fermentation test

OF Basal Medium

Casein	-2g
Sodium chloride	-5g
Dipotassium phosphate	-0.3g
Bromothymol blue	-0.08g
Agar agar	-15g
Distilled water	-1000 mL
pH	-6.8 -7

Sterile liquid paraffin, Glucose, Maltose
Sucrose, Lactose, Xylose, Mannose , Trehalose

Carbohydrate Fermentation Test

Carbohydrate Fermentation Medium

Peptone	–10g
Sodium chloride	-5g
**D.glucose	-5g
Bromo cresolpurple	-0.03g
Agar agar	-13g
Distilled water	-1000mL
pH	–7.1

*carbohydrates are sterilized through filtration.
**it is replased by other sugars.

Oxidase Test

Oxidase Reagent

Tetra methyl P-Phenylene	
diamine hydrochloride	-0.1g
Distilled water	-10 mL

Aminoacid Deaminase Test

Phenylalanine Deaminase Medium

Yeast extract	-3g
Aminoacid	-2g
Sodium chloride	-5g
Disodium hydrogen phosphate	-1g
Agar agar	-15g
Distilled water	-1000 mL
pH	-6.8 -7.2
phenylalanine	-1%

*Should not use meat extract or protein. Because of their varying natural content of phenylalanine. Yeast extract serves as the carbon and nitrogen source.

Ferric Chloride Reagent

Ferric chloride	-5g
Con HCL	-25mL

Distilled water	-10 mL

Decarboxylase Test

Moeller Decarboxylase Medium

Peptone	-5g
Meat extract	-5g
Glucose	-0.5g
Pyridoxol	-5mG
Bromocresol	
purple (1 in 500 mL)	-5 mL
Cresol red (1 in 500 mL)	-2.5 mL
Distilled water	-1000 mL
pH	-6

L-Lysine, L-Ornithine, L-Argnine
Amino acids are added in 1% concentration

Litmus Milk Reduction Test

Skimmed milk powder	-2g
Distilled water	-20mL
Litmus	–trace amount
pH	-6.8

Tween 80 Phosphate Buffered Substrate Medium

Phosphate buffer pH 7	-40mL
Tween 80	-0.2mL
Neutral red(1g/l)	-0.8mL
pH	-6.8-7.2.

Starch Hydrolysis

Starch Agar

Peptone	-5g
Beef extract	-3g
Soluble starch	-2g
Agar agar	-15g
Distilled water	-1000mL
pH	–7

Iodine

Potassium iodide	-20g
Iodine	–10g
Distilled water	-1000mL

Gelatin Hydrolysis

Nutrient Gelatin

Peptone	-5g
Beef extract	-3g
Gelatin	-0.4%
Agar agar	-15
Distilled water	-1000mL
pH	-6.8-7.2

Gelatin Precipitin Reagent

Con HCL	-20mL

Distilled water	-80mL
Mercuric chloride	-15g

Casein Hydrolysis

Skim Agar Medium

Skim milk powder	-100g
Peptone	-5g
Agar agar	-20g
Distilled water	-1000mL
pH	-7.2

Esculin Hydrolysis

Brain heart infusion agar	-40g
Esculin	–1g
Ferric chloride	-0.5g
Distilled water	-1000mL
pH	–6.8-7.2

Melanoate Utilization medium

Yeast extract	-1g
Ammonium sulphate	-2g
Dipotassium hydrogen phosphate	-0.6g
Potassium di hydrogen phosphate	-0.4g
Sodium chloride	-2g
Sodium malonate	-3g
Bromo thymol blue	-0.025g
Distilled water	-1000mL
PH	-7.4

Salt Tolerance Test Medium

6.5% sodium chloride broth

Heart infusion broth	-25g

Sodium chloride	-60g
*Indicator	-1mL

(bromocresol purple in 100mL of 95% ethanol)

Glucose	-1g
Distilled water	-1000mL

*indicator maybe omitted

Chromic acid Preparation

33.768 g of potassium dichromate is dissolved in 350-mL distilled water in standard measuring flask and the flask is kept in an ice bath and slowly added 350mLof concentrated sulfuric acid. The content is made upto 1000mL with distilled water.

O-nitrophenyl-D-Galactoside (ONPG)

0.1M sodium phosphate buffer	-50.0 mL
ONPG (0.0008M)	-12.5 mG

Physiological Saline

Dissolve 9 g of sodium chloride in 1 liter of distilled water

Normal Saline (Buffered)

Sodium chloride (0.85%; 8.5 g in 1 liter of distilled water) pH 7.2

Anthrone reagent

Ref experiment	148 - Page 390

DNS reagent

Refer experiment	149 - Page 391-392

X. Appendix – D - Spotters

1. Antony Van Leeuwenhoek (1632 – 1723)

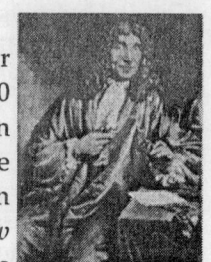

Antony Van Leeuwenhoek is considered as the father **of Microbiology.** He was an amateur lens grinder lived in Delft, Holland from 1632 – 1723. During his lifetime he made more than 250 microscopes consisting of home-ground lenses mounted in brass and silver. It had the magnification power of about 200 – 300 times. His microscopes resembled the compound microscope of today. He communicated his findings to the Royal Society of London and the observations were published in 1677 in the proceedings of the Royal Society as a series of letter. In 1680, he was elected as a *Fellow of the society*. He described his observations as "very little animalcules" which we now recognize as free-living protozoa. He was a qualified surveyor and the town's official wine taster.

He was not an educationalist but had keen mind.

2. Louis Pasteur (1822 – 1895)

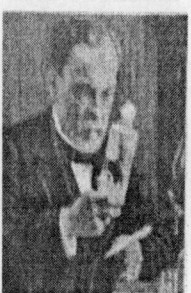

He is the father of **fermentation technology.** He conducted Swan Neck flask experiment to disprove the spontaneous generation theory (1859). He took up the problem of wine industry and introduced Pasteurization (1860). In 1865 he demonstrated that the microscopic germs are responsible for silkworm disease. In 1881- Introduced vaccination against anthrax. In 1885, Pasteur announced to the French Academy of Sciences that he had developed a vaccine for preventing a dread disease, rabies. The term vaccine was given by Pasteur to honour **Edward Jenner.** Pasteur introduced the concept of **pasteurization** in which the microorganisms can be removed without affecting the flavor and taste of grape juice. He discovered causative agent of alcohol fermentation. Life without air, Animals cannot live in the absence of microorganisms were the statements given by him.

3. Robert Koch (1843 – 1910)

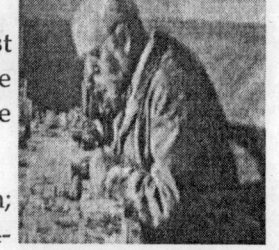

He is the father of Medical Microbiology. He was a German physician. The first demonstration of the role of bacteria in causing disease came from the study of Anthrax by the German physician Robert Koch. In 1876, proposed germ theory of diseases. He established the relationship between *Bacillus anthracis* and anthrax, and published his findings in 1876.

1876- Demonstrated the causative nature of anthrax ; 1881-cultured bacteria on Gelatin; 1881- Used agar to demonstrate pure culture technique; 1882-discovered *tubercle bacilli*; 1884-published postulates; 1883-discovered cholera bacilli

Koch Postulates

The microbes must be present in every case of disease.
The suspected microorganism must be isolated and grown in a pure culture.
The same disease must results when the isolated microbe is inoculated in to the healthy host.
The same organism must be isolated again from the infected host.

4. Joseph Lister (1827 – 1912)

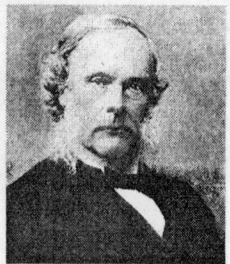

He was a pioneer of **antiseptic surgery.** Joseph Lister developed antiseptic method for preventing infection using carbolic acid (phenol) to treat wounds in 1867. He developed "serial dilution technique" in liquid media. He identified the bacteria, *Bacterium lactis* from milk sample. Lister used bandages soaked in carbolic acid to dress wounds caused by compound fractures.

His discovery of chemicals which prevent infections greatly increased survival rates. His antiseptics principles guide today's modern surgical procedures.

5. Martinus W. Beijerinck (1851 – 1931)

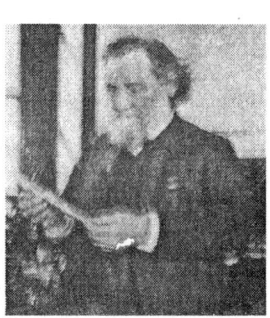

Beijerinck isolated root nodule causing bacteria. After extensive studies he published the results of tobacco mosaic disease in 1898 and 1900. He proposed that the TMV disease is caused by an entity that is entirely different from bacteria, a filterable virus. Beijerinck observed that the virus would multiply only in living plant cells. Beijerinck showed that the viruses could survive for long periods in a dried state. He made fundamental contributions to microbial ecology. He isolated the aerobic nitrogen fixing bacterium *Azatobacter* and sulfate reducing bacterium. He developed enrichment culture technique and proposed the uses of selective media along with winogradsky.

6. Edward Jenner (1749 – 1823)

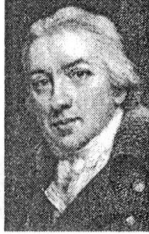

He is the **Father of Immunization.** The significance of immunization against smallpox was come to the light by the work of Edward Jenner. He observed that individual who attended cows with cowpox, a disease of cattle caused by a similar virus, rarely infected by small pox. In May 14, 1796, Jenner extracted the contents of a pustule from the arm of cowpox infected milkmaid, and injected into another person. As he expected, no symptoms were developed when the person was inoculated with smallpox virus. In 1798 Jenner reported to the Royal Society of London on the value of vaccination with cowpox as a means of protecting against smallpox, which is the basis for the immunological prevention of disease.

7. Elie Metchnikoff (1845 – 1916)

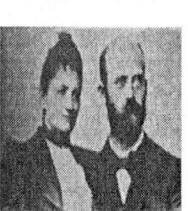

He found out the concept of **Phagocytosis.** His work on antitoxin, provided evidence that, immunity could result from soluble substances in the blood, now known as antibodies. By his work it was clear that blood cells are also important in immunity. He discovered that some blood leukocytes could engulf disease causing bacteria. He called these cells as phagocytes, which is an important process in immunology.

8. Fannie Eilshemius and Walther Hesse (1850 – 1934)

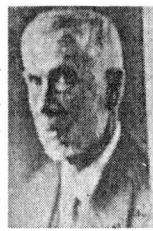

A better alternate for gelatin was provided by Fannie Eilshemius Hesse, the wife of walther hesse, one of Koch's assistant. She suggested the use of agar as a solidifying agent. She showed that agar was not attacked by most bacteria and did not melt until reaching a temperature of above 100^0 C. This development made possible the isolation of pure cultures that contained only one type of bacterium. The discovery of agar directly stimulated progress in all areas of bacteriology.

9. Sergei .N. Winogradsky (1856 – 1953)

The Russian microbiologist Sergei N. Winogradsky made many contributions to soil Microbiology. He discovered that soil bacteria would oxidize iron, sulfur and ammonia to obtain energy. He also showed that many bacteria could incorporate CO_2 into organic matter much like photosynthetic organisms do. Winogradsky also isolated anaerobic nitrogen – fixing soil bacteria and studied the decomposition of cellulose. He developed the enrichment – culture technique and the use of selective media which have been of great importance in microbiology along with Beijerinck

10. Paul Ehrlich (1854 – 1915)

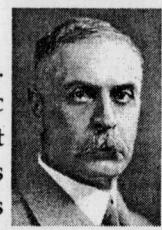

Paul Ehrlich in 1910, worked on Chemotherapy. He used an arsenic based drug called salvarsan to treat syphilis, a sexually transmitted disease, caused by *Treponema pallidum*. In 1898, he proposed that cells possess a wide variety of side chains on their surfaces.

He won the Nobel Prize in 1908 for his work on immunity.

11. Karl Landsteiner (1868 – 1943)

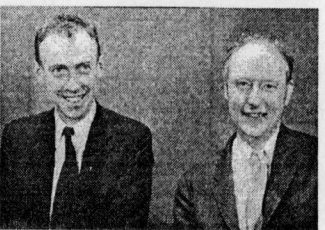

Landsteiner in 1900 discovered blood group antigens and their corresponding agglutinins. Landsteiner was a dominant figure in immunology for 40 years, developing the concept of the antigenic determinant and demonstration. The discovery of blood groups leads to the blood transfusion without provoking reactions. He objected Ehrlich's side chain theory because he was able to make antibodies against substances which were synthetic as well as natural. In 1900, he won the Nobel Prize for his discovery of blood group antigens and antibodies.

12. James Watson and Francis Crick

James Watson and Francis crick proposed the double helical structure of DNA in 1953. They rely on the simple laws of structural chemistry. Watson and crick shared the Noble Prize in 1953 for Medicine with Maurice Wilkins. They explained the model of DNA & how they can transmits hereditary information. The discovery of DNA lead to the development of fields like Genetic engineering, Biotechnology etc., Rapid amplification of DNA by PCR technique is possible nowadays only because of their discovery.

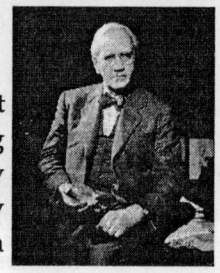

13. Sir Alexander Fleming (1881- 1955)

Sir Alexander Fleming discovered the antibiotic penicillin in 1929. Fleming observed that the mould *Penicillium notatum* killed his cultures of bacterium *Staphylococcus aureus*. After separating the fluid from the cell, Fleming discovered that the cell free liquid was an inhibitor for many bacterial species. He was the first person to demonstrate that a substance produced by microorganisms would inhibit or kill other microorganisms. His discovery made the modern era of drug therapy, and lead to the discovery of therapeutic value of penicillin.

14. Bright Field Microscopy – Refer Experiment No. 4 - Page No. 19
15. Dark Field Microscopy – Refer Experiment No. 4 - Page No. 21
16. Fluorescent Microscopy – Refer Experiment No. 4 - Page No. 21
17. Scanning Electron Microscopy – Refer Experiment No. 4 - Page No. 23
18. Transmission Electron Microscopy – Refer Experiment No. 4 - Page No. 22

19. 40 x objective lens

It is considered as high power objective lens. Its Magnification effect is around 400-450. Numerical aperture is about 0.55-0.65. Focal length of this lens is 4mm. Working distance between stage and lens is 0.5-0.7mm. Resolving power of the lens is 0.35mm.

20. Oil immersion lens

It was first used by Carl abbe. 100 x objective lens is also called oil immersion lens. Cedar wood oil is used as a immersion oil for microscopes. Oil has same refractive index as glass. It prevents the loss of light due to bending of light rays as they pass through air. It enhances the resolving power of the microscope. Open diaphragm during the use of oil immersion lens as much as possible. Blue or green filters are used to enhance the resolving power. Only dirt free optically safe tissue paper is used for lens cleaning. Magnification of Oil immersion lens is 1000-1500; Numerical aperture is 1.25-1.4; Focal length is 1.8-2mm; Working distance is 0.1mm; Resolving power is 0.18mm.

21. pH Meter - Refer Experiment No. 3 - Pg. No. 7
22. Centrifuge - Refer Experiment No. 3 - Pg. No. 8
23. Bunsen burner - Refer Experiment No. 3 - Pg. No. 9
24. Incubator - Refer Experiment No. 3 - Pg. No. 9
25. Morter and Pestel - Refer Experiment No. 3 - Pg. No. 9
26. Magnetic Stirrer - Refer Experiment No. 3 - Pg. No. 9
27. Spectrophotometer - Refer Experiment No. 3 - Pg. No. 10
28. Micro titre plate / ELISA plate - Refer Experiment No. 3 - Pg. No. 10
29. Stir Bar - Refer Experiment No. 3 - Pg. No. 10
30. Vortex Mixer - Refer Experiment No. 3 - Pg. No. 11
31. Ocular Micro meter - Refer Experiment No. 3 - Pg. No. 12
32. Stage Micrometer - Refer Experiment No. 3 - Pg. No. 12
33. Balance - Refer Experiment No. 3 - Pg. No. 12
34. Glass spreader - Refer Experiment No. 3 - Pg. No. 12
35. Water Bath - Refer Experiment No. 3 - Pg. No. 13
36. Haemometer - Refer Experiment No. 3 - Pg. No. 18
37. Refrigerator - Refer Experiment No. 3 - Pg. No. 17
38. Autoclave - Refer Experiment No. 7 - Pg. No. 32
39. Pressure cooker - Refer Experiment No. 7 - Pg. No. 33
40. Hot air overn - Refer Experiment No. 7 - Pg. No. 34
41. Membrane filter - Refer Experiment No. 7 - Pg. No. 34

42. Laminar Flow chamber - Refer Expt. No. 7 - Pg. No. 35
43. Haemocytometer - Refer Expt No. 3 - Pg. No. 13
44. Thermometer - Refer Expt No. 3 - Pg. No. 13
45. Beaker - Refer Expt No. 3 - Pg. No. 13
46. Volumetric flask - Refer Expt No. 3 - Pg. No. 14
47. Pasteur pipettes - Refer Expt No. 3 - Pg. No. 14
48. Pipette - Refer Expt No. 3 - Pg. No. 14
49. Measuring cylinder - Refer Expt No. 3 - Pg. No. 15
50. Cuvette - Refer Expt No. 3 - Pg. No. 15
51. Separating funnel - Refer Expt No. 3 - Pg. No. 15
52. Wash bottle - Refer Expt No. 3 - Pg. No. 15
53. Soxhlet extracter - Refer Expt No. 3 - Pg. No. 15
54. Conical flask - Refer Expt No. 3 - Pg. No. 16
55. Boiling tube - Refer Expt No. 3 - Pg. No. 16
56. Test tube - Refer Expt No. 3 - Pg. No. 16
57. BOD bottle - Refer Expt No. 3 - Pg. No. 17
58. Microscopic slide - Refer Expt No. 3 - Pg. No. 17
59. Cover slip - Refer Expt No. 3 - Pg. No. 17
60. Burette - Refer Expt No. 3 - Pg. No. 17
61. Petridish - Refer Expt No. 3 - Pg. No. 11

62. Inoculation Loop Refer experiment No. 3 - Pg. No. 12

63. Peptone - Refer Experiment No. 6 - Pg. No. 28

64. Sodium Chloride

Sodium chloride is an essential ingredient in most of the culture media. The molecular weight of NaCl is 58. NaCl is an example of an ionic bond. NaCl is neither an acid nor a base. Nacl ions are hydrophilic (Water-loving). It ionizes in water and yield sodium ions and chloride ions. 0.85% NaCl is used for the preparation of Normal saline. 0.9% NaCl is used for the preparation of physiological saline. NaCl is used in the medium for the prevention of osmatic lysis.

65. Yeast extract / Beef or Meat extract - Refer Experiment No. 6 - Page No. 28

66. Agar agar - Refer Experiment No. 6 - Page No. 29

67. Serial dilution set up - Refer Experiment No. 7 - Page No. 39

68. Streak plate technique (Expt. No. 11c) - Page No. 45 & 46

It is a technique used for the purification of microorganisms from mixed population. Pure culture is isolated with the help of this technique. The colonies on a mixed plate are separated on a plate with good spacing among each other using streak plate method. This technique is used for studying cultural, morphological and physiological characters of an individual species. There are different types of streaking methods. They are simple streaking, continuous streaking, Radiant and T streaking.

69. Spread plate technique (Expt. No. 11b)

It is one of the pure culture techniques. Cells are spreaded with the help of L rod throughout the plate. This technique is employed for performing antibiotic assay, mutagenesis activity, enzyme assay and genetic strain isolation. It is based on diluting the mixed culture with liquefied nutrient agar. 0.1mL of inoculum is required for spread plate technique.

70. Pour plate technique (Expt. No. 11a)

It is based on diluting the mixed culture with liquefied nutrient agar. This method has an advantage over streak plate method because it does not need any special skills. Disadvantage of this method is requiring large quantity of media and glasswares. This method is used for the quantitative and qualitative enumeration of microbes from the environment e.g. Isolation of microbes from soil. 1mL of sample is needed to perform pour plate technique.

71. Hanging Drop

It is a simplest method to examine living microorganisms. A special slide with a circular concave depression is called i.e Cavity slide is used to assess microbes present in a living state.

A suspension of microbial specimen is placed on the cover slip, then invert over the concave depression to produce a hanging drop of the specimen. This technique is primarily used to check the motility of bacteria.

E.g: *Pseudomonas aeruginosa* is a motile organism

Staphylococcus aureus is a nonmotile organism

72. Bacterial endospore (Diagram pls. see Page No. 59)

Endospores are thick walled, highly refractive bodies produced by *Bacillus sp.*, *Clostridium* sp. Bacterial spore contain large amounts of dipicolinic acid (DPA) combined with calcium, which may play a role in the heat resistance. Sporulation takes place under unfavorable conditions like heat, irradiation etc., Based on location, spores are classified as terminal spores, subterminal spores and central spores. Spores may be oval, ellipsoid or spherical in shape. The process by which a spore is converted into a vegetative cell is called germination.

73. Biochemical test Media/reagents/photographs of positve or negative reactions (73a - 73K)

Indole test, Methyl red test, Voges Proskauer Test, Citrate Utilization test, TSI test, Urease Test, Nitrate test, Catalse test, Oxidase test, Deaminase test, Decarboxylase test, Carbohydrate fermentation test, OF test, Optochin sensitivity, ONPG test, Starch hydrolysis, Lipid hydrolysis, Casein hydrolysis, Gelatin hydrolysis – **Refer experiment No 25 a to 25 ab and Appendix C**

74. Staining reagents

Crystal Violet, Grams iodine, Safranine, Decolourizer, Nigrosin, Indian Ink, Alberts iodine, alberts stain, Methylene blue, Copper sulphate, malachite green, carbol fuschin, Lactophenol cotton blue, Silver nitrate stain, Waysons stain, Giemsa stain, Wrights stain, Leishmans stain – **Refer experiment No 14 a to 14j, Appendix B and parasitology section.**

75. Aspergillus (Diagram pls. refer Page 233)

Aspergillus is a group of fungus that is frequently isolated from human beings. These organisms cause opportunistic infections. Some species are used in the industry for the production of enzymes. About 167 species are identified , of these 16 species are the etiological agent of Aspergillosis. The organism is found worldwide in soil, air, on mouldy storage grains and on decaying vegetables. Important species are *A.niger, A.flavus,A.fumigatus and A.terreus.*

Identifying features of various agents are,

A.niger - Coarse black granules against the creamy colony.Globose vesicles with biseriate phialids. Large echinulate jet-black conidia in chains.

A.flavus -Yellow to yellow green colonies.Globose to sub globose vesicles with uniseriate or biseriate phialides.Conidial heads that radiate and are loosely formed.

A.fumigatus - Bluish green to grey colonies. Flask shaped vesicles.Uniseriate phialides.

Compact columnar arrangement of conidia

A.terreus - Smallest Aspergilli. Cinnamon to buff brown colonies. Dome shaped vesicles with biseriate phialides. Long and compact conidial heads. Submerged hyphae that may form globose conidia.

76. Penicillium (Diagram pls. refer Page 233)

Penicillium sp are ubiquitous and omnipresent throughout the world. They are found in soil and decaying vegetation. It belonging to the order moniliales and family moniliaceae. Pulmonary infection, keratomycetitis, onchomychosis, cutaneous lesions, bladder infection are due to Penicillium species. Penicillium is one of the most common laboratory contaminants. Penicillin is produced by *Penicillium chrysogenum*. Colony morphology is flat granular that are typically blue green. Modified SDA with chloramphenical is used for cultivation . Phialides are formed as blunt tips. Chains of conidia from the phialides. Phialides may be arranged in whorls.

77. Rhizopus (Diagram pls. refer Page 233)

A genus of rot-causing fungi that includes the common bread mold; some species cause mucormycosis in humans. It belongs to the class zygomycetes; order mucorales and the family Mucoraceae. Rhizopus produce cottony to woolly olive gray colonies that rapidly fill the SDA plate.The surface becomes covered with dark spots when sporangia appear, so Rhizopus is described as *salt and pepper* appearance. On microscopical examination broad irregular hyphae that are aseptate or sparsely septate.Branching sporangiophore with hemispherical columellae arising from nodes adjacent to rhizoids. Grows best at 25 ^{0}C and 37^0 C sometimes up to 50 ^{0} C

78. Mucor (Diagram pls. refer Page 233)

Mucor is a genus of about 40 species of moulds commonly found in soil and on plant surfaces, as well as in rotten vegetable matter. It belongs to the division Zygomycota and family Mucoraceae. On modified SDA it grows at 25°C after 2-4 days. Colonies of Mucor are wooly and rapidly fill the entire petriplate with an abundant matted mycelium. The colony is white at first and becomes grey or yellow. Broad irregular hyphae that are aseptate, septate or sparsely septate. Branching sporangiophores with collumellae supporting sporangia filled with sporangiospores. Absence of rhizoides.

79. Geotrichum (Diagram pls. refer Page 233)

It belongs to kingdom Fungi, Phylum Ascomycota, Order Saccharomycetales, Family Endomycetaceae. It is a normal flora of skin and gastrointestinal tract. It is often isolated from milk and dairy products, vegetables and fruits. It is sensitive to cycloheximide. On the microscopic observation it seen as a septate, hyaline true hyphae with lateral branching. Incubation time is about 2-3 days and the temperature is 25 ° C. On SDA medium it was grown as spreading white yeast like colonies initially, becoming mould like as the colony ages. Arthroconidia germinating in a "hockey stick" arrangement. True hyphae formed.

80. Acremonium (Diagram pls. refer Page 233)

It belongs to kingdom Fungi, phylum Ascomycota, order Hypocreales, family Hypocreaceae. Acremonium species are found in soil, sewage, on vegetation and in food stuffs. This fungus is associated with mycetoma and mycotic keratitis. Corneal scrapings, aspirates, respiratory secretions, pleural fluid, blood, tissue, skin, nail clippings are likely to be submitted for culture. Modified SDA without cycloheximide act as a culture media. Optimum temperature of growth is 30°C. Colonies are smooth and waxy or velvetty and later they may be cottony. The colour varies from white to gray to rose. The hyphae are deligates, thin, hyaline and septate. Conidiophores are hyaline solitary and unbaranched, tapering from the base to the tip. Clusters of conidia at the tips of the phialides.

81. Alternaria (Diagram pls. refer Page 233)

It belongs to the Kingdom Fungi, Phylum Ascomycota, Class Dothideomycetes, Order Pleosporales. Alternaria species are found worldwide as a soil saprophyte and as a plant pathogen. Alteraria species are reported to cause sinusitis, asthma, osteomyelities. Modified SDA is used for cultivation at the temperature between 25-30°C. Dark brown or dark olive-green colony with a white fringe. Produce dematiaceous hypha, conidiophores, and conidia that are , club shaped , and beaked.

82. Curvularia

It belongs to the Kingdom Fungi, Phylum Ascomycota, Class Euascomycetes, Order Pleosporales. It is commonly found in the air and soil as saprophytes. It acts as a opportunistic pathogen and cause mycotic keratitis, allergies, sinusitis etc. Modified SDA used as a culture media and grows best at 25⁰ C to 30⁰C. Velvety or wooly, with dark brown to black to olive green pigmented colonies are formed on SDA media. It produce dark, curved, multicellular conidia resembling cresent rolls, the center cell is swollen and darker than the cells lateral to it. Symphoidal conidiogeny. A dark, protruding helium is seen at the base of conidia.

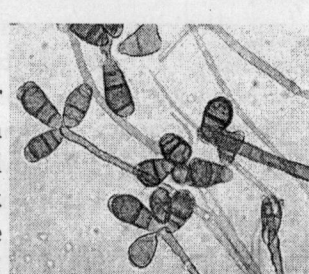

83. Malassezia furfur

The organism is found world wide as a commensal on smooth skin of humans.

It causes **tinea versicolar.** Skin scrapings are submitted for diagnosis. Modified SDA supplemented with olive oil and antibiotics are used for cultivation. *Mallasezia furfur (Petriellidium boydii)* It is lipophilic yeast.

Shiny or pasty white to cream coloured colonies are formed after 1-2 weeks. The phialoconidia are thick walled, round or oval in shape. They typically occur in clusters, individual cells looks like yeast.

84. Piedraia hortae

The organism is a plant parasite. Human infection caused by this parasite is called black piedra. Colour of the colony on SDAis green ish black or black. Asci and ascospores are rarely seen inculture. Hair is used for the diagnosis.

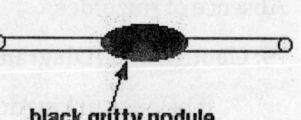

Piedriae hortae

black gritty nodule

85. Cladosporium (Diagram pls. refer page 233)

It is found in soil, on rotting wood and in decaying vegetables. It is worldwide in distribution. *C. carrionii* is one of the etiological agent of chromoblastomycosis. Media used for cultivation are SDA with antimicrobials. It produces characteristic olive green to black colonies. Hyphae is septate in nature. Cladosporium type conidiation in clusters are observed.

86. Helminthosporium

It is found in soil as a saprophyte. It causes mycotic keratitis. SDA with chloramphenicol is used for cultivation. Optimum temperature for growth is 25-30 ⁰C. Dematiaceous hyphae and dark unbranched conidiophores.

Darkly pigmented clavated proconidia produced laterally through pores along the conidiophores.

87. Trichophyton rubrum

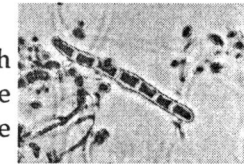

Organisms found thought out the world. This fungus can infect hair and skin of both children and adults, but the nail is not invaded. SDA,DTM are used for cultivation. Colonies are white downy to fluffy or yellow or tinged with red. Hyceliae hyphae is Hyaline, septate hyphae and branched. Hair perforation test negative.

88. Trichophyton verrucosum.

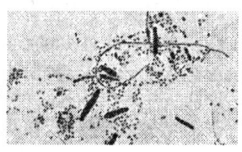

Organisms found throughout the world. It causes ringworm infection in cattle. It causes highly inflammatory infection in human. Best growth at 37 ^{0}C. Hyphae are hyaline, septate and distorted. SDA,DTM are used for cultivation.

89. Trichophyton mentagrophytes

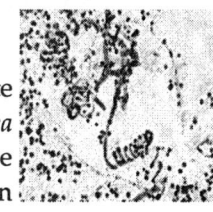

The organism is found throughout the world. It is a most common agent of dermatophyte infection. It is a highly contagious fungus.It is associated with *Tinea cruris, Tinea corporis, Tinea pedis, Tinea capitis, Tinea barbae and Tinea unguium*.DTM, SDA are used for cultivation. Colonies are Flat, granular, creamy yellow to tan or reddish brown with a buff, yellow brown or reddish brown reverse. Hair perforation test positive. Cigar-shaped macroconidia with thin, smooth walls.

90. Sporothrix.

Organisms found throughtout the world. It causes sporotrichosis in humans. SDA,BHIA are used for cultivation. Best growth at 25-37 ^{0}C. At 25-37 ^{0}C, It produces leathery black or mottled black colonies. Thin septate hyphae. Tapering sympoidal conidiophores. At 35- 37 ^{0}C, it produces Cream to tan yeast like colony. Hyaline unicellular budding yeast forms, with a variety of forms. Delicate connection between mother and daughter cells

91. Trichoderma.

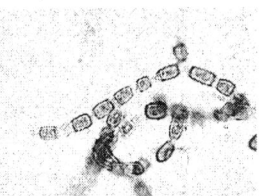

Trichoderma are found in soil throughout the world. They are spread by an airborne route. Modified SDA is used for culture. Subculture is made on Czapek-dox, PDA to enhance conidiation and pigmentation.

It grow best at 35^{0}C . Trichoderma cover the plate with a flat white lawn of hyphal growth. Later the colonies may became velvety to powdery conidiation is heavy. The colour varies from yellow to yellow green. Unicellular hyaline phialoconidia on short plump flask shaped phialophores. Wide angle of branches of the phialophores and philaides. Clusters of sub globose to elliptical conidia in balls at the tip of the phialides.

92. Coccidioides immitis

The pulmonary infection caused by this organism is sometimes called Valley fever. It is a dimorphic fungus.It is most virulent of all the agents of human mycosis. Modified SDA, BHIA are used for cultivation.Optimum temperature for growth is 25^0 C to 30^{0}C. Rapidly growing colonies with early appearance of white cottony aerial mycelium and areas of adherent surface hyphae. Septate hyaline hyphae of varying widths are seen microscopically. Fertile arthroconidiating hyphae are wider than vegetative hyphae. The arthroconidia are usually single celled barrel shaped or rectangular.

93. Histoplasma capsulatum

It is found worldwide and endemic in North America. The pulmonary infections caused by this species are sometimes called *Darlings Disease*. Nickname (a chronic granulomatous infection) of histoplasmosis is *Spelunkers's Disease*. It is a dimorphic fungus.Blood agar plate and SDA are used for cultivation. At 37⁰C, it resembles the cells of *Candida*. Macroconidia are hyaline, unicellular, and relatively large, with spherical or pyriform shaped. As the macroconidia age they become tuberculate, that is, they form finger like projections of the thick wall of the conidium.Mature macroconidia are sometimes described as resembling sunflowers in bloom. It forms waxy, wrinkled light brown colony of yeast at 37⁰C. At 25⁰C they may produce white to brown at first, later they become wooly, as aerial hyphae develop.

94. *Blastomyces dermatidis*

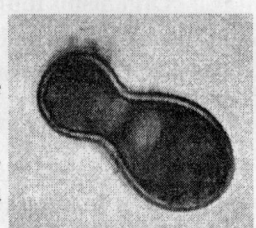

It cause endemic infections. Disease caused by blastomyces is called blastomycosis. Use blood agar plates, BHIA or SDA for cultivation.Optimum temperature for growth is 25-30°C. Globose to pyriform 'lollipops' on conidiophores of varying length at 25-30°C. Waxy, wrinkled, light brown colony of yeast cells at 37°C. Small round or pear shaped conidia grows directly on the septate hyphae.

95. Saccharomyces cerevisiae (Yeast)

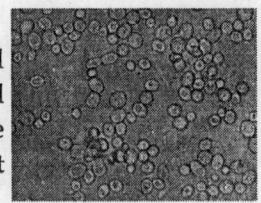

It is a working yeast .Various strains are used in industry to make bread, beer, wine and industrial alcohol. PDA is used for the isolation of *Saccharomyces cerevisiae*. On Rose Bengal agar milky white colonies are formed . It is sensitive to Cycloheximide and produce blastoconidia, but neither germ tube nor chlamydospores. Pseudohyphae may be formed .It produced single multi lateral budding yeast. It is facultative anaerobic one.

96. Cryptococcus neoformans

It is found worldwide .The yeast is able to survive in pigeons gut . It produces Cryptococcosis in human. It produced capsules, capsule production enhanced by inoculating a plate of chocolate agar and incubating it at 37⁰C. It is thin walled globose or oval shaped yeast. It forms smooth mucoid colonies on Sabouraud Dextrose agar.

97. Candida albicans

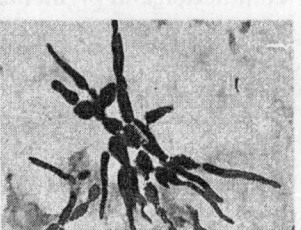

C.clbicans is regonized as the most frequently encountered fungal opportunist and is now regarded as the most common cause of serious fungal disease. The clinical diseases caused by candida are collectively called candidiasis . *C. albicans* is found worldwide on fruits and vegetables. For culture BAP, modified SDA with cycloheximide are used. Candida species develop as entire, white, pasty, convex colonies that initially resemble Staphylococci. The colonies may produce pseudohyphal fringes around the periphery. In a wet preparation *C.albicans* demonstrates blastoconidia on pseudohyphye. Germ tubes formed within 3 hours at 35⁰C.

98. Epidermophyton floccosum

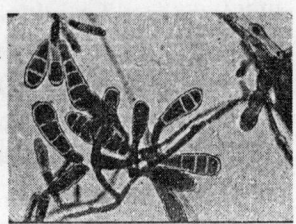

It is an only human pathogen in this genus.Organism is found worldwide in distribution. It is a highly contagious fungus. Skin scraping is a specimen. It produces white, downy somewhat scanty colony.Center of the colony maybe folded. Thin hyaline, Septate and branched hyphae.Absence of microconidia. Abundant characteristic show shoe or paddle shaped macro conidia, with thin smooth walls.

99. Microsporum canis

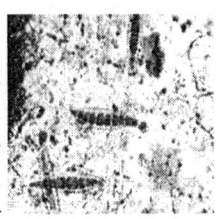

It is found world wide as a zoophilic pathogen. It is highly contagious and easily transmitted from animal to human. It causes *Tinea corporis* and *Tinea capitis*. Modified SDA, DTM, PDA and modified corn meal agar are used for cultivation. It produce hair perforation test positive. Rare microconidia. Characteristic spindle shaped macroconidia with beaked tips. Hyphae are hyaline, septate and branched. Vegetative hyphal structures are racquet hyphae chlamydoconidia. It produces yellow pigmented and good growth and conidiation colony.

100. Pythium

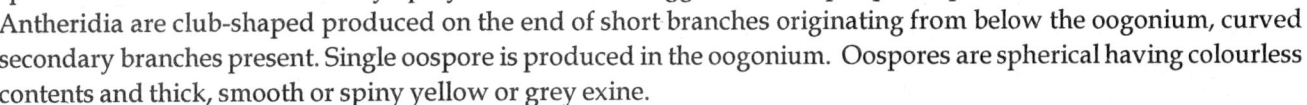

It belongs to class Oomycetes, order peronosporales, family pythiaceae and Genus Pythium. They are aquatic amphibious or terrestrial fungi, saprophytic on plants and insects rotting in water or parasitic on living plants. Thallus is highly branched hyphal network. Mycelium is very thin, aseptate, but septa is formed at the time reproduction of delimit the reproductive organs. Zoosporangia formed at the end of hyphae but not on special branch. Zoospores are kidney shaped with two flagella inserted at the side. Oogonia are small and spherical with colourless or warty-spiny membrane; one egg and a little periplasm present. Antheridia are club-shaped produced on the end of short branches originating from below the oogonium, curved secondary branches present. Single oospore is produced in the oogonium. Oospores are spherical having colourless contents and thick, smooth or spiny yellow or grey exine.

101. Fusarium (Diagram pls. refer page 233)

They are found world wide in soil and on rotting vegetarian and ripe fruit. Fusarium species have been associated with keratitis, onchomycosis, fungemia, invasive nasal infections that spreads on the lungs. Corneal scrapings, aspirates from lesions, respiratory secretions, nail clippings; cerebrospinal fluid and gastric secretions are most likely to be submitted for culture. Sabouraud dextrose agar is used as a culture media. On the media woolly to cottony colonies in a great variety of diffusible colours mostly pink or purple. It can grow best at 25-30 ° C. Both micro conidia and macro conidia, which are cresent shaped with distinct foot cells. The septate hyaline of this organism is 4nm in diameter.

102. Germ Tube (Diagram pls. refer page 232)

It is seen as a long tube like projections extending from the yeast. It is a characteristic feature of *Candia albicans*. It is produced by inoculation of culture on human serum and incubated at 37°C for 2-4 hours. A drop of suspension is examined on a slide under the microscope and observes for pseudohyphae. There is no septum in germ tube.Demonstration of germ tube is known as Reynolds- Braude phenomenon.

103. Anabaena

Group : Cyanobacteria	Order : Nostocales
Family: Nostocaceae	Genus: Anabaena

They are oxygenic photoautotrophic bacteria in which akinetes are usually formed. They are cylindrical, spherical or ovoid forms generally having 2 -10 μm size. The plant body consists of vegetative cells as well as heterocysts and akinetes. The heterocyst are present ether in intercalary or in terminal or both positions. The cells contain slime covering and a distinct individual sheath is absent. The trichomes are normally motile and colonies are not formed. Their species establish symbiotic associations with fungi (lichens), bryophytes (Anthoceros), pteridophytes (Azolla) and gymnosperms (cycas). Examples are *A. azollae, A. cycadae. etc.,*

104. Oscillatoria

Group : Cyanobacteria   Order : Oscillatoriales
Family: Oscillatoriaceae   Genes : Oscillatoria

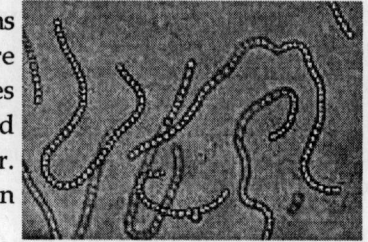

It is a gram-negative, filamentous cyanobacterium which is found in fresh water ponds, pools, lakes and sub-aerial habitats. It is an unbranched filamentous algae. Filaments (trichomes) occur singly or matted together to form thick or thick sheets. The cells exhibit a typical prokaryotic structure and its protoplast is differentiated in to the peripheral pigmented chromoplasm and the central centroplasm. The photosynthetic pigments are found in the surface of the thylakoids. Oscillatoria exhibits intercalary growth. It has G+C% of above 40 – 50.

105. Spirulina

Group : Cyanobacteria   Order: Oscillatoriales
Families: Oscillatoriaceae   Genus: Spirulina

This is an aerobic, fresh, marine cyanobacterium that may found in brackish water inland lakes as well as in hot springs. Generally they grow in closed right-handed or left-handed helix. The cross walls are thin and are invisible or nearly so with light microscopy. They are self pH adjusters that grow between 8.5 and 11. They have gliding motility, consists of a 'turning of the screw' to form continuous helical coil with thin cross walls. These are significant due to their industrial importance in the form of rich protein value (62%). Their colour is variable from blue green to red and mol% G +C contents is 54.

106. Nostoc

They are oxygenic phototrophic bacteria. The trichomes with many constructions at cross walls are present giving the typical contorted appearance. The cells are cylindrical, spherical or ovoid in shape. The heterocysts are intercalary and trichomes present in confluent gel. Some colonies are in ball shaped while few form flattened discs or large sheats. The size of the colonies sometimes reached to 20cm in diameter. Vegetative trichomes are not capable of gliding motility. The hormogonoia are often filled with gas and their width is lessthan that trichomes.

The DNA base composition ranges from 39-45 mol% G+C.

107. Entamoeba histolytica (Diagram pls. refer page 240)

E.histolytica is commonly available in tropical subtropical, temporate regions. Endoparasite. Present in man and other mammals. Alive in mucous layer of colon. Feeds dissolved tissues, bacteria and RBCs. Causes fatal and serious disease. Infected individual discharge mucous and blood in their stool. *E histolytica* has a relatively simple life cycle that alternates between trophozoite and cyst stages.

Trophozoite - The trophozoite is the actively metabolizing, mobile stage. They are alive and actively motile (Unidirectional motility). Amoebas are anaerobic organisms and do not have mitochondria. The finely granular endoplasm contains the nucleus and food vacuoles, which in turn may contain bacteria or red blood cells. Nuclear morphology is best seen in permanent stained preparations. The nucleus has a distinctive central karyosome and a rim of finely beaded chromatin lining the nuclear membrane. Finger like pseudopodia is available.

Cyst - The cyst is a spherical structure, 10-20 μm in diameter, with a thin transparent wall. Fully mature cysts contain four nuclei with the characteristic amoebic morphology. Rod-like structures (chromatoidal bars) are present variably, but are more common in immature cysts. Inclusions in the form of glycogen masses also may be present. A number of non-pathogenic amoebae can parasitize the human gastrointestinal tract and may cause diagnostic confusion. Cyst is dermant stage & resistant to various environmental stress.

108. Giardia lamblia (Diagram pls. refer page 240)

It was first seen by Leewen hoek in 1681 while examining his own stool. It is world wide in distribution. The *Giardia* life cycle involves two stages. The Trophozoite and the Cyst. The *G. lamblia* trophozoite is easily recognized under a microscope. It is about 12 to 15 µm long, shaped like tennis racket.The dorsal surface is convex and the ventral surface is concave with a sucking disc, and has two nuclei that resemble eyes, structures called median bodies that resemble a mouth, and four pairs of flagella that look like hair; these combine to give the stained trophozoite the eerie appearance of a face. The flagella help these organisms to migrate to a given area of the small intestine, where they attach by means of an adhesive disk to epithelial cells and thus maintain their position despite peristalis. It is bilaterally symmetrical. Anterior end is broad and the posterior end is tapers to a sharp point.

The *Giardia* cyst - The form usually seen in the faeces - is ovoid, 6 to 12 µm long, and can often be seen to contain two to four nuclei at one end and prominent diagonal fibrils. Flagella and sucking disc are seen inside of cytoplasm.

109. Ascaris lumbricoides

It causes Ascariasis.It is intestinal nematode. Transmitted by food contaminated with soil containing eggs. Heavy worm burden in intestine can cause intestinal obstruction or malnutrtion. Eggs are visible in faeces. Mebanadazole is used for treatment. Prevention is by proper disposal of human waste. Human is a only host.

110. Schistosoma (Diagram pls. refer page 241)

It causes Schistosomiasis. It is a bisexual blood fluke. Important species are *S.mansoni*-Large lateral spine *S.japanicum*- (Small lateral spine), *S. hematobium*-(Terminal spine). Transmission by penetration of skin by cercariae. Humans are the definite host.Snail is a intermediate host. Eggs in tissue induce inflammation, granuloma, fibrosis and obstruction. Eggs are visible in faeces. Prazigrantel is used for treatment. Proper disposal of waste is a way of prevention.

111. Wuchereria bancrofti

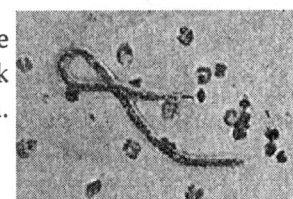

It causes Filariosis. It is a tissue nematode. Bites of female mosquito deposits infective larvae, penetrate wound and produce microfilaria. These circulate in the blood and block lymphatic vessels and cause Elephantiasis. Blood examination reveals microfilaria. Diethylcarbamazine is used for treatment. Mosquito control prevents the infection.

112. Chicken Pox

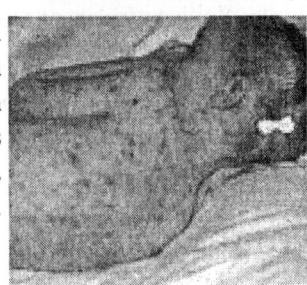

Causative agent of Chicken pox is *Varicella zoster virus*. Small, itchy bumps and blisters over skin and mucous membranes, fever are the symptoms. Virus multiplies in upper respiratory tract and spread via blood to the skin, cytopathic effect of virus in epidermis, induce vesicle formation. Vesicle contain serum, Polymorphonuclear leukocytes and intra nuclear inclusion bodies. Lab diagnosis is by Fluorescent antibody technique, virus isolation in tissue culture. Transmission by respiratory route, highly infectious. Passive immunization with Zoster Immuno Globulin(ZIG) prevents chicken pox.

113. Measles

Causative agent is *measles virus*. Symptoms are Rash, malaise, fever, conjunctivitis, cough and nasal discharge. Virus multiplies in respiratory tract, carried by blood to various parts of the body, notably, skin, lungs, brain and

creates damage to respiratory epithelium leads to secondary infection. Lab diagnosis is by Complement fixation test, haemagglutination inhibition test and cultivation of virus in tissue culture. Acquired by respiratory route. Highly contagious. Prevention by Live attenuated rubella vaccine administered to children at 15 months of age.

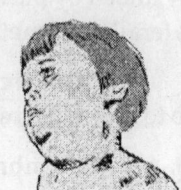

114. Rubella (3 day Measles or German Measles)

Rubella virus is a causative agent. Malaise, headache, fever, rash beginning on forehead and face, enlarged lymph nodes behind the ear are the symptoms. Following replication virus spread to all parts of the body and crosses the placenta. Lab diagnosis is by inoculation of tissue culture with throat samples. Human is the only source of infection.Live attenuated rubella vaccine administered to children at 15 months of age.

115. Mumps

Mumps virus causes it. It is an enveloped virus with helical symmetry. Genome is single stranded negative sense RNA. Respiratory droplet is a source of infection. From upper respiratory tract, the virus spreads to local lymph nodes and then via the blood stream to other organ, especially parotid gland, testes, ovaries, meninges. Virus can be isolated by cell culture .Haemadsorption test is also useful for diagnosis. No antiviral therapy.

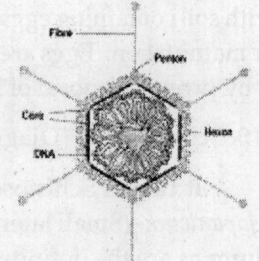

116. Adenovirus

It causes pharyngitis pneumonia, diarrhoea. Some strains cause sarcomas. It is a non-enveloped, icosahedral, Linear DS DNA virus. Disease is transmitted through droplets; Virus infects respiratory epithelium and damages the cells, which cause various symptoms.Virus causes CPE in cell culture. Identified by Fluorescent antibody or Complement Fixation Test. Live vaccine is used for prevention.

117. Rabies Virus

Rabies virus causes rabies infection. It belongs to the family Rhabdovirus and genus Lyssa virus. In Greek Lyssa means rabies. Rabies virus is bullet shaped. Genome is negative sense single stranded RNA. Two layers, matrix layer and outer envelope cover the genome. Matrix is made up of M protein. Outer envelope is made up of lipid-bi- layer as like plasma membrane. External envelope having spike like projections. It is made up of glycoproteins. Spikes are responsible for pathogenic property of

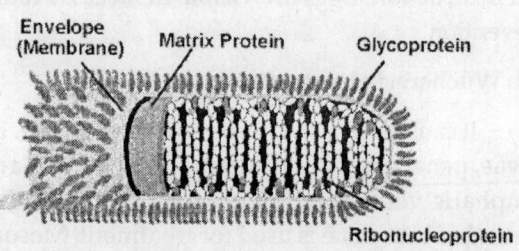

the virus. RNA dependent RNA polymerase is responsible for genome replication. L and P proteins control its activity. Rabies viruses of man and animals allover the world appears to be of a single antigenic type. Antigens of rabies viruses are G protein, M protein, N protein and Hemaglutinin. It is also called street virus.

118. Human Immuno Deficiency Virus (HIV)

It is a lentivirus of the family retroviridae. It is an icosahedral virus containing 72 external spikes. Spikes are made up of Gp120 and Gp 41. It causes Acquired immuno deficiency syndrome in human. The retrovirus genome comprises two identical, plus-sense ssRNA molecules. Retroviruses contain 2 envelope proteins encoded by the env-gene, 4-6 nonglycosylated core proteins and 3 non-structural functional proteins (reverse transcriptase, integrase,

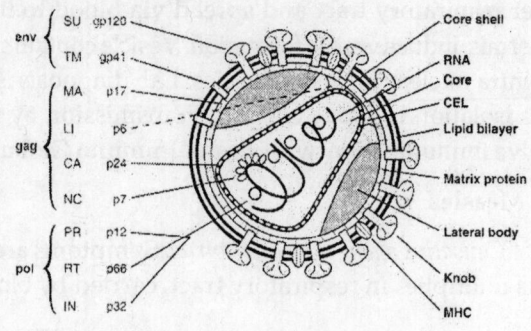

protease: RT, IN, PR) specified by the gag-gene. The RT transcribes the viral ssRNA into double-stranded, circular proviral DNA. This DNA, mediated by the viral integrase, becomes covalently bonded into the DNA of the host cell to make possible the subsequent transcription of the sense strands that eventually give rise to retrovirus progeny. After assembly and budding, retroviruses show structural and functional maturation. In immature virions the structural proteins of the core are present as a large precursor protein shell. After proteolytic processing by the viral protease the proteins of the mature virion are rearranged and form the dense isometric or cone-shaped core typical of the mature virion, and the particle becomes infectious.

119. Hepatitis B Virus

It is the most important virus among hepatitis causing viruses. HBV causing Hepatitis is called serum Hepatitis. In 1965, Blumberg reported protein antigen in the serum of Australian patient. This antigen is called Australian antigen. By 1968, the Australian antigen was shown to be associated with serum hepatitis. This was then considered as Hepatitis surface antigens (HbsAg). HBV is a 42nm spherical virus that posses several antigens. There are three envelope polypeptides that come under the designation HbsAg, HbcAg and HbeAg. HBV belongs to Hepedna viridae. The nucleo capsid of the virion consist of the viral genome surrounded by the core antigen (27nm). Negative strand is complete but

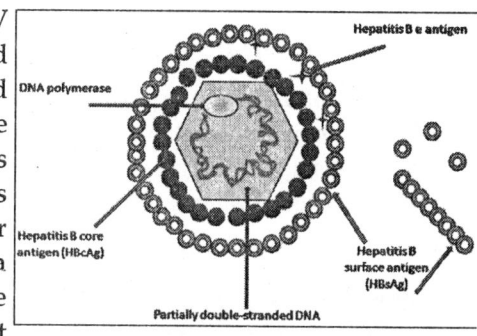

positive strand is incomplete. 3' end of genome is associated with a DNA polymerase molecule. In genome there are 4 major Open reading frame(ORF) . They are ORF-S consists of pre S1, and pre S2 codes for structural proteins of surface and core. ORF-P encodes polymerase that contains DNA polymerase and RNAse H. ORF-X encoded transcriptional activator. ORF-C pre C protein. The virus is stable at 37° C for 60 minutes.

120. Tobaco Mosaic Virus (TMV)

It was first isolated by Dimitri Ivanowski in 1892 with the help of chamberland filter. In 1935, Wendell M.Stanley crystallize the TMV. W.Pirie separated TMV particles into proteins and nucleic acids. TMV is a helical capsid in structure. Capsids are arranged in hollow tube like structure. Single capsid posses 158 amino acids. Individual 17,400-Da protein subunits (protomers) assemble in a helix with an axial repeat of 6.9 nm (49 subunits per three turns). Each turn contains a nonintegral number of subunits (16-1/3), producing a pitch of 2.3 nm. The RNA is sandwiched internally between adjacent turns of capsid protein, forming a RNA helix of the same pitch, 8 nm in diameter, that extends the length of virus, with three nucleotide bases in contact with each subunit. Some 2,130 protomers per virion cover and protect the RNA. The complete virus is 300 nm long and 18 nm in diameter with a hollow cylindrical core 4 nm in diameter.

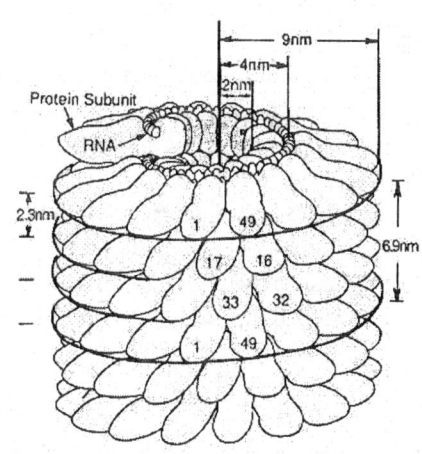

121. Phenol red

Phenol red is an acid base indicator. It is used for serum media, because it detects small changes in pH. Its pH range is 6.8 – 8.4. Colour change is yellow to pink. For use, 5mL of phenol red solution is added to 100mL of the medium to gives final concentration of 0.01%. Phenol red is incorporated in Triple sugar iron test. Used To detect carbohydrate fermentation . It is also used in urease test.

122. Neutrophils (Picture refer page 172)

It is otherwise known as Polymorphonuclear neutrophil granulocyte (PMN). It is formed in the bone marrow; migrate to the blood stream and about 12 hours later move into tissues. Life span is only one day. They are the most abundant leukocytes. They posses a finely granular cytoplasm. Irregular sausage like or segmented nucleus. It contain two types of cytoplasmic granule namely primary granules (electron dense) and secondary granules (less dense). Myeloperoxidase and lysozyme are the major component of primary granule. Secondary granule contains lysozyme, collagenase and lactoferrin. The major function of neutrophils is the capture and destruction of foreign organisms through phagocytosis. Normal value-in blood constituting about 60% to 70% of the blood leucocytes in humans.

123. Eosinophils (Picture refer page 172)

It is one of the Polymorphonuclear granulocyte (PMN). It is stained intensely with eosin. Their halflife in the circulation is only about 30 minutes. Normal values ranges from 2% to 5% in healthy humans. Eosinophils are phagocytic cells that can ingest and destroy foreign material. The granules of eosinophils contain phosphatase and peroxidase and also contain major basic protein (MBP) . MBP is highly toxic for invading parasitic worms (helminthes).

124. Basophils (Picture refer page 172)

Its normal value ranges from >1%. Their cytoplasmic granules are intensely stained with basic dyes such as haematoxylin. They are not normally found in extra vascular tissues. Granules contain vasoactive amines such as histamine and serotonin. It contain single lobe nucleus. Basophils promote acute inflammation.

125. Monocyte (Picture refer page 172)

It is a mononuclear phagocytic cells found in blood. Normal value ranges from 1% to 3%. Half life in circulation is 1-2 days. It is considered as macrophage it is moved to tissues.

126. Monoclonal antibodies or Hybridoma technology

This technique was developed by Kohler and Milstein (1975). Hybridoma technology is used for the production of monoclonal antibodies. Immunized mice spleen cells and myeloma cells are fused with the help of polyethylene glycol (PEG). Fused cells are selected with the help of HAT medium (Hypoxanthine, aminopterin and thymidine). Spleen cells die within few hours, but myeloma cells died because of the absence of the enzyme called Hyphoxanthine phosphoribosyl transferase (HGPRT). Hybridized cells only survive in HAT medium. Antibodies produced in this technique are screened by radioimmunoassay or ELISA technique. Clonal propagation of B lymphocyte is a principle of this technology. (Picture refer page 147)

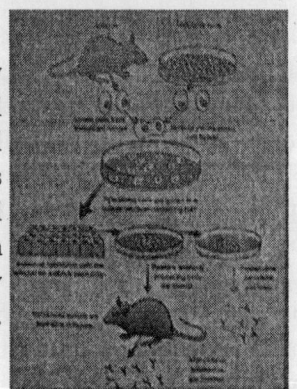

127. Ouchterlony (double diffusion)

It is a precipitation technique in agar, usually accomplished in a slide in which antigen and antibody are allowed to diffuse each other and permit the formation of precipitin line between the sample wells. If two or more sample (antigen) wells are diffused against a single antiserum (antibody) well, the following distinctions can be made : *Lines of identity*: a single precipitin line indicating uniformity and identity of the antigens in the sample wells. *Lines of nonidentity* – two distinct and crossing precipitin lines indicating no cross-reactivity or identity between the antigens in the two sample wells . *Lines of partial identity* – a spur formation, indicating that some of the antigenic determinants (epitopes) are shared between the antigens in the two sample wells.

128. Rocket immunoelectrophoresis

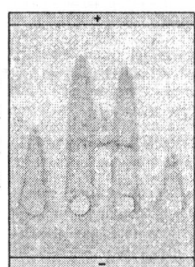

It is a rapid method for the estimation antigen concentration uses the following procedure. Sample wells are punched at one end of a gel plate in which antibody to a specific antigen has been dissolved. Samples are applied and electrophoresed. Rocket – like precipitate lines form; their length depends on the initial antigen sample concentration; a reference line is determined. Unknown concentration is determined by the length of the arc relative to the standard reference.

129. Radial immunodiffusion

It is a method for estimating antigen concentration. Uses the following procedure:Antibody to specific antigen is diffused in an agar gel or slab. Antigen wells are cut, and samples of various known concentrations are applied. Gel is incubated and precipitin rings are developed. The diameter of each precipitin ring is proportional to the initial antigen concentration; a reference line is determined. unknown concentration is determined by the comparison with the reference line.

130. Immunoelectrophoresis (IEP)

It is an antigen-antibody reaction technique developed to resolve highly complex mixtures of antigens. Antigen is placed in agar on a glass slide and subjected to electrophoresis, using an electric current, to separate the serum proteins at a given pH (usually pH 8.4) into their constitutent parts (albumin, and globulin fractions). The separated proteins with their specific antibody are then placed in an antiserum trough, where they form a series of arcs of precipitate.

131. Radio immunoassay (RIA)

It is a sensitive assay for antigen that usually uses a known amount of labeled antigen (Ag) and a known amount of specific antibody for that antigen. A standard inhibition ('quench") curve is generated by reacting increasing known amounts of unlabeled antigen with the constant antiboidy amount and determining the ratio of bound angen. to free angen the more unlabeled antigen present, the less angen will be bound to antibody. unknown concentration is determined by interpolation of the standar inhibition curve.

132. Lymphoid organs – Refer experiment 28

Thymus, bone marrow, Lymph node, Spleen, MALT (Refer pages 126, 127, 128)

133. Spoiled Bread

Most commonly known fermented bakery product is bread. Bread spoilage is more commonly done by Bacillus species leading to ropiness. The chief types of microbial spoilage of baked bread have been noted as Moldiness and ropiness. *Rhizopus stolonifer*, a White cottony mycelium with black dots of sporangia is the chief mold involved in bread spoilage and are commonly called as bread mold. Bread spoilage may be due to warm humid condition, air contaminated with mold presence of 60% milk residual moisture and slicing. Chalky bread caused by *Trichosporon variable, Endomycopsis fibuligera.* Red bread caused by *Monilia sitophila, Geotrichum aurantiacum, Ropiness* of bread caused by *Bacillus subtilis, Bacillus lickeniformis, Bacillus megaterium.*

134. Vitamin B 12

It is also known as cyanocobalamine, antipernicious anaemic factor, castle's extrinisic factor etc.

Riclees et al., 1984 isolated this from liver. Vitamin B12 can be produced commercially by using *Streptomuces olivaceus*, here cobalt chloride acts as a precussor. It is large molecule made up of 63 Carbon atoms. It is a tasteless, odourless, water soluble, thermostable, needle shaped red crystal forming Vitamin. It's deficiency leads to a macrocytic type of anemia known as pernicious anaemia. Helps in synthesis of Thymine, protein, affects mycelin formation etc.

135. Vinegar

The word vinegar is derived from the French word Vinaigre meaning 'sour wine'. Fermentation of carbohydrate to produce ethanol is first step in vinegar production. e.g Fruit juice, a sugar – containing syrup or a hydrolyzed starchy material . Yeast fermentation is used initially for production of alcohol from the substrate. The solutions alcohol concentration is then adjusted between 10 -13 % and acetic acid producing bacterial genus Acetobacter are added. In fringes vinegar generator a dilute solution of alcohol percolates through wood shavings that are covered with growth of Acetobacter. The bacteria oxidize the alcohol to acetic acid.

$$\underset{\text{ethanol}}{2CH_3CH_2OH+2O_2} --------- \underset{\text{Acetic Acid}}{2CH_3COOH+2H_2O}$$

The solution is collected at the bottom of the unit may be re circulated over the shavings to allow more oxidation of alcohol until vinegar of the desired strength is produced.

136. Citric Acid

It is on organic acid. It is used in preparation of medicines, food and candies etc., *Aspergillus niger* is most widely used for commercial production. Molasses act as a raw material for the commercial production. Used in soft drinks, Candies, Medicines, Food industry etc.,

137. Wine - expt. No. 112 - Page No. 321

138. Mushroom - expt. No. 111 - Page No. 318

139. Aflatoxins - expt. No. 107 - Page No. 304

140. Yogurt - expt. No. 101 - Page No. 295

141. Sodium Alginate

Alginate commercially available as alginic acid sodium salt, commonly called sodium alginate. It is a linear polysaccharide normally isolated from many strains of marine brown seaweed. Based on the associated salt alginic acid can be either water soluble or insoluble. Alginate is currently used in food, pharmaceutical, textile and paper industries. Alginate when cross linked with calcium ions forms a gel. It doesn't form covalent bond but is a cross linking and forms calcium alginate.

142. Fermentors

Fermentors are a large cylindrical vessel with controlled environment. The vessel should be capable of being operated aseptically for a number of days. A system of temperature, pH control, sampling facilities should be provided. Parts of fermentors are aseptic inoculation pipe, baffle, impeller, air sparger, sampling point, drain point. Main function of a fermentor is to provide a controlled environment for the growth of microorganisms, to obtain a desired product. The vessel should be designed to require the minimal use of labour in operation, harvesting, cleaning and maintenance.

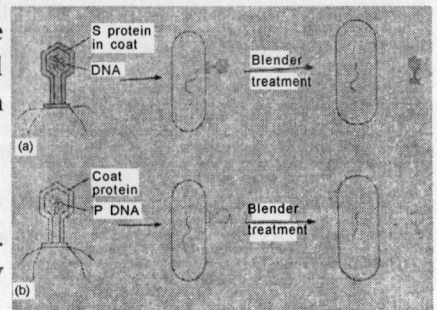

143. Hershey chase experiment

Alfered Hershey and Martha chase demonstrated blender experiment. This experiment is used to demonstrate DNA as a genetic material. They demonstrated that the DNA injected by a phage particle into a bacterium contains all of the information required to synthesize progeny phage particles.

144. Griffith Experiment

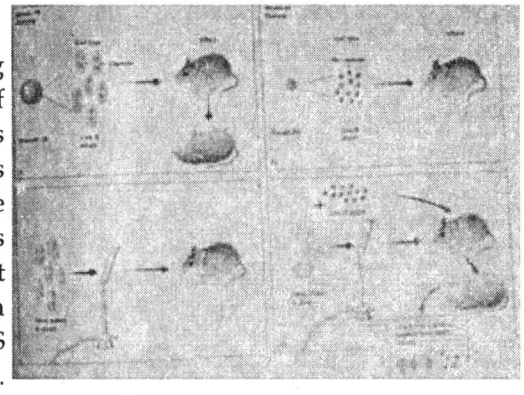

This experiment is performed by Griffith to prove transforming ability of the *Streptococcus pneumoniae* and also for the demonstration of DNA as a genetic material. Two strains of *Streptococcus pneumoniae* is used for this experiment. One is virulent strain (S) another one is avirulent strain(R). S strain of *Streptococcus pneumoniae* is injected to the mice and was died because of pneumonia. Mice are survived when it is injected with R strain of *Streptococcus pneumoniae*. Injection with heat killed strain of *Streptococcus pneumoniae* had no effect. Injection with a Live R strain and a heat killed S strain gave the pneumonia, and Live S strains of *Streptococcus pneumoniae* could be isolated from the dead mice. This confirmed the transformation of virulent DNA from Dead S cells to live avirulent R strains. It leads to conversion of avirulent strain to virulent form. Transformation effect was not observed when the environment is treated with DNase enzyme. Thus DNA carried genetic information required for conversion of R to S strain.

145. EMS (Ethyl methane sulphonate)

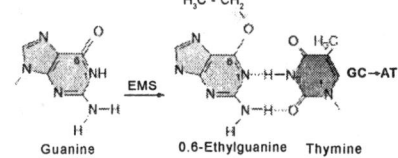

It is an alkylating agent that have been extensively used in genetic research. It induce environmental carcinogenic activity. It is used in chemical warfare and now used in cancer treatment. It will react primarily with guanine, adding an alkyl group to N7 of the purine ring. This alkylation weakens the n-glycosidic bond and greatly increases the depurination. It act as a chemical mutagen. During alkylation DNA base sequence is altered ie.. Conversion of GCGAT, and hydrogen bond is changed.

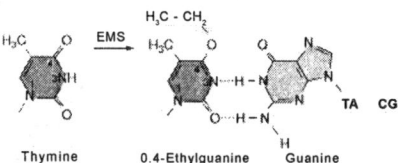

146. Ames test

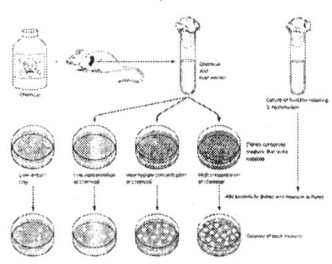

The Ames test developed by Bruce Ames in 1970. It has been widely used to test for cancinogens. The Ames test is a mutational reversion assay employing several special strains of *S.typhimurium* TA 98. The strain of *S.typhimurium* lacks DNA repair system enzymes, which prevent the correction of DNA injury. Mammalian liver enzymes are incorporated into the medium along with the chemical agent. "Plate incorporation test" procedure is adopted to perform Ames test. In this test bacteria, mutagen and liver enzymes are mixed in dilute molter top. Agar is poured on to top of minimal agar plates and incubated for 2 to 3 days at 37⁰C. Histidine also added to the medium". Only revertants that have mutationally regained the ability to synthesize histidine will grow. If the mutagenicity of the chemical is high, the growth of visible colonies is also high. Role of liver enzyme is to induce the mutagenic activity of the test chemical.

147. Replica plating

It is a technique for isolating mutants from a population of microorganisms, grown under non-selective conditions. The culture containing wild type and auxotrophs is plated on complete medium.

After incubation transfer the colonies from the master plate into one or more plates of minimal medium with the help of a disc of sterile velvet. The replica plates are then incubated, only prototrophic cells form colonies. The positions of colonies on the master and replica plates are compared and presumptive auxotrophs are identified by their absence from the replica plates.

148. pBR 322

This plasmid cloning vector is abbreviated as PBR 322 in which P denoted plasmid; B denotes Boliver; R denotes R.Radriguez; 322 denoted the numerial designation. PBR 322 contain 4,361 base pair. It is consist of two resistance gene Amphicillin and Tetracycline. It is also consist Bam HI, HindIII, Sal I recognition site within the tet^r gene. It is also consist of sal PsI recongnition site within Amp^r gene. It is also consist orgin of Replication.

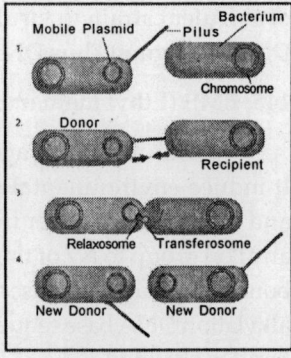

149. Polymerase Chain Reaction (PCR) - Expt. No. 128

150. Conjugation

It is process by which the DNA is transferred from a donar cell to a recepiant cell by cell to cell contact.

It was first discovered in *E.coli* by J.Laderberg and E.L.Tatum in 1951. F plasmid is a plasmid present in conjugative cell. This plasmid is responsible for conjugation. F plasmid has two important genes that are responsible for its character of gene transfer. The genes are Tra+ and Mob+ or nic+. Tra+ - is a transfer gene responsible for the formation of conjugation tube. Mob+ - is a basis of mobilization of gene transfer from cell to cell by conjugation channel . It is naturally occuring process in environment.

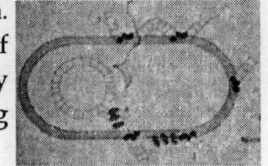

151. Transformation

Transferring of DNA from outside environment to inside of the cell called transformation. Bacterial transformation was first discovered by Griffith (1928) between two strains of *S.pneumoniae* Neisseria, Haemphillus, Bacillus, Staphylococcus, Rhizobium have the capability to accept foreign DNA. naturally. Competence facter play an important role during transformation.

Successful transformation mainly depends on the size of the foreign of DNA

152. Transduction

The transfer of genetic material from one call to another by bacteria phage is called transduction. It was first discovered by Zinder and Lederberg. The infection of bacteriophages is accomplished in several stages such as adsorption, presentation, replication, assembly, lysis and release . Transduction is of two types generalized and specialized. Generalized transduction occurs during the lytic cycle of virulent or temperature phages. Certain temperate phages can also transfer only a few restricted genes of the bacterial chromosome to the recipient bacterial cell. This transfer of bacterial genes adjacent to prophage only to the recipient chromosome is called restricted or specialized transduction . Frequency of transduction based on nature of recipient cell and homologous part of the chromosomes in recipient cell.

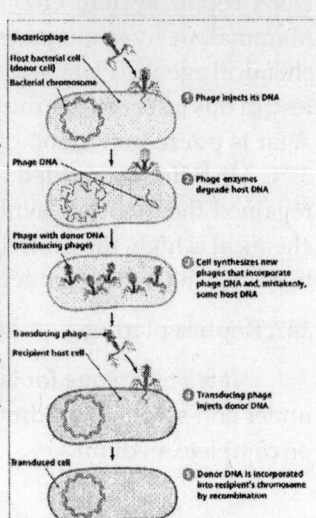

153. Southern Bloting - Refer - Expt. No. 129

154. Western Blotting - Refer - Expt. No. 39 Page 160

155. *Agarobacterium tumefaciens*

It is a gram negative rod shaped bacteria. It causes crown gall disease in plants. The bacterium infects a wound and inserts a short stretch of DNA in to some of the cells around the wound. This bacterium contain Ti plasmid. It mostly affects the dicotyledon plants including grapes, stone fruit trees and roses because their response to wound is compatible with *A.tumefaciens* DNA transfer mechanisms. Transfer of T-DNA help the synthesis of nopaline in plants. This nopaline is used as carbon and nitrogen source for plants . It is cultivated with the help of YEMA medium and the colonies are found as smooth and glistering.

156. Ti plasmid"

Agrobacterium tumifaciens contains a large plasmid which induces Tumour in plant is called Ti plasmid. The size of Ti plasmid ranges between 180 – 250 kb. It contains T – DNA region about 23 – 25 kb which is transferred into plant cells. It can be grouped into these on the basis of opine types, for example, octopine, nopaline, and agropine.

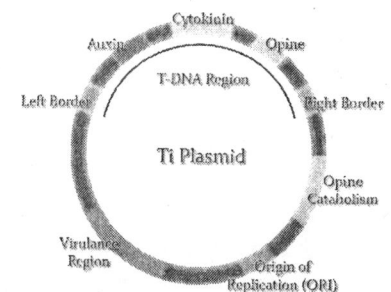

157. Crowngal Disease

Crown gal disease is caused by *Agrobacterium tumefaciens*. This disease occur in plant cell. This disease affects only dicotyledon plants such as grapes, stome fruit trees, sorses. Crowngal formation is the consequence of the transfer, interaction of expression of genes of a specific segment of bacterial plasmid DNA called the T-DNA to the plant cell genome. The T-DNA is actually a tra of the 'tumor inducing' (Ti) plasmid that is carried by most of the strains of *A.tumerfaciens*. Depending on the bacterial strain the Ti plasmid comes from, the length of the T –DNA region can vary from approximately 12 th 20 kb. Strains of *A.trumerfaciens* that do not possess a Tiplasmid cannot induce crown gall tumours.

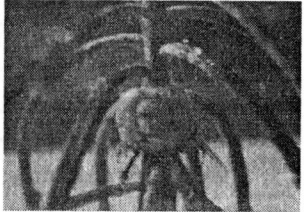

158. Xgal - Refer experiment No - 133 - 362
159. IPTG - Refer experiment No - 133 - 362

160. Lac Operon

The enzymes required for lactose utilization is regulated by lac person. The genes for the 3 enzymes are always transcribed together into a single poly sis tronic lac m RNA. The expression of lac operon is regulated by lac repressor. The lac repressor, a protein having 4 identical subunits of 40,000 daltons each. In E.coli cell there are about 10 lac repressor molecules which are coded by the regulatory gene. The repressor binds strongly and specifically to a short DNA segment called the operator, which is located very close to the start the ß galactosidase gene.

161. Insulin

It is a peptide hormone. It is secreted by the islets of langerhans of pancreas, which catabolizes glucose in blood. It is a boon for the diabetics whose normal function for sugar metabolism generally fails. Insulin consists of two polypepticle chains. Chain A (21 A. A long) and B (30 A. A long). Its precursor is proinsulin which also contains two polypeptide chains A&B. Both A & B are is connected with a third peptide chain – C. Human insulin (humulin) is the first therapeutic product produced by means of recombinant technology by Eli Lilly and Co.

162. Yeast Extract Mannitol Agar Medium

This is a enrichment and selective medium for the isolation of Rhizobium and Agrobacterium. It contains yeast extract; mannitol and congored. Incubation time for Rhizobium growth is 48 – 72 hours. The medium doesn't contain N2 compounds. The Rhizobium produces shiny smooth elevated, glistening colonies. Rhizobium will not use congored but Agrobacterium will use congored and produce pink glistening colonies. PH used for the cultivation of Rhizobium is 7 but for Agrobacterium is 8-9.

163. Bio Film

Microorganisms are grown in solid support and become immobilized, which will produce extracellular polysaccharide. These types of colonization on the surface of the solid support with multilayer are called biofilm. Two methods are available to visualize biofilm that are acrydine orange method and congored staining method.

164. Air sampler

First primitive type of air sampler is pioneered by Wells. A modern version of this sampler is the Reuter Centrifugal air sampler. It is easy to handle and battery powered. It resembles large cylindrical torch with an open-ended drum at one end. The drum encloses impeller blades which can be rotated by battery power when switched on. A plastic strip coated with medium can be inserted along the inner side of the drum. Air is drawn in to the drum and subjected to centrifugal acceleration. This causes the suspended particles to settle on the culture medium. After sampling the strip is removed from the instrument and incubated at 37⁰C for 24 hours and colonies are counted.

165. Eutrophication

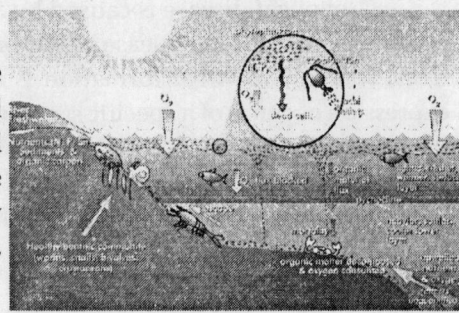

Nutrient enrichment of the environment leads to over growth of algae is called as Eutrophication. The excessive algal growth is referred to as algal bloom. Main effect associated with algal bloom is the production of algal toxin and change of taste and odour. Factors controlling algal bloom are Nutrients, Temperature and Light. Eutrophication is controlled by application of chemical algicide called Copper sulphate, Destratification, Ecological management and advanced water treatment.

166. Oxidation Pond

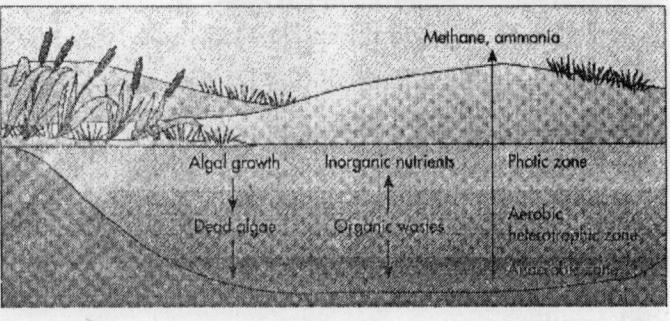

It also called stabilization ponds and lagoons. Aerobic biological oxidation takes place in these ponds, they are classified as facultative, aerobic, anaerobic and maturation ponds. Oxidation ponds are less than 10 feet deep, which maximize algal growth. The pond can be designed to maintain aerobic condition thoughout, but more often decomposition takes place near the surface, which is a aerobic. Oxidation ponds generally are low cost operation but they tend to be inefficient and require large holding capacities and retention times. The effluents containing oxidized products are periodically removed, which are then refilled by raw sewage. Nitrogen is removed by ponds by a number of mechanisms including nitrification, denitrification and ammonification. Ponds remove approximately 40-80% of nitrogen. Oxidation ponds remove significant percentage of indicator and pathogenic bacteria.

167. Activated sludge process

It is a highly efficient system for the aerobic biologic treatment of industrial and municipal wastes. The efficiency of the process depends on the use of high concentration of microorganisms in the form of floc. Sufficient air must be transferred to maintain dissolved oxygen. Aim of this process includes oxidation of biodegradable organic matter and flocculation-separation of newly formed biomass from the treated effluent. Significance of this process is reduction of BOD, reduction of suspended solids, reduction of number of bacteria including pathogens.

168. Trickling filter

It is a simple and relatively inexpensive film-flow type of aerobic sewage treatment method. The film consists of an outer layer of larger fungi, a middle layer of smaller fungi and algae and inner layer with bacteria, algae and fungi. The sewage is distributed by a revolving springler suspended over a bed of porous material. The sewage slowly percolates through the porous bed and the effluent is collected at the bottom. Trickling filters can remove 85-98% of applied BOD and suspended particles and 90-98% of viruses. Fungi used in the system is Fusarium and Bacteria includes Pseudomonas, Flavobacterium, Alkaligens, Zooglea. Algae used are Ulothrix, Chlorella and Euglena. Advantages of this technique are easy operation, low maintanence, cost, reliability and ability to withstand shock loads of toxic inputs

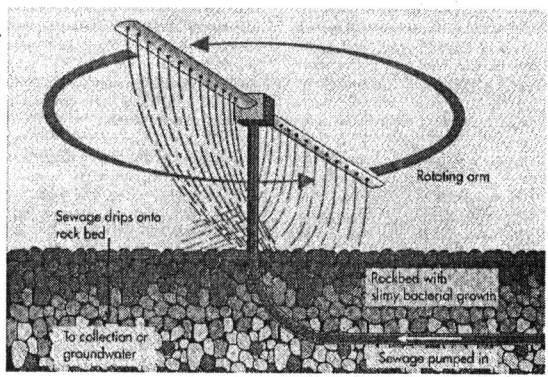

169. Anaerobic digesters

It is a large fermentation tank designed for continuous operation under anaerobic condition. Provision of mechanical mixing, heating, gas collection, sludge addition and draw off of stabilized sludge are incorporated. Anaerobic digestion of wastes can be considered as a two-step process. Complex organic materials are depolymerated and converted into simple form. It is also used for the Production of methane and carbondi oxide. It is a relatively expensive process.

170. Bacteriophage

It is a bacterial virus that contains nucleic acid enclosed in a capsid made up of capsomers. The capsid consists of protein subunits, the protomers. The bacteriophages have hexagonal head, rigid tail with contactile sheath. Most of the bacteriophages are tadpole shaped and consists of 5 important structures such as head, head-tail connection, tail plate and tail fibers. T-even phage contains double stranded (DS) DNA, they multiply with the help of bacteria, use bacterial machinery for multiplication. They infect bacteria resulting into lysis, yield newly synthesized viral particles.

171. Embryonated Eggs - Refer - Expt No. 139 - Page No. 371

172. Escherichia coli

It causes gastroenteritis in human. It is an important cause of acute watery diarrhoea in adults and children. *E.coli* is a common member of the normal flora of the large intestine. As long as these bacteria do not acquire genetic elements encoding for virulence factors, they remain benign commensals. *E.coli* is the head of the large bacterial family, Enterobacteriaceae, the enteric bacteria, which are facultative anaerobic Gram-negative rod. It's nutritional requirement is very simple, grow very fastly and its genome is well known one. *E.coli* can respond to environmental signals such as chemicals, pH, temperature, etc., It is grown on EMB, XLD ,MacConkey and Hektoein enteric agar. Virulence Determinants of Pathogenic *E. coli* are Adhesins, CFAI/CFAII fimbriae , Intimin (non-fimbrial adhesin, Invasins, hemolysins, **flagella, toxins** - LT toxin, ST toxin, Shiga-like toxin, cytotoxins, **endotoxin** (LPS).

Five classes of *E. coli* that cause diarrhoeal diseases are now recognized: EnteroToxigenic *E. coli* (ETEC), EnteroInvasive *E. coli* (EIEC), EnteroHemorrhagic *E. coli* (EHEC), EnteroPathogenic *E. coli* (EPEC), and EnteroAggregative *E. coli* (EAggEC).

173. *Vibrio cholerae*

Vibrio cholerae is a causative agent of cholera. It is a Gram-negative comma shaped bacilli with single polar flagellum. It was first isolated in pure culture by Robert Koch in 1883. Most vibrios have relatively simple growth factor requirements and will grow in synthetic media with glucose as a sole source of carbon and energy. However, since Vibrios are typically marine organisms, most species require large amount of NaCl or seawater base for optimal growth. Vibrios vary in their nutritional versatility, but some species will grow on more than 150 different organic compounds as carbon and energy sources, occupying the same level of metabolic versatility as *Pseudomonas*. In liquid media vibrios are motile by polar flagella. Generation time for *Vibrio cholerae* is less than 30 minutes. In Human it produce a infection called Cholera with a symptom called Diarrhoea (Rice Water Stool). It grows well on TCBS agar and produce yellow colour colonies.

174. *Bordetella pertussis*

Bordetella pertussis was first isolated in pure culture in 1906 by Bordet and Gengou from the sputum of children. Formerly it is called *Hemophillus pertussis*. It is a small ovoid coccobacilli, non motile and non sporing. It is capsulated, but tends to lose the capsule on repeated cultivation. It's bipolar metachromatic granules are demonstrated by toludine blue staining. Bacteria are nutritionally fastidious and are usually cultivated on rich media supplemented with blood. On blood agar, organism grows slowly and requires 3-6 days to form pinpoint colonies. The organisms are strict aerobe and grows best at 35-36°C. It does not ferment sugars, form indole, reduce nitrates, utilize citrate, hydrolyse urea and catalase, oxidase positive. It is a delicate organism being killed readily by heating, drying and disinfectants. Freshly isolated strains have fimbriae. Organism is sensitive to unsaturated fatty acids,sulfides and peroxides.

175. *Neisseria meningitidis*

It is also called Meningococcus. It is a Gram-negative coccus, usually seen in pairs. *Neisseria meningitis* strains are grouped on the basis of their capsular polyscccharide into 12 serogroups. *Neisseria meningitis* is usually cultivated in a peptone blood based medium in a moist chamber containing 5-10 % of CO_2. New York city agar medium and Modified Thayer Martin are agar acts as a selective medium.

176. *Neisseria gonorrhoea*

Gonorrhoea is caused by *Neisseria gonorrhoea*. It is also called Gonococcus. Neisser first described it in gonorrhoeal pus in 1879. Bumm in 1885 cultured the coccus and proved its pathogenecity. It is a Gram negative coccus. It's a fastidious organism, 20% of strains require glutamine for primary isolation. Growth occurs best at pH 7.2-7.6 and at the temperature of 35 – 36°C. Some strains require 5-10 % carbon di oxide. A popular selective medium is the Thayer martin medium, the medium contains Vancomycin, Colistin, Nystatin and Trimethoprim lactate, Vancomycin inhibits gram-positive bacteria. Colistin inhibits gram-negative bacteria except Proteus, Nystatin inhibits yeast cells Trimethoprime lactate inhibits *Proteus*. Gonococci only ferment glucose and not maltose.

177. *Staphylococcus*

Staphylo means grape like clusters, which is due to three-planar cell division. Staphylococci are gram positive spherical bacteria. Von Reckling Heusen first observed it in human pyogenic lesions in 1871. Sir Alexander Ogston demonstrated the causative role of Staphylococcus in 1880.Most significant pathogens of this genus is *S.aureus*. Staphylococci are among the more resistant of non sporing bacteria. Non motile, Non spore former, facultative anaerobe. Fermentation of glucose produce lactic acids Catalase positive, Coagulase positive, Ferment mannitol. It produce golden yellow colony on Nutrient agar. Produce beta hemolysis on blood agar. Utilize Potassium tellurite and reduce it into telluramine and produce black colonies. *S.epidermidis* produce white colonies on Nutrient Agar and Non β hemolytic colony on blood agar.

178. *Streptococcus pneumoniae*

It causes epidemic or even pandemic form of Pneumonia. It remains a leading cause of morbidity and mortality in humans of all ages. Pneumonia is the sixth leading cause of death in the United States. Streptococcus was first isolated by Pasteur and Sternbery independenly during the year 1881 from human saliva. It is a facultative Gram-positive coccus. Also called Diplococcus, often called Pneumococcus. Capsulated, Nonmotile, Alpha haemolytic, sometimes lancet shaped. Inulin fermenter. Bile solubilizer

179. *Corynebacterium diphtheriae*

Corynebacteria are gram-positive, aerobic, nonmotile, rod-shaped bacteria. They have the characteristic of forming irregular shaped, club-shaped or V-shaped arrangements in normal growth. They undergo snapping movements just after cell division, which brings them into characteristic arrangements resembling Chinese letters. **Three strains of *Corynebacterium diphtheriae* are recognized by Mc.Leod on the basis of growth and other characters , gravis, intermedius and mitis. The gravis strain has a generation time (in vitro) of 60 minutes; the intermedius strain has a generation time of about 100 minutes; and the mitis stain has a generation time of about 180 minutes. The faster growing strains typically produce a larger colony on most growth media. It produces a disease called Diphtheria.**

180. *Clostridium perfringens*

It is usually shorter gram positive rods. Capsules may be observed by direct observation of smear from wounds but are not uniformly demonstrable in culture. Spores are central or subterminal but are rarely seen in artificial cultures. It is non motile, aerotolerent anaerobe. In blood agar plate, it produce double zone of haemolysis . They produce invasive enzymes like proteases, DNases, collagenases.. Alpha toxin most important (lecithinase, phospholipase C) and Phage encoded. Lecithin is major lipid in cell membranes. Lecithinase cause Capillary endothelial cells cause leakage, oedema, myonecrosis.

181. *Clostridium tetani*

It is quite long and thin organism. It is usually gram positive and produce terminal spore, so it appears like drumstick. Motility by peritrichous flagella. Obligate anaerobe. Optimum temperature 37°C and pH 7.4. Moderately fastidious requires vitamins and amino acids for growth. Noncapsulated, organisms grows in cooked meat medium with turbidity and some gas formation within 48 hours, there is no digestion of meat., It doesn't ferment any carbohydrate. In horse blood agar, alpha haemolysis is observed first, then beta haemolysis is observed due to prolonged incubation and production of haemolysins. Indole positive, Methyl red and voges proskauer negative. It produce two toxins namely Tetanolysin & Tetanospasmin. Tetanolysin- It disturb the activity of RBC and WBC. It is oxygen labile and heat labile. Tetanospasmin- It is responsible for the symptoms of tetanus. Toxins are released during autolysis of cell.

182. *Mycobacterium tuberculosis*

It is an Acid-Fast Bacilli. It is due to mycolic acid content of the cell wall. It is fairly large nonmotile rod shaped bacterium. Nonspore former, Non capsulated. In tissue it is thin straight rods, occurring singly, in pairs or in clumps. Generation time is 6-12 hours. Optimum temperature is 37°C, pH is 6.4 –7. They only grow in the media containing egg, asparagine, potatoes and serum. Muramyl dipeptide complexed with mycolic acid can cause granuloma formation. Phosphatide induce tubercle formation. Lipid can cause accumulation of macrophages and neutrophils. **Virulent strains of Tubercle bacilli form microscopic serpendine cords in which bacilli are arranged in parellel chains.**

183. *Mycobacterium leprae*

M.leprae causes leprosy. It was the first bacilli isolated from human. It is one of the least understood bacterium. Hanson, a Norwagion physician first observed it. It is a straight or slightly curved rods showing considerable morphological variations. Organisms are found singly or in large masses termed globi. Large numbers of bacilli may be packed in the cells in an arrangement that suggests packets of cigars. It is one of the Acid-Fast Bacilli. The presence of a phenolase in *M.leprae* obtained from lepromatous skin nodule provides simplest test for separating *M.leprae* from other Mycobacterium. It grows well on footpads of ninebanded armadillo at 30°C. This temperature is obtained by controlling air temperatures at 20°C-25°C.

184. *Treponema pallidum*

Syphilis is caused by spirochaete *Treponema pallidum*. *Treponema* is a gram-negative, thin, motile, spiral shaped bacterium in the order *Spirochaetales*. The name *Spirochete* is derived from the Greek words for "coiled hair." The spirochaetes are able to swim in viscous environments (e.g. oral cavity, intestinal tract). *T. pallidum* requires the presence of tissue culture cells, a microaerobic environment and serum components for growth. Its fastidious nature may account for its obligate parasitism. This microorganism is responsible for natural disease in humans only, although rabbits can be infected experimentally. *T. pallidum* cannot be grown in cell free cultures.

185. Blood Agar

Blood agar is used for the differentiation of *Staphylococcus, Streptococcus* and others based on haemolysis.5% defibrinated sheep blood is recommended for the preparation of blood agar. Three haemolytic patterns are described in blood agar, Alpha hemolysis- Partial hemolysis; Beta hemolysis- Complete hemolysis; Gamma hemolysis- No hemolysis. Coagulase positive *Staphylococcus aureus* produce beta haemolysis. *Streptococcus pyogenes* produce beta haemolysis when it is incubated anaerobically. Based on the type of supplements added to the blood agar its name will vary, they are Neomycin blood agar, Ampicillin blood agar, Tellurite ceffixime blood agar, Kanamycin blood agar. Supplements are used to select particular species from the human body. Satellism pattern is described when *H.influenzae* is cross inoculated with *Staphylococcus aureus*.

186. EMB AGAR(Eosin Methylene Blue agar)

It is a selective cum differential medium used for the isolation of Gram-negative enteric organisms. Eosin and methylene blue used as a indicator in EMB medium. Gram-positive organisms are inhibited by the action of eosin and methylene blue mixture. Those organisms that ferment one or two sugars appear as black or dark centered colonies e.g. Enterobacter.*E.coli* produce metallic sheen colonies because of it ferments all sugars available in the medium and reduce the pH of the medium, acidic pH precipitates the both dyes and observe metallic sheen. Colonies that don't ferment lactose or sucrose is transparent. Adding 5% agar inhibits Proteus swarming motility. *Pseudomonas aeruginosa* produce umbonate colonies with filamentous margin, usually violet in appearance.

187. Hektoein Enteric Agar

HE agar is recommended for the isolation of Salmonella and Shigella from faecal specimens. It contains lactose, sucrose and salicin. Bromothymol blue and acid fuchsin acts as an indicator. Salmonella and Shigella do not ferment any of the sugars available in the medium and produce blue or green colour colonies.In the presence of acid bromothymol blue produce yellow colour, and the acid fuchsin produces red colour. The combination of yellow and red produces orange or pink or salmon colour.

Salmonella - Produce Blue green with black centers,

Shigella - Produce Small greenish colonies

E.coli Enterobacter,Klebsiella - Produce Salmon colour colonies.

188. XLD Agar

Xylose Lysine Deoxycholate Agar. It is a selective cum differential media used for the isolation of enteric pathogens. Selectivity nature is increased through the addition of deoxycholate. Lysine is incorporated into the medium to offset the acid production. If the organism is only ferments xylose the colour of the colony is pink, depletion of xylose leads to lysine decarboxlation which cause reversion of pH. Phenol red acts as a indicator.Lactose and sucrose fermentors produce yellow colonies. Sodium thiosulphate is a sulphur source.Ferric ions acts as a indicator for the hydrogen sulphide production.

Colony appearance on XLD agar.
Yellow colony:*Escherichia.coli, Enterobacter, Klebsiella, Serratia and Citroba*cter.
Yellow colony with black center:*Citrobacter freundii, Proteus*
Red colony:*Shigella,Pseudomonas*
Red colony with black center :*Salmonella and Edwardsiella.*

189. Mac Conkey Agar

It is used for the differentiation of enteric organisms. Lactose is the main carbohydrate, which acts as a differential source based on lactose utilization. Lactose utilizing microorganisms produce pink colour colonies , which are referred to as LF colonies. Non lactose fermenting colonies produce yellowish colonies and are called NLF colonies. Gram positive organisms are inhibited by bile salts in the medium.

Escherichia coli — Pink colour rough colonies
Klebsiella –Pink colour mucoid colonies
Salmonella , Shigella, Pseudomonas produce NLF colonies.

190. Chocolate Agar

It is sometimes called CHOC agar. It is used for the cultivation of fastidious microorganisms like *H.influenzae*, *N. meningititis* and *N.gonorrhoea*.It provides X and V factor for the growth of fastidious microorganisms. It is prepared heating blood agar at 100^0C for 10-minutes in-water bath. Because of its colour after heating, the name was given. Additional enrichment and inhibitory substances are added to the medium to enhance the growth of specific microorganisms.

191. CLED agar

It is an acronym of Cystine Lactose Electrolyte Deficiency medium. CLED agar with bromothymol blue is recommend for the isolation, enumeration and identification of urinary pathogens on the basis of lactose fermentation. The nutrients in CLED Agar are supplied by peptones, pancreatic digests of gelatin casein, and beef extract. Lactose is included to provide an energy source for organisms capable of utilizing it by a fermentative mechanism. The cystine permits the growth of "dwarf colony" coliforms. Bromthymol blue is used as a pH indicator to differentiate lactose fermenters from lactose nonfermenters. Organisms that ferment lactose will lower the pH and change the colour of the medium from green to yellow. Electrolyte sources are reduced in order to restrict the swarming of *Proteus* species.

Typical colonial morphology on CLED Agar is as follows:
Escherichia coli : Yellow colonies, opaque, center slightly deeper yellow
Klebsiella : Yellow to whitish-blue colonies, extremely mucoid
Proteus : Translucent blue colonies
Pseudomonas aeruginosa : Green colonies with typical matted surface and rough periphery
Enterococci : Small yellow colonies, about 0.5 mm in diameter
Staphylococcus aureus : Deep yellow colonies, uniform in colour
Staphylococci coagulase-negative : Pale yellow colonies, more opaque than *E. faecalis*

192. Cooked Meat Medium

In 1916, Robertson developed a cooked meat medium for use in the cultivation of certain anaerobe. Cooked Meat Medium is still widely used for the cultivation and maintenance of Clostridia and for determining proteolytic activity of anaerobes. Cooked Meat Medium provides a favourable environment for the growth of anaerobes, since the muscle protein in the heart tissue granules is a source of amino acids and other nutrients. The muscle tissue also provides reducing substances, particularly glutathione, which permits the growth of strict anaerobes. During the cultivation of clostridia, saccharolytic organisms usually produce acid and gas. Growth of proteolytic organisms is generally characterized by blackening and dissolution of the meat particles. *Clostridium tetani* produces proteolytic reaction; *Clostridium perfringens* produce saccharolytic reaction

193. Cetrimide Agar

It is a selective medium used for the isolation of *Pseudomonas aeruginosa* from pus, sputum, drains etc.It is also used for determining the ability of an organism to produce fluorescein and pycocyanin. Cetrimide (Cetyllrimethyl ammonium bromide) is incorporated in the medium to inhibit microbes other than *P.aeruginosa*. *P.aeruginosa* colonies may appear pigmented blue, blue green or non-pigmented. Cetrimide act as a quaternary ammonium compound, which cause release of N_2, phosphorus from bacterial cells other than *P.aeruginosa*.

194. TCBS agar

It is recommended for the isolation and cultivation of Vibrio. TCBS Agar is highly selective for the isolation of *V. cholerae* and *V. parahaemolyticus* as well as other vibrios. Inhibition of gram-positive bacteria is achieved by the incorporation of oxgall, which is a naturally occurring substance containing a mixture of bile salts, and sodium cholate, a pure bile salt. Sodium thiosulfate serves as a sulfur source and, in combination with ferric citrate, detects hydrogen sulfide production. Saccharose (sucrose) is included as a fermentable carbohydrate for the metabolism of vibrios. The alkaline pH of the medium enhances the recovery of *V. cholerae*. Thymol blue and bromthymol blue are included as indicators of pH changes.

Typical colonial morphology on TCBS Agar is as follows:
V. cholerae .... Large yellow colonies.
V. parahaemolyticus .... Colonies with blue to green centers.
V. alginolyticus .... Large yellow colonies.

195. Baired Parker Agar

It is a selective medium for the isolation of coagulase positive *Staphylococous aureus*. It was developed by Baired Parker. Lithium chloride and Potassium tellurite is incorporated into the medium as a selective agent. Glycin is added to the medium to enhance the growth of *Staphylococus*. Egg yolk emulsion is used to identify the proteolytic character of the isolate. During growth *S. aureus* utilize potassium tellurite, convert it into telluramine and produce black colonies.

X. Appendix E – Sources of Microorganisms

American Type Culture Collection
12301 Parklawn Drive
Rockville, MD 20852–1776
USA/Canada 1-800-638-6597
Outside USA/Canada 1-301-881-2600
FAX 1-301-231-5826
www.atcc.org

REMEL
PO Box 14428
12076 Santa Fe Drive
Lenexa, KA 66215–3594
1-800-255-6730
FAX 1-800-447-3643
www.remelinc.org

Difco Laboratories
Division of Becton Dickinson Company
Becton Drive
Franklin Lakes, NJ 07417
1-202-847-6800
FAX 1-410-584-7121
www.bd.com/microbiology

ICN Pharmaceuticals Inc.
1263 South Chillicothe
Aura, Ohio 44202
1-800-854-0530
FAX 1-800-334-6999
www.biomark@icnbiomed.com

Thomas Scientific
PO Box 99
Swedesboro, NJ 08085
1-800-345-2100
FAX 1-800-345-5232
www.thomassci.com

VWR Scientific Products
Educational Division
1310 Goshen Parkway
West Chester, PA 19380–5985
1-800-932-5000
FAX 1-610-436-1761
www.vwrsp.com

Becton Dickinson
Microbiological Systems
PO Box 243
Cockeysville, MD 21030–0248
1-201-818-8900
FAX 410-584-7121
www.bd.com

Curator
Microbial Type Culture Collection & Gene Bank
Institute of Microbial TechnologySector 39-A,
Chandigarh-160036
India
Phones 2690562,2695215,2695216
Fax: 2690632/2690585
Telegram: IMTECH
E.mail: tapan@imtech.res.in
www.imtech.res.in

X. Appendix F – Sources of Media, Chemicals and Glasswares

Himedia Laboratories
A-406, Bhaveshwar Plaza, LBS Marg, Mumbai - 400 086, India
Phone: 91-022-2500 0970, 2500 3747, 2500 1607, 2500 0653
Fax: 91-022-2500 5764, 2500 2468, 2500 2286
www.himedialabs.com

Difco Laboratories
Division of Becton Dickinson Company
Becton Drive
Franklin Lakes, NJ 07417
1-202-847-6800
FAX 1-410-584-7121
www.bd.com/microbiology

ICN Pharmaceuticals Inc.
1263 South Chillicothe
Aura, Ohio 44202
1-800-854-0530
FAX 1-800-334-6999
www.biomark@icnbiomed.com

Thomas Scientific
PO Box 99
Swedesboro, NJ 08085
1-800-345-2100
FAX 1-800-345-5232
www.thomassci.com

EM Science
480 Democrat Road
Gibbstown, NJ 08027
1-800-222-0342
FAX 1-856-423-4389
www.emscience.com

Qualigens Fine Chemicals
Dr. Annie Basant Road, Worli,
Near Doordarshan, Mumbai 110 04,
Maharashtra
P: +(91)-(22)-24959268 .

GENEI Industries, Inc.
1930 South 23rd St.
Saginaw, MI 48601
Phone:(989)752-6424
Fax: (989)752-1546
www.genei.com

Borosil Glass Works Limited
Khanna Construction House, 44,
R.G. Thadani Marg, Worli,
Mumbai- 400706 (India)
Ph : +91 22 24930362 / 24930366
Fax : +91 22 24950561
www.borosil.com

X. Appendix G –Calculations

Atomic weight

The average mass of atoms of an element, calculated using the relative abundance of isotopes in a naturally occurring element. It is the weighted average of the masses of naturally occurring isotopes. Also Known As: Atomic Mass. Examples: The atomic mass of carbon is 12.011; the atomic mass of hydrogen is 1.0079.

Molecular Mass (Molecular Weight)

In theory, the relative molecular mass or molecular weight of a compound is the mass of a molecule of the compound relative to the mass of a carbon atom taken as exactly 12. In practice, the molecular mass, MM, (molecular weight, MW) of a compound is the sum of the atomic masses (atomic weights) of the atomic species as given in the molecular formula.

Calculate the Molecular Mass (MM) of the compound ammonium sulfate, $(NH_4)_2SO_4$

The formula of ammonium sulfate is composed of two atoms of nitrogen, eight atoms of hydrogen, one atom of sulfur and four atoms of oxygen

Atomic mass nitrogen = 14.01 (from the Periodic Table)
Atomic mass hydrogen = 1.008 (from the Periodic Table)
Atomic mass of sulfur = 32.06 (from the Periodic Table)
Atomic mass of oxygen = 16.00 (from the Periodic Table)

Molecular Mass (MM) for ammonium sulfate $(NH_4)_2SO_4$

= (2 x atomic mass nitrogen) + (8 x atomic mass hydrogen) + atomic mass sulfur + (4 x atomic mass oxygen)

Molecular Mass (MM) = (2 x 14.01) + (8 x 1.008) + 32.06 + (4 x 16.00)

= 28.02 + 8.064 + 32.06 + 64.00
= 132.144g/mole

Alternatively, Molecular Mass (MM) = [2 x molecular mass ammonium ions (NH_4)] + atomic mass sulfur + (4 x atomic mass oxygen)

Molecular Mass (MM) = {2 x [14.01 + (4 x 1.008)]} + 32.06 + (4 x 16.00)

= {2 x [14.01 + 4.032]} + 32.06 + 64.00
= {2 x 18.042} + 32.06 + 64.00
= 36.084 + 32.06 + 64.00
= 132.144g/mol

Percent Composition (Percentage Composition)

The percent composition (percentage composition) of a compound is a relative measure of the mass of each different element present in the compound.

To calculate the percent composition (percentage composition) of a compound

Calculate the <u>molecular mass</u> (molecular weight, formula mass, formula weight), MM, of the compound

Calculate the total mass of each element present in the formula of the compound

Calculate the percent compositon (percentage composition): % by weight (mass) of element

= (total mass of element present ÷ molecular mass) x 100

Calculate the percent by weight of sodium (Na) and chlorine (Cl) in sodium chloride (NaCl)

Calculate the molecular mass (MM):

MM = 22.99 + 35.45 = 58.44

Calculate the total mass of Na present:

1 Na is present in the formula, mass = 22.99

Calculate the percent by weight of Na in NaCl:

%Na = (mass Na ÷ MM) x 100 = (22.99 ÷ 58.44) x 100 = 39.34%

Calculate the total mass of Cl present:

1 Cl is present in the formula, mass = 35.45

Calculate the percent by weight of Cl in NaCl:

%Cl = (mass Cl ÷ MM) x 100 = (35.45 ÷ 58.44) x 100 = 60.66%

The answers above are probably correct if %Na + %Cl = 100, that is, 39.34 + 60.66 = 100.

Equivalent weight

The equivalent weight of an element or radical is equal to its atomic weight or formula weight divided by the <u>valence</u> it assumes in compounds. The unit of equivalent weight is the atomic mass unit ; the amount of a substance in grams numerically equal to the equivalent weight is called a gram equivalent. Hydrogen has atomic weight 1.008 and always assumes valence 1 in compounds, so its equivalent weight is 1.008. Oxygen has an atomic weight of 15.9994 and always assumes valence 2 in compounds, so its equivalent weight is 7.9997. Iron (atomic weight 55.845) has an equivalent weight of 27.9225 in ferrous compounds (valence 2) and 18.615 in ferric compounds (valence 3).

Molar Solutions

A 1 molar solution is a solution in which 1 mole of a compound is dissolved in a total volume of 1 litre.

For example: The molecular weight of sodium chloride (NaCl) is 58.44, so one gram molecular weight (= 1 mole) is 58.44g. If you dissolve 58.44g of NaCl in a final volume of 1 litre, you have made a 1M NaCl solution.

To make a 0.1M NaCl solution, you could weigh 5.844g of NaCl and dissolve it in 1 litre of water; OR 0.5844g of NaCl in 100mL of water (see animation below); OR make a 1:10 dilution of a 1M sample.

$$\text{Molarity (M)} = \frac{\text{Number of Moles of Solute}}{\text{Solution Volume (Liter/s)}}$$

Solutions made using percentage by weight (w/v)

The number of grams in 100mL of solution is indicated by the percentage. For example, a 1% solution has one gram of solid dissolved in 100mL of solvent. To make this type of solution properly, you should weight 1g and dissolve it in slightly less than 100mL. Once the solids have dissolved, you can bring the volume up to the final 100mL (see animation below).

Solutions made using percentage by volume (v/v)

In this case, the percentage indicates the volume of the full strength solution in 100mL of dilute solution.

Normal solution

A solution that contains one gram-equivalent of replaceable hydrogen per litre of solution, multiples of this concentration being expressed as like multiples of N. Thus one litre of solution containing 1 gram relative molecular mass of HCl would be an N solution, but the like of H_2SO_4, because of the two hydrogen atoms per molecule, would be a 2N solution.

Units of measurements Metric Prefixes

To help the SI units apply to a wide range of phenomena, the 19th General Conference on Weights and Measures in 1991 extended the list of metric prefixes so that it reaches from yotta- at 10^{24} (one septillion) to yocto- at 10^{-24} (one septillionth). Here are the metric prefixes, with their numerical equivalents stated in the American system for naming large numbers:

yotta- (Y-)	10^{24}	1 septillion
zetta- (Z-)	10^{21}	1 sextillion
exa- (E-)	10^{18}	1 quintillion
peta- (P-)	10^{15}	1 quadrillion
tera- (T-)	10^{12}	1 trillion
giga- (G-)	10^{9}	1 billion
mega- (M-)	10^{6}	1 million
kilo- (k-)	10^{3}	1 thousand
hecto- (h-)	10^{2}	1 hundred
deka- (da-)**	10	1 ten
deci- (d-)	10^{-1}	1 tenth
centi- (c-)	10^{-2}	1 hundredth
milli- (m-)	10^{-3}	1 thousandth
micro- (μ-)	10^{-6}	1 millionth
nano- (n-)	10^{-9}	1 billionth
pico- (p-)	10^{-12}	1 trillionth
femto- (f-)	10^{-15}	1 quadrillionth
atto- (a-)	10^{-18}	1 quintillionth
zepto- (z-)	10^{-21}	1 sextillionth
yocto- (y-)	10^{-24}	1 septillionth

ISO Standard Paper Sizes

A Series Formats		B Series Formats		C Series Formats	
4A0	1682 × 2378	-	-	-	-
2A0	1189 × 1682	-	-	-	-
A0	841 × 1189	B0	1000 × 1414	C0	917 × 1297
A1	594 × 841	B1	707 × 1000	C1	648 × 917
A2	420 × 594	B2	500 × 707	C2	458 × 648
A3	297 × 420	B3	353 × 500	C3	324 × 458
A4	210 × 297	B4	250 × 353	C4	229 × 324
A5	148 × 210	B5	176 × 250	C5	162 × 229
A6	105 × 148	B6	125 × 176	C6	114 × 162
A7	74 × 105	B7	88 × 125	C7	81 × 114
A8	52 × 74	B8	62 × 88	C8	57 × 81
A9	37 × 52	B9	44 × 62	C9	40 × 57
A10	26 × 37	B10	31 × 44	C10	28 × 40

Note: To convert the dimensions to inches, divide by 25.4. Thus an A4 sheet measures 8.27 by 11.69 inches, making it a little taller and narrower than an 8.5 by 11 inch sheet.

Derived Units of the International System (SI)

Derived Unit	Measures	Derivation	Formal Definition
hertz (Hz)	frequency	/s	s^{-1}
newton (N)	force	$kg \cdot (m/s^2)$	$kg \cdot m \cdot s^{-2}$
pascal (Pa)	pressure	N/m^2	$kg \cdot m^{-1} \cdot s^{-2}$
joule (J)	energy or work	$N \cdot m$	$kg \cdot m^2 \cdot s^{-2}$
watt (W)	power	J/s	$kg \cdot m^2 \cdot s^{-3}$
coulomb (C)	electric charge	$A \cdot s$	$A \cdot s$
volt (V)	electric potential	W/A	$kg \cdot m^2 \cdot s^{-3} \cdot A^{-1}$
farad (F)	electric capacitance	C/V	$kg^{-1} \cdot m^{-2} \cdot s^4 \cdot A^2$
ohm (omega)	electric resistance	V/A	$kg \cdot m^2 \cdot s^{-3} \cdot A^{-2}$
siemens (S)	electric conductance	A/V	$kg^{-1} \cdot m^{-2} \cdot s^3 \cdot A^2$
weber (Wb)	magnetic flux	$V \cdot s$	$kg \cdot m^2 \cdot s^{-2} \cdot A^{-1}$
tesla (T)	magnetic flux density	Wb/m^2	$kg \cdot s^{-2} \cdot A^{-1}$
henry (H)	inductance	Wb/A	$kg \cdot m^2 \cdot s^{-2} \cdot A^{-2}$
degree Celsius (°C)	temperature	K - 273.15	K
radian (rad)	plane angle		$m \cdot m^{-1}$
steradian (sr)	solid angle		$m^2 \cdot m^{-2}$
lumen (lm)	luminous flux	$cd \cdot sr$	$cd \cdot sr$
lux (lx)	illuminance	lm/m^2	$m^{-2} \cdot cd \cdot sr^{-1}$
becquerel (Bq)	activity	/s	s^{-1}
gray (Gy)	absorbed dose	J/kg	$m^2 \cdot s^{-2}$
sievert (Sv)	dose equivalent	$Gy \cdot (multiplier)$	$m^2 \cdot s^{-2}$
katal (kat)	catalytic activity	mol/s	$mol \cdot s^{-1}$

The term *derived unit* covers any algebraic combination of the base units, but it is only the 22 combinations listed above that have approved special names. For example, the SI derived unit of momentum (mass times velocity) has no special name; momentum is stated in kilogram meters per second (kg·m/s) or in newton seconds (N·s). A few SI derived units do have special names that have been defined but not approved. Here are some examples:

Units of Length

10 millimeters (mm) = 1 centimeter (cm)
10 centimeters = 1 decimeter (dm) = 100 millimeters
10 decimeters = 1 meter (m) = 1000 millimeters
10 meters = 1 dekameter (dam)
10 dekameters = 1 hectometer (hm) = 100 meters
10 hectometers = 1 kilometer (km) = 1000 meters

Units of Area

100 square millimeters (mm2) = 1 square centimeter (cm2)
100 square centimeters = 1 square decimeter (dm2)
100 square decimeters = 1 square meter (m2)
100 square meters = 1 square dekameter (dam2) = 1 are

100 square decameters = 1 square hectometer (hm2) = 1 hectare (ha)
100 square hectometers = 1 square kilometer (km2)

Units of Liquid Volume

10 milliliters (mL) = 1 centiliter (cL)
10 centiliters= 1 deciliter (dL) = 100 milliliters
10 deciliters= 1 liter[1] = 1000 milliliters
10 liters= 1 dekaliter (daL)
10 dekaliters= 1 hectoliter (hL) = 100 liters
10 hectoliters= 1 kiloliter (kL) = 1000 liters
1 galon =U.S. 3.785 liters= British 4.546 liters.

Units of Volume

1000 cubic millimeters (mm3) = 1 cubic centimeter (cm3)
1000 cubic centimeters= 1 cubic decimeter (dm3)= 1 000 000 cubic millimeters
1000 cubic decimeters= 1 cubic meter (m3)= 1 000 000 cubic centimeters= 1 000 000 000 cubic millimeters

Units of Mass

 10 milligrams (mG)= 1 centigram (cg)
10 centigrams= 1 decigram (dg) = 100 milligrams
10 decigrams= 1 gram (g) = 1000 milligrams
10 grams= 1 dekagram (dag)
10 dekagrams= 1 hectogram (hg) = 100 grams
10 hectograms= 1 kilogram (kg) = 1000 grams
1000 kilograms= 1 megagram (Mg) or 1 metric ton(t)

A confusing unit of measure is a barrel. A barrel's capacity is determined often by who uses the term, or what it contains. For example:

1 barrel (bbl) of petroleum or related products = 42 gallons.
1 barrel of Portland cement is 376 pounds.
1 barrel of flour - 196 pounds.
1 barrel of pork or fish - 200 pounds.
1 barrel of (US) dry measure is 3.29122 bushels or 4.2104 cubic feet

How to convert Celsius temperatures to Fahrenheit

Multiply the Celsius temperature by 9/5.
Add 32° to adjust for the offset in the Fahrenheit scale.
Example: convert 37° C to Fahrenheit.
37 * 9/5 = 333/5 = 66.6
66.6 + 32 = 98.6° F

How to convert Fahrenheit temperatures to Celsius

Subtract 32° to adjust for the offset in the Fahrenheit scale.
Multiply the result by 5/9.
Example: convert 98.6° Fahrenheit to Celsius.
98.6 - 32 = 66.6
66.6 * 5/9 = 333/9 = 37° C.

Temperature Scales			
Fahrenheit	**Celsius**	**Kelvin**	
212	100	373	Boiling point of water at sea-level
194	90	363	
176	80	353	
158	70	343	
140	60	333	
122	50	323	
104	40	313	
86	30	303	
68	20	293	Average room temperature
50	10	283	
32	0	273	Melting (freezing) point of ice (water) at sea-level
14	-10	263	
-4	-20	253	
-22	-30	243	
-40	-40	233	
-58	-50	223	
-76	-60	213	
-94	-70	203	
-112	-80	193	-89°C (-129 °F) Lowest recorded temperature. Vostok, Antarctica July, 1983
-130	-90	183	
-148	-100	173	

Reference: Ahrens (1994)

Department of Atmospheric Sciences
University of Illinois at Urbana-Champaign

X. Appendix H – pH and pH Indicators

pH is a measure of hydrogen ion (H+) activity. In dilute solutions, the H+ activity is essentially equal to the concentration.

pH Indicator	pH Range	Full Acidic Colour	Full Basic Colour
Brilliant green	0.0–2.6	Yellow	Green
Bromcresol green	3.8–5.4	Yellow	Blue-green
Bromcresol purple	5.2–6.8	Yellow	Purple
Bromophenol blue	3.0–4.6	Yellow	Blue
Bromothymol blue	6.0–7.6	Yellow	Blue
Congo red	3.0–5.0	Blue-violet	Red
Cresol red	2.3–8.8	Orange	Red
Cresolphthalein	8.2–9.8	Colourless	Red
2,4-dinitrophenol	2.8–4.0	Colourless	Red
Ethyl violet	0.0–2.4	Yellow	Blue
Litmus	4.5–8.3	Red	Blue
Malachite green	0.2–1.8	Yellow	Blue-green
Methyl green	0.2–1.8	Yellow	Blue
Methyl red	4.4–6.4	Red	Yellow
Neutral red	6.8–8.0	Red	Amber
Phenolphthalein	8.2–10.0	Colourless	Pink
Phenol red	6.8–8.4	Yellow	Red
Resazurin	3.8–6.4	Orange	Violet
Thymol blue	8.0–9.6	Yellow	Blue

All of the above indicators can be made by

(1) Dissolving 0.04 g of indicator in 500 mL of 95% ethanol,

(2) Adding 500 mL of distilled water and

(3) Filtering through Whatman No. 1 filter paper. Indicators should be stored in a dark, tightly closed bottle.

X. Appendix I – Glossary

Absorption- movement of ions and water into an organism as a result of metabolic processes, frequently against an electrochemical potential gradient (active) or as a result of diffusion along an activity gradient (passive).

Acid dyes- dyes that are anionic or have negatively charged groups such as carboxyls.

Acid-fast staining- a staining procedure that differentiates between bacteria based on their ability to retain a dye when washed with an acid alcohol solution.

Acidophile- a microorganism that has its growth optimum between about ph 0 and 5.5.

Actinobacteria- a group of gram-positive bacteria containing the actinomycetes and their high G C relatives.

Actinomycete- an aerobic, gram-positive bacterium that forms branching filaments (hyphae) and asexual spores.

Actinorhizae- associations between actinomycetes and plant roots.

Activated sludge- solid matter or sediment composed of actively growing microorganisms that participate in the aerobic portion of a biological sewage treatment process. The microbes readily use dissolved organic substrates and transform them into additional microbial cells and carbon dioxide.

Adjuvant- material added to an antigen to increase its immunogenicity. Common examples are alum, killed *Bordetella pertussis,* and an oil emulsion of the antigen, either alone (freund's incomplete adjuvant) or with killed mycobacteria (freund's complete adjuvant).

Aerobe- an organism that grows in the presence of atmospheric oxygen.

Aerotolerant anaerobes- microorganisms that grow equally well whether or not oxygen is present.

Aflatoxin- a polyketide secondary fungal metabolite that can cause cancer.

Agar- complex polysaccharide derived from certain marine algae that is a gelling agent for solid or semisolid microbiological media. Agar consists of about 70% agarose and 30% agaropectin. Agar can be melted at temperature above 100°C; gelling temperature is 40-50°C.

Agarose- nonsulfated linear polymer consisting of alternating residues of d-galactose and 3,6-anhydro-l-galactose. Agarose is extracted from seaweed, and agarose gels are often used as the resolving medium in electrophoresis.

Agglutinates- the visible aggregates or clumps formed by an agglutination reaction.

Agglutination reaction- the formation of an insoluble immune complex by the cross-linking of cells or particles.

Agglutinin- the antibody responsible for an agglutination reaction.

Airborne transmission- the type of infectious organism transmission in which the pathogen is truly suspended in the air and travels over a meter or more from the source to the host.

Akinetes- specialized, nonmotile, dormant, thick-walled resting cells formed by some cyanobacteria.

Alga- a common term for a series of unrelated groups of photosynthetic eucaryotic microorganisms lacking multicellular sex organs (except for the charophytes) and conducting vessels.

Algology- the scientific study of algae.

Aliphatic- organic compound in which the main carbon structure is a straight chain.

Alkalophile- a microorganism that grows best at phs from about 8.5 to 11.5.

Alkane- straight chain or branched organic structure that lacks double bonds.

Alkene- straight chain or branched organic structure that contains at least one double bond.

Alleles: Alternative forms of a genetic *locus*; a single allele for each locus is inherited separately from each parent (e.g., at a locus for eye color the allele might result in blue or brown eyes).

Allergen- a substance capable of inducing allergy or specific susceptibility.

Allochthonous flora- organisms that are not indigenous to the soil but that enter soil by precipitation, diseased tissues, manure, and sewage. They may persist for some time but do not contribute in a significant way to ecologically significant transformations or interactions.

Allosteric site- site on the enzyme other than the active site to which a nonsubstrate compound binds. Binding may result in a conformational change at the active site so that the normal substrate cannot bind to it.

Alpha hemolysis- a greenish zone of partial clearing around a bacterial colony growing on blood agar.

Amensalism (antagonism)- interaction between organisms where one organism is adversely affected and the other organism is unaffected, like antibiosis and allelopathy.

Ames test- a test that uses a special salmonella strain to test chemicals for mutagenicity and potential carcinogenicity.

Amino group- an $-NH_2$ group attached to a carbon skeleton as in the amines and amino acids.

Ammonification- liberation of ammonium (ammonia) from organic nitrogenous compounds by the action of microorganisms.

Amphitrichous- a cell with a single flagellum at each end.

Amplification: An increase in the number of copies of a specific DNA fragment; can be in vivo or in vitro.

Anaerobe- an organism that grows in the absence of free oxygen.

Anaerobic digestion- the microbiological treatment of sewage wastes under anaerobic conditions to produce methane.

Antagonist- biological agent that reduces the number or disease-producing activities of a pathogen.

Antibiosis- inhibition or lysis of an organism mediated by metabolic products of the antagonist; these products include lytic agents, enzymes, volatile compounds, and other toxic substances.

Antibiotic- a microbial product or its derivative that kills susceptible microorganisms or inhibits their growth.

Antibody (immunoglobulin)- a glycoprotein produced in response to the introduction of an antigen; it has the ability to combine with the antigen that stimulated its production. Also known as an immunoglobulin (ig).

Antigen- a foreign (nonself) substance (such as a protein, nucleoprotein, polysaccharide, or sometimes a glycolipid) to which lymphocytes respond; also known as an immunogen because it induces the immune response.

Antigenic drift- a small change in the antigenic character of an organism that allows it to avoid attack by the immune system.

Antigenic shift- a major change in the antigenic character of an organism that alters it to an antigenic strain unrecognized by host immune mechanisms.

Antimicrobial agent- an agent that kills microorganisms or inhibits their growth.

Antisepsis- the prevention of infection or sepsis.

Antiseptic- chemical agents applied to tissue to prevent infection by killing or inhibiting pathogens.

Antiserum- serum containing induced antibodies.

Antitoxin- an antibody to a microbial toxin, usually a bacterial exotoxin, that combines specifically with the toxin, in vivo and in vitro, neutralizing the toxin.

Arbuscular mycorrhizal fungi- the mycorrhizal fungi in a symbiotic fungus-root association that penetrate the outer layer of the root, grow intracellularly, and form characteristic much-branched hyphal structures called arbuscules.

Arbuscules- branched, treelike structures formed in cells of plant roots colonized by endotrophic mycorrhizal fungi.

Aromatic- organic compounds which contain a benzene ring, or a ring with similar chemical characteristics.

Arthroconidium- a thallic conidium released by the fragmentation or lysis of hypha. It is not notably larger than the parental hypha, and separation occurs at a septum.

Arthrospore- a spore resulting from the fragmentation of a hypha.

Ascocarp- a multicellular structure in ascomycetes lined with specialized cells called asci in which nuclear fusion and meiosis produce ascospores. An ascocarp can be open or closed and may be referred to as a fruiting body.

Ascogenous hypha- a specialized hypha that gives rise to one or more asci.

Ascogonium- the receiving (female) organ in ascomycetous fungi which, after fertilization, gives rise to ascogenous hyphae and later to asci and ascospores.

Ascomycetes- a division of fungi that form ascospores.

Ascospore- a spore contained or produced in an ascus.

Ascus- a specialized cell, characteristic of the ascomycetes, in which two haploid nuclei fuse to produce a zygote, which immediately divides by meiosis; at maturity an ascus will contain ascospores.

Aseptic technique- manipulating sterile instruments or culture media in such a way as to maintain sterility.

Autoclave- an apparatus for sterilizing objects by the use of steam under pressure. Its development tremendously stimulated the growth of microbiology.

Autoradiography: A technique that uses X- ray film to visualize radioactively labeled molecules or fragments of molecules; used in analyzing length and number of DNA fragments after they are separated by gel *electrophoresis*.

Autosome: A *chromosome* not involved in sex determination. The *diploid* human *genome* consists of 46 chromosomes, 22 pairs of autosomes, and 1 pair of *sex chromosomes* (the X and Y chromosomes).

Autotroph- organism which uses carbon dioxide as the sole carbon source.

Bacteremia- the presence of viable bacteria in the blood.

Bactericide- an agent that kills bacteria.

Bacteriocin- agent produced by certain bacteria that inhibits or kills closely related isolates and species.

Bacteriophage (phage) typing- a technique in which strains of bacteria are identified based on their susceptibility to a variety of bacteriophages.

Bacteriophage- virus that infects bacteria, often with destruction or lysis of the host cell.

Bacteriostatic- inhibiting the growth and reproduction of bacteria.

Barophilic or barophile- organisms that prefer or require high pressures for growth and reproduction.

Barotolerant- organisms that can grow and reproduce at high pressures but do not require them.

Base sequence analysis: A method, sometimes automated, for determining the *base sequence*.

Base sequence: The order of *nucleotide* bases in a DNA molecule.

Basic dyes- dyes that are cationic, or have positively charged groups, and bind to negatively charged cell structures. Usually sold as chloride salts.

Basidiocarp- the fruiting body of a basidiomycete that contains the basidia.

Basidioma (plural, basidiomata)- fruiting body that produces basidia; also termed a basidiocarp.

Basidiomycetes- a division of fungi in which the spores are born on club-shaped organs called basidia.

Basidiospore- a spore born on the outside of a basidium following karyogamy and meiosis.

Basidium- a structure that bears on its surface a definite number of basidiospores (typically four) that are formed following karyogamy and meiosis. Basidia are found in the basidiomycetes and are usually club-shaped.

Batch culture- a culture of microorganisms produced by inoculating a closed culture vessel containing a single batch of medium.

Beta haemolysis- a zone of complete clearing around a bacterial colony growing on blood agar. The zone does not change significantly in colour.

Binary fission- division of one cell into two cells by the formation of a septum. It is the most common form of cell division in bacteria.

Bioaccumulation-accumulation of a chemical substance in living tissue.

Biochemical oxygen demand (BOD)- the amount of oxygen used by organisms in water under certain standard conditions; it provides an index of the amount of microbially oxidizable organic matter present.

Biodegradation- the breakdown of a complex chemical through biological processes that can result in minor loss of functional groups, fragmentation into larger constitutents, or complete breakdown to carbon dioxide and minerals. Often the term refers to the undesired microbial-mediated destruction of materials such as paper, paint, and textiles.

Biofilms- organized microbial systems consisting of layers of microbial cells associated with surfaces, often with complex structural and functional characteristics. Biofilms have physical/chemical gradients that influence microbial metabolic processes. They can form on inanimate devices (catheters, medical prosthetic devices) and also cause fouling (e.g., of ships' hulls, water pipes, cooling towers).

Biogeochemical cycling- the oxidation and reduction of substances carried out by living organisms and/or abiotic processes that results in the cycling of elements within and between different parts of the ecosystem (the soil, aquatic environment, and atmosphere).

Bioinsecticide- a pathogen that is used to kill or disable unwanted insect pests. Bacteria, fungi, or viruses are used, either directly or after manipulation, to control insect populations.

Biomagnification- the increase in concentration of a substance in higher-level consumer organisms.

Biopesticide- the use of a microorganism or another biological agent to control a specific pest.

Bioremediation- the use of biologically mediated processes to remove or degrade pollutants from specific environments. Bioremediation can be carried out by modification of the environment to accelerate biological processes, either with or without the addition of specific microorganisms.

Biosensor- the coupling of a biological process with production of an electrical signal or light to detect the presence of particular substances.

Biosphere- zone incorporating all forms of life on earth. The biosphere extends from deep in sediment below the ocean to several thousand meters elevation in high mountains.

Bioterrorism- the intentional or threatened use of viruses, bacteria, fungi, or toxins from living organisms to produce death or disease in humans, animals, and plants.

Biotransformation or microbial transformation- the use of living organisms to modify substances that are not normally used for growth.

Blastospore- a spore formed by budding from a hypha.

Broad-spectrum drugs- chemotherapeutic agents that are effective against many different kinds of pathogens.

Budding- a vegetative outgrowth of yeast and some bacteria as a means of asexual reproduction; the daughter cell is smaller than the parent.

Bursa of fabricius- found in birds; the blind saclike structure located on the posterior wall of the cloaca; it performs a thymuslike function. A primary lymphoid organ where b-cell maturation occurs. Bone marrow is the equivalent in mammals.

Burst size- the number of phages released by a host cell during the lytic life cycle.

Capsule- a layer of well-organized material, not easily washed off, lying outside the bacterial cell wall.

Carcinogen- substance which causes the initiation of tumor formation. Frequently a mutagen.

Catalyst- substance that promotes a chemical reaction by lowering the activation energy without itself being changed in the end. Enzymes are a type of catalyst.

Catheter- a tubular surgical instrument for withdrawing fluids from a cavity of the body, especially one for introduction into the bladder through the urethra for the withdrawal of urine.

Cellulose- glucose polysaccharide (with beta-1,4-linkage) that is the main component of plant cell walls. Most abundant polysaccharide on earth.

Centimorgan (cM): A unit of measure of *recombination* frequency. One centimorgan is equal to a 1% chance that a marker at one genetic *locus* will be separated from a marker at a second locus due to *crossing over* in a single generation. In human beings, 1 centimorgan is equivalent, on average, to 1 million *base pairs*.

Centromere: A specialized *chromosome* region to which spindle fibers attach during cell division.

Chelate (chelator)- organic chemical that forms ring compound in which a metal is held between two or more atoms strongly enough to diminish the rate at which it becomes fixed by soil, thereby making it more available for plant and microbial uptake.

Chemical oxygen demand (COD)- the amount of chemical oxidation required to convert organic matter in water and wastewater to Co_2.

Chemoautotroph- organism that obtains energy from the oxidation of reduced inorganic compounds or elements and obtains carbon from carbon dioxide.

Chemoheterotroph- organism that obtains energy and carbon from the oxidation of organic compounds.

Chemolithotroph- organism that obtains energy from the oxidation of inorganic compounds and uses inorganic compounds as electron donors.

Chemoorganotroph- organism that obtains energy and electrons (reducing power) from the oxidation of organic compounds.

Chemostat- continuous culture device usually controlled by the concentration of limiting nutrient and dilution rate.

Chlamydospore- an asexually produced, thick-walled resting spore formed by some fungi.

Chloramphenicol- a broad-spectrum antibiotic that is produced by streptomyces venezuelae or synthetically; it binds to the large ribosomal subunit and inhibits the peptidyl transferase reaction.

Chromatography- any technique used to separate different species of molecules (or ions) by subjecting them to two different carrier phases: mobile and stationary phases.

Chromogen- a colourless substrate that is acted on by an enzyme to produce a coloured end product.

Chromophore group- a chemical group with double bonds that absorbs visible light and gives a dye its colour.

Chromosomes: The self- replicating genetic structures of cells containing the cellular DNA that bears in its *nucleotide* sequence the linear array of *genes*. In *prokaryotes*, chromosomal DNA is circular, and the entire genome is carried on one chromosome. *Eukaryotic* genomes consist of a number of chromosomes whose DNA is associated with different kinds of *proteins*.

Clone- (i) population of cells all descended from a single cell. (ii) number of copies of a dna fragment to be replicated by a phage or plasmid.

Cloning vector- DNA molecule that is able to bring about the replication of foreign dna fragments.

Cloning: The process of asexually producing a group of cells (clones), all genetically identical, from a single ancestor. In *recombinant DNA technology*, the use of DNA manipulation procedures to produce multiple copies of a single *gene* or segment of DNA is referred to as cloning DNA.

Coagulase- an enzyme that induces blood clotting; it is characteristically produced by pathogenic staphylococci.

Codon- a sequence of three nucleotides in mrna that directs the incorporation of an amino acid during protein synthesis or signals the start or stop of translation.

Coenzyme- low-molecular-weight chemical which participates in an enzymatic reaction by accepting and donating electrons or functional groups.

Coliform- a gram-negative, nonsporing, facultative rod that ferments lactose with gas formation within 48 hours at 35°C.

Colony forming units (CFU)- the number of microorganisms that can form colonies when cultured using spread plates or pour plates, an indication of the number of viable microorganisms in a sample.

Colony- a cluster or assemblage of microorganisms growing on a solid surface such as the surface of an agar culture medium; the assemblage often is directly visible, but also may be seen only microscopically.

Commensalism- interaction between organisms where one organism benefits from the association while the second organism remains unaffected.

Comminution- reduction in the size of organic materials as a result of feeding by soil organisms; shredding is one form of comminution.

Community- all organisms that occupy a common habitat and interact with one another.

Compensatory growth- accelerated population growth in response to grazing or predation.

Competent- a bacterial cell that can take up free dna fragments and incorporate them into its genome during transformation.

Competition- rivalry between two or more species for a limiting factor in the environment that usually results in reduced growth of participating organisms.

Complementary DNA (cDNA): DNA that is synthesized from a *messenger RNA* template; the single-stranded form is often used as a *probe* in *physical mapping*.

Complementary sequences: *Nucleic acid base sequences* that can form a double-stranded structure by matching *base pairs*; the complementary sequence to G- T- A- C is C- A- T- G.

Compost- organic residues which have been mixed, piled, and moistened, with or without addition of fertilizer and lime, and generally allowed to undergo thermophilic decomposition until the original organic materials are substantially altered or decomposed.

Conidiophore- aerial hypha bearing conidia.

Conidium - nonmotile, asexual spore resulting from mitotic nuclear division and formed from the ends or sides of a hypha; produced in abundant numbers by the asexual phase of soil fungi in the phyla ascomycota and basidiomycota.

Conjugation- 1. The form of gene transfer and recombination in bacteria that requires direct cell-to-cell contact. 2. A complex form of sexual reproduction commonly employed by protozoa.

Conjugative plasmid- self-transmissible plasmid; a plasmid that encodes all the functions needed for its own intercellular transmission by conjugation.

Conserved sequence: A *base sequence* in a DNA molecule (or an *amino acid* sequence in a *protein*) that has remained essentially unchanged throughout evolution.

Contig map: A map depicting the relative order of a linked *library* of small overlapping clones representing a complete chromosomal segment.

Contigs: Groups of *clones* representing overlapping regions of a *genome*.

Cosmid- a plasmid vector with lambda phage cos sites that can be packaged in a phage capsid; it is useful for cloning large DNA fragments.

Crossing over: The breaking during *meiosis* of one maternal and one paternal *chromosome*, the exchange of corresponding sections of DNA, and the rejoining of the chromosomes. This process can result in an exchange of alleles between chromosomes. Compare *recombination*.

Culture- population of microorganisms cultivated in an artificial growth medium. A pure culture is grown from a single cell; a mixed culture consists of two or more microbial species or strains growing together.

Cyanobacteria- a large group of bacteria that carry out oxygenic photosynthesis using a system like that present in photosynthetic eucaryotes.

Cyst- a general term used for a specialized microbial cell enclosed in a wall. Cysts are formed by protozoa and a few bacteria. They may be dormant, resistant structures formed in response to adverse conditions or reproductive cysts that are a normal stage in the life cycle.

Cytopathic effect- the observable change that occurs in cells as a result of viral replication. Examples include ballooning, binding together, clustering, or even death of the cultured cells.

Deamination- the removal of amino groups from amino acids.

Decomposer- heterotrophic organism that breaks down organic compounds.

Decomposition- chemical breakdown of a compound into simpler compounds, often accomplished by microbial metabolism.

Degradation- process whereby a compound is usually transformed into simpler compounds.

Diatomaceous earth-geologic deposit of fine, grayish siliceous material composed chiefly or wholly of the remains of diatoms. It may occur as a powder or as a porous, rigid material.

Diauxic growth- a biphasic growth pattern or response in which a microorganism, when exposed to two nutrients, initially uses one of them for growth and then alters its metabolism to make use of the second.

Diazotroph- organism that can use dinitrogen as its sole nitrogen source, i.e. Capable of n_2 fixation.

Diffusion (nutrient)- movement of nutrients in soil that results from a concentration gradient.

Dilution plate count method- method for estimating the viable numbers of microorganisms in a sample. The sample is diluted serially and then transferred to agar plates to permit growth and quantification of colony-forming units.

Diploid: A full set of genetic material, consisting of paired *chromosomes* one chromosome from each parental set. Most animal cells except the *gametes* have a diploid set of chromosomes. The diploid human *genome* has 46 chromosomes. Compare *haploid*.

Direct count- method of estimating the total number of microorganisms in a given mass of soil by direct microscopic examination.

Disinfectant- agent that kills microorganisms.

DNA fingerprinting- molecular genetic techniques to assess possible differences among dna in a samples.

DNA library- collection of cloned dna fragments which in total contain genes from the entire genome of an organism; also called a gene library.

DNA replication: The use of existing DNA as a template for the synthesis of new DNA strands. In humans and other *eukaryotes*, replication occurs in the cell *nucleus*.

DNA sequence: The relative order of *base pairs*, whether in a fragment of DNA, a *gene*, a *chromosome*, or an entire *genome*. See *base sequence analysis*.

Domain: A discrete portion of a *protein* with its own function. The combination of domains in a single protein determines its overall function.

Double helix: The shape that two linear strands of DNA assume when bonded together.

Doubling time- time needed for a population to double in number or biomass.

Droplet nuclei- small particles (1 to 4 mm in diameter) that represent what is left from the evaporation of larger particles (10 mm or more in diameter) called droplets.

Ectomycorrhiza- mycorrhizal type in which the fungal mycelia extend inward, between root cortical cells, to form a network (hartig net) and outward into the surrounding soil. Usually the fungal hyphae also form a mantle on the surface of the root.

Electrophoresis- separation of charged molecules, such as nucleic acids, in an electrical field.

Electrophoresis- a technique that separates substances through differences in their migration rate in an electrical field due to variations in the number and kinds of charged groups they have.

Embrane is sometimes considered part of the pellicle.

Endomycorrhiza- referring to a mutualistic association of fungi and plant roots in which the fungus penetrates into the root cells and arbuscules and vesicles are formed.

Endonuclease- endoenzyme that cleaves phosphodiester bonds within a nucleic acid molecule.

Endospore- differentiated cell formed within the cells of certain gram-positive bacteria and extremely resistant to heat and other harmful agents.

Endosymbiont- an organism that lives within the body of another organism in a symbiotic association.

Enrichment culture- technique in which environmental (including nutritional) conditions are controlled to favor the development of a specific organism or group of organisms.

Enteric bacteria- general term for a group of bacteria that inhabit the intestinal tract of humans and other animals. Among this group are pathogenic bacteria such as *salmonella* and *shigella*.

Enzyme: A *protein* that acts as a catalyst, speeding the rate at which a biochemical reaction proceeds but not altering the direction or nature of the reaction.

Enzyme-linked immunosorbent assay (ELISA)- a technique used for detecting and quantifying specific antibodies and antigens.

Episome- plasmid that replicates by inserting itself into the bacterial chromosome.

Ericoid mycorrhiza- type of mycorrhiza found on plants in the ericales. The hyphae in the root are able to penetrate cortical cells (endomycorrhizal habit); however, no arbuscules are formed. Major forms are ericoid, arbutoid, and monotropoid.

Eutrophication- enrichment of natural waters with excess nutrients that leads to algae blooms and subsequent oxygen deficiency when the algae die and bacteria degrade them.

Exogenous DNA: DNA originating outside an organism.

Exons: The *protein-* coding DNA sequences of a *gene*. Compare *introns*.

Exonuclease: An *enzyme* that cleaves *nucleotides* sequentially from free ends of a linear nucleic acid substrate.

Extreme barophilic bacteria- bacteria that require a high-pressure environment to function.

Extreme environment- an environment in which physical factors such as temperature, ph, salinity, and pressure are outside of the normal range for growth of most microorganisms; these conditions allow unique organisms to survive and function.

Extremophiles- microorganisms that grow under harsh or extreme environmental conditions such as very high temperatures or low phs.

Exudate- low molecular weight metabolites that leak from plant roots into soil.

F plasmid- an F plasmid that carries some bacterial genes and transmits them to recipient cells when the f cell carries out conjugation; the transfer of bacterial genes in this way is often called sexduction.

Facultative anaerobes- microorganisms that do not require oxygen for growth, but do grow better in its presence.

Faecal coliform- coliforms whose normal habitat is the intestinal tract and that can grow at 44.5°c.

Faecal enterococci- enterococci found in the intestine of humans and other warm-blooded animals. They are used as indicators of the fecal pollution of water.

Feedback inhibition- inhibition by an end product of the biosynthetic pathway involved in its synthesis.

Fermentation- an energy-yielding process in which an energy substrate is oxidized without an exogenous electron acceptor. Usually organic molecules serve as both electron donors and acceptors.

Fermentation- metabolic process in which organic compounds serve as both electron donors and electron acceptors.

Fertilizer- any organic or inorganic material of natural or synthetic origin (other than liming materials) added to a soil to supply one or more elements essential to plant growth.

Filamentous- in the form of very long rods, many times longer than wide (for bacteria), in the form of long branching strands (for fungi).

FISH (fluorescence in situ hybridization): A *physical mapping* approach that uses fluorescein tags to detect *hybridization* of *probes* with *metaphase chromosomes* and with the less- condensed *somatic interphase* chromatin.

Fixation- the process in which the internal and external structures of cells and organisms are preserved and fixed in position.

Flow cytometry: Analysis of biological material by detection of the light- absorbing or fluorescing properties of cells or subcellular fractions (i.e., *chromosomes*) passing in a narrow stream through a laser beam. An absorbance or fluorescence profile of the sample is produced. Automated sorting devices, used to fractionate samples, sort successive droplets of the analyzed stream into different fractions depending on the fluorescence emitted by each droplet.

Flow karyotyping: Use of flow cytometry to analyze and/or separate *chromosomes* on the basis of their DNA content.

Fluorescent- able to emit light of a certain wavelength when activated by light of a shorter wavelength.

Fluorescent antibody- antiserum conjugated with a fluorescent dye, such as fluorescein or rhodamine.

Fruiting body- macroscopic reproductive structure produced by some fungi, such as mushrooms, and some bacteria, including myxobacteria. Fruiting bodies are distinctive in size, shape, and colouration for each species.

Fungistasis- suppression of germination of fungal spores or other resting structures in natural soils as a result of competition for available nutrients, presence of inhibitory compounds, or both.

Gamete: Mature male or female reproductive cell (sperm or ovum) with a *haploid* set of *chromosomes* (23 for humans).

Gel- inert polymer, usually made of agarose or polyacrylamide, that separates macromolecules such as nucleic acids or proteins during electrophoresis.

Gene cloning- isolation of a desired gene from one organism and its incorporation into a suitable vector for the production of large amounts of the gene.

Gene expression: The process by which a *genes* coded information is converted into the structures present and operating in the cell. Expressed genes include those that are transcribed into *mRNA* and then translated into *protein* and those that are transcribed into *RNA* but not translated into protein (e.g., *transfer* and *ribosomal RNAs*).

Gene families: Groups of closely related *genes* that make similar products.

Gene mapping: Determination of the relative positions of *genes* on a DNA molecule (*chromosome* or *plasmid*) and of the distance, in *linkage* units or physical units, between them.

Gene probe- a strand of nucleic acid which can be labeled and hybridized to a complementary molecule from a mixture of other nucleic acids.

Gene product: The biochemical material, either *RNA* or *protein*, resulting from expression of a gene. The amount of gene product is used to measure how active a gene is; abnormal amounts can be correlated with disease- causing alleles.

Gene- unit of heredity; a segment of dna specifying a particular protein or polypeptide chain, a tRNA or an mrna.

Generation time- time needed for a population to double in number or biomass.

Genetic code- information for the synthesis of proteins contained in the nucleotide sequence of a DNA molecule (or in certain viruses, of an rna molecule).

Genetic engineering- *in vitro* techniques for the isolation, manipulation, recombination, and expression of DNA.

Genome- complete set of genes present in an organism.

Genomic library: A collection of *clones* made from a set of randomly generated overlapping DNA fragments representing the entire *genome* of an organism. Compare *library, arrayed library*.

Genomics- the study of the molecular organization of genomes, their information content, and the gene products they encode.

Genotype- precise genetic constitution of an organism.

Genus (plural, genera)- the first name of the scientific name (binomial); the taxon between family and species.

Gliding motility- a type of motility in which a microbial cell glides along when in contact with a solid surface.

Growth factor- organic compound necessary for growth because it is an essential cell component or precursor of such components and cannot be synthesized by the organism itself. Usually required in trace amounts.

Habitat- place where an organism lives.

Haemadsorption- the adherence of red blood cells to the surface of something, such as another cell or a virus.

Haemagglutination- the agglutination of red blood cells by antibodies.

Haemagglutinin- the antibody responsible for a hemagglutination reaction.

Halogen- any of the five elements F, CL, BR, I, and at that form part of group vii a of the periodic table.

Halophile- organism requiring or tolerating a saline environment

Haploid: A single set of *chromosomes* (half the full set of genetic material), present in the egg and sperm cells of animals and in the egg and pollen cells of plants. Human beings have 23 chromosomes in their reproductive cells. Compare *diploid*.

Heavy metals- those metals which have densities > 5.0 mG m^{-3}. These include the metallic elements cu, fe, mn, mo, co, zn, cd, hg, ni, and pb. Al and se have densities < 5 but are also considered heavy metals.

Hermaphroditic- containing both male and female sex organs.

Heterocysts- specialized cells produced by cyanobacteria that are the sites of nitrogen fixation.

Heteropolysaccharide- the class name for polysaccharides composed of two or more different kinds of monomeric units.

Heterotroph- organism capable of deriving carbon and energy for growth and cell synthesis from organic compounds; generally also obtain energy and reducing power equivalents from organic compounds.

Heterozygosity: The presence of different *alleles* at one or more *loci* on *homologous chromosomes*.

Hfr strain- a bacterial strain that donates its genes with high frequency to a recipient cell during conjugation because the f factor is integrated into the bacterial chromosome.

Homeobox: A short stretch of *nucleotides* whose *base sequence* is virtually identical in all the *genes* that contain it. It has been found in many organisms from fruit flies to human beings. In the fruit fly, a homeobox appears to determine when particular groups of genes are expressed during development.

Homologies: Similarities in DNA or *protein* sequences between individuals of the same species or among different species.

Homologous chromosomes: A pair of *chromosomes* containing the same linear *gene* sequences, each derived from one parent.

Human gene therapy: Insertion of normal DNA directly into cells to correct a genetic defect.

Humus- total of the organic compounds in soil exclusive of undecayed plant and animal tissues, their "partial decomposition" products, and the soil biomass. The term is often used synonymously with soil organic matter.

Hybridization- natural formation or artificial construction of a duplex nucleic acid molecule by complementary base pairing between two nucleic acid strands derived from different sources.

Hydrogen bond- chemical bond between a hydrogen atom of one molecule and two unshared electrons of another molecule.

Hydrogen-oxidizing bacterium-facultative lithotrophs that, in the absence of an oxidizable organic source, oxidize H_2 for energy and synthesize carbohydrates with carbon dioxide as their source of carbon.

Hygroscopic water- water adsorbed by a dry soil from an atmosphere of high relative humidity.

Hymenium-layer of hyphae which are fertile in producing asci (fungi in the phylum ascomycota) or basidia (fungi in the phylum basidiomycota) from the process of meiosis.

Hyperparasite-parasite that feeds on another parasite.

Hyperthermophile- an organism that has its growth optimum above 80°C.

Hypha (plural, hyphae)-long and often branched tubular filament that constitutes the vegetative body of many fungi and funguslike organisms. Bacteria of the order actinomycetes also produce branched hyphae.

Hypoxic- insufficient availability of oxygen in an environment to support aerobic respiration.

IgA- immunoglobulin a; the class of immunoglobulins that is present in dimeric form in many body secretions (e.g., saliva, tears, and bronchial and intestinal secretions) and protects body surfaces. IgA also is present in serum.

IgD- immunoglobulin D; the class of immunoglobulins found on the surface of many b lymphocytes; thought to serve as an antigen receptor in the stimulation of antibody synthesis.

IgE- immunoglobulin E; the immunoglobulin class that binds to mast cells and basophils, and is responsible for type I or anaphylactic hypersensitivity reactions such as hay fever and asthma. Ige is also involved in resistance to helminth parasites.

IgG- immunoglobulin G; the predominant immunoglobulin class in serum. Has functions such as neutralizing toxins, opsonizing bacteria, activating complement, and crossing the placenta to protect the fetus and neonate.

IgM- immunoglobulin M; the class of serum antibody first produced during an infection. It is a large, pentameric molecule that is active in agglutinating pathogens and activating complement. The monomeric form is present on the surface of some B lymphocytes.

Immobilization- the incorporation of a simple, soluble substance into the body of an organism, making it unavailable for use by other organisms.

Immunity- the ability of a human or animal body to resist infection by microorganisms or their harmful products such as toxins.

Immunoblot (western blot)-detection of proteins immobilized on a filter by complementary reaction with specific antibody.

immunodiffusion- a technique involving the diffusion of antigen and/or antibody within a semisolid gel to produce a precipitin reaction where they meet in proper proportions. Often both the antibody and antigen diffuse through the gel; sometimes an antigen diffuses through a gel containing antibody.

Immunoelectrophoresis- the electrophoretic separation of protein antigens followed by diffusion and precipitation in gels using antibodies against the separated proteins.

Immunofluorescence- a technique used to identify particular antigens microscopically in cells or tissues by the binding of a fluorescent antibody conjugate.

Immunogen- substance which is capable of eliciting immune response. An immunogen usually has a fairly high molecular weight (usually greater than 10,000), thus, a variety of macromolecules such as proteins, lipoprotein, polysaccharides, and some nucleic acids can act as immunogens.

In situ hybridization: Use of a DNA or RNA probe to detect the presence of the *complementary DNA* sequence in cloned bacterial or cultured *eukaryotic* cells.

In vitro- literally "in glass"; it describes whatever happens in a test tube or other receptacle, as opposed to *in vivo*. When a study or an experiment is done outside the living organism, in test tube, it is done *in vitro*.

In vitro: Outside a living organism.

In vivo- in the body, in a living organism, as opposed to *in vitro*; when a study or an experiment is done in the living organism, it is done *in vivo*.

Indicator organism- an organism whose presence indicates the condition of a substance or environment, for example, the potential presence of pathogens. Coliforms are used as indicators of fecal pollution.

Infrared (IR)- the portion of the electromagnetic spectrum with wavelengths from about 0.75 μm to 1 mm.

Inhibition- prevention of growth or function.

Inoculate- to treat with microorganisms for the purpose of creating a favorable response. For example, treatment of legume seeds with rhizobia to stimulate n_2 fixation.

Inoculum- material used to introduce a microorganism into a suitable situation for growth.

Insertion- genetic mutation in which one or more nucleotides are added to dna.

Insertion sequence (IS element)- simplest type of transposable element. Has only genes involved in transposition.

Integration- process by which a dna molecule becomes incorporated into another genome.

Intercalating agents- molecules that can be inserted between the stacked bases of a dna double helix, thereby distorting the dna and inducing insertion and deletion mutations.

Interphase: The period in the cell cycle when DNA is replicated in the nucleus; followed by *mitosis*.

Intracellular- inside the cell.

Introns: The DNA *base sequences* interrupting the *protein-* coding sequences of a *gene;* these sequences are *transcribed* into *RNA* but are cut out of the message before it is *translated* into protein. Compare *exons.*

Isolation- any procedure in which an organism present in a particular sample or environment, is obtained in pure culture.

Isotope- different form of the same element containing the same number of protons and electrons, but differing in the number of neutrons.

Karyotype: A photomicrograph of an individuals *chromosomes* arranged in a standard format showing the number, size, and shape of each chromosome type; used in low- resolution *physical mapping* to correlate gross chromosomal abnormalities with the characteristics of specific diseases.

Kilobase (kb): Unit of length for DNA fragments equal to 1000 *nucleotides.*

Kirby-bauer method- a disk diffusion test to determine the susceptibility of a microorganism to chemotherapeutic agents.

Koch's postulates-set of laws formulated by robert koch to prove that an organism is the causal agent of disease.

Lag phase-period after inoculation of fresh growth medium during which population numbers do not increase.

Leaching- (i) removal of valuable metals from ores by microbial action. (ii) the removal of materials in solution from the soil.

Lectins- plant proteins with a high affinity for specific sugar residues.

Leghemoglobin- iron-containing, red pigment(s) produced in root nodules during the symbiotic association between rhizobia and leguminous plants. The pigment is similar but not identical to mammalian hemoglobin.

Library: An unordered collection of *clones* (i.e., cloned DNA from a particular organism), whose relationship to each other can be established by *physical mapping.* Compare *genomic library, arrayed library.*

Linkage map: A map of the relative positions of genetic *loci* on a *chromosome,* determined on the basis of how often the loci are inherited together. Distance is measured in *centimorgans (cM).*

Linkage: The proximity of two or more *markers* (e.g., *genes, RFLP* markers) on a *chromosome;* the closer together the markers are, the lower the probability that they will be separated during DNA repair or replication processes (binary fission in *prokaryotes, mitosis* or *meiosis* in *eukaryotes*), and hence the greater the probability that they will be inherited together.

Lipophilic- having an affinity for fat.

Lipopolysaccharide (LPS)-complex lipid structure containing unusual sugars and fatty acids found in many gram-negative bacteria.

Lithotroph- organism that uses an inorganic substrate such as ammonia or hydrogen as an electron donor in energy metabolism. There are two types of lithotrophs: chemolithotroph and photolithotroph.

Litter- surface layer of the forest floor consisting of freshly fallen leaves, needles, twigs, stems, bark, and fruits.

Localize: Determination of the original position *(locus)* of a *gene* or other *marker* on a chromosome.

Locus (pl. loci): The position on a *chromosome* of a *gene* or other chromosome *marker;* also, the DNA at that position. The use of *locus* is sometimes restricted to mean regions of DNA that are *expressed.* See *gene expression.*

Lophotrichous- having a tuft of polar flagella.

Luminescence- production of light.

Lysogeny- an association where a prokaryote contains a prophage and the virus genome is replicated in synchrony with the host chromosome.

Macromolecule- large molecule formed from the connection of a number of small molecules.

Macronutrient- a substance required in large amounts for growth, usually attaining a concentration of > 500 mG kg^1 in mature plants. Usually refers to n, p, k, ca, mG, and s.

Macrorestriction map: Map depicting the order of and distance between sites at which *restriction enzymes* cleave *chromosomes*.

Marker: An identifiable physical location on a *chromosome* (e.g., *restriction enzyme cutting site, gene*) whose inheritance can be monitored. Markers can be expressed regions of DNA (genes) or some segment of DNA with no known coding function but whose pattern of inheritance can be determined. See *RFLP, restriction fragment length polymorphism*.

Medium - any liquid or solid material prepared for the growth, maintenance, or storage of microorganisms.

Megabase (Mb): Unit of length for DNA fragments equal to 1 million *nucleotides* and roughly equal to 1 *cM*.

Meiosis- in eukaryotes, reduction division, the process by which the change from diploid to haploid occurs.

Mesophile- organism whose optimum temperature for growth falls in an intermediate range of approximately 15 to 40°c.

Metachromatic granules- granules of polyphosphate in the cytoplasm of some bacteria that appear a different colour when stained with a blue basic dye. They are storage reservoirs for phosphate. Sometimes called volutin granules.

Metaphase: A stage in *mitosis* or *meiosis* during which the *chromosomes* are aligned along the equatorial plane of the cell.

Methanogenesis- biological production of methane.

Methanotroph- organism capable of oxidizing methane.

Microaerophile- a microorganism that requires low levels of oxygen for growth, around 2 to 10%, but is damaged by normal atmospheric oxygen levels.

Microaggregate- clustering of clay packets stabilized by organic matter and precipitated inorganic materials.

Microbial biomass- total mass of microorganism alive in a given volume or mass of soil.

Microbial mat- a firm structure of layered microorganisms with complementary physiological activities.

Microbial population- total number of living microorganisms in a given volume or mass of soil.

Micrometer- one-millionth of a meter, or 10^{-6} meter, the unit usually used for measuring microorganisms.

Micronutrients- nutrients such as zinc, manganese, and copper that are required in very small quantities for growth and reproduction. Also called trace elements.

Mineralization- conversion of an element from an organic form to an inorganic state as a result of microbial decomposition.

Minimal inhibitory concentration (MIC)- he lowest concentration of a drug that will prevent the growth of a particular microorganism.

Minimal lethal concentration (MLC)- the lowest concentration of a drug that will kill a particular microorganism.

Mixed acid fermentation- a type of fermentation carried out by members of the family enterobacteriaceae in which ethanol and a complex mixture of organic acids are produced.

Mixotroph- organism able to assimilate organic compounds as carbon sources while using inorganic compounds as electron donors. Compare with autotroph and heterotroph.

Mold- any of a large group of fungi that cause mold or moldiness and that exist as multicellular filamentous colonies; also the deposit or growth caused by such fungi. Molds typically do not produce macroscopic fruiting bodies.

Monoclonal antibody- antibody produced from a single clone of cells. This antibody has uniform structure and specificity.

monotrichous- having a single flagellum.

Mordant- a substance that helps fix dye on or in a cell.

Most probable number (MPN)- the statistical estimation of the probable population in a liquid by diluting and determining end points for microbial growth.

Motility- movement of a cell under its own power.

Multiplexing: A *sequencing* approach that uses several pooled samples simultaneously, greatly increasing sequencing speed.

Municipal solid waste- combined consumer and commercial waste generated within a defined geographic area

Mushroom- large, sometimes edible, fruiting body produced by some fungi.

Mutagen -substance that causes the mutation of genes.

Mutant- organism, population, gene, or chromosome that differs from the corresponding wild type by one or more base pairs.

Mutation- a permanent, heritable change in the genetic material.

Mutation: Any heritable change in DNA *sequence*. Compare *polymorphism*.

Mutualism- interaction between organisms where both organisms benefit from the association.

Mycorrhizosphere- unique microbial community that forms around a mycorrhiza.

Mycovirus- virus that infects fungi.

Necrosis- damage of living tissues because of infection or injury.

Necrotrophic- nutritional mechanism by which an organism produces a battery of hydrolytic enzymes to kill and break down host cells and then absorb nutritional compounds from the dead organic matter.

Negative staining- a staining procedure in which a dye is used to make the background dark while the specimen is unstained.

Neutralism- lack of interaction between two organisms in the same habitat.

Niche- functional role of a given organism within its habitat.

Nicotinamide adenine dinucleotide (NAD$^+$)- important coenzyme, functioning as a hydrogen and electron carrier in a wide range of redox reactions; the oxidized form of the coenzyme is written nad$^+$, the reduced form as nadh.

Nicotinamide adenine dinucleotide phosphate (NADP$^+$)- important coenzyme, functioning as a hydrogen and electron carrier in a wide range of redox reactions; the oxidized form of the coenzyme is written nadp$^+$, the reduced form as nadph.

Nitrate reduction (biological)- process whereby nitrate is reduced by plants and microorganisms to ammonium for cell synthesis (nitrate assimilation, assimilatory nitrate reduction) or to various lower oxidation states (n_2, n_2o, no,) by bacteria using nitrate as the terminal electron acceptor in anaerobic respiration.

Nitrification- biological oxidation of ammonium to nitrite and nitrate, or a biologically induced increase in the oxidation state of nitrogen.

Nitrogen fixation (ecology)- process by which a few bacteria in the soil convert gaseous nitrogen ($n2$) to ammonia, which can be used by living organisms.

Nitrogenous base: A nitrogen- containing molecule having the chemical properties of a base.

Nodulins- unique proteins produced in root hairs or nodules in response to rhizobial infection.

Nonpolar- possessing hydrophobic (water repelling) characteristics and not easily dissolved in water.

Northern blot- hybridization of single-stranded nucleic acid (dna or rna) to rna fragments immobilized on a filter.

Nosocomial infection- an infection that develops within a hospital (or other type of clinical care facility) and is produced by an infectious organism acquired during the stay of the patient.

Nucleic acid- polymer of nucleotides.

Nucleic acid: A large molecule composed of *nucleotide* subunits.

Nucleoid- aggregated mass of dna that makes up the chromosome of prokaryotic cells.

Nucleoside- nucleotide without the phosphate group.

Nucleotide- monomeric unit of nucleic acid, consisting of a sugar (pentose), a phosphate, and a nitrogenous base.

Nucleotide: A subunit of DNA or RNA consisting of a nitrogenous base (*adenine, guanine, thymine,* or *cytosine* in DNA; adenine, guanine, *uracil,* or cytosine in RNA), a phosphate molecule, and a sugar molecule (deoxyribose in DNA and ribose in RNA). Thousands of *nucleotides* are linked to form a

Nucleus: The cellular organelle in *eukaryotes* that contains the genetic material.

Obligate- (i) adjective referring to an environmental factor (for example, oxygen) that is always required for growth. (ii) organism that can grow and reproduce only by obtaining carbon and other nutrients from a living host, such as obligate symbiont.

Oligonucleotide- short nucleic acid chain, either obtained from an organism or synthesized chemically.

Oligotroph- microorganism specifically adapted to grow under low nutrient supply. Thought to subsist on the more resistant soil organic matter and be little affected by the addition of fresh organic materials. Sometimes a synonym for autochthonous.

Oligotrophic environment- an environment containing low levels of nutrients, particularly nutrients that support microbial growth.

Oncogene: A *gene,* one or more forms of which is associated with cancer. Many oncogenes are involved, directly or indirectly, in controlling the rate of cell growth.

Operon- cluster of genes whose expression is controlled by a single operator; typical in prokaryotic cells.

Organelle- membrane-enclosed body specialized for carrying out certain functions; found only in eukaryotic cells.

Organotroph- organism that obtains reducing equivalents (stored electrons) and carbon from organic substrates.

Osmosis- diffusion of water through a membrane from a region of low solute concentration to one of higher concentration.

Osmotic potential- portion of total soil water potential due to the presence of solutes in soil water.

Osmotolerent- organisms that grow over a wide range of salt concentration.

Pasteur effect- the decrease in the rate of sugar catabolism and change to aerobic respiration that occurs when microorganisms are switched from anaerobic to aerobic conditions.

Pasteurization- process using mild heat to reduce microbial numbers in heat-sensitive materials.

Pasteurization- the process of heating milk and other liquids to destroy microorganisms that can cause spoilage or disease.

Pathogenicity island- a large segment of dna in some pathogens that contains the genes responsible for virulence; often it codes for the type iii secretion system that allows the pathogen to secrete virulence proteins and damage host cells. A pathogen may have more than one pathogenicity island.

Pellicle- relatively rigid layer of proteinaceous elements just beneath the cell membrane in many protozoa and algae.

Periplasmic space- area between the cell membrane and the cell wall in gram-negative bacteria, containing certain enzymes involved in nutrition.

Peritrichous flagellation- having flagella attached to many places on the cell surface.

Petri dish- a shallow dish consisting of two round, overlapping halves that is used to grow microorganisms on solid culture medium; the top is larger than the bottom of the dish to prevent contamination of the culture.

pH- negative logarithm of the hydrogen ion activity. The degree of acidity (or alkalinity) of a soil as determined by means of a glass or other suitable electrode or indicator at a specified moisture content or soil-water ratio, and expressed in terms of the ph scale.

Phagotrophic- form of feeding where animals, such as protozoans, engulf particulate nutrients, such as bacterial cells or detritus.

Phenotype- observable properties of an organism.

Phosphobacterium- bacterium that is especially good at solubilizing the insoluble inorganic phosphate in soil.

Photoautotroph- organism able to use light as its sole source of energy and carbon dioxide as sole carbon source.

Photoheterotroph- organism able to use light as a source of energy and organic materials as carbon source.

Photophosphorylation- synthesis of high-energy phosphate bonds, as atp, using light energy.

Photoreactivation- the process in which blue light is used by a photoreactivating enzyme to repair thymine dimers in dna by splitting them apart.

Photosynthesis- process of using light energy to synthesize carbohydrates from carbon dioxide.

Phototaxis- movement toward light.

Phototrophs- organisms that use light as their energy source.

Phycobiont- the algal or cyanobacterial partner in a lichen.

Phylogeny- ordering of species into higher taxa and the construction of evolutionary trees based on evolutionary (genetic) relationships.

Physical map: A map of the locations of identifiable landmarks on DNA (e.g., *restriction enzyme cutting sites, genes*), regardless of inheritance. Distance is measured in *base pairs*. For the human *genome,* the lowest- resolution *physical map* is the banding patterns on the 24 different *chromosomes*; the highest- resolution map would be the complete *nucleotide* sequence of the chromosomes.

Pilus - fimbria-like structure that is present on fertile cells and is involved in dna transfer during conjugation. Sometimes called sex pilus.

Plaque- localized area of lysis or cell inhibition caused by virus infection on a lawn of cells.

plasmid- a double-stranded dna molecule that can exist and replicate independently of the chromosome or may be integrated with it. A plasmid is stably inherited, but is not required for the host cell's growth and reproduction.

Plasmid- covalently closed, circular piece of dna which, as an extrachromosomal genetic element, is not essential for growth.

Plasmid fingerprinting- a technique used to identify microbial isolates as belonging to the same strain because they contain the same number of plasmids with the identical molecular weights and similar phenotypes.

Plasmolysis- the process in which water osmotically leaves a cell, which causes the cytoplasm to shrivel up and pull the plasma membrane away from the cell wall.

Plate count- number of colonies formed on a solid culture medium when uniformly inoculated with a known amount of soil, generally as a dilute soil suspension. The technique estimates the number of certain organisms present in the soil sample.

Poly-beta-hydroxybutyrate (PHB)- common storage material of prokaryotic cells consisting of beta-hydroxybutyrate or other beta-alkanoic acids.

Polyclonal antiserum- mixture of antibodies to a variety of antigens or to a variety of determinants on a single antigen.

Polygenic disorders: Genetic disorders resulting from the combined action of *alleles* of more than one *gene* (e.g., heart disease, diabetes, and some cancers). Although such disorders are inherited, they depend on the simultaneous presence of several alleles; thus the hereditary patterns are usually more complex than those of *single- gene disorders*. Compare single- gene disorders.

Polymerase chain reaction (PCR)- an in vitro technique used to synthesize large quantities of specific nucleotide sequences from small amounts of dna. It employs oligonucleotide primers complementary to specific sequences in the target gene and special heat-stable dna polymerases.

Polymerase, DNA or RNA: *Enzymes* that catalyze the synthesis of *nucleic acids* on preexisting nucleic acid templates, assembling RNA from ribonucleotides or DNA from deoxyribonucleotides.

Polymorphism: Difference in DNA sequence among individuals. Genetic variations occurring in more than 1% of a population would be considered useful polymorphisms for genetic *linkage* analysis. Compare *mutation*.

Pour plate- a petri dish of solid culture medium with isolated microbial colonies growing both on its surface and within the medium, which has been prepared by mixing microorganisms with cooled, still liquid medium and then allowing the medium to harden.

Precipitation (or precipitin) reaction- the reaction of an antibody with a soluble antigen to form an insoluble precipitate.

Precipitin- the antibody responsible for a precipitation reaction.

Predation- relationship between two organisms whereby one organism (predator) engulfs or captures and digests the second organism (prey).

Pribnow boxa- special base sequence in the promoter that is recognized by the rna polymerase and is the site of initial polymerase binding.

Primary producer- organism that adds biomass to the ecosystem by synthesizing organic molecules from carbon dioxide and simple inorganic nutrients.

Primer- molecule (usually a polynucleotide) to which dna polymerase can attach the first nucleotide during dna replication.

Primer: Short preexisting polynucleotide chain to which new deoxyribonucleotides can be added by DNA *polymerase*.

Probe- a short, labeled nucleic acid segment complementary in base sequence to part of another nucleic acid, which is used to identify or isolate the particular nucleic acid from a mixture through its ability to bind specifically with the target nucleic acid.

Probe: Single- stranded DNA or RNA molecules of specific base *sequence*, labeled either radioactively or immunologically, that are used to detect the *complementary* base sequence by *hybridization*.

Probiotic- (1) the oral administration of either living microorganisms or substances to promote the health and growth of an animal or human. (2) a living organism that may provide health benefits beyond its nutritional value when it is ingested.

Prokaryote: Cell or organism lacking a membrane- bound, structurally discrete *nucleus* and other subcellular compartments. Bacteria are prokaryotes. Compare *eukaryote*. See *chromosomes*.

Promoter- site on dna where the rna polymerase binds and begins transcription.

Proton motive force (PMF)- energized state of a membrane created by expulsion of protons through action of an electron transport chain.

Protoplasm- complete cellular contents, cytoplasmic membrane, cytoplasm, and nucleus; usually considered the living portion of the cell, thus excluding those layers peripheral to the cell membrane.

Protoplast fusion- the joining of cells that have had their walls weakened or completely removed.

Protoplast- a bacterial or fungal cell with its cell wall completely removed. It is spherical in shape and osmotically sensitive.

Prototropha- microorganism that requires the same nutrients as the majority of naturally occurring members of its species.

Psychrophile- a microorganism that grows well at 0°c and has an optimum growth temperature of 15°C or lower and a temperature maximum around 20°C.

Psychrotroph- a microorganism that grows at 0°c, but has a growth optimum between 20 and 30°C, and a maximum of about 35°C.

Pure culture- a population of cells that are identical because they arise from a single cell.

Putrefaction- the microbial decomposition of organic matter, especially the anaerobic breakdown of proteins, with the production of foul-smelling compounds such as hydrogen sulfide and amines.

Quellung reaction- the increase in visibility or the swelling of the capsule of a microorganism in the presence of antibodies against capsular antigens.

R factors or r plasmids- plasmids bearing one or more drug resistant genes.

Radappertization- the use of gamma rays from a cobalt source for control of microorganisms in foods.

Radioimmunoassaya- very sensitive assay technique that uses a purified radioisotope-labeled antigen or antibody to compete for antibody or antigen with unlabeled standard and samples to determine the concentration of a substance in the samples.

Reagin- antibody that mediates immediate hypersensitivity reactions. Ige is the major reagin in humans.

Recalcitrant- resistant to microbial attack.

Recombinant clones: *Clones* containing *recombinant DNA molecules*. See *recombinant DNA technologies*.

Recombinant DNA- DNA molecule containing dna originating from two or more sources.

Recombinant DNA molecules: A combination of DNA molecules of different origin that are joined using *recombinant DNA technologies*.

Recombination- process by which genetic elements in two separate genomes are brought together in one unit.

Recombination repair- a DNA repair process that repairs damaged DNA when there is no remaining template; a piece of dna from a sister molecule is used.

Recombination: The process by which progeny derive a combination of *genes* different from that of either parent. In higher organisms, this can occur by *crossing over*.

Red tides- red tides occur frequently in coastal areas and often are associated with population blooms of dinoflagellates. Dinoflagellate pigments are responsible for the red colour of the water. Under these conditions, the dinoflagellates often produce saxitoxin, which can lead to paralytic shellfish poisoning.

Refractive index- the ratio of the velocity of light in the first of two media to that in the second as it passes from the first to the second.

5

Regulatory regions or sequences: A DNA *base sequence* that controls *gene expression.*

Replica plating- a technique for isolating mutants from a population by plating cells from each colony growing on a nonselective agar medium onto plates with selective media or environmental conditions, such as the lack of a nutrient or the presence of an antibiotic or a phage; the location of mutants on the original plate can be determined from growth patterns on the replica plates.

Replication-conversion of one double-stranded dna molecule into two identical double-stranded dna molecules.

Repression-process by which the synthesis of an enzyme is inhibited by the presence of an external substance (the repressor).

Reservoir- in the context of human pathogens, a place where disease-causing organisms reside when they are not living in a human host.

Resolution- the ability of a microscope to separate or distinguish between small objects that are close together.

Resolution: Degree of molecular detail on a *physical map* of DNA, ranging from low to high.

Restriction endonuclease (restriction enzyme)- enzyme that recognizes and cleaves specific DNA sequence, generating either blunt or single-stranded (sticky) ends.

Restriction enzyme cutting site: A specific *nucleotide sequence* of DNA at which a particular *restriction enzyme* cuts the DNA. Some sites occur frequently in DNA (e.g., every several hundred *base pairs*), others much less frequently (*rare-cutter*; e.g., every 10,000 base pairs).

Restriction enzyme, endonuclease: A *protein* that recognizes specific, short *nucleotide sequences* and cuts DNA at those sites. Bacteria contain over 400 such *enzymes* that recognize and cut over 100 different DNA sequences. See *restriction enzyme cutting site.*

Restriction enzymes- enzymes produced by host cells that cleave virus dna at specific points and thus protect the cell from virus infection; they are used in carrying out genetic engineering.

Restriction fragment length polymorphism (RFLP)- method to identify differences between similar genes from different organisms. Digestion of genes with restriction endonucleases followed by separation of the resulting fragments by gel electrophoresis yields banding patterns that are characteristic of the individual gene.

Restriction fragment length polymorphism (RFLP): Variation between individuals in DNA fragment sizes cut by specific *restriction enzymes; polymorphic sequences* that result in RFLPs are used as *markers* on both *physical maps* and genetic *linkage maps.* RFLPs are usually caused by *mutation* at a cutting site. See *marker.*

Reverse transcription- process of copying information found in rna into dna.

Rhizobacteria- bacteria that aggressively colonize roots.

Rhizobia- bacteria capable of living symbiotically in roots of leguminous plants, from which they receive energy and often fix molecular dinitrogen. Collective common name for *Rhizobium* and closely related genera.

Rhizoid- rootlike structure that helps to hold an organism to a substrate.

Rhizomorph- mass of fungal hyphae organized into long, thick strands usually with a darkly pigmented outer rind and containing specialized tissues for absorption and water transport.

Rhizoplane- plant root surfaces and usually strongly adhering soil particles.

Rhizosphere competence- ability of an organism to colonize the rhizosphere.

Rhizosphere- zone of soil under the influence of plant roots in which the kinds, numbers, or activities of microorganisms differ from that of the bulk soil.

Rhizosphere- a region around the plant root where materials released from the root increase the microbial population and its activities.

Ribotyping- ribotyping is the use of E. Coli rRNA to probe chromosomal dna in southern blots for typing bacterial strains. This method is based on the fact that rRNA genes are scattered throughout the chromosome of most bacteria and therefore polymorphic restriction endonuclease patterns result when chromosomes are digested and probed with rrna.

Root nodule- specialized structure occurring on roots, especially of leguminous plants, in which bacteria fix dinitrogen and make it available for the plant.

Root nodule- gall-like structures on roots that contain endosymbiotic nitrogen-fixing bacteria (e.g., Rhizobium or bradyrhizobium is present in legume nodules).

Sanitization- elimination of pathogenic or deleterious organisms, insect larvae, intestinal parasites, and weed seeds.

Saprophyte- an organism that takes up nonliving organic nutrients in dissolved form and usually grows on decomposing organic matter.

Saprophyte- nonparasitic nutritional mechanism by which an organism obtains its food exclusively from the degradation of nonliving organic material.

Secondary metabolite- product of intermediary metabolism released from a cell, such as an antibiotic.

Septate- divided by a septum or cross wall; also with more or less regular occurring cross walls.

Septic tank- a tank used to process small quantities of domestic sewage. Solid material settles out and is partially degraded by anaerobic bacteria as sewage slowly flows through the tank. The outflow is further treated or dispersed in aerobic soil.

Septicemia- a disease associated with the presence in the blood of pathogens or bacterial toxins.

Sequence tagged site (STS): Short (200 to 500 *base pairs*) DNA sequence that has a single occurrence in the human genome and whose location and base sequence are known. Detectable by *polymerase chain reaction*, STSs are useful for localizing and orienting the mapping and sequence data reported from many different laboratories and serve as landmarks on the developing *physical map* of the human genome. Expressed sequence tags (ESTs) are STSs derived from cDNAs.

Sequencing: Determination of the order of *nucleotides (base sequences)* in a DNA or *RNA* molecule or the order of *amino acids* in a *protein*.

Serial dilution- series of stepwise dilutions (usually in sterile water) performed to reduce the populations of microorganisms in a sample to manageable numbers.

Serology- the branch of immunology that is concerned with in vitro reactions involving one or more serum constituents (e.g., antibodies and complement).

Serotyping- a technique or serological procedure that is used to differentiate between strains (serovars or serotypes) of microorganisms that have differences in the antigenic composition of a structure or product.

Serum resistance- the type of resistance that occurs with bacteria such as *Neisseria gonorrhoeae* because the pathogen interferes with membrane attack complex formation during the complement cascade.

Serum- the clear, fluid portion of blood lacking both blood cells and fibrinogen. It is the fluid remaining after coagulation of plasma, the noncellular liquid faction of blood.

Sex chromosomes: The X and Y *chromosomes* in human beings that determine the sex of an individual. Females have two X chromosomes in diploid cells; males have an X and a Y chromosome. The sex chromosomes comprise the 23rd chromosome pair in a *karyotype*. Compare *autosome*.

Sex pilus- a thin protein appendage required for bacterial mating or conjugation. The cell with sex pili donates DNA to recipient cells.

Shine-dalgarno sequence- a segment in the leader of procaryotic mrna that binds to a special sequence on the 16s rRNA of the small ribosomal subunit. This helps properly orient the mrna on the ribosome.

Siderophore- a small molecule that complexes with ferric iron and supplies it to a cell by aiding in its transport across the plasma membrane.

Sigma factor- a protein that helps the rna polymerase core enzyme recognize the promoter at the start of a gene.

Silage- fermented plant material with increased palatability and nutritional value for animals, which can be stored for extended periods.

Silent mutation- a mutation that does not result in a change in the organism's proteins or phenotype even though the dna base sequence has been changed.

Single- gene disorder: Hereditary disorder caused by a *mutant* allele of a single *gene* (e.g., Duchenne muscular dystrophy, retinoblastoma, sickle cell disease). Compare *polygenic disorders*.

Single radial immunodiffusion (RID) assay- an immunodiffusion technique that quantitates antigens by following their diffusion through a gel containing antibodies directed against the test antigens.

Site-directed mutagenesis- insertion of a different nucleotide at a specific site in a molecule using recombinant dna methodology.

Slime- the viscous extracellular glycoproteins or glycolipids produced by staphylococci and pseudomonas aeruginosa bacteria that allows them to adhere to smooth surfaces such as prosthetic medical devices and catheters. More generally, the term often refers to an easily removed, diffuse, unorganized layer of extracellular material that surrounds a bacterial cell.

Sludge- a general term for the precipitated solid matter produced during water and sewage treatment; solid particles composed of organic matter and microorganisms that are involved in aerobic sewage treatment (activated sludge).

Snapping division- a distinctive type of binary fission resulting in an angular or a palisade arrangement of cells, which is characteristic of the genera arthrobacter and corynebacterium.

SOS repair- a complex, inducible repair process that is used to repair DNA when extensive damage has occurred.

Southern blotting technique- the procedure used to isolate and identify dna fragments from a complex mixture. The isolated, denatured fragments are transferred from an agarose electrophoretic gel to a nitrocellulose filter and identified by hybridization with probes.

Species- species of higher organisms are groups of interbreeding or potentially interbreeding natural populations that are reproductively isolated. Bacterial species are collections of strains that have many stable properties in common and differ significantly from other groups of strains.

Spheroplast- a relatively spherical cell formed by the weakening or partial removal of the rigid cell wall component (e.g., by penicillin treatment of gram-negative bacteria). Spheroplasts are usually osmotically sensitive.

Sporangiospore- spore formed within a sporangium by fungi in the phylum zygomycota.

Sporangium- fungal structure which converts its cytoplasm into a variable number of sporangiospores; formed by fungi in the phylum zygomycota.

Spore- a differentiated, specialized form that can be used for dissemination, for survival of adverse conditions because of its heat and dessication resistance, and/or for reproduction. Spores are usually unicellular and may develop into vegetative organisms or gametes. They may be produced asexually or sexually and are of many types.

Sporulation- the process of spore formation.

Spread plate- a petri dish of solid culture medium with isolated microbial colonies growing on its surface, which has been prepared by spreading a dilute microbial suspension evenly over the agar surface.

Sterilization- rendering an object or substance free of viable microbes.

Sterilization- the process by which all living cells, viable spores, viruses, and viroids are either destroyed or removed from an object or habitat.

Strain- a population of organisms that descends from a single organism or pure culture isolate.

Streak plate- a petri dish of solid culture medium with isolated microbial colonies growing on its surface, which has been prepared by spreading a microbial mixture over the agar surface, using an inoculating loop.

Streptolysin-O (SLO)- a specific hemolysin produced by *Streptococcus pyogenes* that is inactivated by oxygen (hence the "o" in its name). SLO causes beta-hemolysis of blood cells on agar plates incubated anaerobically.

Streptolysin-S (SLS)- a product produced by *Streptococcus pyogenes* that is bound to the bacterial cell but may sometimes be released. SLS causes beta hemolysis on aerobically incubated blood-agar plates and can act as a leukocidin by killing leukocytes that phagocytose the bacterial cell to which it is bound.

Succession- gradual process brought about by the change in the number of individuals of each species of a community and by the establishment of new species that gradually replace the original inhabitants.

Superantigen- superantigens are bacterial proteins that stimulate the immune system much more extensively than do normal antigens. They stimulate t cells to proliferate nonspecifically through simultaneous interaction with class II MHC proteins on antigen-presenting cells and variable regions on the b chain of the t-cell receptor complex. Examples include streptococcal scarlet fever toxins, staphylococcal toxic shock syndrome toxin-1, and streptococcal m protein.

Superinfection- a new bacterial or fungal infection of a patient that is resistant to the drug(s) being used for treatment.

Suppressor mutation- a mutation that overcomes the effect of another mutation and produces the normal phenotype.

Surfactant- a substance that lowers the surface tension of a liquid.

Swab- a wad of absorbent material usually wound around one end of a small stick and used for applying medication or for removing material from an area; also, a dacron-tipped polystyrene applicator.

Symbiosis- living together in intimate association of two dissimilar organisms. The interactions between the organisms can be commensal or mutualistic.

Symbiosis- the living together or close association of two dissimilar organisms, each of these organisms being known as a symbiont.

Synergism- association between organisms that is mutually beneficial. Both populations, however, are capable of surviving in their natural environment on their own.

Tandem repeat sequences: Multiple copies of the same *base sequence* on a *chromosome*; used as a marker in *physical mapping*.

Technology transfer: The process of converting scientific findings from research laboratories into useful products by the commercial sector.

Telomere: The ends of *chromosomes*. These specialized structures are involved in the replication and stability of linear DNA molecules.

Thallus- vegetative body that is not differentiated into tissue systems or organs.

Thermal death time (TDT)- the shortest period of time needed to kill all the organisms in a microbial population at a specified temperature and under defined conditions.

Thermophile- a microorganism that can grow at temperatures of 55°C or higher; the minimum is usually around 45°C.

Thermophile- organism whose optimum temperature for growth is between 45 and 85°C.

Ti plasmid- conjugative tumor-inducing plasmid present in the bacterium *agrobacterium tunefaciens* which can transfer genes into plants.

Transcription: The synthesis of an *RNA* copy from a *sequence* of DNA (a *gene*); the first step in *gene expression*. Compare *translation*.

Transduction the transfer of genes between bacteria by bacteriophages.

Transformation- a mode of gene transfer in bacteria in which a piece of free dna is taken up by a bacterial cell and integrated into the recipient genome.

Transgenic- describes genetically modified plants or animals containing foreign genes inserted by means of recombinant dna techniques.

Transition mutations- mutations that involve the substitution of a different purine base for the purine present at the site of the mutation or the substitution of a different pyrimidine for the normal pyrimidine.

Transposition- the movement of a piece of dna around the chromosome.

Transposon a DNA segment- that carries the genes required for transposition and moves about the chromosome; if it contains genes other than those required for transposition, it may be called a composite transposon. Often the name is reserved only for transposable elements that also contain genes unrelated to transposition.

Transversion mutations- mutations that result from the substitution of a purine base for the normal pyrimidine or a pyrimidine for the normal purine.

Trichome- row of cells which have remained attached to one another following successive cell divisions. Trichomes are formed by many cyanobacteria and by species of *beggiatoa*.

Trickling filter- a bed of rocks covered with a microbial film that aerobically degrades organic waste during secondary sewage treatment.

Trophozoite- the active, motile feeding stage of a protozoan organism; in the malarial parasite, the stage of schizogony between the ring stage and the schizont.

Ultraviolet (UV) radiation- radiation of fairly short wavelength, about 10 to 400 nm, and high energy.

Vector- (i) plasmid or virus used in genetic engineering to insert genes into a cell. (ii) agent, usually an insect or other animal, able to carry pathogens from one host to another.

Vesicles- spherical structures, formed intracellularly, by some arbuscular mycorrhizal fungi.

Viable- alive; able to reproduce.

Viable but nonculturable- organisms that are alive but cannot be cultured on laboratory media.

Viable count- measurement of the number of live cells in a microbial population.

Virion- virus particle; the virus nucleic acid surrounded by protein coat and in some cases other material.

Virulence- degree of pathogenicity of a parasite.

Wastewater treatment- the use of physical and biological processes to remove particulate and dissolved material from sewage and to control pathogens.

Widal test- a test involving agglutination of typhoid bacilli when they are mixed with serum containing typhoid antibodies from an individual having typhoid fever; used to detect the presence of salmonella typhi and s. Paratyphi.

Wild type- strain of microorganism isolated from nature. The usual or native form of a gene or organism.

Winogradsky column- glass column with an anaerobic lower zone and an aerobic upper zone, which allows growth of microorganisms under conditions similar to those found in nutrient-rich water and sediment.

Xenobiotic- compound foreign to biological systems. Often refers to human-made compounds that are resistant or recalcitrant to biodegradation and decomposition.

Xerophile- organism adapted to grow at low water potential, i.e., very dry habitats.

Yeast artificial chromosome (YAC): A vector used to clone DNA fragments (up to 400 kb); it is constructed from the telomeric, centromeric, and replication origin sequences needed for replication in yeast cells. Compare *cloning vector, cosmid.*

Yeast- fungus whose thallus consists of single cells that multiply by budding or fission.

YM shift- the change in shape by dimorphic fungi when they shift from the yeast (y) form in the animal body to the mold or mycelial form (m) in the environment.

Zymogenous organism- refers to an often transient or alien microorganism that grows rapidly when high energy-containing nutrients become available. Also called copiotroph.

•••

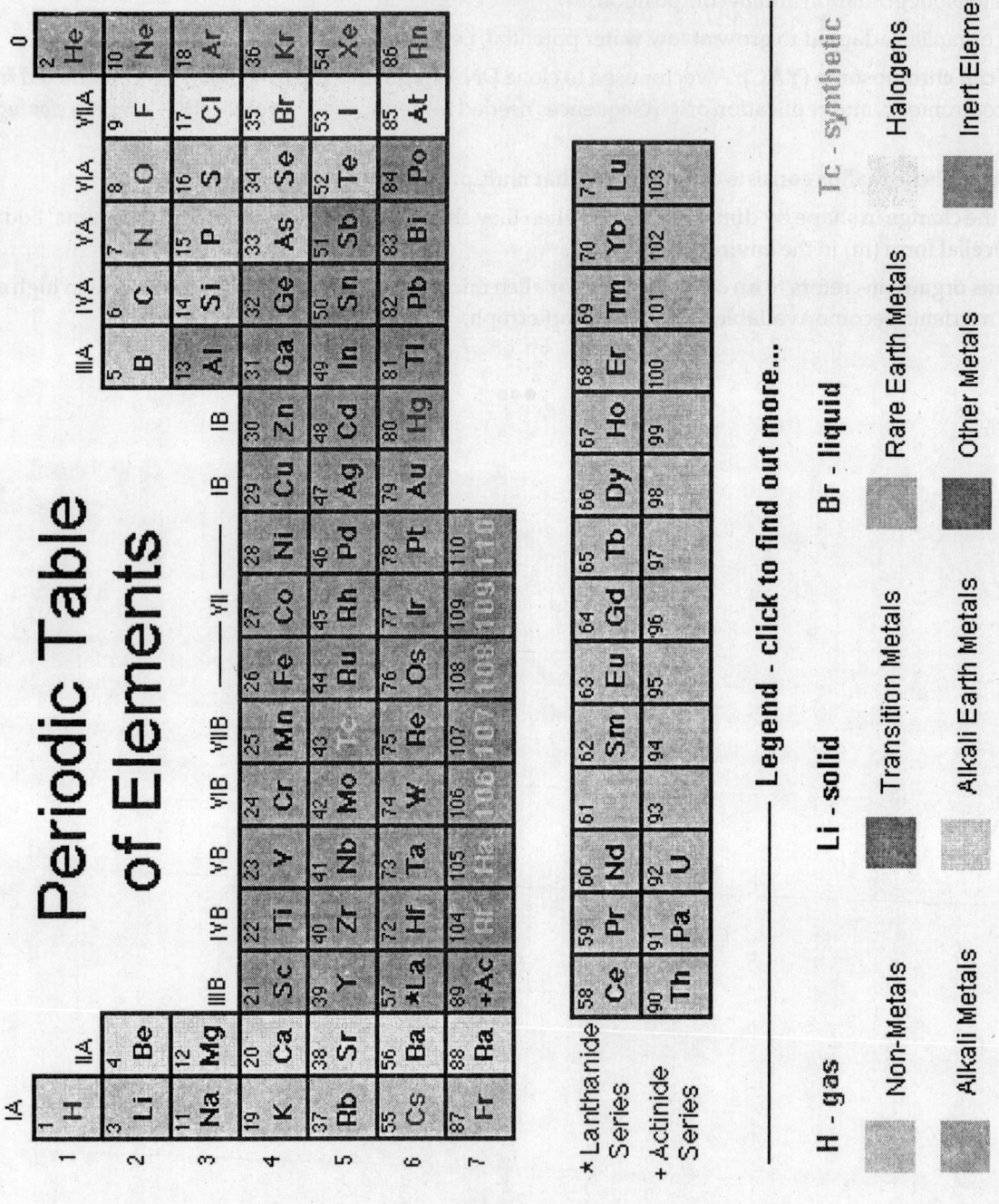

Periodic Table of Elements

	IA																		0
1	1 H	IIA											IIIA	IVA	VA	VIA	VIIA		2 He
2	3 Li	4 Be											5 B	6 C	7 N	8 O	9 F		10 Ne
3	11 Na	12 Mg	IIIB	IVB	VB	VIB	VIIB	———— VIII ————		IB	IB		13 Al	14 Si	15 P	16 S	17 Cl		18 Ar
4	19 K	20 Ca	21 Sc	22 Ti	23 V	24 Cr	25 Mn	26 Fe	27 Co	28 Ni	29 Cu	30 Zn	31 Ga	32 Ge	33 As	34 Se	35 Br	36 Kr
5	37 Rb	38 Sr	39 Y	40 Zr	41 Nb	42 Mo	43 Tc	44 Ru	45 Rh	46 Pd	47 Ag	48 Cd	49 In	50 Sn	51 Sb	52 Te	53 I	54 Xe
6	55 Cs	56 Ba	57 *La	72 Hf	73 Ta	74 W	75 Re	76 Os	77 Ir	78 Pt	79 Au	80 Hg	81 Tl	82 Pb	83 Bi	84 Po	85 At	86 Rn
7	87 Fr	88 Ra	89 +Ac	104 Hf	105 Ha	106	107	108	109	110								

* Lanthanide Series	58 Ce	59 Pr	60 Nd	61	62 Sm	63 Eu	64 Gd	65 Tb	66 Dy	67 Ho	68 Er	69 Tm	70 Yb	71 Lu
+ Actinide Series	90 Th	91 Pa	92 U	93	94	95	96	97	98	99	100	101	102	103

Tc - synthetic

Legend - click to find out more...

H - gas   Li - solid   Br - liquid

	Non-Metals		Transition Metals		Rare Earth Metals		Halogens
	Alkali Metals		Alkali Earth Metals		Other Metals		Inert Elements

Appendix . K – Bibliography

Ian Freshney. A. 2005. Culture of Animal cells – A manual of basic techniques. 5th edi. John Wiley & Sons., Inc., Publication.

Elmer W.Koneman, Stephen D.Allen, William M.Janda, Paul C. Schreckenberger, Washington C.Winn, Jr. Introduction to Diagnostic Microbiology, J.B. Lippincott Company, 1994.

Elmer W.Koneman, Stephen D.Allen, William M.Janda, Paul C.Schreckenberger, Wasihington C.Winn,Jr .Color atlas and Text book of Diagnostic Microbiology, 5th Ed, J.B.Lippincott Philadelphia, New York, 1997.

Henry D. Isenberg. Essential Procedure for Clinical Microbiology, A.S.M. Press Washington, 1998.

Joklik, Willott,Amus, Wilfert. Zinsser Microbiology, Appleton & Lance Publication, 20th Ed,1992.

Kanai L.Mukharjee, Medical laboratory technology, Tata McGraw - Hill ,Volume II,1986.

Kathleen Talaro, Arthur Talaro. Foundations in Microbiology, 2nd Ed, W.M.C.Brown Publishers Chigago,1996.

Lansing M. Prescott, John P.Harley, Donald A.Klein. Microbiology, 4th Ed, W.C.B McGraw-Hill, 1999.

Lansing M. Prescott, John P.Harley, Donald A.Klein. Microbiology, 5th Ed, W.C.B Mcgraw-Hill, 2001.

Michael J. Pelczar, Jr.E.C.S.Chan, Noel .R Kreig, Microbiology concepts & Applications, McGraw - Hill, 1993.

Monica chesbrough. Medical laboratory manual for Tropical Countries, Educational low priced books scheme, volume II, 1984.

Ronold M.Atlas, Principles of Microbiology, 2nd Ed, Wm. C. Brown Puplishers,1977.

Samuel Baron . Medical microbiology, 2nd Ed, Addison- Wesley Publication & Co, New York.1986.

Tortora.J, Funke.R Case.L. Microbiology an Introduction. 6th Ed, Addison Wesley Longman 1997.

Markus R. Wenk; Aaron Z. Fernandis. Manuals in Biomedical Research — Vol. 3 A Manual For Biochemistry Protocols. 2007. World Scientific Publishing Co. Pte. Ltd.

John P. Harley, Lansing M. Prescott. Laboratory Exercises in Microbiology, Fifth Edition The McGraw"Hill Companies, 2002.

APPENDIX - L - INDEX

• • •